THE PRIMATE ENDOMETRIUM

ANNALS OF THE NEW YORK ACADEMY OF SCIENCES
Volume 622

THE PRIMATE ENDOMETRIUM

Edited by Carlo Bulletti and Erlio Gurpide

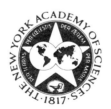

The New York Academy of Sciences
New York, New York
1991

The art that appears on the softcover version of this volume was provided by Prof. Hans Ludwig, MD, FRCOG, FACOG (hon.) and the originals appear in the paper by H. Ludwig and U. M. Spornitz on pages 28–46 of this volume.

Library of Congress Cataloging-in-Publication Data

The Primate Endometrium / edited by Carlo Bulletti and Erlio Gurpide.
    p. cm. – (Annals of the New York Academy of Sciences ; v. 622)
    Includes bibliographical references and index.
    ISBN 0-89766-665-8. – ISBN 0-89766-666-6 (pbk.)
    1. Endometrium – Congresses. I. Bulletti, Carlo. II. Gurpide,
    Erlio, 1927- . III. Series.
    QP262.P75 1991
    599.80416 – dc20   91-8449
                                           CIP

CCP
Printed in the United States of America
ISBN 0-89766-665-8 (cloth)
ISBN 0-89766-666-6 (paper)
ISSN 0077-8923

ANNALS OF THE NEW YORK ACADEMY OF SCIENCES

Volume 622
May 15, 1991

THE PRIMATE ENDOMETRIUM[a]

Editors
CARLO BULLETTI and ERLIO GURPIDE

Conference Organizers
CARLO BULLETTI, CARLO FLAMIGNI, ERLIO GURPIDE, and VALERIO MARIA JASONNI

Conference Advisory Board
PAUL C. MACDONALD, ROBERT M. BRENNER, and ROGER J. B. KING

CONTENTS

[a] This volume is the result of a conference entitled **First Conference on the Primate Endometrium** sponsored by The University of Bologna, Bologna, Italy and Mount Sinai School of Medicine, New York, New York, and held in New York City on 28–30 May, 1990.

Part III. Interaction among Cells of Different Types

Part IV. Implantation

Part V. Endometriosis

Part VI. Steroid Replacement Therapy

Part VII. Onset of Labor

Part VIII. Endometrial Cancer—Basic

Part IX. Endometrial Cancer—Clinical

Financial assistance was provided by the following:

MAJOR CONTRIBUTORS
- ICI-Pharma Italia SpA
- Maggioni-Winthrop SpA

OTHER CONTRIBUTORS
- Ciba-Geigy Corp. (USA)
- National Institute of Child Health and Human Development (USA)
- National Research Council (CNR, Italy)
- Poli Industria Chimica SpA
- Serono Laboratories (USA)
- University of Bologna
- Wyeth-Ayerst Laboratories (USA)
- Wyeth SpA

Acknowledgments

The First International Conference on the Primate Endometrium was made possible through the initiative and effort of several collaborators, especially Drs. C. Flamigni and V. M. Jasonni, Chairman and Vice-Chairman, respectively, of the Reproductive Medicine Unit of the Department of Obstetrics & Gynecology, University of Bologna, and the Program Committee, which included Drs. R. Brenner, R. J. B. King, and P. C. MacDonald. The various sessions were chaired by Drs. D. Amadori, R. Berkowitz, L. Castagnetta, C. Cohen, L. Deligdisch, C. Flamigni, S. B. Gusberg, V. Reyniak, R. Scott, and L. Tseng. The Dean of Mount Sinai Medical School, Dr. N. Kase, the Director of the Postgraduate School of Medicine, Dr. K. Smith, the Chairman of the Department of Obstetrics, Gynecology & Reproductive Science, Dr. R. Berkowitz, and Dr. R. Litwak (Department of Surgery) provided most helpful support. The staff of the Postgraduate School, working in collaboration with Mrs. A. Rogers (Dept. of Ob., Gyn & Reprod. Sci, MSSM) and Mrs. R. Furegato (Dept. of Ob. Gyn., Univ. of Bologna) contributed in a very important manner to the organization of the Conference. Ms. Joyce Hitchcock, Associate Editor at the New York Academy of Sciences, effectively edited and directed the production of this volume of the *Annals*.

E. GURPIDE AND C. BULLETTI, *Editors*

Introduction:
Research on the Human Endometrium

ERLIO GURPIDE

Department of Obstetrics, Gynecology & Reproductive Science
Mount Sinai School of Medicine
New York, New York 10029

CARLO BULLETTI

Reproductive Medicine Unit
Department of Obstetrics & Gynecology
University of Bologna
Via Massarenti 13
40138 Bologna, Italy

This volume of the *Annals of the New York Academy of Sciences* is the proceedings of an International Conference on the Primate Endometrium, held at the Mount Sinai Medical Center, New York City, May 28–30, 1990 in response to the accelerated increase in the number of reports describing novel, often surprising, properties of this tissue.

Early fundamental experiments revealed uterotropic actions of estrogens and effects of progestins on the endometrium of rodents, rabbits and primates.[1-4] Although the human tissue is strongly affected by these hormones, it differs from the endometrium of rabbits and rodents in several aspects regarding hormonal regulation of enzymatic activities, secretory products and decidua formation, as could be expected from species differences in reproductive strategies and temporal patterns of ovarian hormone production. In contrast, the Rhesus monkey has menstrual cycles similar to those of humans and has been successfully used as an experimental model providing conditions which cannot be reproduced in women. Hence the focus of the Conference on the primate endometrium.

The attractiveness of endometrial research derives from both its clinical relevance and the opportunity it offers to investigate topics of fundamental importance in cell biology. TABLE 1 outlines some of the clinical and biological topics relevant to endometrial research, most of which are expertly covered in this volume.

There are characteristics of the human endometrium which make this tissue unique as a research model. Endometrial tissue is commonly available as surgical specimens obtained by curettage or after hysterectomies. The endogenous hormonal environment at which the portion of tissue available for *in vitro* research was exposed *in vivo* can be determined from histologic features or from analysis of blood samples at the time of surgery. In fact, regulation of biochemical parameters by either estradiol or progesterone, or lack of hormonal regulation, is suggested by changes observed in tissue samples obtained at different days of the menstrual cycle. Another attractive feature of endometrial research is the variety of endometrial samples that can be collected. Although most of the curettage specimens are histologically normal,[5] samples of

1

TABLE 1. Clinical and Biological Topics Relevant to Endometrial Research

CLINICAL RELEVANCE OF STUDIES ON HUMAN ENDOMETRIUM

- Infertility
- *In vitro* fertilization
- Contraception
- Menstruation, dysfunctional uterine bleeding
- Endometriosis
- Hormonal replacement therapy
- Preterm labor/delivery
- Endometrial cancer

TOPICS OF CELL BIOLOGY/BIOCHEMISTRY RELEVANT TO ENDOMETRIAL STUDIES

- Differentiation
- Stromal-epithelial interactions
- Embryo-endometrium interactions
- Extracellular matrix functions
- Mechanisms of steroid hormone actions
- Cell proliferation; growth factors
- Cytokines, eicosanoids, polyamines
- Autocrine and paracrine regulatory mechanisms
- Tumorigenesis, invasiveness, progression
- Immunology

hyperplastic and neoplastic tissue can also be obtained, allowing interesting biochemical comparisons with normal tissue exposed to similar endogenous hormonal environments. Furthermore, endometrium of pregnancy can be collected during surgical abortions or by scraping fetal membranes obtained after vaginal or cesarean deliveries.

Development of procedures for the separation and culture of stromal and epithelial cells allowed the identification of drastic differences in the characteristics and hormonal responsiveness of these endometrial cell types. Highly homogeneous preparation of decidual cells from gestational endometrium were also obtained, making possible studies in which their properties and secretory capabilities could be compared with those of the stromal cells of proliferative or early secretory endometrium. In fact, stromal cells isolated from proliferative endometrium can now be decidualized *in vitro* to yield morphologically distinct cells showing, as far as currently tested, the same products of differentiation detected in decidual cells of pregnancy. Of great interest are recent findings on cells of bone marrow origin which reside, and can even proliferate, in the endometrium.

Various endometrial adenocarcinoma cell lines, some of them responsive to steroid hormones and growth factors, are widely used for studies on regulation of cancer cell proliferation, providing information which might be relevant to normal epithelial endometrial cells and useful in the evaluation of possible aberrations associated with neoplastic transformation.

Most of the experimental results presented by the contributors to these proceedings have been generated either by direct analysis of endometrial tissue, collected at various physiologic or drug-induced *in vivo* conditions, or by *in vitro* manipulation of endometrial tissue. Different preparations are available for *in vitro* studies to suit specific experimental purposes. For instance, realization of the importance of paracrine communication among the various types of endometrial cells indicates that preservation of the cellular architecture of the tissue during *in vitro* studies is desirable when the emphasis is placed on physiologic relevance. The preparation that may be most appropriate for this purpose is based on extracorporeal perfusion of whole uteri through arterial vessels catheterized after hysterectomy, and collection of effluents and endometrial samples. Such perfusions can be prolonged from 48–72 h with retention of endometrial viability, as evaluated by morphologic and biochemical parameters,[6,7] and applied to test for actions of agents added to the perfusion medium, to evaluate synthetic and metabolic activities and to study interactions with human trophoblastic cells in attempts to simulate endometrial interactions with the trophectoderm during embryo implantation.

Endometrial fragments offer another acceptable level of preservation of tissular structure and have been successfully used to test for hormonal effects, as in the early experiments on actions of progestins on polarized glycogen accumulation in glandular epithelial cells[8] or quantitative studies on estrogen metabolism.[9,10] Tissue fragments placed on grids at the surface of the medium in culture dishes, retain morphologic viability and responsiveness to hormones for 2 to 4 days, or longer if appropriate hormonal support is provided. Products secreted into the culture medium can be identified, rates of production can be measured and cells of origin can be determined by using immunochemical techniques, Northern blot analysis of mRNA extracted from the tissue, labeled thymidine incorporation into nucleic acids, and *in situ* hybridization procedures.

Structurally preserved endometrial glands, isolated from tissue fragments by enzymatic dispersion and removal of stromal cells, offer a well-defined system for biochemical studies, albeit at the expense of losing information on possible influences of stromal cells. Dispersion and resolution of endometrial cells, leading to near homogeneous cell preparations, allow the identification of biochemical characteristics and responsiveness to bioactive agents specific to each cell type.

It has been recognized, however, that the behavior of cells depends on the culture conditions and most particularly on the nature of the substrate to which they are attached. Stromal cells grown on plastic surfaces show a distorted cytoskeletal distribution; epithelial cells, which also become flat when attached to the plastic surface, lose the ability to establish their characteristic intercellular junctional structures. In contrast, cells cultured on collagen or other extracellular matrix components maintain their morphologic and functional polarity. Co-cultures of cells of different types, including decidual cells, provide reasonable models to study paracrine intercellular communications and the postulated role of the stroma as a mediator in actions of estradiol on epithelial cells.

Of particular current interest, reflected by several contributions in these proceedings, is the study of decidual cells of the luteal phase endometrium and of the decidua parietalis. These cells have unique properties, made evident more than a decade ago by the recognition that they were a source of prolactin[11,12] and, more recently, by reports on their capability to produce cytokines.[13,14] Furthermore, the effects of prolactin, cytokines and neuropeptides of decidual origin on neighboring cells and fetal tissues may be important in the regulation of processes related to the onset of labor. The design of experimental conditions under which stromal cells isolated from proliferative endometrium can be "decidualized" *in vitro* under the influence of ovarian hormones[15] has provided an important experimental tool for the study of the decidual differentiation process and for the distinction of true decidual cells from endometrial granulated lymphocytes, macrophages and other resident lymphoid cells, also capable of producing cytokines.

Specimens of primary endometrial adenocarcinoma, collected after hysterectomy for determination of grade, hormone receptor status, ploidy, oncogene expression and the presence of marker antigens, are also available for research purposes. Direct tests for responsiveness of cancer tissue to progestins and estrogens provide information of potential prognostic value and are possibly useful in the prediction of responses to hormonal treatment or cytotoxic therapy.[16] Tumor tissue fragments may be used for *in vitro* studies, may be implanted into nude mice to form tumors or may serve to start cell cultures, some of which can lead to the establishment of endometrial cancer cell lines. Such preparations have been useful for research purposes, particularly in studies on cell proliferation and its regulation by hormones, growth factors, cytokines and other mitogenic or growth supporting agents. Although similar studies have been conducted for many years using human breast cancer cell lines and breast tumors transplanted into nude mice, biochemical differences between human breast and endometrial adenocarcinoma cells, such as their responses to tamoxifen and hydroxytamoxifen,[17] justify and enhance the interest in studies with cells from both sites.

The studies on the endometrium presented in this volume exemplify the mutual dependence of the "basic science" and "clinical" approaches to research, each providing to the other the stimulus, inspiration, rationale and methodology that make progress possible.

REFERENCES

1. CORNER, G. W. & W. M. ALLEN. 1929. Physiology of the corpus luteum. II. Production of a special uterine reaction (progestational proliferation) by extracts of the corpus lutem. Am. J. Physiol. **88**: 326.
2. HISAW, F. L. & F. L. HISAW JR. 1961. Action of estrogens and progesterone on the reproductive tract of lower primates. *In* Sex and Internal Secretions, W. C. Young & G. W. Corner, Eds. Vol. I: 556–589. The Williams & Williams Co.
3. PSYCHOYOS, A. 1973. Endocrine control of egg implantation. *In* Handbook of Physiology, R. O. Greep & E. B. Astwood, Eds. Section 7, Part 2: 187–216. Am. Physiol. Soc.
4. KATZENELLENBOGEN, B. S. & J. GORSKI. 1975. Estrogen actions and synthesis of macromolecules in target cells. *In* Biochemical Actions of Hormones. G. Litwack, Ed. Vol. III: 188–238, Academic Press.
5. VELLIOS, F. 1984. Endometrial hyperplasia and carcinoma in-situ. Gynecol. Oncol. **2**: 152.
6. BULLETTI, C., V. M. JASSONI, L. LUBICZ, C. FLAMIGNI & E. GURPIDE. 1986. Extracorporeal perfusion of the human uterus. Am. J. Obstet. Gynecol. **154**: 683.
7. BULLETTI, C., V. M. JASSONI, P. M. CIOTTI, S. TABANELLI, S. NALDI & C. FLAMIGNI. 1988. Extraction of estrogens by human perfused uterus. Effect of membrane permeability and binding by serum proteins on differential influx into endometrium and myometrium. Am. J. Obstet. Gynecol. **159**: 509.
8. CSERMELY, T., L. M. DEMERS & E. C. HUGHES. 1969. Organ culture of human endometrium. Effects of progesterone. Obstet. Gynecol. **34**: 252.
9. GURPIDE, E. & M. WELCH. 1969. Dynamics of uptake of estrogens and androgens by human endometrium. J. Biol. Chem. **244**: 5159.
10. TSENG, L., A. STOLEE & E. GURPIDE. 1972. Quantitative studies on the uptake and metabolism of estrogens and progesterone by human endometrium. Endocrinology **90**: 390.
11. RIDDICK, D. H. & M. A. KUSMIK. 1977. Decidua: A possible source of amniotic fluid prolactin. Am. J. Obstet. Gynecol. **127**: 187.

12. GOLLANDER, A., HURLEY, T., BARRET, J. & S. HANDWERGER. 1979. Synthesis of prolactin by human decidua in vitro. J. Endocrinol. **82**: 263.

13. CASEY, M. L., S. M. COX, B. BEUTLER, L. MILEWICH & P. C. MACDONALD. 1989. Cachectin/tumor necrosis factor-alpha formation in human decidua: Potential role of cytokines in infection-induced preterm labor. J. Clin. Invest. **83**: 430.

14. ROMERO, R., Y. K. WU, D. T. BRODY, E. OTARZUN, G. W. DUFF & S. K. DURUM. 1989. Human decidua: A source of interleukin-1. Obstet. Gynecol. **73**: 31.

15. HUANG, J. R., L. TSENG, P. BISCHOF & O. A. JANNE. 1987. Regulation of prolactin production by progestin, estrogen and relaxin in human endometrial stromal cells. Endocrinology **121**: 2011.

16. KAUPPILA, A., H. E. ISOTALO, T. KIVINBEN & R. J. VIHKO. 1986. Prediction of clinical outcome with estrogen and progestin receptor concentrations and their relationships to clinical and histopathological variables in endometrial cancer. Cancer Res. **46**: 5380.

17. GOTTARDIS, M. M., S. P. ROBINSON, P. G. SATYASWAROOP & V. C. JORDAN. 1988. Contrasting actions of tamoxifen on endometrial and breast tumor growth in the athymic mouse. Cancer Res. **48**: 812.

Histology of the Human Endometrium: From Birth to Senescence

ALEX FERENCZY

Departments of Pathology and Obstetrics & Gynecology
The Sir Mortimer B. Davis Jewish General Hospital
Montreal, Quebec, Canada H3T 1E2

CHRISTINE BERGERON

Institut de Pathologie et Cytologie Appliqueés
Paris, France

INTRODUCTION

The intriguingly complex yet intimately inter-related biomorphologic phenomena in the human endometrium are geared to assist the developing conceptus and have been the subject of extensive investigations by students interested in this fascinating reproductive target tissue. One of the earliest students of the endometrium was Soranus of Ephesus, who in A.D. 200 was the first to provide a comprehensive description of the human uterus.[1] However, it was not until the XVth century when Leonardo da Vinci and Vesalius, who, on the basis of their experience in dissecting cadavers, correctly described the endometrial cavity as a single chamber system.[1] In the early 20th century, the embryonic development of the endometrium has been thoroughly studied by means of morphology by R. Muller and later by others[2,3] and has been directly related to that of the Mullerian ducts *per se*. Today, most investigators favor a common histogenetic origin for both the endometrial epithelium and its supportive mesenchyme, *i.e.*, from the primitive mesoderm.[3] This common derivation may explain cellular interconversions of human endometrial cells in certain situations.[4] For example, histology, ultrastructure and tissue culture experience with various cell lines demonstrated conversion of mesenchymal cells to epithelial cells in neoplastic conditions.[5] However, the contrary, *i.e.*, conversion of epithelial cells to mesenchymal cells, is much more frequently observed, both in non-neoplastic and malignant conditions *in vitro*[5,6] and *in vivo*.[7] Proliferation, differentiation and the eventual invagination of this primitive epithelial-mesenchymal system (including the myometrium) into the pelvic region during embryonic development result in the Mullerian tissue complex in adulthood. The influence of gonadal sex-steroid hormones on the development of the Mullerian duct is not clear.[8] However, estradiol (E_2R) and progesterone (PR) receptors are present in the fetal uterus of guinea pigs,[9] and at ultrastructural levels progesterone-related predecidua-like cells have been observed in human fetal endometrial specimens.[10] Also, high levels of estradiol preserve the Mullerian ducts in the male chick by its direct action on the ducts themselves[11] or by inhibiting the Mullerian inhibitor factor (MIF),[12] a glycoprotein produced by fetal Sertoli cells in the male and the granulosa cells in the female.[13]

In the adult, endometrial morphology and cellular functions are strongly influenced both directly and indirectly by sex-steroids. Indeed, steroid control of endometrial cells is mediated by estradiol (E_2) and progesterone (P) via their respective intranuclear receptors[14-18] and peptide growth factors and their receptors.[19-21] Cell culture studies of several weeks duration failed to demonstrate proliferative or secretory response of either the epithelial or stromal cells to estradiol or progesterone despite appreciable levels of steroid receptor concentration.[22] This experience may suggest that growth factors and their receptors or regulatory genes[23,24] may be involved in stimulating growth of the endometrium via an autocrine or paracrine pathway in *in vivo* situations. For example, epidermal growth factor (EGF) via its receptors acts as a mitogen for a variety of cells and participates in cell differentiation as well.[19] EGF binds to endometrium[20,25] and E_2 enhances binding of EGF to uterine cells *in vitro*.[26] Also, by immunohistochemistry and electron microscopy, serotonin and somatostin containing endocrine type cells have been found in normal cyclic endometrium.[27] Both hormones are considered to be related to growth-promoting cellular phenomena. Tenascin, an extracellular matrix protein has been immunolocalized around proliferative phase endometrial glands but not in secretory phase endometrium except around the proliferative vascular system.[28] These observations are in agreement with the concept that tenascin mediates epithelial/mesenchymal interactions, particularly cell migration and proliferation during embryonic development as well as during normal physiologic and neoplastic conditions by inhibiting cell attachment to fibronectin. In MCF-7 breast cancer cells, production of tenascin may be stimulated by hormonally regulated growth factors.[29] Recently, it has been speculated that heat shock protein (HSP-84 and HSP-86) in the rodent's uterus are synthesized in response to E_2 rather than stress and may be mediators of E_2-dependent uterine growth.[30] This interplay between ovarian sex steroids, peptide growth factors and structure/function makes the endometrium a highly sensitive indicator of the hypothalamic-pituitary-ovarian axis. Indeed, the morphologic evaluation of the endometrium (dating) is considered useful in the diagnostic work-up of the infertile patient (FIG. 1). It also serves for better understanding the mechanisms of hormonal interactions at the cellular level.

Morphologically, the human endometrium contains two tissue layers with distinct response to hormonal stimuli and physiologic functions.[31,32] These are the upper two-third "functionalis" layer and the lower one-third "basalis" layer (FIG. 2).

CYCLIC PROLIFERATIVE ENDOMETRIUM

The histologic changes that occur during the pre-ovulatory phase of the menstrual cycle are neither specific of a given day nor of ovulation and are thus not useful for dating the endometrium. Indeed, all of the tissue components including the glands, stromal cells and endothelial cells demonstrate proliferation which peaks on cycle days 8 to 10.[31] The morphologic hallmarks of these alterations are increased mitotic activity and nuclear DNA and cytoplasmic RNA synthesis (FIG. 3, A and B). Labeling intensity of the nucleoprotein precursor radiothymidine is increased and DNA-S phase is shortened (FIG. 4).[33] The very large number of mitotic figures in gland cells of proliferative endometrium and the short DNA-S phase correlate well with high levels of nuclear organizing regions (NORs) as determined by histochemical tracing with silver stain.[34] NORs are found on chromosomes 13–15, 21 and 22 as loops of DNA, are transcribed to ribosomal RNA and are an index of cell proliferation.[35]

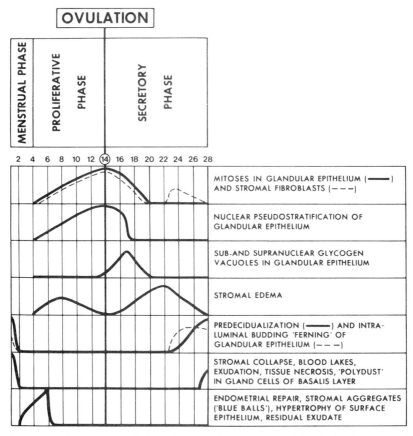

FIGURE 1. The major morphologic characteristics of the endometrium during the menstrual cycle. (*From* Ferenczy, A. 1987. Anatomy and histology of the uterine corpus. *In* Blaustein's Pathology of the Female Genital Tract. Third Edition. Springer-Verlag. New York, p. 257.)

The proliferative changes are significantly more pronounced in the functionalis than the basalis layer.[31] The biologic rationale for the geographic variation in proliferative indices may lie in the different physiologic functions of the functionalis vs. the basalis layer. The former is the seat of blastocyst implantation, whereas the latter provides origin for the regenerative endometrium following menstrual degeneration of the functionalis.[33]

Ultrastructural evidence of tissue proliferation is evidenced by an increase in free and bound ribosomes, mitochondria, Golgi and primary lysosomes in gland cells and stromal fibroblasts. Biochemically, these organelles provide for protein matrix, energy and synthesis of enzymes. Most of these are involved in carbohydrate metabolism and include glucose-6 phosphate dehydrogenase, isocitric dehydrogenase, pyruvate kinase and lactate dehydrogenase. Other enzymes are related to lytic processes at the time of implantation or if conception has not occurred menstrual degeneration.[31,32]

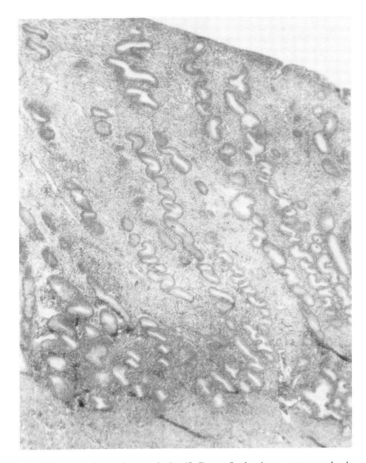

FIGURE 2. Proliferative endometrium, cycle day 12. Rows of voluminous, tortuous glands, arranged at regular intervals characterize the preovulatory endometrium. The glands have an S-shaped configuration, are closely apposed, and the lining cells have pseudostratified nuclei. The somewhat edematous stroma of the functionalis layer contrasts with the dense, compact stroma of the lower basal layer (H&E ×120). (*From* Ferenczy, A. 1987. Anatomy and histology of the uterine corpus. *In* Blaustein's Pathology of the Female Genital Tract. Third Edition. Springer-Verlag. New York, p. 257.)

A typical feature of proliferative endometrium in epithelial cells is increased cilio- and microvillogenesis (FIG. 5A). This is considerably decreased in endometrial cells that are exposed to endogenous or exogenous progestogens but are increased in hyperplastic endometria associated with hyperestrogenism.[31] The data suggest that endometrial ciliogenesis and microvillogenesis are estrogen-dependent.[31] The strong forward and slow recovery ciliary beat pattern and their concentration around gland openings (FIG. 5B) facilitate mobilization and distribution of endometrial secretions during the luteal phase of the cycle.[33]

Intranuclear E_2R and PR concentrations are the highest[14-18] during the preovula-

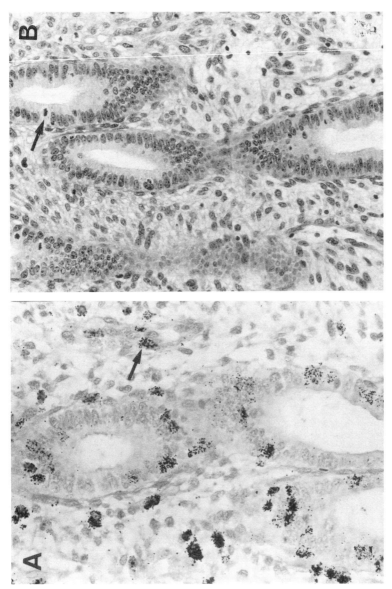

FIGURE 3. Proliferative endometrium. A. *Cycle day 12.* Radiothymidine granules are heavily incorporated into nuclei of endometrial gland cells, stromal fibroblasts and capillary endothelium (*arrow*) (H&E ×250). B. *Cycle day 7.* Straight glands with narrow lumens, pseudostratified nuclei of gland cells and mitoses (*arrows*). The stroma is edematous and well vascularized (H&E ×200). (*From* Ferenczy, A. & M. Guralnick. 1983. Endometrial microstructure: structure-function relationships throughout the menstrual cycle. Semin. Reprod. Endocrinol. **1:** 205.)

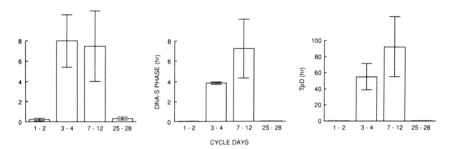

FIGURE 4. Kinetic characteristics of the endometrium during the menstrual cycle by *in vitro* histoautoradiography using the double-labeling technique with ^{3}H-thymidine. Labeling index (LI), DNA synthesis phase (DNA-S phase), and potential doubling time (TpD) are negligible during the premenstrual and early menstrual periods. Note the sudden increase in LI and shortening of the DNA-S phase and tissue turnover time during the regenerative period on cycle days 3–4. The postregenerative period (cycle day 5 on) is characterized by prolongation of both the DNA-S phase and tissue turnover time. (*From* Ferenczy, A. 1987. Anatomy and histology of the uterine corpus. *In* Blaustein's Pathology of the Female Genital Tract. Third Edition. Springer-Verlag. New York, p. 257.)

tory period of the menstrual cycle by immunohistochemical tracing with monoclonal antibodies against E_2R and PR (FIG. 6, A and B) confirming the fact that PR synthesis is mainly induced by E_2 in target cells via the E_2-receptor complex mechanism. The presence of PR in the proliferative phase is thus a good marker of endometrial E_2-sensitivity.

SECRETORY PHASE ENDOMETRIUM

After ovulation, the E_2-primed endometrium undergoes progestational secretory differentiation[31,32] and the daily changes are specific of post-ovulatory endometrium. Only these alterations are useful to date the endometrium (FIG. 1) and to determine whether ovulation has taken place. The gland cells acquire subnuclear intracytoplasmic glycogenization, the first histologic sign that ovulation has taken place (FIG. 7, A and B). Ultrastructurally giant mitochondria and the so-called nucleolar channel system (NCS) appear in gland cells.[32] NCSs are unique to women and occur mainly during the post-ovulatory period (FIG. 8, A and B). They are presumably produced by the infolding of the nuclear membranes under P stimulation and may facilitate transport of nuclear RNA to the cytoplasmic substance. The development of these fine structural alterations in gland cells is followed by active extracellular (apocrine) secretion of glycoproteins. This is characterized by protrusions and eventual detachment of the apical portion of cells containing glycoproteins (FIG. 8C). Post-ovulatory type endometrial glands also secrete the so-called uteroglobin-like protein, progestogen-associated endometrial protein (PEP)[36] and the pregnancy-associated endometrial α_2-globulin (α_2-PEG).[37] The precise physiologic role of these apparently P-dependent proteins is not clear, but they may be related to implantation and PEP to reflect corpus luteum function. Transudation of plasma from circulating blood in the endometrial mucosa also contributes to uterine secretory fluids.[31,32] Intraglandular secretions achieve maximum level on cycle day 21 and coincide with the time of blastocyst im-

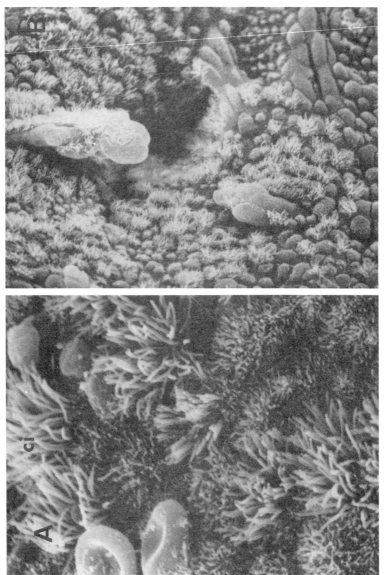

FIGURE 5. Proliferative endometrium, cycle day 12. A. Scanning electron microscopy of surface epithelium with ciliated cells (ci) and microvillous cells. Red blood cells 7μ in size are seen (×3000). B. On cycle days 5 to 6 the surface is completely repaired and the gland openings are surrounded by ciliated cells (×1000). (*From* Ferenczy, A. & M. Guralnick. 1983. Endometrial microstructure: Structure-function relationships throughout the menstrual cycle. Semin. Reprod. Endocrinol. 1: 205.)

plantation, if in fact, fertilization takes place in this cycle. As apocrine secretory activity is initiated in gland cells, DNA synthesis and mitoses decrease and disappear, respectively.[31,32] Inhibition of mitosis has been attributed to rising levels of postovulatory P, which down-regulate E_2 action.[38] This concept is supported by recent immunohistochemical studies in which E_2R and PR were significantly reduced or absent in endometrial glands soon after the time of implantation.[15-18] Another mechanism contributing to progesterone stimulated arrest of epithelial growth may be via the P specific enzyme 17β hydroxydehydrogenase (E_2DH). This enzyme converts E_2 into estrone (E_1) which leaves the target cell without stimulating the nucleus.[39]

By the time of implantation, on cycle days 21–22, the predominant morphologic alteration is edema of the endometrial stroma (FIG. 9A). This is possibly mediated by prostaglandin E_2 (PGE_2) and prostaglandin $F_{2\alpha}$ ($PGF_{2\alpha}$) and coincides also with rising E_2 and P levels. Estradiol stimulates the production of $PGF_{2\alpha}$, whereas progesterone stimulates the synthesis of both $PGF_{2\alpha}$ and E_2 in *in vitro* conditions.[40] PGE_2 presumably promotes capillary permeability either directly or by increasing histamine release resulting in stromal edema. Receptors for E_2 and P have been immunolocalized in the muscular wall of endometrial vessels,[41] and sex steroids may also play a role in vascular proliferation in the endometrium. The endothelial lining of endometrial vessels is uniformly free of sex steriod receptors.[15,16,41] The arachidonic acidprostaglandin related cyclooxygenase has been localized in smooth muscle cells and endothelium of endometrial arterioles in the human by immunohistochemistry.[42] Prostaglandins are likely to be the primary stimulator of vascular mitotic activity, which leads to coiling of the arteriolar/capillary system.

The stroma of the endometrium is composed of highly specialized stromal cells. They are not simply fibroblasts, but respond to hormonal stimuli and have receptors for both E_2 and P.[14-18] In addition, they synthesize prostaglandins,[43] and when transformed into decidual cells actively secrete prolactin, immunosuppressive substances and a variety of serum proteins,[44] in particular pregnancy-associated endometrial α_1-globulin (α_1-PEG)[45] components of the basement membrane.[46] The latter resembles other basement membranes in the body such as found in glomeruli for example. Interestingly, the so-called Nitabuch's fibrinoid layer at the placental implantation site is made of laminin-rich, fibrillar basement membrane-like material.[31] This is presumably of decidual rather than trophoblastic origin. Although endometrial stromal cells were suggested to derive from the bone marrow,[47] at present most consider their origin from the primitive uterine mesenchymal stem cells.[10]

The *raison d'être* of endometrial stromal fibroblasts is their potential transformation into gestational decidual cells (decidua vera) via their precursor form, the predecidual cells (FIG. 9B). Predecidualization occurs after implantation on cycle day 23 and consists of cytonuclear enlargement with increased nuclear DNA synthesis (polyploidy), mitotic activity, and the formation of pericellular laminin rich basement membrane.[47] The latter is typical of epithelial cells, although basement membrane surrounds other mesenchymal type cells as well, including adipocytes and muscle cells. Similarly, predecidual cells akin to epithelial cells contain cytokeratin positive intermediate filaments by immunohistochemistry.[48] Growth factors responsible for polyploidy and mitoses in predecidual cells are not fully known or understood.[49,50] Immunohistochemically, predecidual cells are devoid of E_2R.[16-18] As a result, E_2 acts either directly without its receptors or stromal cell proliferation in the mid-secretory endometrium or via growth-related peptides[25] or via prostaglandins[34] or E_2 has no action on post-ovulatory stromal cell replication. Curiously, predecidual cells have

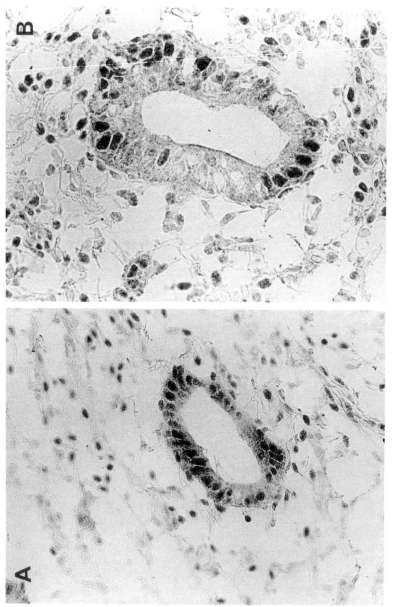

FIGURE 6. Immunocytolocalization of E_2R (A) and PR (B) during the proliferative phase. **A.** There is strong intranuclear staining with ER-ICA in both the endometrial glands and stromal fibroblasts (no counterstain, ×450.) (*From* Bergeron, C., A. Ferenczy & G. Shyamala. 1988. Distribution of estrogen receptors in various cell types of normal, hyperplastic and neoplastic human endometrial tissues. Lab. Invest. **58:** 338.) **B.** The nuclei of most gland cells and stromal fibroblasts demonstrate strong staining reaction with Mab α- PR6 (no counterstain, ×450). Figure shown at 90% of original size.

PRs by immunohistochemistry,[16-18] and in the absence of E_2R, they may be constitutively synthesized.[16] PRs together with the high levels of mid-secretory progesterone are likely to influence cytoplasmic differentiation of endometrial stromal fibroblasts and the secretory functions of decidual cells. For example, the production of prolactin in pre-decidual and particularly gestational decidual cells is regulated by progesterone and the peptide hormone relaxin.[51] Decidual transformation is not unique to endometrial stromal cells for similar alterations may occur in the subcoelomic mesenchyme of the pelvis, ovary and abdomen in association with progestational stimulation, particularly during pregnancy.[52] Decidualization can be produced also, by electrical, mechanical or chemical stimulation in progesterone-primed uteri of rodents.[53] In the gestational endometrium, decidual cells control the invasive nature of the implanting trophoblasts. Indeed, in the absence of decidua, the trophoblast deeply invades the myometrium leading to placenta accreta, increta and percreta. These phenomena in turn produce intractable post-partum hemorrhage which must be treated by hysterectomy. Prolactin, identical to pituitary prolactin, was demonstrated *in vitro* in both predecidual and gestational decidual cells by immunoblotting, and its production is regulated by the combined effects of progesterone and the peptide hormone relaxin.[51]

In the non-gestational endometrium, predecidual transformation expands after the 23rd day of the cycle and forms the so-called compacta layer in the upper strata of the functionalis of the endometrium by cycle day 25. Transmission electron microscopy and enzyme tracing found Golgi-derived acid phosphatase rich primary lysosomes in the epithelial, stromal and endothelial cells of the endometrium.[31,32] In the first half of the secretory phase, acid phosphatase and other potent lytic enzymes are confined to the lysosomes (FIG. 10A). Progesterone inhibits their release by stabilizing lysosomal membranes. During the second half of the secretory phase of the menstrual cycle, both E_2 and P are withdrawn; as a result the lysosomal membrane integrity is no longer maintained, and the enzymes are released into autophagic bodies (FIG. 10B), and later into the cytoplasmic substance and intracellular space. The lytic enzymes will digest all cellular elements including desmosomes and surface membranes. In the vascular endothelium, this will lead to platelet deposition and further release of prostaglandins, vascular thrombosis, extravasation of red blood cells and tissue necrosis.[31-33] Coinciding with the dramatic increase of polymorphonuclear leukocytes, prostaglandins both $F_{2\alpha}$ and E_2 increase significantly in the secretory endometrium and the levels are higher in the menstrual endometrium.[36,40,43] PGs are produced via sex steroids[43] in *in vivo* experiments and endometrial stromal fibroblasts contain PG synthesizing enzymes, whereas gland cells may process and degrade PGs.[54] It is possible that $PGF_{2\alpha}$ stimulates vasoconstriction and myometrial contraction at the endomyometrial level which leads to ischemia of the functionalis. That vasoconstriction is prostaglandin rather than hormone-related is supported further by immunohistochemical studies which failed to trace E_2R and PR in myometrial vessels in the human.[15,16]

From the time of implantation on, the so-called metrial cells or granulocytes (also termed kornchenzellen or K cells) appear and are also present in early gestational endometrium.[31,32] These cells have phloxinophilic cytoplasmic granules and non-lobulated nucleus (FIG. 10C). These cells were believed to secrete relaxin and contribute to the destruction of the reticulum network of the endometrium at the implantation site or prior to menstruation via lytic enzymes.[32] Today, the most widely held hypothesis, however, is that metrial cells have an immunoprotective influence on blastocyst implantation[55] by suppressing cytotoxic lymphocytes. Indeed, recent immuno-

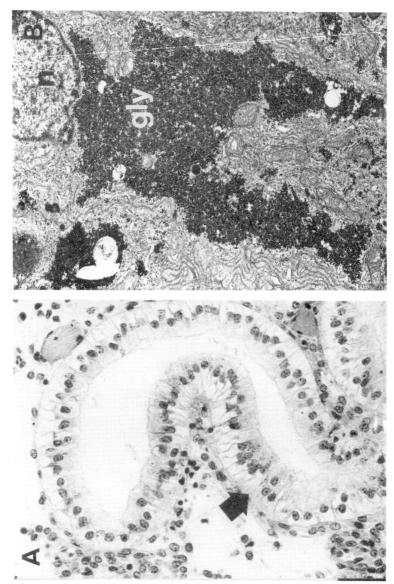

FIGURE 7. Secretory endometrium, cycle day 17. A. Secretory endometrial glands have "S"-shaped configuration, subnuclear vacuolization (*arrow*) and palisading of nuclei in the middle of the lining epithelium (H&E ×250). B. Subnuclear vacuoles correspond at the electron microscopic level to massive accumulation of electron-dense glycogen granules (gly). (×15000). (*From* Ferenczy, A. & M. Guralnick. 1983. Endometrial microstructure: structure-function relationships throughout the menstrual cycle. Semin. Reprod. Endocrinol. **1:** 205.)

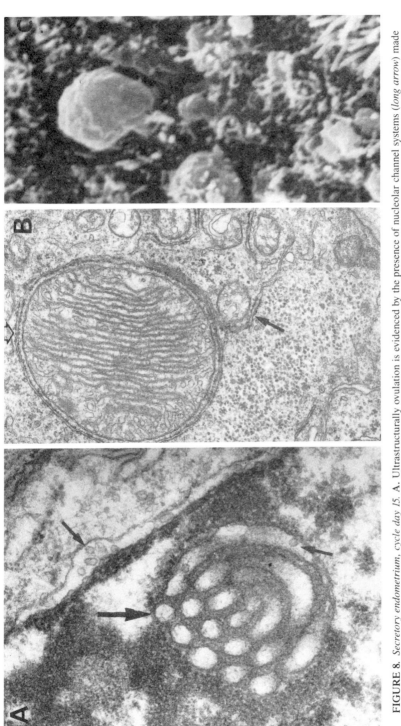

FIGURE 8. *Secretory endometrium, cycle day 15.* **A.** Ultrastructurally ovulation is evidenced by the presence of nucleolar channel systems (*long arrow*) made of large hollow, membrane-bound tubules 600 to 1000 Å in size. Note vesicular structures between the inner and outer nuclear membranes and NCS tubules (*short arrows*) (×30,000). **B.** Energy-rich giant mitochondrion packed with cristae, intimately surrounded by parallel membranes of granular endoplasmic reticulum (*arrow*) and glycogen granules (×20,000). **C.** *Secretory endometrium, cycle day 19.* Epithelial cells with prominent cytoplasmic budding, representing apocrine secretory protuberance. Hair-like microvilli cover surface membrane of cell (×32,000). (*From* Ferenczy, A. & M. Guralnick. 1983. Endometrial microstructure: Structure-function relationships throughout the menstrual cycle. Semin. Reprod. Endocrinol. **1:** 205.)

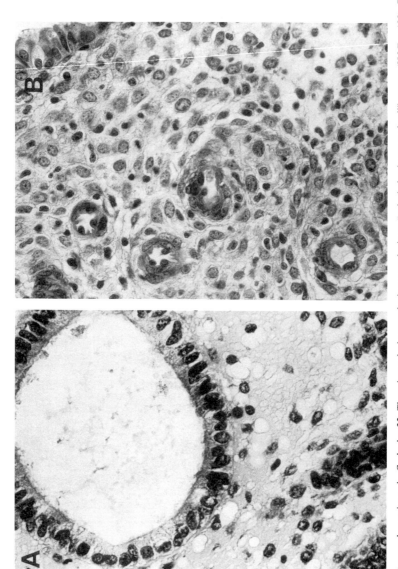

FIGURE 9. Secretory endometrium. A. *Cycle day 22.* There is marked stromal edema producing a "naked glands–stromal cell" pattern (H&E ×400). B. *Cycle day 24.* Liver cell-like predecidual stromal cells with large nucleus and cytoplasmic substance delimited by well-formed cytoplasmic membranes (H&E ×400).

histochemical studies identified them as granulated lymphocytes, for they react with leukocyte common antigen (CD-4), T cell antigens (CD-2,7,38), CHL, MT-1 and NKH-1.[56] Their perivascular location and increased incidence in the late secretory phase of the menstrual cycle suggest a derivation directly from blood rather than intra-endometrial lymphoid aggregates. Supernatants from cultures of secretory phase endo-metrium have shown a marked hormone and nutrient-independent suppressive effect of lymphocyte response to phytohemaglutinin M stimulation and the mixed lympho-cyte reaction. Suppression was significantly greater by secretory than proliferative endometrial tissue and was suspected to be due to as yet uncharacterized, soluble, diffusible and immunosuppressive factors.[57] The extent of participation of metrial cells in implantation seems to be limited, however, for ectopic tubal implantation sites are often devoid of metrial cells.

MENSTRUAL PHASE ENDOMETRIUM

Its accurate histologic interpretation confirms that bleeding has occurred as a result of ovulation. Also, since the duration of the luteal phase is generally constant it pro-vides information of the approximate date of ovulation. On the basis of present his-tologic, histochemical and immunohistochemical data, it appears that the menstrual tissue is the result of the enzymatic autodigestion and prostaglandin related ischemic necrosis of non-gestational estrogen/progestogen primed endometrium. The menstrual fluid is made of autolysed functionalis devoid of nuclear DNA synthesis[33] and sex steroid receptors,[15,16] inflammatory exudate, red blood cells, and proteolytic enzymes (FIG. 11A). One of the latter, blood protease plasmin, presumably prevents clotting of menstrual blood. Plasminogen activators, which convert plasminogen into plasmin, are also found in late secretory and menstrual endometrium and are released from degenerated endometrial vascular endothelium.[31]

REGENERATIVE PHASE ENDOMETRIUM

Nuclear DNA tracing studies have shown increased DNA synthesis in the basalis of the fundus and body of the uterus and the adjacent isthmic and peritubal ostial endometrium, all of which remain intact throughout the menstrual cycle. Interestingly, DNA synthesis occurs only in those areas of the basalis which have been completely denuded by cycle days 2 and 3.[33] Nuclear DNA synthesis is correlated with rapid re-epithelialization by proliferating gland cells from the basalis layer and the surface epithelium of peritubal/isthmic regions of the endometrial cavity.[33] The newly formed resurfacing cells are flattened to spindle shape resembling fibroblasts (FIG. 11B). How-ever, they are in direct contact with epithelial surface and gland cells and their ultra-structure, including basement membrane formation, intercellular desmosomes are in keeping with their epithelial nature. They are rich in intracellular microfilamentous/microtubular systems and pseudopodial projections (FIG. 11C), features that are con-sistent with ameboid contraction/expansion/migration.[33] Post-menstrual epithelial re-pair is closely related to the underlying stromal fibroblasts. These typically aggregate under the resurfacing epithelium and form a compact cell mass over which the epi-thelial cells migrate (FIG. 11B). Experimental studies demonstrated that epithelial growth may be triggered and sustained by the adjacent supportive fibroblasts.[4,29] Whether

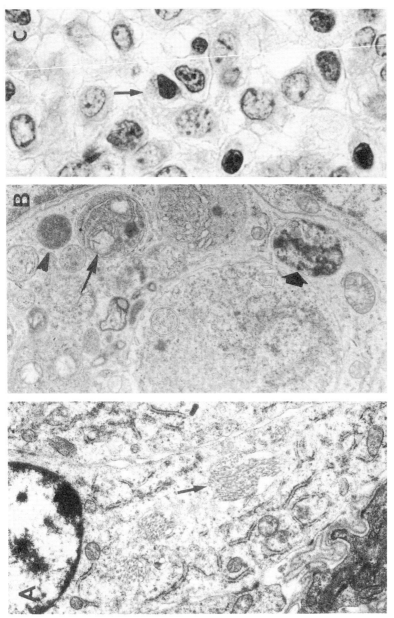

FIGURE 10. Secretory endometrium, cycle day 25. A. Ultrastructure of predecidual stromal cells with membrane-bound heterophagolysosomes (*arrow*) containing extracellular collagen fibers (×7000). B. Intracytoplasmic, membrane-bound primary lysosomes (*arrowhead*) flanked by autocytophagolysosomes (*arrow*) with incorporated cytoplasmic organelles (*arrowhead*) in varying stages of enzymatic digestion (×18000). (*From* Ferenczy, A. & M. Guralnick. 1983. Endometrial microstructure: Structure-function relationships throughout the menstrual cycle. Semin. Reprod. Endocrinol. **1**: 205.) C. Metrial cell (*arrow*) with granular cytoplasm surrounded by predecidual cells (H&E ×500). Figure shown at 90% of original size.

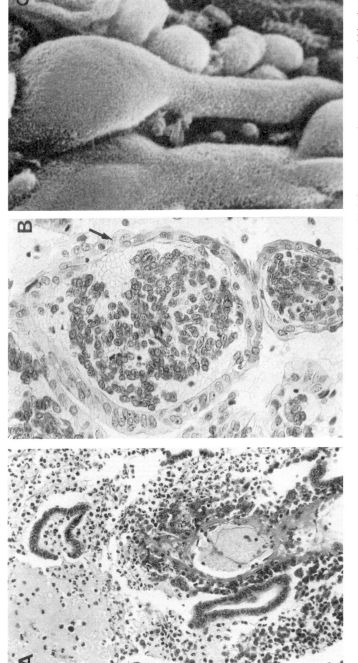

FIGURE 11. Menstrual endometrium, cycle day 1. **A.** The stroma and glands are collapsed, admixed with inflammatory exudate, extravasated red blood cells and thrombosed vessels (*middle*) (H&E ×300). **B.** Endometrial stromal fibroblasts forming aggregates over resurfacing regenerative epithelial cells, which typically have flattened cytoplasm (*arrow*), enlarged nuclei and nucleoli consistent with repair and nuclear polyploidy (H&E ×300). (*From* Ferenczy, A. 1987. Anatomy and histology of the uterine corpus. *In* Blaustein's Pathology of the Female Genital Tract. Third Edition. Springer-Verlag. New York, p. 257.) **C.** *Menstrual endometrium, cycle days 3–4.* The regenerative surface epithelial membrane contains voluminous, flattened epithelial cells with pseudopodial extensions (×2000). (*From* Ferenczy, A. & M. Guralnick. 1983. Endometrial microstructure: structure–function relationships throughout the menstrual cycle. Semin. Reprod. Endocrinol. **1**: 205.) Figure shown at 80% of original size.

this close interaction is simply mechanical, providing surface on which migration may occur, or exchange of substances that regulate growth, *i.e.*, EGF also occurs between the two cell systems is not clear. The fact that endometrial stromal fibroblasts produce a fibronectin inhibitor, tenascin,[29] which in turn facilitates epithelial migration is in favor of a complex physical/chemical inter-relationship during the process of endometrial regeneration.

Also, the participation of E_2 to endometrial regeneration *per se* is unclear. Since plasma levels are low during the menstrual period, tissue repair *per se* is suspected to be injury- rather than hormone-dependent. Migration and short DNA synthesis phase of the regenerative epithelial cells explain the spectacularly rapid wound healing capability of the human endometrium (FIG. 4). Furthermore, the presently available data are inconsistent with previous postulate that the regenerative endometrium derives directly from persistent or residual secretory endometrium or stromal fibroblasts of the endometrium.[31] Indeed, neither ultrastructural nor immunohistochemical evidence is provided for conversion of epithelial cells from stromal cells during periods of endometrial regeneration. Also, in experimental endometrial regeneration in the rabbit, proliferation kinetics and morphologic alterations of the regenerative but estrogen-deprived atrophic endometrium associated with ovariectomy were similar to those animals with intact ovaries.[33] Following the initial epithelial spread, cell division increases and the subsequent inter-anastomosis between converging epithelial membranes lead to complete reconstruction of a new surface epithelium by cycle day 5.[33] From cycle day 5 on, there is a sudden increase in nuclear DNA synthesis and mitoses in all cell components of the regenerated endometrium (FIG. 4). These changes are accompanied by an increase in plasma E_2 and endometrial E_2 receptor concentrations.[14,15] The basalis endometrium contains high levels of E_2R but is immunonegative for PR during periods of menstruation.[15,16] It is of interest to note that in menstruating primates (rhesus monkeys) the origin of postmenstrual endometrium is also the basalis layer, which akin to its human counterpart retains DNA synthesis and receptors for E_2 during the entire menstrual cycle.[58]

SENESCENT ENDOMETRIUM

In the absence of sufficiently elevated estrogenic concentrations, either of endogenous or exogenous sources that are required to stimulate endometrial growth, the endometrium undergoes progressive involution from proliferative to inactive in the mid-50s to atrophy (senescence) in the late-60s. Histologically, the inactive endometrium contains glands that resemble architecturally those of the premenopausal proliferative phase; however, they are devoid of mitoses and the supportive stroma, which lacks mitoses, is more compact than its cyclic counterpart. The atrophic endometrium consists mainly of the basalis layer with few glands oriented parallel to the surface; the stroma is fibrotic and the vessels are often obliterated by fibrosis (FIG. 12, A and B). Although mitotic activity is absent, nuclear synthesis and E_2Rs are maintained in the senescent, inactive but not in the severely atrophic endometrium.[14] This phenomenon explains why upon estrogenic stimulation, the inactive (but not the severely atrophic) endometrium may be *rejuvenated* to a proliferative type tissue and both gland cells and stromal fibroblasts acquire receptors for progesterone which if exposed to progestogens may undergo secretory transformation including decidualization of the stroma.[59] Alternatively, high doses of sustained exogenous estrogenic stimulation un-

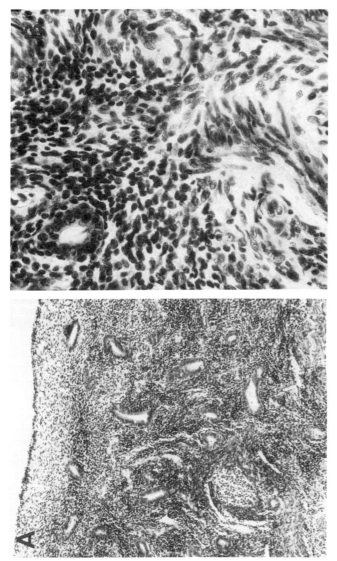

FIGURE 12. Atrophic endometrium. A. The endometrial mucosa is retracted, containing few atrophic glands with narrow lumen (H&E ×120). B. Higher magnification of atrophic glands compressed by fibrocellular stroma. The vessels are partly obliterated by fibrosis (*lower*) (H&E ×300).

opposed by progestogens may lead to the development of hyperplasia,[60] whereas progestational therapy either prevents hyperplasia or reverts hyperplastic endometrium into a secretory tissue.[61]

CONCLUSION

Knowledge and understanding of the morphologic alterations that occur in the human endometrium during the normal menstrual cycle are significant inasmuch as they reflect normal physiologic functions of the hypothalamic pituitary ovarian axis which in turn are the prerequisite for the successful implantation of the conceptus. Also, normal morphology serves as baseline information for recognizing endometrium in pathologic states.

Further studies with immunohistochemistry using growth- and immunosuppressive-related substances may shed insight into our understanding of the cellular mechanisms that operate endometrial epithelial/stromal interactions in relation to hormonal stimuli.

SUMMARY

Embryologically, the human endometrium is of mesodermal origin, and constitutes the mucosal lining of the fused Mullerian ducts of the uterus. In the adult, premenopausal woman, the endometrium follows a precisely programmed series of morphologic and physiologic events, characterized by growth, secretory differentiation, and in the absence of conception, degeneration and regeneration. Proliferation, secretion and degeneration are confined to the upper functionalis layer, whereas the lower basalis layer is the seat of regenerative endometrium. In the postmenopausal years, absence of biologically significant estrogenic stimulation leads to progressive endometrial involution, from proliferative to inactive in the mid-50s to atrophy in the late-60s.

Cyclic endometrial alterations are controlled by the ovarian estrogens and progesterone via their respective endometrial intranuclear receptors, and possibly other peptides and enzymes. They provide appropriate environment for the implanting conceptus. The intimate inter-relationship between endometrial structure/function and steroid hormones during the premenopausal period serves as an indicator of the hypothalamo-pituitary-ovarian axis as related to ovulatory states.

REFERENCES

1. RAMSEY, E. M. 1989. History. In Biology of the Uterus. 2nd edit. R. M. Wynn & W. P. Jollie, Eds.: 1–17. Plenum Publishing Corp. New York, NY.
2. HUNTER, R. H. 1930. Observations on the development of the human female genital tract. Contributions to Embryology 22: 91–107.
3. O'RAHILLY, R. 1977. Prenatal human development. In Biology of the Uterus. R. M. Wynn, Ed.: 35–57. Plenum Publishing Corp. New York, NY.
4. COOKE, P. S., F. B. A. UCHIMA, D. K. FUJII, H. A. BERN & G. R. CUNHA. 1986. Restoration of normal morphology and estrogen responsiveness in cultured vaginal and uterine epithelia transplanted with stroma. Proc. Natl. Acad. Sci. USA 83: 2109–2113.
5. MASUDA, A., A. TAKEDA, H. FUKAMI, C. YAMADA & M. MATSUYAMA. 1987. Characteristics of cell lines established from a mixed mesodermal tumor of the human ovary. Cancer 60: 2696–2703.

6. CONNELL, N. D. & J. G. RHEINWALD. 1983. Regulation of the cytoskeleton in mesothelial cells: Reversible loss of keratin and increase in vimentin during rapid growth in culture. Cell **34:** 245–253.

7. DAWE, C. J., J. WHANG-PENG, W. D. MORGAN, E. C. HEARON & T. KNUTSEN. 1971. Epithelial origin of polyoma salivary tumors in mice: Evidence based on chromosome-marked cells. Science **171:** 394–397.

8. PELLINIEMI, L. J. & M. DYM. 1980. The fetal gonad and sexual differentiation. In Maternal-fetal Endocrinology. D. Tulchinsky & K. J. Ryan, Eds. W. B. Saunders. Philadelphia, PA.

9. PASQUALINI, J. R., C. SUMIDA, A. GULINO, J. TARDY, B. L. NGUYEN, C. GELLY & C. COSQUER-CLAVREUL. 1983. Progesterone receptor during fetal development. In Progesterone and Progestins. C. W. Bardin, E. Milgrom & P. Mauvais-Jarvis, Eds. Raven Press. New York, NY.

10. KONISHI, I., S. FUJII, H. OKAMURA & T. MORI. 1984. Development of smooth muscle in the human fetal uterus: An ultrastructural study. J. Anat. **11:** 1–14.

11. MACLAUGHLIN, D. T., J. M. HUTSON & P. K. DONAHOE. 1983. Specific estradiol binding in embryonic Mullerian ducts: a potential modulator of regression in the male and female chick. Endocrinology **113:** 141–145.

12. DRISCOLL, S. G. & S. H. TAYLOR. 1980. Effects of prenatal maternal estrogen on the male urogenital system. Obstet. Gynecol. **56:** 537–542.

13. VOUTILAINEN, R. & W. L. MILLER. 1989. Potential relevance of Mullerian inhibiting substance to ovarian physiology. Semin. Reprod. Endocrinol. **7:** 88–93.

14. PRESS, M. F., N. NOUSEK-GOEBL, W. J. KING, A. L. HERBST & G. L. GREENE. 1984. Immunohistochemical assessment of estrogen receptor distribution in the human endometrium throughout the menstrual cycle. Lab. Invest. **51:** 495–503.

15. BERGERON, C., A. FERENCZY & G. SHYAMALA. 1988. Distribution of estrogen receptors in various cell types of normal, hyperplastic and neoplastic human endometrial tissues. Lab. Invest. **58:** 338–345.

16. BERGERON, C., A. FERENCZY, D. O. TOFT, W. SCHNEIDER & G. SHYAMALA. 1988. Immunocytochemical study of progesterone receptors in the human endometrium during the menstrual cycle. Lab. Invest. **59:** 862–869.

17. LESSEY, B. A., A. P. KELLAM, D. A. METZGER, A. F. HANEY, G. L. GREENE & K. S. MCCARTY. 1988. Immunohistochemical analysis of human uterine estrogen and progesterone receptors throughout the menstrual cycle. J. Clin. Endocrinol. Metab. **67:** 334–340.

18. GARCIA, E., P. BOUCHARD, J. DE BRUX, J. BERDAN, R. FRYDMAN, G. SCHAISON, E. MILGROM & M. PERROT-APPLANAT. 1988. Use of immunocytochemistry of progesterone and estrogen receptors for endometrial dating. J. Clin. Endocrinol. Metab. **67:** 80–87.

19. CARPENTER, G. & J. G. ZENDEGUI. 1986. Epidermal growth factor, its receptor and related proteins. Exp. Cell Res. **164:** 1–10.

20. HOFMANN, G. E., C. V. RAO, G. H. BARROWS, G. S. SHULTZ & J. S. SANFILIPPO. 1984. Binding sites for epidermal growth factor in human uterine tissues and leiomyomas. J. Clin. Endocrinol. Metab. **58:** 880–884.

21. KOUTSILIERIS, M. 1989. Human uterus-derived growth substances for rat bone cells and fibroblasts. Am. J. Obstet. Gynecol. **161:** 1313–1317.

22. KLEINMAN, D., Y. SHARON, I. SAROV & V. INSLER. 1983. Human endometrium in cell culture: A new method for culturing human endometrium as separate epithelial and stromal components. Arch. Gynecol. **234:** 103–112.

23. MURPHY, L. J., L. C. MURPHY & H. G. FRIESEN. 1987. Estrogen induction of N-myc and c myc proto-oncogene expression in the rat uterus. Endocrinol **120:** 1882–1888.

24. UDOM, L. D., J. M. BARRETT, C. G. PANTAZIS, L. D.. STODDARD & P. G. MCDONOUGH. 1989. Immunocytochemical study of ras and myc proto-oncogene polypeptide expression in the human menstrual cycle. Am. J. Obstet. Gynecol. **161:** 1663–1668.

25. BERCHUCK, A., A. P. SOISSON, G. J. OLT, J. T. SOPER, D. L. CLARKE-PEARSON, R. C. BAST JR. & K. S. MCCARTY JR. 1989. Reactivity of epidermal growth factor receptor monoclonal antibodies with human uterine tissues. Arch. Pathol. Lab. Med. **113:** 1155–1158.

26. MUKKU, V. R. & G. M. STANCEL. 1985. Regulation of epidermal growth factor receptor by estrogen. J. Biol. Chem. **260:** 9820–9824.

27. SATAKE, T. & M. MATSUYAMA. 1987. Argyrophil cells in normal endometrial glands. Virchows Arch. A. **410:** 449–454.

28. VOLLMER, G., G. P. SIEGAL, R. CHIQUET-EHRISMANN, V. A. LIGHTNER, H. ARNHOLDT & R.
     KNUPPEN. 1990. Tenascin expression in the human endometrium and in endometrial adeno-
     carcinomas. Lab. Invest. **62**: 725–730.
29. CHIQUET-EHRISMANN, R., P. KALLA & C. A. PEARSON. 1989. Participation of tenascin and TGF-
     beta in reciprocal epithelial-mesenchymal interactions of MCF 7 cells and fibroblasts. Cancer
     Res. **49**: 4322–4325.
30. SHYAMALA, G., Y. GAUTHIER, S. K. MOORE, M. G. CATELLI & S. J. ULLRICH. 1989. Estrogenic
     regulation of murine uterine 90-kilodalton heat shock protein gene expression. Mol. Cell.
     Biol. **9**: 3567–3570.
31. FERENCZY, A. & M. GURALNICK. 1983. Endometrial microstructure: Structure-function rela-
     tionships throughout the menstrual cycle. Semin. Reprod. Endocrinol. **1**: 205–219.
32. WYNN, R. M. 1989. The human endometrium. Cyclic and gestational changes. *In* Biology of
     the Uterus. 2nd edit. R. M. Wynn & W. P. Jollie, Eds.: 289–331. Plenum Publishing Corp.
     New York, NY.
33. FERENCZY, A. 1980. Regeneration of the human endometrium. *In* Progress in Surgical Pathology.
     C. M. Fenoglio & M. Wolff, Eds. Vol. 1: 157–173, Masson Publ. Inc. New York, NY.
34. WILKINSON, N., C. H. BUCKLEY, L. CHAWNER & H. FOX. 1990. Nucleolar organiser regions
     in normal, hyperplastic and neoplastic endometria. Int. J. Gynecol. Pathol. **9**: 55–59.
35. CROCKER, J., J. C. MACARTNEY & P. J. SMITH. 1988. Correlation between DNA flow cytometric
     and nucleolar organiser regions in non-Hodgkin's lymphoma. J. Pathol. **154**: 1–6.
36. JOSHI, S. G. 1983. Progestin-regulated proteins of the human endometrium. Semin. Reprod.
     Endocrinol. **1**: 221–236.
37. WAITES, G. T., P. L. WOOD, R. A. WALKER & S. C. BELL. 1988. Immunohistological localization
     of human endometrial secretory protein, pregnancy-associated endometrial α_2-globulin (α_2-
     PEG) during the menstrual cycle. J. Reprod. Fertil. **82**: 665–672.
38. KATZENELLENBOGEN, B. S. 1980. Dynamics of steroid hormone receptor action. Ann. Rev. Physiol.
     42: 17–35.
39. GURPIDE, E., L. TSENG & S. B. GUSBERG. 1977. Estrogen metabolism in normal and neoplastic
     endometrium. Am. J. Obstet. Gynecol. **129**: 809–816.
40. NEULEN, J., H. P. ZAHRADNIK, U. FLECKEN & M. BRECKWOLDT. 1988. Effects of estradiol-17β
     and progesterone on the synthesis of prostaglandin $F_{2\alpha}$, prostaglandin E_2 and prostaglandin
     I_2 by fibroblasts from human endometrium in vitro. Prostaglandins **36**: 17–30.
41. PERROT-APPLANAT, M., M. T. GROYER-PICARD, E. GARCIA, F. LORENZO & E. MILGROM. 1988.
     Immunocytochemical demonstration of estrogen and progesterone receptors in muscle cells
     of uterine arteries in rabbits and humans. Endocrinology **123**: 1511–1519.
42. RAO, C. V., N. CHEGINI & Z. M. LEI. 1989. Immunocytochemical localization of 5- and
     12-lipoxygenases and cyclooxygenase in nonpregnant human uteri. *In* New Trends in Lipid
     Mediators Research. Reproductive Biology and Endocrine System. U. Zor, Z. Naor & A.
     Danon, Eds. **3**: 283–286. S. Karger. Basel.
43. SMITH, S. K., M. H. ABEL & D. T. BAIRD. 1984. Effect of 17β-estradiol and progesterone on
     the levels of prostaglandin $F_{2\alpha}$ and E_2 in human endometrium. Prostaglandins **27**: 591–597.
44. RIDDICK, D. H., D. C. DALY & C. A. WALTERS. 1983. The uterus as an endocrine compartment.
     Clinics Perinatol. **10**: 627–639.
45. WAITES, G. T., R. F. L. JAMES & S. C. BELL. 1988. Immunohistological localization of the human
     endometrial secretory protein pregnancy-associated endometrial α_1-globulin, an insulin like
     growth factor-binding protein during the menstrual cycle. J. Clin. Endocrinol. Metab. **67**:
     1100–1104.
46. WEWER, U. M., M. FABER, L. A. LIOTTA & R. ALBRECHTSEN. 1985. Immunochemical and
     ultrastructural assessment of the nature of the pericellular basement membrane of human de-
     cidual cells. Lab. Invest. **53**: 624–633.
47. KEARNS, M. 1983. Life history of decidual cells: A review. Am. J. Reprod. Immunol. **3**:
     78–82.
48. WINTER, S., E. D. YARRASCH, E. SCHMID & W. W. FRANKE. 1980. Differences in polypeptide
     composition of cytokeratin filaments, including filaments from different epithelial tissues and
     cells. Eur. J. Cell Biol. **22**: 371.
49. KING, R. S. B., P. T. TOWNSEND, M. I. WHITEHEAD, O. YOUNG & R. W. TAYLOR. 1981. Bio-

chemical analysis of separated epithelium and stroma from endometria of premenopausal and postmenopausal women receiving estrogen and progestin. J. Steroid. Biochem. **14:** 979–987.

50. SATYASWAROOP, P. G., D. J. WARTELL & R. MORTEL. 1982. Distribution of progesterone receptor, estradiol dehydrogenase and 20α-dehydroprogesterone dehydrogenase activities in human endometrial glands and stroma. Progestin induction of steroid dehydrogenase activities in vitro, is restricted to the glandular epithelium. Endocrinology **111:** 743–749.

51. HUANG, J. R., L. TSENG, P. BISCHOF & O. A. JANNE. 1987. Regulation of prolactin production by progestin, estrogen and relaxin in human endometrial stromal cells. Endocrinology **121:** 2011–2017.

52. HERR, J. 1978. Decidual cells in the human ovary at term. Am. J. Anat. **152:** 7–28.

53. ZAYTSEV, P. & J. B. TAXY. 1987. Pregnancy-associated ectopic decidua. Am. J. Surg. Pathol. **11:** 526–530.

54. CASEY, M. L., D. GAL, K. KORTE, J. R. OKITA, P. C. MACDONALD & M. D. MITCHELL. 1986. Metabolism of arachidonic acid by human endometrial glands and stromal cells maintained in monolayer cultures. *In* Mechanism of Menstrual Bleeding. D. T. Baird & E. A. Michie, Eds. Raven Press. New York, NY.

55. BULMER, J. N. & P. M. JOHNSON. 1985. Immunohistochemical characterization of the decidual leucocyte infiltrate related to endometrial gland epithelium in early human pregnancy. Immunology **55:** 35–44.

56. PACE, D., L. MORRISON & J. N. BULMER. 1989. Proliferative activity in endometrial stromal granulocytes throughout menstrual cycle and early pregnancy. J. Clin. Pathol. **42:** 35–39.

57. WANG, H. S., H. KANZAKI, M. YOSHIDA, S. SATO, M. TOKUSHIGE & T. MORI. 1987. Suppression of lymphocyte reactivity in vitro by supernatants of explants of human endometrium. Am. J. Obstet. Gynecol. **157:** 956–963.

58. PADYKULA, H. A. 1989. Regeneration in the primate uterus. The role of stem cells. *In* Biology of the Uterus. 2nd edit. R. M. Wynn & W. P. Jollie, Eds. Plenum Publishing Corp. New York, NY.

59. CLEMENT, P. B. & R. E. SCULLY. 1988. Idiopathic postmenopausal decidual reaction of the endometrium. Int. J. Gynecol. Pathol. **7:** 152–161.

60. GELFAND, M. M. & A. FERENCZY. 1989. A prospective 1-year study of estrogen and progestin in postmenopausal women: Effects on the endometrium. Obstet. Gynecol. **74:** 398–402.

61. FERENCZY, A. & M. GELFAND. 1989. The biologic significance of cytologic atypia in progestogen-treated endometrial hyperplasia. Am. J. Obstet. Gynecol. **160:** 126–131.

Microarchitecture of the Human Endometrium by Scanning Electron Microscopy: Menstrual Desquamation and Remodeling

H. LUDWIG[a] AND U. M. SPORNITZ[b]

[a] Department of Obstetrics and Gynecology
[b] Department of Anatomy
University of Basel
4052 Basel, Switzerland

Using specimens from twenty-two uteri, collected by vaginal or abdominal hysterectomy (TABLE 1), we investigated the surface of the normal human endometrium in order to follow by scanning electron microscopy the shape-change of the endometrial surface in the course of menstrual desquamation. The medical indication of those hysterectomies were cervical pathology in most cases, malposition of the uterus or elective procedures in some. During the period of investigation the surgery was strictly dated according to the menstrual cycle of the patient. Cases with known endometrial pathology or those with gross uterine pathology were not included into the study group. The paper is concentrating on the morphology of the normal endometrium. The surface-morphology of cases with irregular uterine bleeding and of those with IUD in place were also investigated. The results will be reported separately. The details of the preparation method are published elsewhere.[1]

There is some controversy whether or not the endometrium desquamates completely during menstruation. On the basis of biopsies Flowers and Wilborn stated in 1978[2] that the most striking feature of menstruating endometrium was "its vigorous attempt to survive." Lysosomal activity, lipid accumulation, expulsion of glycoproteins and the uptake of stromal debris by epithelial cells was found. The authors stated that regression rather than cell death was the chief event of menstruation. In contrast to this we found a rather complete break-down of the functional endometrium when investigating the entire fundal portion of the uterus removed during the first three days after the onset of menstrual bleeding. Anatomical preparations of a menstruating uterus show the rather uniqueness of bleeding signs at the fundal uterine cavity. Restoration of the endometrial surface starts parallel to the endometrial shedding and will — under normal cyclic conditions — be completed at the latest around the 6th day of the cycle. This statement is in agreement with Nogales-Ortiz et al.[3]

On the first day of menstrual bleeding some areas of the fundal endometrium are already devoid the lining surface epithelium. Occasionally tiny sections of capillary

[a] Address for correspondence: Prof. Hans Ludwig, MD, FRCOG, FACOG (hon.),· University of Basel, Wartenbergstrasse 9, CH 4052 Basel.

TABLE 1. Materials and Methods

Material

    Range of age: 24–50 years

    Dating: basal body temperature, serum-estradiol histology of endometrial biopsy (NOYES)

    Number examined: 22 hysterectomy specimens
                           156 tissue specimens

Preparation

1. Uterus (corpus and cervix) cut longitudinally upper fundal cavity additional transverse cut immediately after surgery
2. Rinsing of the endometrial cavity with 0.1 M phosphate buffer solution pH 7.4 (osmolarity 300 mOsm)
3. Selection and pinning of tissue samples
4. Fixation of pinned tissue samples in 2.5% glutaraldehyde for 24 hours
5. Repinning of samples, second fixation 8 hours
6. Dehydration in graded alcohol series
7. Critical point drying CO_2
8. Gold sputtering

vessels running parallel to the surface of the fundal endometrium are observed to be open (FIG. 1). These are the spots where continuous menstrual bleeding starts. On the second and the third day of the regular menstrual bleeding the glandular stumps of the layer basalis withstanding menstrual desquamation of the functionalis are sticking out from the stroma. Their margins produce small processes of horizontally outgrowing epithelium (FIGS. 2 & 3). Very rapidly the superficial parts of the endometrial glands are transformed into small cones (FIGS. 4 & 5), and it is from flanks of those cones of the glandular stumps that the new lining surface epithelium emanates. The spiral-shaped growth pattern perpetuated from the circular structure of the glandular column. The direction of growth is vertical when forming the increasing length of the glands into the depths of the functional endometrium (FIG. 7), but it is horizontal when the new lining epithelium is built in between the gland openings (FIGS. 8 & 9). All glands within the central portion of the fundal endometrium open in round-shaped mouths, only laterally and later in the midluteal phase do more of them show lengthy fissures instead of openly rounded mouths. The dynamics of the remodeling process are quite fast. The growth of the newly formed lining surface epithelium is directed towards the denuded area covered with stromal debris, where one can detect fibers surrounded by white blood cells or macrophages and lysosomes (FIG. 6) lined up along fibrous or epithelial remnants.

A fibrin mesh partly covers the menstrual wound. This mesh must rapidly be degraded (FIG. 10), because it is only seen in preparations of day one to day four of the cycle. Local fibrinolytic activity is known to be high at that time. The activity of the clearing process within and underneath the menstrual slough seems to be at its peak around the third and fourth days. At the fourth day the newly formed lining surface epithelium already covers more than 2/3 of the entire fundal area (FIG. 11). Some of the proliferating endometrial glands show small excessive outgrows of the

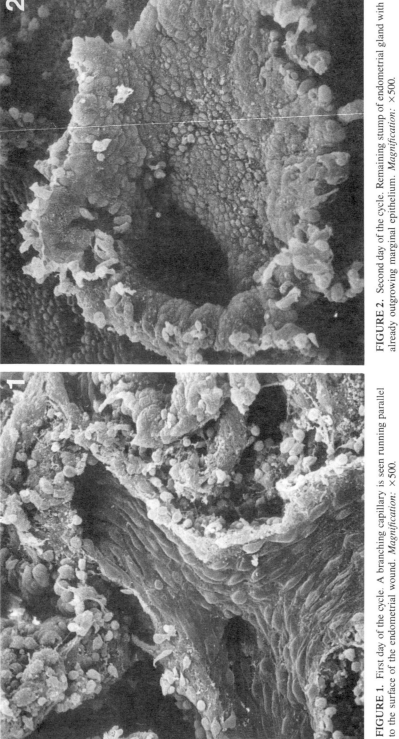

FIGURE 1. First day of the cycle. A branching capillary is seen running parallel to the surface of the endometrial wound. *Magnification:* ×500.

FIGURE 2. Second day of the cycle. Remaining stump of endometrial gland with already outgrowing marginal epithelium. *Magnification:* ×500.

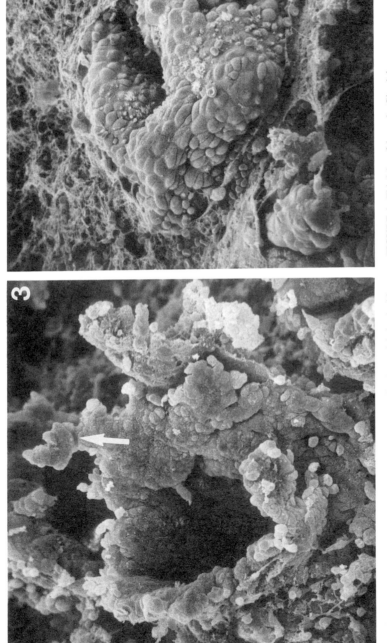

FIGURE 3. Second day of the cycle. Remaining stump of endometrial gland with lacerations and outgrowing epithelial tongues (*arrow*). *Magnification:* ×500.

FIGURE 4. Third day of the cycle. Glandular stumps are seen to form cone-shaped bulgings within the menstrual wound. The level of the surrounding tissue is not yet epithelized but covered by a network of fibrin (*f*) and blood cells. *Magnification:* ×500.

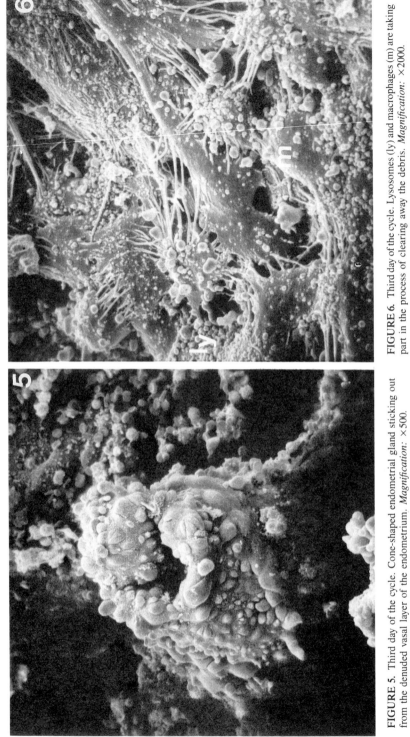

FIGURE 5. Third day of the cycle. Cone-shaped endometrial gland sticking out from the denuded vasal layer of the endometrium. *Magnification:* ×500.

FIGURE 6. Third day of the cycle. Lysosomes (ly) and macrophages (m) are taking part in the process of clearing away the debris. *Magnification:* ×2000.

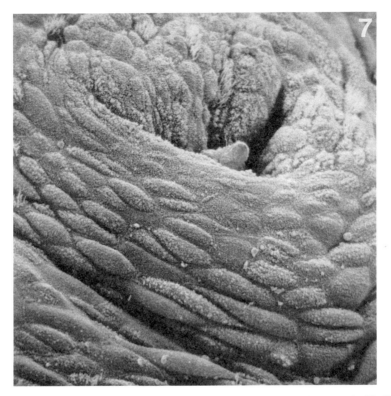

FIGURE 7. Fourth day of the cycle. New lining epithelium is formed by spiralling growth of fusiform epithelial cells. *Magnification:* × 1000.

new epithelium. Those micropolyps are avascular at the beginning (FIG. 12). Most of those polypous formations will survive only for a few days and then be rejected, but a few might remain. Those micropolyps will soon get vascularized, but they are still unstable formations. They are supposedly the source of intermenstrual bleeding when destroyed and shed from the reestablished endometrial surface later in the cycle (FIG. 13).

On the fifth and sixth day of the menstrual cycle, the endometrial wound is completely re-epithelized and it is not before then that the stromal tissue starts to grow and to remodel the internal bolsterous shape of the uterine cavity.[4] The thickening of the endometrial layer will not start before the completion of the restoration of the lining surface epithelium. After that the speed of growth of the stromal tissue obviously exceeds that of the endometrial glands, the interrelation resulting in a slight prominence of the interglandular areas in comparison to the level of the glandular openings (FIGS. 14 & 15). The surface of the fundal endometrium gradually reaches the smooth appearance known from midcycle (FIGS. 16–18). Exactly this shape persists from the periovulatory phase to the midluteal phase. Obviously, this process ends in creating the most favorable environment for nidation.

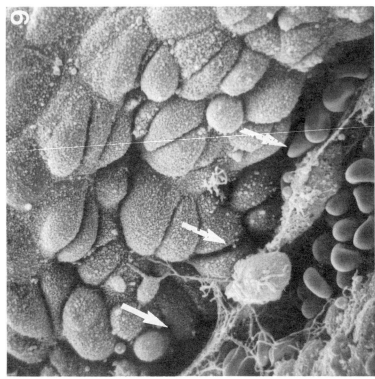

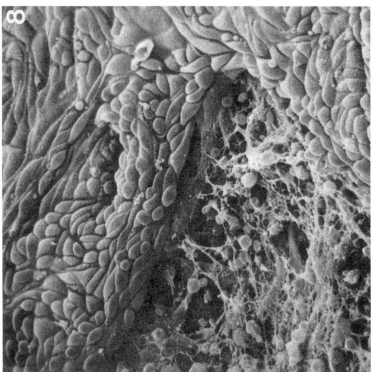

FIGURES 8 and 9. Fourth day of the cycle. The newly formed lining surface epithelium is progressing towards (*arrows* in FIG. 9) the last denuded areas. Those denuded spots are still covered with a tiny fibrin mesh. White blood cells and macrophages are interspersed. *Magnifications:* FIGURE 8, ×500; FIGURE 9, ×2000.

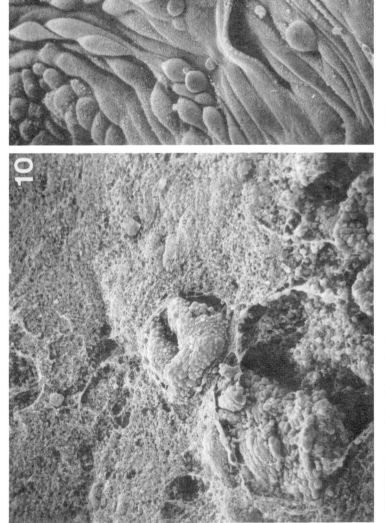

FIGURE 11. Fourth day of the cycle. Rapid proliferation of new lining surface epithelium covering the denuded surface. *Magnification:* ×1000.

FIGURE 10. Fourth day of the cycle. Cone-shaped endometrial gland surrounded by fibrin mesh (*f*). *Magnification:* ×200.

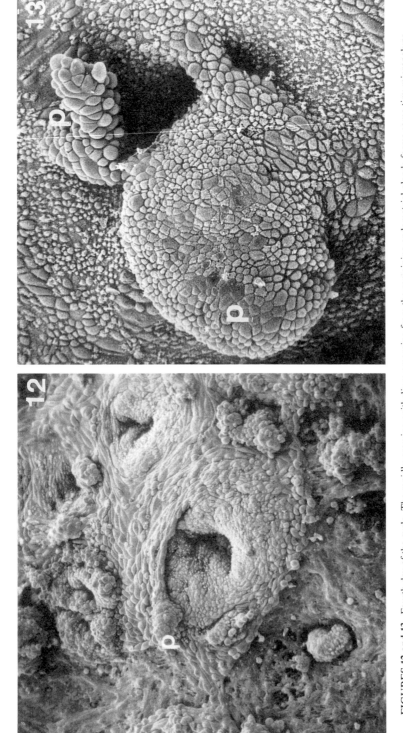

FIGURES 12 and 13. Fourth day of the cycle. The rapidly growing epithelium emerging from the remaining endometrial glands forms some tiny micropolyps. They are always situated adjacent to the glands. Those micropolyps will soon disappear. Only a few persist and will then grow larger and become vascularized. *Magnifications:* FIGURE 12, ×200; FIGURE 13, ×500.

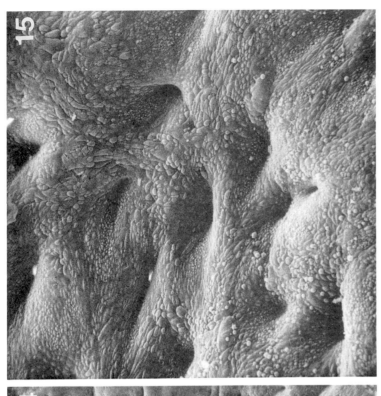

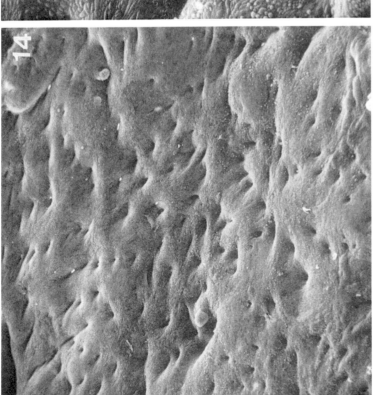

FIGURES 14 and 15. Seventh day of the cycle. The endometrial stroma starts to grow after the re-epithelization of the endometrium is completed. In the mid-proliferative phase of the cycle the endometrial surface of the fundal portion appears slightly uneven owing to the enhanced stroma proliferation in between the glands. The gland openings are seen depressed. This process results in bulging of the interglandular tissue fields. The young lining surface epithelium is polymorphous (FIG. 15). The circular pattern of growth around the glands can still be followed at survey magnifications. *Magnifications:* FIGURE 14, ×50; FIGURE 15, ×200.

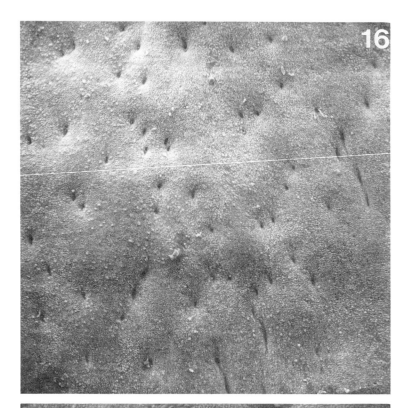

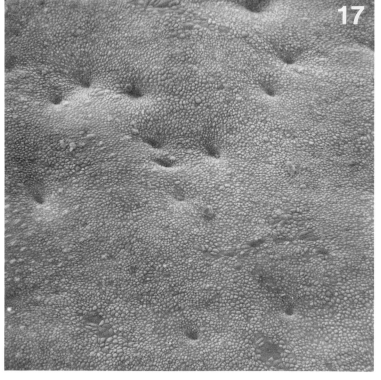

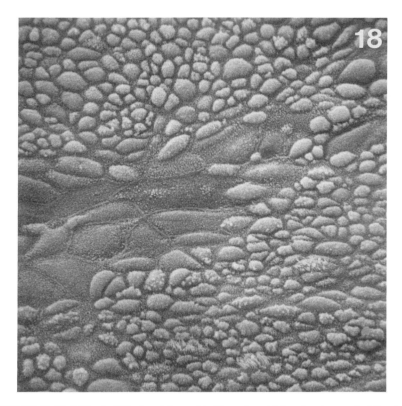

FIGURES 16–18. Midcycle (15th day of the cycle). The endometrial surface is smooth. The gland openings of the fundal portion are rounded; at more lateral sites the orifices are elongated. The lining surface epithelium is completed as an uninterrupted monolayer. A few fields with larger polygonal cells are interspersed (FIG. 18), representing the most recent parts of the lining surface. *Magnifications:* FIGURE 16, ×50; FIGURE 17, ×200; FIGURE 18, ×1000.

Ciliogenesis starts around the 7th and 8th day of the menstrual cycle. Ciliated cells which are seen before that date are cells growing out from the remaining glands (FIG. 19), not those newly formed. The cilioneogenesis (FIG. 20) in the lining surface epithelium can best be followed by scanning electron microscopy.

The transitional area between the endometrium and the endosalpinx is characterized by a marked increase in the number of ciliated cells.[5] Once fully developed ciliated cells of tubal or endometrial origin (among the latter are two types, persisting from glandular epithelium and others newly formed) cannot be differentiated from one another (FIG. 21). It has been suggested that human endometrial ciliated cells represent a developmental overlap with the uterine (interstitial) tube epithelium and that the high incidence of ciliary abnormality might be related to a relatively high turnover rate caused by menstruation. Abnormal cilia were interpreted as being due to a defect of ciliogenesis probably occurring after the formation of the basal bodies.[6] This interpretation is doubtful and possibly caused methodologically by the small number

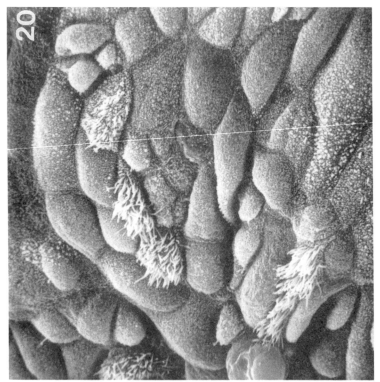

FIGURE 20. Eighth day of the cycle. Within the lining surface epithelium new ciliated cells are created. Different stages of ciliogenesis can be observed. *Magnification:* ×2000.

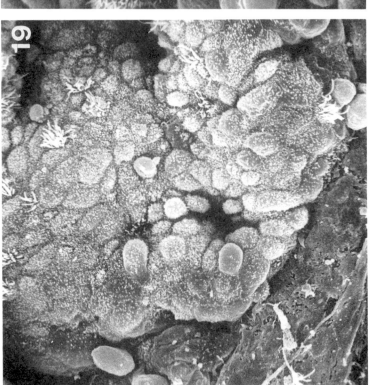

FIGURE 19. Second day of the cycle. Ciliated cells emanate within the epithelial growth from the depths of the glands. Those are surviving glandular ciliated cells. *Magnification:* ×2000.

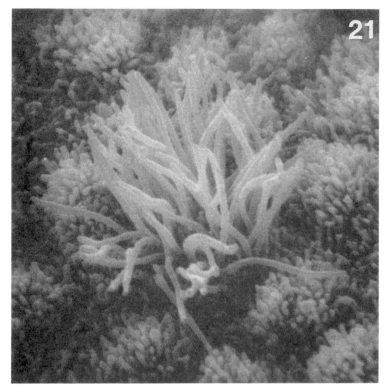

FIGURE 21. Midcycle. Most of the ciliated cells are fully developed. From days 15 to 22 the microvillous patterns of the nonciliated cells of the lining surface epithelium is considerably expressive. *Magnification:* ×10,000.

TABLE 2. Remodeling of the Endometrium after Menstrual Desquamation: Sequence of Events Observed by SEM

Day of Cycle	Characteristics of Surface Morphology
24 h after onset of menstruation	Desquamation of the superficial endometrium (zona compacta) under the preservation of stumps of endometrial glands; bleeding from torn endometrial vessels, washing away of menstrual debris.
2nd + 3rd day	Stumps of endometrial glands transformed into cones; lining epithelium grows out from endometrial glands. Fibrin mesh formed covering part of the menstrual wound. Start of re-epithelization. Lysosomes, macrophages take part in the process of clearing tissue debris.
4th day	Rapid proliferation of new lining surface epithelium, fibrin mesh replaced by epithelium; epithelial excess proliferation: occasional appearing of micropolyps.
5th + 6th day	Postmenstrual uterine wound closed by re-epithelization; new ciliated cells formed; micropolyps disappear. Start of stromal growth.
7th + 8th day	Final clearing of the uterine cavity, uninterrupted layer of the lining surface epithelium and ciliogenesis. Enhanced stroma formation (leading to bulging interglandular tissue cushions). Apical differentiation of non-ciliated cells (microvilli).

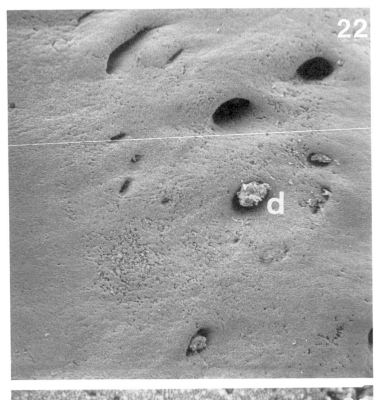

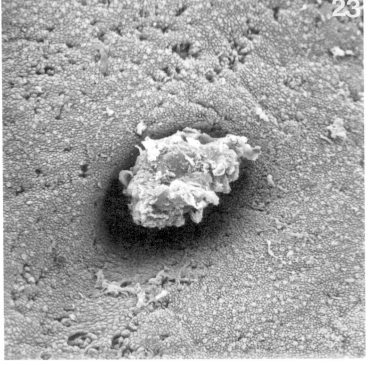

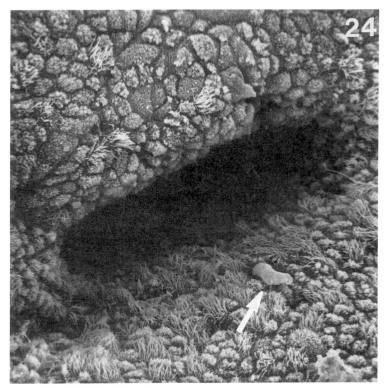

FIGURES 22–24. Twenty-eighth day of the cycle. Before menstrual break-down the lining surface epithelium shows focal disruptions. Some glandular openings are filled with secretory material and cellular debris (*d* in FIG. 22). White blood cells and macrophages have immigrated into the stroma. Only a few of them appear at surface level (*arrow* in FIG. 24).

of samples examined. By comparing different stages of endometrial restoration in a series of specimens it seems probable that the endometrial cilia within the lining surface epithelium are undergoing a rapid development according to the progress of the cyclic maturation of the endometrium. They are not quite the same type of cell as ciliated cells of the tubal epithelium or of the glandular epithelium of the basal endometrial layer. Ciliogenesis was not observed in the latter types of ciliated cells.

The sequence of events as briefly described is summarized (TABLE 2) and illustrated by micrographs taken from samples of the collected specimens, each representing one consecutive day of the normal cycle.

The menstrual breakdown announces itself by some morphological features: around day 22 the immigration of white blood cells and macrophages into the stroma of the endometrium starts. This is interpreted as a sign of the establishment of a cellular immunological response to the nidation.[7] In case of non-conception and imminent menstrual break-down, the integrity of cells of the lining surface epithelium will weaken, and clefts will appear between groups of lining cells. Small fissures and some surface defects out of the loss of several epithelial cells are typical signs of the late luteal

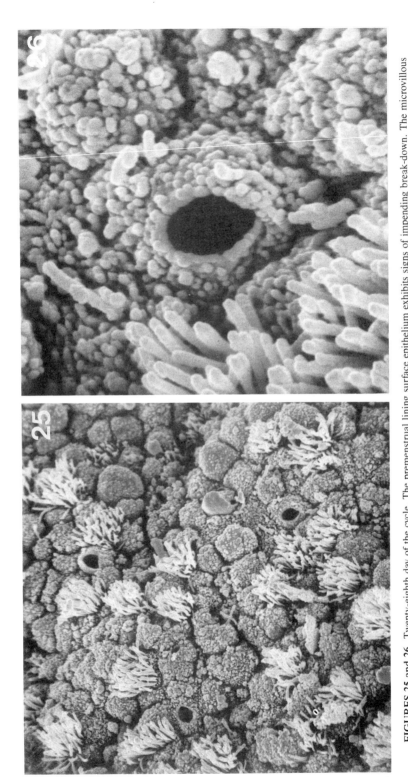

FIGURES 25 and 26. Twenty-eighth day of the cycle. The premenstrual lining surface epithelium exhibits signs of impending break-down. The microvillous pattern is flat or even lacking in some cells. Others have produced remarkable apical defects. The ciliated cells appear unchanged. *Magnifications:* FIGURE 25, ×2000; FIGURE 26, ×10,000.

phase endometrium (FIGS. 22–24); some cells are seen with apical membrane defects (FIGS. 25 & 26). White blood cells emerge within the disruptures of the lining surface epithelium (*arrow* in FIG. 24).

The onset of bleeding is triggered by a rather complicated interference of vascular, paracrine, and endocrinological factors. The process is as yet not fully understood. As the result, a sudden destruction of the superficial layer of the endometrium occurs with liberation of glandular stumps within the epithelial debris, accompanied by an accumulation of white and red blood cells. The local fibrinolytic and lysosomal activity increases and vascular ruptures create the non-coagulable menstrual flow.

SUMMARY

Twenty-two hysterectomy specimens were collected over a period of two decades in order to investigate the morphological sequence of menstrual desquamation and its consecutive remodeling of the endometrium. The technique used was described earlier by H. Ludwig and H. Metzger (1976).[1] Scanning electron microscopy is the only way to illustrate and describe the microarchitecture of the endometrial surface. At the beginning of the menstrual bleeding, glandular stumps surviving the desquamation of the layer functionalis stick out from the debris at the top of the basal layer. Fibrin mesh formation, the liberation of lysosomes, and the emigration of white blood cells and macrophages, both being already present in the midluteal endometrial stroma, can be observed. They are interrelated with the clearance of the menstrual wound. Coincidentally with the process of desquamation the re-epithelization starts and takes the first four to six days of the normal cycle. The events are illustrated by selecting specimens of uteri from women with comparable data but from different days of the normal cycle. Surprisingly transitory excess formation of epithelial outgrows (micropolyps) are observed. They disappear later in the cycle. some might persist and form micropolyps, which will be the source of occasional intermenstrual bleeding – so far the polyps are vascularized. The endometrial surface is covered *de novo* by a lining surface epithelium at the sixth day. Ciliogenesis occurs within this epithelium. Other ciliated cells emanate from the glandular epithelium. In early stages of menstrual regeneration the growth pattern of the epithelial monolayer forming the lining surface in spiral traces according to their origination from the circle-structures of the endometrial glands. Before the incoming menstrual break-down small crevices, clefts or defects appear within the lining surface endometrium, a few white blood cells, enriched in the stroma around the vessels, might even reach the surface. The apical membranes of several non-ciliated cells exhibit rounded leaks, others show ruptures. It is the tissue break-down around the superficial endometrial vessels, what creates the onset of menstrual blood flow. In the very early preparations of the bleeding endometrium those opened capillary vessels could be identified.

REFERENCES

1. LUDWIG, H. & H. METZGER. 1976. The re-epithelization of endometrium after menstrual desquamation. Arch. Gynecol. 221: 51–60.
2. FLOWERS, C. E. & W. H. WILBORN. 1978. New observations on the physiology of menstruation. Obstet. Gynecol. 51: 16–24.

3. NOGALES-ORTIZ, F., J. PUERTA & F. F. NOGALES, JR. 1978. The normal menstrual cycle. Chronology and mechanism of endometrial desquamation. Obstet. Gynecol. **51:** 259–264.
4. BAGGISH, M. S., C. J. PAUERSTEIN & J. D. WOODRUFF. 1967. Role of stroma in regeneration of endometrial epithelium. Am. J. Obstet. Gynecol. **99:** 459–465.
5. FADEL, H. E., D. BERNS, L. J. ZANEVELD, G. D. WILBANKS & E. E. BRUESCHKE. 1976. The human uterotubal junction: A scanning electron microscope study during different phases of the menstrual cycle. Fertil. Steril. **27:** 1176–1186.
6. DENHOLM, R. B. & I. A. MORE. 1980. Atypical cilia of the human endometrial epithelium. J. Anat. **131:** 309–315.
7. KELLY, J. K. & H. FOX. 1979. The local immunologic defence system of the human endometrium. J. Reprod. Immunol. **1:** 39–45.

Regeneration in the Primate Uterus: The Role of Stem Cells

HELEN A. PADYKULA

Department of Cell Biology
University of Massachusetts Medical School
Worcester, Massachusetts 01655

INTRODUCTION

Artificial programming of the menstrual cycle in rhesus monkeys is a remarkable advance in primate uterine biology.[1] Ovariectomized mature monkeys received subcutaneous silastic implants of estradiol and progesterone that mimic the serum steroidal hormonal profile of a natural 28-day menstrual cycle. Transfer of surrogate preimplantation embryos into the ampulla of the fallopian tube during artificial cycles resulted in successful pregnancies and birth of normal offspring. This achievement was followed by production of fertile cycles in women who had been ovariectomized or had primary ovarian failure.[2,3] These fundamental demonstrations established that primate uterine cyclic growth depends primarily on an appropriate pattern of systemic estradiol and progesterone secretion.

These basic experiments united the primate uterus with the uteri of subprimates in mutual dependence on ovarian steroids for cyclicity. They have also provided an important primate model in the rhesus monkey for experimentation that will ultimately lead to better understanding of the control mechanisms that guide cyclic endometrial growth and differentiation in women and other menstruating primates. Recently, another important parameter related to the control of endometrial mitotic activity has been identified in the rat endometrium. Although cell proliferation is under control of serum and tissue estradiol, its mitogenic action is effected through the mediation of epidermal growth factor (EGF) binding to endometrial tissue EGF receptors.[4] This observation provides an avenue for identifying control mechanisms that produce differential intratissue mitotic patterns. A new era is upon us that will center on localization of tissue growth factors, such as angiogenic factor (AGF), fibroblastic growth factor (FGF), *etc.*

Besides systemic ovarian steroidal secretion, an essential intrinsic endometrial tissue mechanism consists of an omnipresent small pool of multipotential stem cells that divide slowly. It is assumed that, at the outset of puberty or of a new menstrual cycle, stem cells give rise to progenitor cells that divide more rapidly and become committed to specific pathways of differentiation to give rise to characteristic endogenous endometrial cell types. That is, initial estrogen-stimulated cell growth involves mitotic recruitment and differentiation of luminal and glandular epithelial cells, stromal fibroblasts, endometrial granular cells, and the cellular components of the endometrial microvasculature. The synthesis of the endometrial extracellular matrix is also under steroidal control through cellular activity.

ENDOMETRIECTOMY AND THE LOCATION OF THE ENDOMETRIAL STEM CELLS

From primate reproductive biology and human clinical practice, it has long been known that removal of all visible endometrial tissue by curettage in women and monkeys is followed, after a short delay, by rapid reconstruction of a new endometrium that can support pregnancy. Since the basal portions of the endometrial glands interdigitate with myometrial stroma and smooth muscle at the endometrial-myometrial junction, it may be inferred that endometrial stem cells for epithelial, stromal, and vascular components are located near or within the endometrial-myometrial junction.

Carl Hartman (1944)[5] provided graphic evidence of the effects of repeated regeneration of the rhesus monkey uterus after endometriectomy (FIG. 1), as expressed in the following excerpts selected by Dr. John McCracken from Hartman's fundamental publication:

> Endometriectomy, as I practiced it, consisted of removal of most of the endometrium, including the basalis. In six experiments, the endometrium was wiped out as clean as possible with a cotton sponge, so that no vestige of mucosa was visible to the naked eye—yet perfect regeneration occurred.
>
> More than 200 endometriectomies were performed on intact rhesus monkeys, both cycling and in early pregnancy. The greatest number of hysterotomies in one animal was four. However, five animals had endometriectomies performed three times at intervals of two to four months. Twenty-eight animals were operated upon twice. The purpose of using this approach was to obtain implanting embryos and also to conserve the animals for further use and to obtain additional specimens from the same animal. Coincidentally using the endometriectomy technique, an unsurpassed opportunity was provided to study the regenerative powers of the endometrium.

Quantitative analyses of estrogen and progesterone receptors in the monkey endometrium were performed during the luteal phase between days 17–22 to obtain enough tissue for analysis.[6] Repeated endometriectomies were performed on several monkeys to obtain adequate endometrial tissue without negative consequences. After curretage of the rabbit endometrium, regeneration of the luminal epithelium was rapidly initiated at 3 hours; at 72 hours, regeneration of the endometrium was complete and the endometrium resembled the control.[7]

Thus, the regenerative capacity of the mammalian endometrium is impressive. It resembles that of the epidermis in that a relatively small number of the stem cells can reconstruct the original structure quite effectively. Human epidermal stem cells have been identified within the basal and immediate suprabasal cells.[8] Moreover, isolated human epidermal stem cells of an individual will proliferate and form sheets in culture that can be transferred to sites of severe burns in the same individual to promote healing without immunologic rejection. As for the endometrium, it remains to be determined whether or not the most basal endometrial region is the only site of multipotential stem cells.

Cyclic endometrial renewal consists of a small pool of multipotential stem cells that divide slowly (FIG. 2). Under systemic hormonal changes, such as the cyclic increase in the serum level of estradiol, it can be postulated that stem cells migrate and give rise to a group of progenitor cells that become committed to specific types of cell differentiation, e.g. epithelial, stromal, and vascular, within certain microenvironments.[9] Progenitor cells have higher mitotic rates than stem cells and thus the result

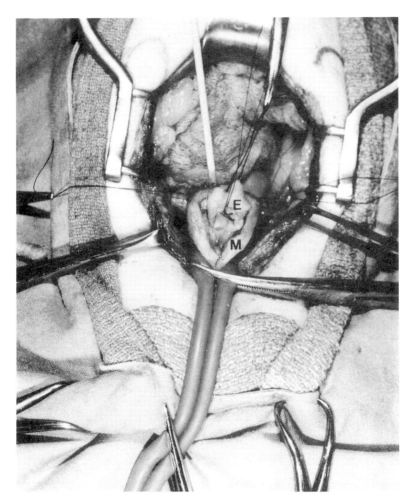

FIGURE 1. Surgical endometriectomy, mature rhesus monkey. The endometrium is removed by cutting along the endometrial-myometrial junction with a scalpel. A suture through the endometrial tissue (E) serves to lift as it is being separated from the myometrium (M). Dr. John A. McCracken of the Worcester Foundation for Experimental Biology derived this technique from C. G. Hartman's (1944)[24] original description of endometriectomy.

is progressive endometrial growth. The "options" for progenitor cells are: (1) continued mitotic activity with concomitant differentiation, or (2) to become postmitotic and thus transient. In relation to primate endometrial regeneration, the destination of migrating stem-progenitor cells may be the four zones or microenvironments of the primate endometrium.

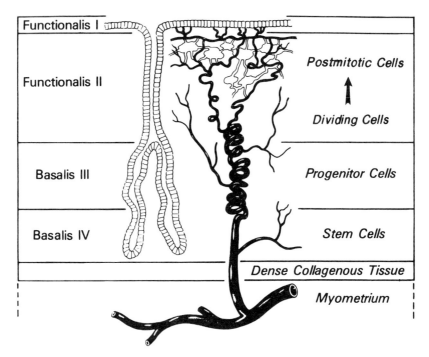

FIGURE 2. Endometrial zonation of the rhesus monkey adapted from Bartelmez.[12] The primate endo-metrium consists of four structurally distinct zones. The germinal basalis consists of two zones, basalis III and basalis IV. The functionalis is composed of two zones, functionalis I and functionalis II. Endo-metrial regeneration after endometriectomy proceeds from the remains of basalis IV and after the menses from basalis III and IV.

COMPARTMENTALIZATION OF THE PRIMATE ENDOMETRIUM

The uterine endometrium of mammals possesses a germinal compartment that per-sists from cycle to cycle during reproductive life. The germinal compartment gives rise to a transient compartment for the purpose of accommodating implantation of the blastocyst as well as to provide for the maternal component of the placenta if preg-nancy should occur. Thus, after a menstrual cycle or the close of pregnancy, the tran-sient component is eliminated, only to be repeated (FIGS. 2 and 3).

In subprimate mammals, it is difficult to distinguish between the germinal and transient endometrial compartments because cell death and regression of the transient tissue occurs *in situ*.[10] However, in menstruating primates, the endometrial function-alis is the transient compartment that is shed by tissue sloughing accompanied with bleeding. At the close of menses, the germinal basalis remains and enters into the hormonal environment of the next cycle to produce a new functionalis. Thus the rhesus monkey provides a natural system for analysis of the germinal and transient endo-metrial compartments because of the clear cut separation of the transient cells at the

Day 19 Normal Human Uterus
zone I   zone II

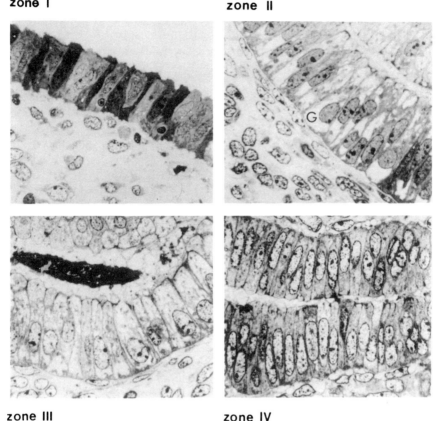

zone III   zone IV

FIGURE 3. Histologic zonation of the human endometrium, day 19 of the menstrual cycle. The epithelia of the four zones were photographed at the same magnification. Note the zonal variation in epithelial cell height, shape, and degree of glycogen storage (G).

close of menses. Then, during the subsequent menstrual cycle, it is possible to trace the origin of the transient compartment from the germinal compartment during estrogen and progesterone dominance.

The neuroendocrine features of the rhesus hypothalamic-ovarian circuit have been carefully defined and are comparable to that of women.[11] In women and monkeys, the menstrual cycles are approximately 28 days in length, with ovulation occurring approximately 38 hours after the LH surge. Thus, the rhesus monkey is an appropriate model for identifying intraendometrial control mechanisms that make provision for the possibility of pregnancy during a cycle by preparing a transient "home" for an embryo within the functionalis. In addition, the control mechanisms should insure that the germinal basalis will persist from cycle to cycle. These control mechanisms remain to be defined.

Our recent studies on [³H]thymidine ([³H]TdR) incorporation during the natural menstrual cycle have provided data that may lead to definition of the cyclic origin of the functionalis as well as the germinal mechanisms within the basalis. To interpret the pattern of [³H]TdR incorporation into endometrial tissue, it is necessary to consider the zonal subcompartmentalization of the functionalis and basalis of the rhesus and human endometria, as defined histologically by Bartelmez,[12,13] and ultrastructure.[14]

ZONATION OF THE PRIMATE ENDOMETRIUM

Compartmentalization extends beyond the major subdivision of germinal basalis and transient functionalis. Bartelmez[12,13] identified four histologically different horizontal zones in the rhesus and human endometria as follows (FIGS. 2 and 3):

FUNCTIONALIS: Zone I   ⟶   luminal epithelium and subjacent stroma
                 Zone II   ⟶   upper endometrium in which the straight region of the glands course and are widely separated by stroma

BASALIS: Zone III ⟶   midregions of the glands that are widely separated by stroma
                 Zone IV   ⟶   basal regions of the glands in a fibrous stroma adjacent to the endometrial-myometrial junction

This endometrial quadripartite zonation had been largely ignored until functional differences were identified among the four zones by radioautography.[15] A single intravenous injection of [³H]thymidine was made on a specific day of the menstrual cycle. At one hour later endometrial biopsies were obtained by hysterotomy. Plastic sections (2μm) were used to prepare radioautographs from which the zonal labeling indices for the luminal and glandular epithelia were determined (TABLES 1 and 2). At that time, other

TABLE 1. Midcycle Zonal Distribution of Mitotic Activity Rhesus Monkey Endometrium Epithelial Labeling-Index[a]

Day of Cycle	Zone			
	I	II	III	IV
−2	11% (841)	10% (5023)	6% (3969)	1% (3293)
−1	10% (1630)	10% (4897)	5% (4522)	2% (3564)
−1	–	14% (2945)	7% (4279)	3% (4383)
0	11% (856)	7% (3005)	5% (2947)	4% (2974)
+1	11% (2103)	11% (8579)	5% (2020)	5% (1806)
+2	12% (12055)	13% (19870)	7% (2746)	4% (11785)
+3	9% (1429)	11% (5141)	6% (4878)	7% (4472)
OVEX[b]	5% (2122)	2% (2702)	1% (2157)	1% (2024)

From Padykula et al.[15]

 [a] Endometrial biopsies taken at 1 h after ³H-thymidine injection. A minimum of 2,000 cells/zone/specimen was used to determine L.I.

 [b] Endometrial biopsy obtained 1 month after removal of ovaries.

TABLE 2. Zonal Labeling Index of Endometrial Luminal and Glandular Epithelia and Fibroblasts of the Endometrial Stroma during the Periovulatory and Luteal Phases of the Menstrual Cycle in the Rhesus Monkey

	Labeling Index (%)	
	Periovulatory[a]	Luteal[b]
Luminal and glandular epithelia		
Zone I	10.0 ± 0.3	4.3 ± 1.9[c]
II	9.8 ± 1.0	0.8 ± 0.2[c]
III	5.8 ± 0.2[1,2]	1.4 ± 0.5[c]
IV	3.7 ± 0.8[1,2]	8.8 ± 1.4[c,2,3]
Stromal fibroblasts		
Zone I	4.3 ± 1.2	4.6 ± 0.4
II	4.9 ± 1.0	3.1 ± 0.9
III	3.7 ± 1.0	2.3 ± 0.8
IV	0.8 ± 0.1[1,2,3]	1.1 ± 0.2[1]

[a] Values for periovulatory endometrium were determined on Days -2, -1, 0, $+1$, and $+3$ from the luteinizing peak.

[b] Values for luteal endometrium were determined on Days $+5$, $+6$, and $+10$.

[c] Denotes statistical significance between periovulatory and luteal phases for each zone as determined by Student's t-test.

[1-3] Numbers indicate statistically significant differences between the zones during either the periovulatory or luteal phase: 1 vs. Zone I; 2 vs. Zone II; 3 vs. Zone III. All values are the mean ± SEM; $p < 0.05$ was considered statistically significant.

laboratories were localizing estrogen receptors through immunocytochemistry in the cynomologous monkey.[16,17] Zonal differences were observed also in the distribution of these receptors in human endometria during the menstrual cycle.[18-20]

CYCLIC CHANGES IN ENDOMETRIAL ZONAL UPTAKE OF [³H]TdR

Although current understanding of cyclic renewal of the primate endometrium is fragmentary, it is possible to construct an hypothesis of cyclic endometrial growth derived from the data on [³H]thymidine incorporation during the natural menstrual cycle. The pioneer effort in this approach was made by Ferenczy *et al.*[21] who incubated slices of human endometrium *in vitro* with [³H]TdR. Labeling of nuclei occurred only at the surface of the slices and thus the data were limited and did not permit functional interpretation. Thus, it was necessary to use an appropriate animal model, such as the mature female rhesus monkey, to effect *in vivo* labeling on specific days during the 28-day rhesus menstrual cycle.[15,22] Initial [³H]TdR labeling centered around the estradiol peak on the premise that estrogen is a mitogen for epithelial, stromal, and vascular cells during the proliferative phase, *i.e.*, estrogen dominance. A single intravenous injection of [³H]TdR was made and an endometrial biopsy was taken one hour later and prepared for plastic sections (2μm) for light microscopy and ultrathin sections for electron microscopy. Radioautographs were prepared with an effort to obtain a plane-of-section that runs parallel to the endometrial glands and coiled arterioles to provide accurate recognition of the four zones.

EPITHELIAL MITOTIC ACTIVITY IN THE TRANSIENT COMPARTMENT DURING ESTROGEN DOMINANCE

Zonal variation in the [³H]TdR labeling indices was visually evident in the radio-autographs. As the data in TABLES 1 and 2 indicate, high epithelial proliferative activity in the functionalis was evident from −2 to +3 days of estrogen dominance. In contrast, epithelial cells of the basalis had lower labeling indices. Overall, the epithelial LI of the functionalis was approximately 10%, whereas that of the basalis III was 5–6% and that of basalis IV progressively increased from 1 to 11%. Thus, during estrogen dominance, the epithelial [³H]TdR LI of the functionalis is approximately twice that of the basalis.

GERMINAL MECHANISMS IN THE ENDOMETRIAL BASALIS

During the postovulatory period of progesterone dominance, the zonal pattern of [³H]TdR uptake was identifiable on day +5 by the antiestrogenic action of progesterone as an inhibitor of epithelial proliferation in the functionalis I and II and basalis III (TABLE 2).[22] In contrast, basalis IV escapes progesterone inhibition, as the [³H]TdR labeling index from −2 to +10 days continues to increase to 11%. Here it is possible to make an important correlation between the radioautographic data and the immuno-cytochemical distribution of the estrogen receptor in the cyclic human and monkey (artificial menstrual cycles).[18,19] During the preovulatory (proliferative) phase, nuclear estrogen receptor is localized in all 4 zones of the glandular and luminal epithelia. However, this reactivity decreased steadily in Zones I, II and III during the postovulatory period of progesterone dominance, except in the deep basalis (Zone IV). Hence, this persistence of estrogen receptor correlates with the steadily increasing mitotic activity of epithelial cells in Zone IV.

Thus, in the most basal regions of the preovulatory endometrium, high epithelial activity persists along with nuclear binding of the estrogen receptor. In other words, Zone IV epithelial cells "escape progesterone mitotic inhibition." Thus, the deep endometrium contains unique germinal cells that differentiate under the control of a distinctly different mechanism from that of the functionalis and basalis III. Histologists have long recognized increasing epithelial pseudostratification in the basalis during the late luteal phase. Pseudostratification reflects the crowding of columnar glandular cells that are being rapidly produced.

Continued high epithelial proliferation in the basalis IV during progesterone dominance requires special comment. Progesterone is used clinically in human endometrial cancer to suppress abnormal mitotic activity. It is likely that basalis IV of the human endometrium may also "escape progesterone inhibition", and thus clinicians should be aware of this possibility until the mitotic control mechanisms for germinal basalis IV have been identified.

HYPOTHESIS: CYCLIC ENDOMETRIAL RENEWAL IN MENSTRUATING PRIMATES

1. The basalis is a bifunctional germinal compartment that will reconstruct a new functionalis.

2. The transient functionalis expands rapidly during the mitogenic stimulus of estrogen dominance. A fundamental functional and structural dichotomy exists within the basalis. During postovulatory rising serum progesterone, epithelial proliferation is inhibited in basalis III and functionalis I & II. In contrast, proliferation in basalis IV continues to increase at least to day 12 or 20.

3. The basalis expands primarily by heightened epithelial cell proliferation in basalis IV which "escapes inhibition by progesterone." Simultaneously, the nuclear estrogen receptor persists in high concentration only in basalis IV during progesterone dominance.

4. The heightened postovulatory rate of production of basalis IV epithelial cells contributes to intracyclic growth for the possibility of pregnancy as well as for inter-cycle stem cell continuity.

5. After menses, the program of basalis III includes rapid covering of the men-strual wound and reinitiation of mitotic activity to recreate the zonal microenviron-ments in the new functionalis.

6. The program for postmenstrual reconstruction or for pregnancy is most likely prepared during the cellular expansion that occurs during progesterone dominance of the preceding menstrual cycle.

7. By day + 14, epithelial proliferation is inhibited in all zones of the premenstrual endometrium[12,23,24] (TABLE 2). Intercycle mitotic quiescence persists until day 4–5 of the next cycle as a new group of stem-progenitor cells is activated.[17]

REFERENCES

1. HODGEN, G. D. 1983. Surrogate embryo transfer combined with estrogen-progesterone therapy in monkeys. JAMA 250: 2167–2171.
2. LUTJEN, P., A. TROUNSON, J. LEETON, J. FINDLAY, C. WOOD & P. RENOU. 1984. The estab-lishment and maintenance of pregnancy using in vitro fertilization and embryo donation in a patient with primary ovarian failure. Nature 307: 174–175.
3. NAVOT, D., N. LAUFER, J. KOPOLOVIC, R. RABINOWITZ, A. BIRKENFELD, A. LEWIN, M. GRANAT, E. J. MARGALIOTH & J. G. SCHENKER. 1986. Artificially induced endometrial cycles and es-tablishment of pregnancies in the absence of ovaries. N. Engl. J. Med. 315: 806–811.
4. MUKKU, V. R. & G. M. STANCEL. 1985. Regulation of epidermal growth factor receptor by estrogen. J. Biol. Chem. 260: 9820–9824.
5. HARTMAN, C. G. 1944. Regeneration of the monkey uterus after surgical removal of the endo-metrium and accidental endometriosis. West J. Surg. Obstet. Gynecol. 52: 87–102.
6. KREITMANN-GIMBAL, B., F. BAYARD, W. E. NIXON & G. D. HODGEN. 1980. Patterns of estrogen and progesterone receptors in monkey endometrium during the normal menstrual cycle. Steroids 35: 471–475.
7. SCHENKER, J. G., M. I. SACKS & W. Z. PLISHUK. I. Regeneration of rabbit endometrium fol-lowing curettage. Am. J. Obstet. Gynecol. 111: 970–978.
8. LAVKER, R. M. & T. T. SUN. 1983. Epidermal stem cells. J. Invest. Dermatol. (Suppl.): 1215–1275.
9. HALL, A. K. 1983. Stem cell is a stem cell is a stem cell. Cell 33: 11–12.
10. PADYKULA, H. A. 1981. Shifts in uterine stromal cell populations during pregnancy and regres-sion. In Cellular and Molecular Aspects of Implantation. S. R. Glasser & D. W. Bullock, Eds.: 197–216. Plenum Plublishing Corporation, New York.
11. KNOBIL, E. 1980. The neuroendocrine control of the menstrual cycle. Rec. Prog. Horm. Res. 36: 53–88.
12. BARTELMEZ, G. W. 1951. Cyclic changes in the endometrium of the rhesus monkey (Macaca mulatta), Contrib. Embryol., Carnegie Institute 34: 99–146.
13. BARTELMEZ, G. W. 1957. The phases of the menstrual cycle and their interpretation in terms of pregnancy cycle. Am. J. Obstet. Gynecol. 74: 931–955.
14. KAISERMAN-ABRAMOF, I. R. & H. A. PADYKULA. 1989. Ultrastructural epithelial zonation of the primate endometrium (rhesus monkey). Am. J. Anat. 184: 13–31.

15. PADYKULA, H. A., L. G. COLES, J. A. McCRACKEN, N. W. KING, C. LONGCOPE & I. R. KAISERMAN-ABRAMOF. 1984. A zonal pattern of cell proliferation and differentiation in the rhesus endometrium during the estrogen surge. Biol. Reprod. **31:** 1103–1118.
16. WEST, N. B. & R. M. BRENNER. 1983. Estrogen receptor levels in the oviduct and endometria of cynomologus macaques during the menstrual cycle. Biol. Reprod. **29:** 1303–1312.
17. McCLELLAN, M., N. B. WEST & R. M. BRENNER. 1986. Immunocytochemical localization of estrogen receptors in the macaque endometrium during the luteal-follicular transition. Endocrinology. **19:** 2467–2475.
18. PRESS, M. F. 1984. Immunocytochemical assessment of estrogen receptor in the human endometrium throughout the menstrual cycle. Lab. Invest. **50:** 490–486.
19. PRESS, M. F., N. NOUSEK-GOEBEL, A. L. HERBST & G. GREENE. 1985. Immunocytochemical microscopic localization of estrogen receptor with monoclonal estrophilin antibodies. J. Histochem. Cytochem. **33:** 915–924.
20. PRESS, M. F., N. NOUSEK-GOEBEL, M. BUR & G. GREENE. 1986. Estrogen receptor localization in the female genital tract. Am. J. Pathol. **123:** 280–292.
21. FERENCZY, A., G. BERTRAND & M. M. GELFAND. 1979. Proliferation kinetics of human endometrium during the normal menstrual cycle. Am. J. Obstet. Gynecol. **133:** 859–867.
22. PADYKULA, H. A., L. G. COLES, W. C. OKULICZ, S. I. RAPAPORT, J. A. McCRACKEN, N. W. KING, JR., C. LONGCOPE & I. R. KAISERMAN-ABRAMOF. 1989. The basalis of the primate endometrium: A bifunctional germinal compartment. Biol. Reprod. **40:** 681–690.
23. NOYES, R. W., A. T. HERTIG & J. ROCK. 1950. Dating the endometrial biopsy. Fertil. Steril. **1:** 3–25.
24. NOYES, R. W. 1973. Normal phases of the endometrium. *In* The Uterus. H. J. Norris & A. T. Hertig, Eds. The William & Wilkins Company, Baltimore MD.

Leukocytes and Resident Blood Cells in Endometrium[a]

JUDITH N. BULMER,[b] MARGARET LONGFELLOW,
AND ANNE RITSON

Department of Pathology
University of Leeds
Leeds, LS2 9JT, England

INTRODUCTION

Considerable research effort has recently been directed towards elucidation of local immunological interactions between fetal and maternal cells in the pregnant uterus. Functional studies of decidual cell suspensions have inevitably focused attention on the constituent cells of decidua in humans and experimental animals, and hence on leukocyte populations in human nonpregnant endometrium. Thorough phenotypic and functional characterization of leukocytes in normal endometrium will improve understanding of implantation and placentation and will allow investigation of the pathogenetic mechanisms underlying pregancy pathology.

IMMUNOHISTOCHEMICAL CHARACTERIZATION OF HUMAN ENDOMETRIAL LEUKOCYTES

Leukocytes in Nonpregnant Endometrium

Immunohistochemical techniques have been used to characterize leukocytes in both nonpregnant and decidualized human endometrium. The antigenic phenotype of the various leukocyte populations has become clearer as the range of monoclonal antibodies directed against leukocyte surface antigens has increased. In nonpregnant endometrium, leukocytes are present within the stroma of the stratum basalis and stratum functionalis and also in an intraepithelial position.[1-4] In basalis, leukocytes are scattered individually or form aggregates comprising B cells, T cells and macrophages. Leukocytes in basalis do not vary according to menstrual cycle stage. Intraepithelial lymphocytes (IEL) may be detected in surface and gland epithelium and include CD3 + CD8 + T cells and CD56 + CD16 − granulated lymphocytes; the proportion of granulated IEL increases in the late secretory phase and in early pregnancy.[5]

Leukocytes are a prominent stromal component in the stratum functionalis and the relative proportions of various cell types varies according to menstrual cycle stage. B lymphocytes and "classic" CD16 + natural killer (NK) cells are rare throughout the

[a] This work was supported by grants from the Yorkshire Regional Health Authority and Birthright.
[b] Author to whom correspondence should be addressed.

cycle. In proliferative endometrium three major populations of stromal leukocytes have been identified: CD3+ T lymphocytes, most of which are also CD8+, CD14+ macrophages and CD56+ CD3− CD16− lymphocytes. Leukocytes in the early secretory phase are present in similar proportions to those in proliferative endometrium. In the late secretory phase of the menstrual cycle, the number of endometrial stromal leukocytes increases, predominantly due to a rise in the number of CD56+ CD3− CD16− lymphocytes from day 23–24 onwards,[3,4,6] although there may also be a rise in the number of macrophages premenstrually.[2] The dramatic increase in the number of CD56+ CD3− CD16− cells has caused speculation that these cells may play a role in implantation and establishment of the fetoplacental unit.

Leukocytes in Human Decidua

Early immunohistochemical studies indicated that leukocytes are a major component of human decidua throughout pregnancy[7] and, in common with nonpregnant endometrium, there are three major populations. T lymphocytes account for less than 20% of leukocytes in first trimester decidua. Most are CD8+ and express the αβ heterodimeric form of T cell receptor; T cells expressing the γδ heterodimer are rare and usually identified in an intraepithelial position.[8] T cells account for an increased proportion of decidual leukocytes in late pregnancy as the number of CD56+ CD3− CD16− cells declines after the first trimester.[9,10]

CD14+ decidual macrophages are present in decidua parietalis and decidua basalis throughout gestation and are often closely associated with extravillous trophoblast in decidua basalis.[10] Most are intensely class II MHC+ and many express CD11c. The role of decidual macrophages is uncertain and production of a purified population has proved difficult in our experience. Immunosuppression due to secretion of prostaglandin E_2 has been attributed to decidual macrophages[11] as has antigen presenting capacity.[12] These cells may also be concerned with phagocytosis of tissue debris consequent on trophoblastic invasion of decidua.[13]

CD56+ CD3− CD16− leukocytes are detected predominantly in first trimester decidua. These phenotypically unusual cells were initially described in early pregnancy decidua[9,14] and a comparable population was later described in nonpregnant endometrial stroma in the late secretory phase of the menstrual cycle.[3,4] They are intensely positive for CD56 but do not express other NK lineage markers such as CD16, CD57 and CD11b. Sixty to seventy percent also express the E-rosette receptor, CD2, and a lower number are CD7+.[9,15] They are present scattered throughout decidua (FIG. 1) but aggregate around endometrial glands and arterioles. Although abundant in the first trimester of pregnancy, accounting for at least 50% of decidual leukocytes, they decline in numbers in the second half of pregnancy and are uncommon at term. Immunohistochemical studies of cell suspensions and formalin-fixed paraffin-embedded sections have provided substantial evidence that these cells are the so-called "endometrial stromal granulocytes."[16]

ENDOMETRIAL STROMAL GRANULOCYTES

Weill[17] noted a population of cells with acidophilic granules in human decidua. Later studies showed that these cells were uncommon in proliferative endometrium

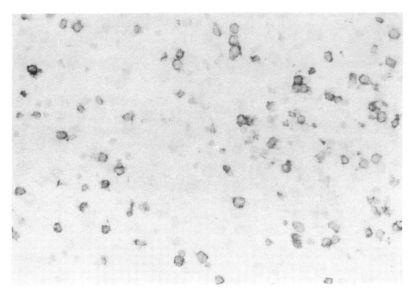

FIGURE 1. Frozen section of first trimester human decidua labeled with anti-CD56 (NKH1) using an indirect immunoperoxidase technique. Note positive cells scattered throughout the tissue. *Magnification*: ×250.

but increased in the secretory phase; they were termed "Körnchenzellen," "K" cells or granular endometrial stromal cells.[18,19] The cells were 10–12µm diameter and the cytoplasmic granules were phloxinophilic with a phloxine tartrazine stain and also stained with Giemsa, toluidine blue, eosin and methyl violet.[19] Dallenbach-Hellweg[20] termed them "endometrial stromal granulocytes" and considered that these and the proposed analogues in rat uterus, the granulated metrial gland (GMG) cells, derived from undifferentiated endometrial stromal cells and secreted relaxin. However, rat metrial gland is not a significant source of biologically active relaxin.[21] Recent studies have provided conclusive evidence that mouse GMG cells derive from bone marrow[22] and that human endometrial stromal granulocytes express the leukocyte common antigen, CD45, and the NK lineage marker, CD56.[16]

Although commonly detected with phloxine tartrazine, other stains can be used to demonstrate "endometrial stromal granulocytes." No significant difference was noted in the number of granulated cells in formalin-fixed paraffin-embedded sections of human endometrium stained with phloxine tartrazine, low pH alcian blue (FIG. 2) and low pH toluidine blue.[23] However, whereas the granules were variable in size and often large when stained with phloxine, in sections stained with toluidine blue the granules appeared smaller and uniform.

There is increasing evidence from phenotypic and functional studies that human endometrial stromal granulocytes and their rodent analogues, GMG cells, are granulated leukocytes, most probably within the NK lineage group. It may therefore be more appropriate to term these cells endometrial granulated lymphocytes (eGL).

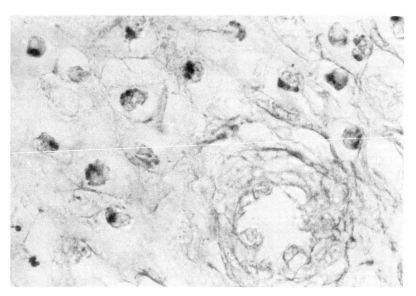

FIGURE 2. Paraffin-embedded section of first trimester human decidua stained with low pH alcian blue and counterstained with eosin, showing numerous cells with cytoplasmic granules clustered around a small vessel. *Magnification:* ×1000.

ENDOMETRIAL GRANULATED LYMPHOCYTES IN NON-HUMAN PRIMATES

Granulated cells have also been detected in the uterine lining of non-human primates in the late secretory phase of the menstrual cycle and early pregnancy and these appear to be ultrastructurally similar to granulated cells in rat and human endometrium.[24] In our own studies granulated cells were abundant in early pregnancy decidua from Cynomolgus monkeys and showed similar staining characteristics to those in human decidua.

We have recently had the opportunity to examine frozen sections of day 45 pregnant baboon decidua. Antibodies directed against human CD2, CD56 and class II MHC antigens cross-reacted with baboon tissue. Abundant CD56+ cells were detected in baboon decidua (FIG. 3). Fewer CD2+ cells were present in a similar distribution. Class II MHC+ cells were also abundant (FIG. 3) and appeared more numerous than macrophages in human decidua. Non-human primates may provide a useful model of normal implantation and placentation.

KINETICS OF ENDOMETRIAL GRANULATED LYMPHOCYTES

The increased number of CD56+ and CD3− CD16− cells in late secretory phase endometrium and early pregnancy decidua can be accounted for, at least partly, by

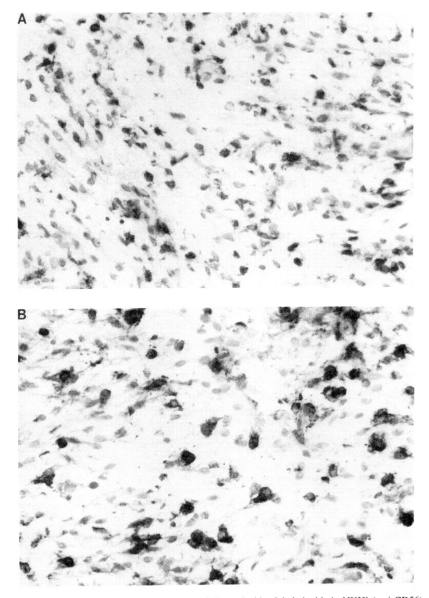

FIGURE 3. Frozen sections of 45 day pregnant baboon decidua labeled with A. NKH1 (anti-CD56); B. anti-class II MHC. Note the presence of numerous positive cells with both antibodies. *Magnification*: ×250.

local proliferation. In premenstrual endometrium eGL are often in mitosis and a substantial proportion of CD56+ cells in late secretory phase endometrium express the nuclear proliferation antigen detected by the monoclonal antibody, Ki67.[25] Fluctuations in the number of CD56+ eGL according to menstrual cycle stage could reflect expression of steroid hormone receptors by these cells. Although estrogen receptors were reported on CD3+ T cells in basal lymphoid aggregates, progesterone receptors were not detected on any endometrial leukocytes.[26] However, these authors did not use an anti-CD56 antibody; further studies are underway to determine whether CD56+ eGL express progesterone receptor. Progesterone does not, however, improve the viability of purified eGL *in vitro* (unpublished data).

In Vitro *Decidualization of Endometrial Explants*

Endometrial explants were subject to *in vitro* decidualization[27] in an attempt to determine whether eGL influx into endometrium directly from peripheral blood on a particular day of the menstrual cycle or whether they differentiate *in situ* from precursors. In the latter case, it should be possible to cause precursors present in endometrium at an early stage of the cycle to differentiate in explants undergoing decidualization *in vitro* under the influence of added progesterone.

Twenty specimens of endometrium were washed in RPMI 1640 and carefully cut into 1mm^3 fragments. Explants were cultured on filter paper squares supported on stainless steel grids in organ culture dishes. Control explants were cultured in Trowell's T8 nutrient medium (Gibco, Paisley, UK) containing 20% heat inactivated fetal bovine serum (FBS), 10mM L-glutamine, 100 iu/ml penicillin and 100μg/ml streptomycin. Other explants were subjected to *in vitro* decidualization by addition of 0.2ng/ml 17β estradiol and 50ng/ml progesterone to the culture medium. Explants were removed after 2, 4, 6, 8 and 10 days *in vitro* and either frozen in liquid nitrogen-cooled isopentane or fixed for 24 hours in 10% formol saline and embedded in paraffin wax.

This system allowed culture of explants for up to 10 days with good preservation of tissue structure. Addition of progesterone resulted in secretory changes in glands and predecidual change in stroma. However, this system did not prove useful for study of eGL differentiation. Although CD45+ cells were often abundant in day 0 control endometrium, after only two days *in vitro* CD45+ cells could only be detected at the edges of the explants and occasionally round endometrial glands. Antibodies to CD2, CD3, CD38 and CD56 did not label any cells in explants even after only two days *in vitro*. Similarly, eGL were rarely detected in cultured explants stained with phloxine tartrazine, even if numerous eGL were detected in day 0 samples. No evidence of proliferation of eGL was seen in any specimens. Although the number of CD45+ cells and eGL decreased sharply after two days of culture, there was no morphological evidence of necrosis of these cell types in explants. It is possible that leukocytes in the explants migrated out of the tissue into the culture medium.

FUNCTIONAL STUDIES OF ENDOMETRIAL LEUKOCYTES

There have been many functional studies of human decidua and endometrium but characterization of cells under investigation has often been incomplete. Different techniques have been used for tissue dispersal and these yield cell suspensions which differ significantly in their composition.[28] Varying methods of further purification also affect the cell populations in functional studies.

Immunosuppressive Activity in Human Decidua and Non-pregnant Endometrium

The capacity of decidual supernatants to suppress lymphocyte proliferation and cytotoxicity has led to the suggestion that local immunosuppression within the placental bed may explain the survival of the fetoplacental unit. The cell types responsible for immunosuppression in human and murine decidua remain unclear. In the mouse, decidual suppressor activity has been attributed to granulated non-T, non-B lymphocytes which have been reported to mediate immunosuppression by secretion of transforming growth factor β (TGFβ).[29] Immunosuppression in murine decidua has also been attributed to prostaglandin E2 secreted by macrophages[11] or true decidualized stromal cells.[30]

Explants of first trimester human decidua are also immunosuppressive but the cells responsible are again not well defined. "Large" and "small" suppressor cells have been described[31] and TFGβ has been implicated as a suppressor factor in human decidua.[29] Prostaglandin E2 has also been implicated and may be produced by decidual cells and macrophages.[32] Johnson *et al.*[33] reported suppression of mixed lymphocyte responses by supernatants of endometrial epithelial cell cultures.

Clark *et al.*[34] suggested that varying results in studies of immunosuppressive activity could be explained by the use of mechanical versus enzymatic techniques of tissue dispersal and reported that disaggregation with certain collagenase types may cause loss of suppressor function. In order to determine whether this is true for human decidua, we examined the immunosuppressive effect of supernatants produced by decidual explants and by various cell suspensions. Cell suspensions from first trimester human decidua were prepared by (1) sieving through a 100µm sieve; (2) digestion of 0.1% type II collagenase/DNase (Sigma); (3) digestion in 0.1% pronase (Sigma); (4) digestion in 0.1% dispase (Sigma). Culture supernatants were harvested after 24, 48 and 72 hours of culture and from explant cultures of normal human decidua. The ability of the supernatants to suppress peripheral blood lymphocyte responses to phytohemagglutinin (PHA) at 10µg/ml and Concanavalin A (Con A) at 50µg/ml was assessed by standard techniques.

The mean results of suppression of lymphocyte PHA responses from five experiments are shown in TABLE 1. No significant difference in suppressor activity was noted between the different techniques of decidual tissue dispersal and none of these differed significantly from explant culture supernatants. Thus, collagenase or protease digestion did not appear to alter the immunosuppressive activity of supernatants. It is known that there are major differences in the composition of suspensions prepared by these dispersal methods.[28] These data therefore suggest that many cell types may be responsible for the suppressor activity in human decidua.

The suppressor function of culture supernatants from eGL enriched by centrifugation over a 5%/10%/20% Nycodenz gradient and from adherent cells in first trimester human decidua was also investigated. Supernatants were collected at 24, 48 and 72 hours and their effect on the PBL response to PHA and ConA and in the mixed lymphocyte reaction (MLR) was assessed. The immunosuppressive activity of enriched eGL supernatants in shown in TABLE 2. In all cases, suppression by enriched eGL

TABLE 1. Suppression of PBL Response to PHA

Preparation of Decidual Supernatant	Percent Suppression					
	24 Hour		48 Hour		72 Hour	
	Mean	SEM	Mean	SEM	Mean	SEM
Explant	48.0	10.8	60.4	7.5	73.0	6.8
Sieved	61.6	17.2	78.4	7.9	78.6	12.4
Collagenase II	63.8	14.6	82.2	7.9	77.8	8.5
Pronase	72.7	17.5	81.8	9.1	93.6	2.8
Dispase	45.8	11.0	73.6	8.5	81.6	10.3

was lower than that by unfractionated decidual cell suspensions. Although eGL supernatants suppressed PBL responses to PHA, some specimens had a stimulatory effect on ConA and MLR responses. Culture supernatants from adherent cells also produced a stimulatory effect on PBL responses to PHA (3 of 10 specimens), ConA (4 of 5 specimens) and in the MLR (4 of 5 specimens). This stimulatory effect may be due to the presence of cytokines in culture supernatants. Immunosuppression in human decidua may be partly due to eGL and adherent cells but clearly other cell types must also play a role.

Wang et al.[35] examined suppressor activity of supernatants from explant cultures of human endometrium and reported increased immunosuppression of PBL responses to PHA and in a MLR by secretory phase endometrium compared with proliferative endometrium. Johnson et al.[33] also reported greater suppressor activity by epithelial cultures prepared from secretory endometrial glands. We assayed suppressor activity in supernatants from explant cultures of five proliferative and six secretory specimens of normal human endometrium. The ability of these supernatants to suppress lymphocyte responses to PHA is shown in TABLE 3. Although there was a tendency to increased suppression by secretory phase samples, the results did not reach significance. Furthermore, supernatants from proliferative and secretory endometrium often stimulated the PBL response to ConA. This may also be due to production of cytokines by endometrium. Tabibzadeh et al.[36] have recently reported production of interleukin 6

TABLE 2. Suppression of PBL Proliferation by eGL Supernatants

Mitogen	Specimen No.	24 Hour	48 Hour	72 Hour
PHA	1	9	3	3
	2	49	35	99
	3	47	53	98
	4	38	52	69
	5	19	29	35
MLR	1	58	36	48
	2	124[a]	54[a]	28[a]
	3	27[a]	6[a]	34[a]
	4	97[a]	50	50
	5	25[a]	38	57

[a] Stimulation of response.

TABLE 3. Suppression of PBL Response to PHA

Specimen	24 Hour	48 Hour	72 Hour
Day 7	21	31	48
Day 7	39	50	76
Day 8	34	55	51
Day 9	26	44	36
Day 12	41	81	85
Mean	37	60	73
Day 19	54	70	79
Day 21	48	40	52
Day 22	43	43	73
Day 22	47	51	77
Day 24	40	66	70
Day 30	40	40	56
Mean	45	51	68

by human endometrial stromal cells. The precise identity of the immunosuppressive cells in human decidua and endometrium remains unknown and it is likely that this *in vitro* effect can be attributed to many cell types.

Functional Studies of Endometrial Granulated Lymphocytes

Endometrial granulated lymphocytes (eGL) have been purified from first trimester human decidua by labeling with anti-CD56 and panning onto immunoglobulin-coated plates. This approach has yielded populations of 93% CD38+, 84% CD2+ and 88% CD56+ cells, most of which contain 5–10 cytoplasmic granules of varying size.[37] The purified population responded poorly to PHA, ConA, phorbol 12, 13 dibutyrate/ionomycin, IL1, IL2 and IFNγ; a small rise in tritiated thymidine uptake was considered to be due to proliferation of contaminating CD3+ T cells.

In view of their morphological similarity to peripheral blood NK cells, decidual cells and purified eGL have been tested for NK activity. In a standard 4 hour K562 chromium release assay purified eGL showed NK activity comparable with that of peripheral blood lymphocytes and this cytotoxic effect was not enhanced by IL2 or IFNγ.[37] At effector:target ratios of 50:1, cytotoxicity was in the region of 30–40%. There was no killing of two LAK targets, Daudi and Colo 320, and attempts to generate LAK cells was unsuccessful.

Decidual NK activity has been investigated in other studies but the proportion of CD56+ cells in cell populations has differed. King *et al.*[38] reported killing of K562 cells but no cytotoxicity against first trimester trophoblast cells. Manaseki and Searle[39] also noted NK activity against K562 targets by decidual lymphocyte preparations, which was enhanced with IL2. In both these studies decidual lymphocytes were prepared by centrifugation over Lymphoprep; the population studied in the latter report included 10% CD16+ cells and 10% CD3+ cells[39] whilst the cell population employed in the former study was characterized only for CD45, CD56 and CD2.[38]

The ability of mouse GMG cells to lyse trophoblast targets has been demonstrated using time-lapse video recordings of GMG cells and labyrinthine trophoblast.[40] It may be necessary to adopt a similar approach to study killing of trophoblast targets by human eGL since chromium release assays detect short-term killing and may not be

TABLE 4. Composition of Nonpregnant Endometrial Cell Suspensions

Specimen	Percent Cells Labeled						
	CD45	CD56	CD38	CD2	CD3	CD14	CAM 5.2
Day 6	22	5	3	20	19	2	32
Day 7	20	7	9	21	15	3	40
Day 16	43	17	19	44	22	2	30
Day 20	96	40	45	80	57	7	3
Day 25	92	45	47	71	42	10	3
Day 25	98	51	49	80	50	5	11

sufficiently sensitive to detect lysis of individual cells. eGL can be extracted from decidual suspensions by labeling with anti-CD56 followed by panning or treatment with magnetic Dynabeads (Dynal) and interactions of these cells with trophoblast cultures can be studied by time-lapse video recording, and scanning or transmission electron microscopy.

Functional Studies of eGL in Nonpregnant Endometrium

Croy et al.[41] failed to demonstrate NK activity in nonpregnant pig endometrium and suggested that the presence of an embryo may be necessary for NK activation. We have performed a preliminary investigation of NK activity in nonpregnant human endometrium. Samples of normal human endometrium were obtained from hysterectomies performed for nonendometrial pathology. Tissues were digested in 0.1% type II collagenase/0.1% DNase for 2.5 hours using gentle agitation. This long dispersal procedure was necessary because cell yields were low using our standard 30 minute serial digest technique,[37] possibly because leukocytes were more firmly bound within the tissue. The percentage of the various cell types in suspensions prepared from samples at various stages of the menstrual cycle is shown in TABLE 4. Leukocytes increased in number in secretory phase samples and in the late secretory phase 40–50% of cells in suspensions were CD56+. The proportion of CD3+ T cells was much higher than in decidual cell suspensions.

Endometrial cell suspensions from six specimens were cultured overnight to remove adherent cells and the nonadherent fraction was then tested in a 4-hour K562 chromium release assay. The results are shown in TABLE 5. None of the specimens showed cytotoxicity greater than 13% specific lysis, and most specimens exhibited lower lytic activity. Although suspensions from day 25 endometrium contained 45–50% CD56+ cells, no significant NK activity could be demonstrated. Thus, it is possible that, as has been suggested for porcine endometrium,[41] NK activity in human endometrium requires the presence of an embryo for activation or, alternatively, is activated by the specific hormonal milieu of pregnancy.

CONCLUSIONS

Although there has been considerable progress in characterization and functional analysis of human endometrial leukocytes, much work still needs to be done. The

TABLE 5. NK Activity of Nonpregnant Endometrial Cells against K562 Targets

Specimen	% Specific Killing			
	$50:1^a$	$25:1^a$	$12.5:1^a$	$6.25:1^a$
Day 6	10	3	2	1
Day 7	13	8	9	4
Day 16	1	0	0	0
Day 20	0	0	0	0
Day 25	2	1	0	0
Day 25	10	4	1	0
PBL	42	34	27	12

[a] Effector:target ratio.

role of macrophages in nonpregnant endometrium and decidua is uncertain. The *in vivo* importance of local immunosuppression in implantation and placentation also remains to be established. Although several studies have indicated that decidual CD56+ eGL are capable of NK activity, their function *in vivo* may be unrelated to this. In particular, eGL may be involved in production of cytokines which may have a role in immunosuppression or placental growth regulation.

ACKNOWLEDGMENT

We are grateful to Professor P. M. Johnson for providing sections of baboon decidua.

REFERENCES

1. MORRIS, H., J. EDWARDS, A. TILTMAN & M. EMMS. 1985. J. Clin. Pathol. **38:** 644–652.
2. KAMAT, B. & P. G. ISAACSON. 1987. Am. J. Pathol. **127:** 66–73.
3. BULMER, J. N., D. P. LUNNY & S. V. HAGIN. 1988. Am. J. Reprod. Immunol. Microbiol. **17:** 83–90.
4. MARSHALL, R. J. & D. B. JONES. 1988. Int. J. Gynecol. Pathol. **7:** 225–235.
5. PACE, E., M. LONGFELLOW & J. N. BULMER. 1991. J. Reprod. Fertil. **91:** 165–174.
6. KING, A., V. WELLINGS, L. GARDNER & Y. W. LOKE. 1989. Human Immunol. **24:** 195–205.
7. BULMER, J. N. & C. A. SUNDERLAND. 1983. J. Reprod. Immunol. **5:** 383–387.
8. BULMER, J. N., L. MORRISON, A. RITSON, D. PACE & A. W. BOYLSTON. In preparation.
9. BULMER, J. N. & C. A. SUNDERLAND. 1984. Immunology **52:** 349–357.
10. BULMER, J. N., J. C. SMITH, L. MORRISON & M. WELLS. 1988. Placenta **9:** 237–246.
11. TAWFIK, O. W., J. S. HUNT & G. W. WOOD. 1986. Am. J. Reprod. Immunol. Microbiol. **12:** 111–117.
12. OKSENBERG, J. R., S. MOR-YOSEF, E. PERSITZ, Y. SCHENKER, E. MOZES & C. BRAUTBAR. 1986. Am. J. Reprod. Immunol. Microbiol. **11:** 82–88.
13. BULMER, J. N. & P. M. JOHNSON. 1985. Clin. Exp. Immunol. **57:** 393–403.
14. RITSON, A., & J. N. BULMER. 1987. Immunology **62:** 329–331.
15. BULMER, J. N., P. M. JOHNSON & D. BULMER. 1987. Leukocyte populations in human decidua and endometrium. *In* Immunoregulation and Fetal Survival. T. J. Gill III & T. G. Wegmann, Eds.: 111–134. Oxford University Press. New York, NY.
16. BULMER, J. N., D. HOLLINGS & A. RITSON. 1987. J. Pathol. **153:** 281–287.
17. WEILL, P. 1921. Arch. Anat. Microsc. **17:** 77–82.
18. NUMERS, C. V. 1953. Acta Pathol. Microbiol. Scand. **33:** 250–256.
19. HAMPERL, H. & G. HELLWEG. 1958. Obstet. Gynecol. **11:** 379–387.
20. DALLENBACH-HELLWEG, G. 1987. The normal histology of the endometrium. *In* Histopathology of the Endometrium.:25–92. Springer-Verlag. Berlin, FRG.

21. LARKIN, L. H. 1974. Endocrinology **94:** 567–570.
22. PEEL, S., I. STEWART & D. BULMER. 1983. Cell Tiss. Res. **233:** 647–656.
23. BULMER, J. N., L. MORRISON, M. LONGFELLOW, A. RITSON & D. PACE. Submitted.
24. CARDELL, R. R., F. L. HISAW & A. B. DAWSON. 1969. Am. J. Anat. **124:** 307–340.
25. PACE, D., L. MORRISON & J. N. BULMER. 1989. J. Clin. Pathol. **42:** 35–39.
26. TABIBZADEH, S. S. & P. G. SATYASWAROOP. 1989. Am. J. Clin. Pathol. **91:** 656–663.
27. DALY, D. C., I. A. MASLAR & D. H. RIDDICK. 1983. Am. J. Obstet. Gynecol. **145:** 672–678.
28. RITSON, A. & J. N. BULMER. 1987. J. Immunol. Methods. **104:** 231–236.
29. CLARK, D. A., M. FALBO, R. B. ROWLEY, D. BANWATT & Y. STEDRONSKA-CLARK. 1988. J. Immunol. **141:** 3833–3840.
30. LALA, P. K., R. S. PARHAR, M. KEARNS, S. JOHNSON & J. M. SCODRAS. 1986. Immunological aspects of the decidual response. *In* Reproductive Immunology 1986. D. A. Clark & B. A. Croy, Eds.: 190–198. Elsevier Science Publishers. Amsterdam.
31. DAYA, S., D. A. CLARK, C. DEVLIN, J. JARRELL & A. CHAPUT. 1985. Fertil. Steril. **44:** 778–785.
32. PARHAR, R. S., T. G. KENNEDY & P. K. LALA. 1988. Cell Immunol. **116:** 392–410.
33. JOHNSON, P. M., J. M. RISK, J. N. BULMER, Z. NIEWOLA & I. KIMBER. 1987. Antigen expression at materno-fetal interfaces. *In* Immunoregulation and Fetal Survival. T. J. Gill III & T. G. Wegmann, Eds.: 181–196. Oxford University Press. New York, NY.
34. CLARK, D. A., J. BRIERLEY, R. SLAPSYS, S. DAYA, N. DAMJI, A. CHAPUT & K. ROSENTHAL. 1986. Trophoblast-dependent and trophoblast-independent suppressor cells of maternal origin in murine and human decidua. *In* Reproductive Immunology 1986. D. A. Clark & B. A. Croy, Eds.: 219–226. Elsevier Science Publishers. Amersterdam.
35. WANG, H., H. KANZAKI, M. YOSHIDA, S. SATO, M. TOKUSHIGE & T. MORI. 1987. Am. J. Obstet. Gynecol. **157:** 956–963.
36. TABIBZADEH, S. S., U. SANTHANAM, P. B. SEHGAL & L. T. MAY. 1989. J. Immunol. **142:** 3134–3139.
37. RITSON, A. & J. N. BULMER. 1989. Clin. Exp. Immunol. **77:** 263–268.
38. KING, A., C. BIRKBY & Y. W. LOKE. 1989. Cell Immunol. **118:** 337–344.
39. MANASEKI, S. & R. F. SEARLE. 1989. Cell Immunol. **121:** 166–173.
40. STEWART, I. J. & D. D. Y. MAKHTAR. 1988. Placenta **9:** 417–426.
41. CROY, B. A., A. WATERFIELD, W. WOOD & G. J. KING. 1988. Cell Immunol. **115:** 471–480.

Expression of the Uteroglobin Promoter in Epithelial Cell Lines from Endometrium[a]

GERD HELFTENBEIN, ANASTASIA MISSEYANNI,
GUSTAV HAGEN, WERNER PETER,
EMILY P. SLATER, RONALD D. WIEHLE,[b]
GUNTRAM SUSKE, AND MIGUEL BEATO

Institut für Molekularbiologie und Tumorforschung (IMT)
Emil-Mannkopff-Str. 2
D-3550 Marburg, Federal Republic of Germany

INTRODUCTION

Understanding the mechanism by which differentiated cells restrict the expression of their genetic potential to a selected subset of genetic programs is one of the main challenges of modern molecular biology. The prevailing concept in the field is that the differentiated phenotype is attained by a series of differential decisions, probably taking place during cell division, and resulting in the equipment of individual cells with a different set of transregulatory proteins. A particular combination of regulatory proteins will switch off a fraction of the inherited genetic messages and switch on other segments of the genetic information. According to this concept defining the differentiation state of a particular cell implies the identification of its particular array of transregulatory proteins. Although this reductionistic approach is certainly over-simplified, it has been very useful as a working hypothesis in the study of development. In *Drosophilia*, starting with the fertilized egg, a network of regulatory inter-actions is established by the sequential induction and/or repression of genes encoding transregulatory proteins. Initial insight into mouse embryogenesis supports the validity of these concepts for mammalian development.

In line with this model, terminally differentiated cells are endowed with specific regulatory proteins able to interact with particular sequences in the promoter or enhancer regions of tissue-specific genes. For example, the transcription factor Oct-2, also known as OTF-2, is responsible for the expression of immunoglobulin genes in lymphoid cells, and this effect is mediated by the presence of specific binding sites for this factor in the enhancer and the promoter region of the immunoglobulin genes.[1,2] Similar findings have been described for liver, pancreas, muscle and pituitary gene expression.

[a] The experimental work summarized in this chapter was performed with financial help from the Deutsche Forschungsgemeinschaft and the Fond der Chemischen Industrie.
[b] *Present address:* J. G. Brown Cancer Center, Louisville, KY 40219.

Along these lines, we have decided to study the factors responsible for maintenance of the differentiate state of mammalian endometrium. Our particular interest in this tissue stems from the fact that its growth and differentiation are modulated by steroid hormones, and that this tissue undergoes very dramatic differentiation changes in adult life. Ovarian hormones influence the morphology and function of endometrial cells during the female cycle, and are responsible for the transformation of the endometrium into the so-called uterine decidua during the initial phase of pregnancy. Our goal is to understand how steroid hormones influence the complex processes leading to proliferation and differentiation of endometrial cells during the normal cycle and during early pregnancy. Although ovarian hormones exert their effects on epithelial as well as on mesenchymal cells of the endometrium, we have initiated our studies with epithelial cells for purely strategic reasons. Some years ago, we initiated studies directed to elucidate the mechanism responsible for induction of the uteroglobin gene in epithelial cells of rabbit endometrium.[3] As a product of these studies we have cloned and sequenced the uteroglobin gene region of the rabbit genome,[4,5] and can now use this knowledge to analyze the expression of the uteroglobin gene in the endometrial epithelial cells.

Rabbit uteroglobin is a small globular protein composed of two identical subunits of 70 amino acids each, held together by two disulfide bridges and non-covalent interactions.[6] The protein was originally detected in the uterine fluid of pregnant rabbits during the preimplantation phase. Subsequently, the same protein was found in the lung of male and female rabbits and in the male genital organs. Though originally detected in rabbits and other members of the genus lagomorpha,[7] uteroglobin-like proteins have also been found in rat[8] and human tissues.[9]

The physiological function of uteroglobin is unclear. It has been postulated that the protein could serve as a protease inhibitor,[10] as an immunosuppressor,[11,12] and as an antiflammin,[13] by virtue of its ability to inhibit phospholipase A2. None of these functions has been demonstrated conclusively. The only activity of the protein that can be detected after extensive purification *in vitro* is its ability to selectively bind progestins[14] and methyl/sulfonyl metabolites of polychlorinated biphenyls (PCB).[15] We have recently produced recombinant uteroglobin, that upon expression in *E. coli* is able to form dimers and to efficiently bind progesterone.[16] These results clearly prove that the high affinity binding of these ligands is an intrinsic property of uteroglobin, rather than a contaminating activity of the partially purified protein preparations. Whether the affinity for these low molecular weight compounds is related to the physiological role of the protein remains to be established.

Independently of its physiological role, uteroglobin has been useful as a marker for following hormone response in mammalian epithelial cells. Induction of uteroglobin gene expression is observed in epithelial cells of the rabbit endometrium following estrogen treatment, but maximal induction requires administration of progesterone. Induction by both hormones takes place at the level of transcription of the uteroglobin gene,[17] although a possible influence of ovarian hormones on the stability of the uteroglobin messenger RNA cannot be excluded. In the lung, the inducing hormone seems to be hydrocortisone,[18] but the effects are far less dramatic than in the uterus, and expression of the uteroglobin gene in the *Clara* cells is high in the absence of glucocorticoids. There are also indications that expression of the uteroglobin gene in the male genital tract is dependent upon androgens.[19,20] Thus, the uteroglobin system offers the possibility to study multi-hormonal control of gene expression in a tissue-specific fashion.

STRUCTURE OF THE RABBIT UTEROGLOBIN GENE REGION

The rabbit uteroglobin gene encompasses some 3 kb of the rabbit genome and its composed of 3 short exons and 2 introns of different length (FIG. 1). We have sequenced the complete uteroglobin gene, 4 kb of the 5'-flanking region and 1 kb of the 3'-flanking region. Contrary to what is found in many other hormonally regulated genes, no binding sites for glucocorticoid or progesterone receptors were found in the proximity of the uteroglobin promoter. Instead, a set of six binding sites for these receptors were found 2.5 kb upstream of the start of transcription.[21,22] In an attempt to understand the physiological significance of these elements, we analyzed the chromatin structure of the uteroglobin gene in endometrial cells during the course of hormonal induction. We found a DNase I hypersensitive site 1 kb 3' of the uteroglobin gene (FIG. 1). This site is observed constitutively in endometrium and even in tissues that do not express the gene, such as the liver.[22] Upstream of the uteroglobin gene no DNase I hypersensitive region was detected in non-expressing tissues or in the endometrial chromatin prior to hormone induction. Following estrogen and progesterone treatment three additional hypersensitive regions appear in the chromatin of endometrial cells.[22] One of these regions, the main DNase I hypersensitive site after combined treatment with estrogens and progesterone, coincides with the cluster of receptor binding side at −2.5 kb, suggesting that these elements play a role in hormone induction *in vivo*. In addition, DNase I hypersensitive sites particularly sensitive to estrogen administration occur in the promoter region and at −3.7 kb (FIG. 1). We know that these two sites overlap potential binding sites for the estrogen receptor. In the promoter region we have identified a binding site for the estrogen receptor that is able to confer estrogen inducibility to the thymidine kinase promoter of the herpes simplex virus, and is most likely involved in the physiological estrogen induction of uteroglobin gene expression in endometrium.[23]

TISSUE-SPECIFIC EXPRESSION OF THE RABBIT UTEROGLOBIN PROMOTER *IN VIVO* AND *IN VITRO*

To test the ability of the uteroglobin promoter to confer tissue-specific expression to heterologous coding sequences, we constructed hybrid genes containing different regions of the uteroglobin promoter linked to the chloramphenicol acetyl transferase (CAT) gene of *E. coli*, followed by the splicing and polyadenylation signals of SV40, and a duplication of the SV40 enhancer. These hybrid constructions were transfected into different cell lines including the Ishikawa cell line, a clone derived from a human endometrial adenocarcinoma.[24] The transcripts originating from the uteroglobin promoter were quantified by contransfection of the internal control gene containing the SV40 early promoter/enhancer unit, or the Rous sarcoma virus (RSV) promoter/enhancer region, linked to the CAT gene. The results clearly demonstrate that the uteroglobin promoter is relatively more efficiently transcribed in Ishikawa cells than in HeLa cells (TABLE 1) or in T47D cells, derived from a mammary carcinoma.

These gene transfer experiments were confirmed in cell-free transcription assays performed with nuclear extracts derived from the different cell lines. Here again, the extract derived from Ishikawa cells transcribes the uteroglobin promoter more efficiently than does the HeLa cell extract, relative to the SV40 enhancer/promoter com-

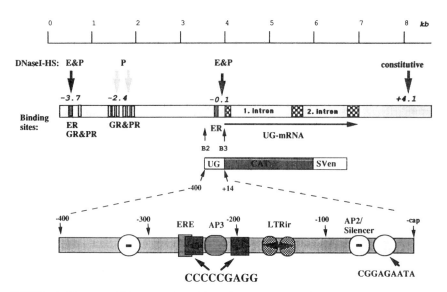

FIGURE 1. The uteroglobin gene region. Schematic representation of the uteroglobin gene region. The transcribed region is indicated by the horizontal arrow labeled Ug-mRNA. The DNaseI hypersensitive sites (DNaseI-HS) are shown above the gene; E indicates estrogen inducibility and P, progesterone inducibility. The binding sites for estrogen receptor (ER), glucocorticoid receptor (GR) and progesterone receptor (PR) are shown underneath the gene. Also shown is the type of construction used for gene transfer experiments with the B2/B3 fragment of the uteroglobin promoter (UG) linked to the chloramphenicol acetyl transferase of *E. coli* (CAT) and the SV40 enhancer (SVen). A more detailed representation of the B2/B3 region is shown at the bottom, with the position of relevant element indicated: estrogen responsive element (ERE), AP3 binding site with the flanking palindrome, the palindrome found in the LTR of retroviruses (LTRir), the AP2/silencer region and the TATA box region.

bination (TABLE 1). Other promoters such as the thymidine kinase promoter or the RSV promoter were less efficiently transcribed in Ishikawa cells than in HeLa cells. Thus, it seems that Ishikawa cells contain a set of factors that enables them to utilize the uteroglobin promoter efficiently.

To map the regions of the uteroglobin promoter that are responsible for the selective transcription in Ishikawa cells, we generated a series of 5'-deletion mutants and tested them *in vivo* and *in vitro*. The results of the quantitative analysis of these data enabled the identification of at least three regions in the uteroglobin promoter relevant for expression in Ishikawa cells (TABLE 1). The region between −395 and −258 is not essential for promoter efficiency, but deletion of the region between −258 and −220 leads to a reduction of the promoter activity *in vivo* and *in vitro* in endometrial cells. A similar decrease in activity is found upon deletion of the region between −205 and −177. The constructions with only 177 nucleotides upstream of the transcription start point are poorly expressed in gene transfer experiments in Ishikawa as well as in HeLa cells. The low expression level precludes further analysis of sequences closer to the promoter *in vivo*. However, relative to the SV40 promoter, the −177 promoter deletion is still considerably more efficient in Ishikawa extracts than

TABLE 1. Analysis of 5'-Deletion Mutants of the Uteroglobin Promoter in Gene Transfer and Cell-free Transcription Experiments[a]

Deletion Endpoint	(UG/SV2) %			
	Ishikawa		HeLa	
	In Vivo	*In Vitro*	*In Vivo*	*In Vitro*
−395	(44)	(3.2)	(4.1)	(0.62)
	100	100	100	100
−376	120	131	75	94
−346	108	111	80	129
−301	153	128	200	120
−283	−	131	−	127
−258	105	131	90	82
−220	25	91	80	57
−205	25	86	62	61
−177	5	45	46	24
−159	4.7	53	100	25
−126	5.7	60	−	24
−96	9.4	59	103	24
−47	4.6	43	−	22
−35	4.5	11	43	11

[a] The values of the −395 deletion are expressed as a ratio of activity of the uteroglobin promoter over the SV40 enhancer/promoter, and taken as 100%. The values for the other deletions are expressed as % of the −395 deletion.

in HeLa cell extracts. Further deletion of the region between −96 and −35 leads to reduction of the Ishikawa preference of the uteroglobin promoter, suggesting that this area contains other elements important for endometrium-specific transcription. Deletion of the region between −96 and −47 has little effect but deletion of the sequences between −47 and −35, abolishes endometrium-specific transcription of the promoter, in agreement with the observed Ishikawa specific DNaseI footprint over the TATA box region. This latter result suggests that an endometrium specific factor binds to the TATA box region and may be responsible for the observed preferential transcription of the uteroglobin promoter in Ishikawa nuclear extracts.

DNA BINDING EXPERIMENTS WITH NUCLEAR EXTRACTS

To identify possible factors responsible for the observed behavior of the 5'-deletion series, we performed DNaseI footprinting experiments with extracts from either Ishikawa or HeLa cells. We found a complex pattern of DNaseI protection, with at least eight individual footprints exhibiting quantitative and qualitative differences between the two cell types (FIG. 2). Over the promoter distal region between −280 and −177 there are three DNaseI protected regions, that are observed with extracts from both cell lines. However, the relative intensity of the individual projections is different in both cell lines. In the most distal promoter region between −280 and −250 (VIII) protection is stronger in HeLa extracts. In the region between −177 or −140 a footprint (V) is observed with both cell extracts, but protection is stronger in Ishikawa cell extracts. Both cell extracts generate two additional footprints of similar intensity between −140

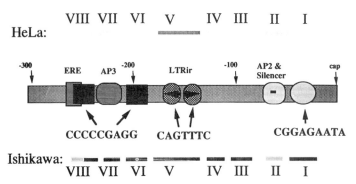

FIGURE 2. DNaseI footprints over the uteroglobin promoter. Schematic representation of the utero-globin promoter region –300/ + 1 with the relevant regions indicated (see legend to Fɪɢ. 1). The foot-print generated with HeLa extracts are shown above the promoter and those obtained with Ishikawa extracts are indicated underneath.

and –90 (III and IV). In addition, we find two differential footprints in the region between –96 and –20. One footprint around –70 (II) is detected exclusively with ex-tracts from HeLa cells, whereas over the region of the TATA box, between –40 to –20, there is a footprint (I) observed exclusively with Ishikawa cell extracts.

A comparison of the nucleotide sequence within the two relevant footprints at –255/–240 and –205/–180 reveals a conserved 14 bp sequence: CCCTCGGGGGCAGG, that has not been previously reported (Fɪɢ. 3). In the region –173/–147 there is a palin-drome with the structure CAGTTTCA, that is frequently found in the LTR of retro-viruses. The function of this palindrome is unclear as its deletion does not show a phenotype in transfection experiments, but there is a clear footprint over this region in Ishikawa nuclear extracts. The region around –70 that yields a footprint only with HeLa nuclear extracts shows strong homology to the AP2 site of the SV40 enhancer. Finally, the footprint over the TATA box covers a sequence CGGAGA, that is also found in the rat uteroglobin gene, and in the uteroferrin promoter, another endometrium-specific gene (Fɪɢ. 3).

We interpret these data to be indicative of the existence of a combination of ubi-quitous and specific factors that by interaction with different sequence elements in the uteroglobin promoter are responsible for its selective transcription in endometrium.

COMPARISON OF THE 5'-FLANKING SEQUENCES OF RAT AND RABBIT UTEROGLOBIN GENES

The tissue expression patterns of rabbit and rat uteroglobin are qualitatively similar but quantitatively different, in that the rat protein is preferentially expressed in *Clara* cells of the lung, whereas the rabbit protein is preferentially expressed in epithelial cells of the endometrium. To analyze the reasons for this difference we cloned the uteroglobin gene from the rat genome and compared the nucleotide sequence in its 5'-flanking region with that of the rabbit gene.[25] This comparison shows that the first 900 base pairs upstream of the start of transcription are well conserved among the two genes, although the estrogen responsive element at –260 of the rabbit uteroglobin

UGUE-Element

```
UG    -240  (<----):     CCTGCCCCCGAGG
UG    -200  (---->):     CCTCCCCCCGAGG
rUG   -417  (<----):     CCTCCCTCCAAGG
UF    -158  (<----):     CCTGCCCCACAGC

Consensus:               CCTSCCcCcgAGG
```

AP3

```
SV40  -251  (---->):     GGGTGTGGAAAG
UG    -223  (<----):     GGGTGTGGCAAG
```

LTR-Palindrome

```
UG    -169  (---->):     CAGTTTCAAT
UG    -148  (<----):     CAGTTTCCAT
rUG   -162  (---->):     CAGTTTCAAT
rUG   -140  (<----):     CAGTTTCTTT
MLV   -171  (---->):     CAGTTTCAAT
MLV   -148  (<----):     CAGTTTCCAT

Consensus:               CAGTTTC-MT
```

TATA Box

```
UG    -40/-20       CCGGAGAATACAAAAAGGCAC
UF    -40/-20       GCGGAGAAACTGCATCATCCT
rUG   -35/-15       CAGGAACATATAAAAAGCCAC

UTERINE TATA        ccGGAgaAtataaAaag-Caa
                      : : : :   :
ChLYS-42/-22        GTGGAGGAAGTTAAAAGAAGA
```

FIGURE 3. **A.** Nucleotide sequence of the uteroglobin promoter from –400 to +10. **B.** Sequence motifs of the uteroglobin promoter found in other endometrium-specific genes. **Abbreviations:** UGUE = uteroglobin upstream element; UG = rabbit uteroglobin gene; rUG = rat uteroglobin gene; UF = pig uteroferrin gene;[27] MLV = Moloney murine leukemia virus; and ChLys = chicken lysozyme gene.[28]

gene is not found in the rat gene (FIG. 4). There are two other regions of homology, one found between –900 and –1.1 kb of the rat gene and between –1.2 and –1.4 kb of the rabbit gene, and the other located between –1.2 and –1.6 kb in the rat and between –3.9 and –3.4 in the rabbit uteroglobin gene (FIG. 4). Thus, the –2.4 kb region of the rabbit uteroglobin gene containing the main set of hormone-responsive sites

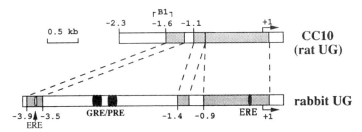

FIGURE 4. Comparison of the 5'-flanking region of the rat and rabbit uteroglobin genes. Schematic representation of the 5'-flanking regions of the uteroglobin genes from rat and rabbit with the conserved regions indicated in gray. The binding sites for estrogen receptor (ERE) glucocorticoid receptor (GRE) and progesterone receptor (PRE) are indicated.

for glucocorticoids and progesterone is lacking in the rat gene. This difference may be responsible for the differential behavior of the two genes in terms of tissue-specificity. Whether this difference is the consequence of an insertion introduced into the rabbit genome by a viral transposon, or whether it results from a deletion of the rat utero-globin 5'-flanking region is not known.

In the promoter region, the sequence immediately adjacent to the TATA box, that has been shown to be relevant for endometrium specific expression of the rabbit utero-globin gene, is conserved in the rat uteroglobin promoter. In addition, some of the other factor binding sites in the upstream region are also present in the rat promoter. The functional significance of any of these elements remains to be determined in the gene transfer experiments.

ESTABLISHMENT OF RAT ENDOMETRIAL CELL LINES

Because the human *Ishikawa* cell line was derived from an adenocarcinoma and no other established endometrial cell lines are available for comparison, we decided to establish endometrial cell lines derived from rabbit, rat or mouse primary cultures. After initial difficulties with rabbit endometrial cells, we tried to establish cell lines from rat endometrium. To this end, we used a series of murine leukemia virus based retroviral vectors containing different viral oncogenes and the positive selection marker *neo*, that confers neomycin resistance.[26] The following oncogenes were utilized: the wild-type or a temperature-sensitive mutant of the SV40 large T-antigen, the adeno-virus E1A gene or the Harvey-*ras* oncogene. In a first step we immortalized several cell lines with either the adenovirus E1A or the SV40 large T-antigen, and we obtained several cell lines that have been maintained in culture now for more than one year. In a later step, a few of these immortalized cells were superinfected with a second retrovirus carrying the Ha-*ras* oncogene. A description of some properties of these cell lines is shown in TABLE 2.

The morphology of these endometrial cell lines is indicative of their epithelial origin, and partly depends upon the tissue culture support. The two cell lines trans-formed by the Ha-*ras* oncogene exhibit a differential expression of cytokeratins de-pendent upon whether the cells are grown on plastic or on a substrate of NIH-3T3 cells. When grown on a monolayer of formalin-fixed fibroblasts, these cells appear

TABLE 2. Equipment of Endometrial Cell Lines with Intermediate Filaments and Hormone Receptors

Cell Line	CK1		CK8		CK18		CK19		Vimentin		PR n/cell	GR n/cell (×1000)	ER
	P[d]	F[e]	P	F	P	F	P	F	P	F			
Ishikawa	+	?	−	−/+	−/+	+++	+	+++	−	+	3.7	12	5
RENE 1[a]	−	?	−	−/+	−	−/+	−	−	+	++	10.6	0	2
RENE 2[a]	−	?	−	−	−	−	−	−	?	++	8	53	−
RENT 4[b]	−	?	−	−	−	−	−	−	+	++	1.6	23	10
RENTR 01[c]	?	?	+	++	−	++	−	+++	?	+++	0.7	22.3	−
RENTR 03[c]	?	?	−	++	−	++	−	++	?	++	0.3	100	−

[a] Immortalized with adenovirus E1A.
[b] Immortalized with SV40 large T antigen.
[c] Immortalized with SV40 large T antigen followed by transformation with Ha-*ras*.
[d] P: Plastic.
[e] F: Fixed NIH-3T3-Cells.

to differentiate in culture. Individual islands of cells with epithelial pattern of intermediate filaments are found surrounded by cells that express vimentin and are localized to the external areas of the islands.[26] It seems, therefore, that these cell lines could be interesting to study the process of epithelial differentiation in culture.

We also have established two cell lines by transformation with a retrovirus containing a temperature-sensitive mutant of the SV40 large T-antigen. These two cell lines show a temperature-sensitive phenotype. At 34°C the cells grow exponentially with a doubling time of 48 h, and exhibit an elongated morphology with small cytoplasm and high density of growth. A few hours after shifting to 39°C, the cells start to differentiate and, after two days, they stop growing and the cytoplasm becomes larger and flatter. If these cells are now shifted again to 34°C, after a lag phase, the cells start to grow again and resume the transformed phenotype.

The various cell lines established with wild type immortalizing or transforming oncogenes, as well as the temperature-sensitive cell lines derived from rat endometrium, should be very useful to analyze the steps responsible for differentiation of the epithelial phenotype. Gene transfer experiments will determine whether we are able to reproduce the tissue specificity of uteroglobin gene transcription with any of the cell lines we have established from rat endometrium.

SUMMARY

To understand the molecular mechanism of endometrial differentiation we have initiated an analysis of the uteroglobin promoter. Uteroglobin is normally expressed in endometrial tissues under the control of ovarian hormones. In gene transfer experiments with the Ishikawa cell line, derived from a human endometrial adenocarcinoma, we have identified several regions in the promoter of the uteroglobin gene that are responsible for its endometrium-specific expression. To evaluate the generality of these findings, we have begun cloning the promoter regions of potential endometrial markers, including the rat, mouse, and human uteroglobin gene. In the rat, expression of the uteroglobin-like gene, CC10, is dominant in the lung but is also observed in the endometrium of progesterone treated animals. A comparison of the

5'-flanking sequence of the rat and rabbit uteroglobin gene resulted in the detection of similarities and differences that could explain their differential expression *in vivo*. To substantiate these findings we have established several cell lines from rat endometrium using murine retroviral vectors containing a positive selection marker and various viral oncogenes, such as SV40 large T antigen, adenovirus E1A, and Ha-*ras*. Cell lines immortalized by SV40 T-antigen were subsequently transformed with the Ha-*ras* oncogene. Several cell lines exhibit properties of epithelial endometrial cells. Two cell lines generated with a temperature sensitive mutant of the SV40 large T-antigen grow as transformed cells at the permissive temperature, but differentiate upon shifting to the non-permissive temperature. These rat endometrial cell lines should be useful for the analysis of endometrium-specific gene expression and as model systems for endometrial carcinoma.

REFERENCES

1. FALKNER, F. G. & H. G. ZACHAU. 1984. Correct transcription of an immunoglobin *k* gene requires an upstream fragment containing conserved sequence elements. Nature **310:** 71–74.
2. KEMLER, I., E. SCHREIBER, M. M. MÜLLER, P. MATTHIAS & W. SCHAFFNER 1989. Octamer transcription factors bind to two different sequence motifs of the immonoglobulin heavy chain promoter. EMBO J **8:** 2001–2008.
3. BEATO, M., J. ARNEMANN, C. MENNE, H. MÜLLER, G. SUSKE & M. WENZ. 1983. Regulation of the expression of the uteroglobin gene by ovarian hormones. *In* Regulation of Gene Expression by Hormones. K. W. McKerns, Ed.: 151–175. Plenum Publishing Corp. New York, NY.
4. MENNE, C., G. SUSKE, J. ARNEMANN, A. C. B. CATO & M. BEATO. 1982. Isolation and structure of the gene for the progesterone inducible protein uteroglobin. Proc. Natl. Acad. Sci. USA **79:** 4853–4857.
5. SUSKE, G., M. WENZ, A. C. B. CATO & M. BEATO. 1983. The uteroglobin gene region: Hormonal regulation, repetitive elements and complete nucleotide sequence. Nucl. Acids Res. **11:** 2257–2271.
6. POSTINGL, H., A. NIETO & M. BEATO. 1978. Amino acid sequence of progesterone-induced rabbit uteroglobin. Biochemistry **17:** 3908–3912.
7. LOPEZ DE HARO, M. S. & A. NIETO. 1983. Isolation and characterization of uteroglobin from the lung of the hare. Arch. Biochem. Biophys. **226:** 539–547.
8. SINGH, G., S. SINGAL, S. L. KATYAL, W. E. BROWN & S. A. GOTTRON. 1987. Exp. Lung Res. **13:** 299–309.
9. SINGH, G., S. L. KATYAL, W. E. BROWN, S. PHILIPS, A. L. KENNEDY, J. ANTHONY & N. SQUEGLIA. 1988. Amino-acid and cDNA nucleotide sequences of human Clara cell 10 kDa protein. Biochim. Biophys. Acta **950:** 329–337.
10. BEIER, H. M. 1976. Uteroglobin and related biochemical changes in the reproductive tract during early pregnancy in the rabbit. J. Reprod. Fert., Suppl. **25:** 53–69.
11. MUKHERJEE, D. C., A. K. AGRAWAL, R. MANJUNATH & A. B. MUKHERJEE. 1983. Suppression of epididymal sperm antigenicity in the rabbit by uteroglobin and transglutaminase. Science **219:** 989–991.
12. MUKHERJEE, A. B., R. E. ULANE & A. K. AGRAWAL. 1982. Role of uteroglobin and transglutaminase in masking the antigenicity of implanting rabbit embryos. Am. J. Reprod. Immunol. **2:** 135–141.
13. LEVIN, S. W., J. DE B. BUTLER, U. K. SCHUMACHER, P. D. WIGHTMAN & A. B. MUKHERJEE. 1986. Uteroglobin inhibits phospholipase A2 activity. Life Sci. **38:** 1813–1819.
14. BEATO, M. & R. BAIER. 1975. Binding of progesterone to uteroglobin. Biochim. Biophys. Acta **392:** 346–356.
15. LUND, J., I. BRANDT, L. POELLINGER, A. BERGMAN, E. KLASSON-WEHLER & J.-A. GUSTAFSSON. 1985. Target cells for the polychlorinated biphenyl metabolite 4,4'-Bis(methylsulfonyl)-2,2',5,5'-tetrachlorobiphenyl. Characterization of high affinity binding in rat and mouse lung cytosol. Mol. Pharmacol. **27:** 314–323.

16. PETER, W., M. BEATO & G. SUSKE. 1989. Recombinant rabbit uteroglobin expressed at high levels in E. coli forms stable dimers and binds progesterone. Protein Eng. **3**: 61–66.
17. MÜLLER, H. & M. BEATO. 1980. RNA synthesis in rabbit endometrial nuclei. Hormonal regulation of transcription of the uteroglobin gene. Eur. J. Biochem. **112**: 235–241.
18. LOMBARDERO, M. & A. NIETO. 1981. Glucocorticoid and developmental regulation of uteroglobin synthesis in rabbit lung. Biochem. J. **200**: 487–494.
19. LOPEZ DE HARO, M. S., L. ALVAREZ & A. NIETO. 1988. Testosterone induces the expression of the uteroglobin gene in rabbit epididymis. Biochem. J. **250**: 647–651.
20. NOSKE, I. G. & M. FEIGELSON. 1976. Immunological evidence of uteroglobin (blastokinin) in the male reproductive tract and in nonreproductive ductal tissues and their secretions. Biol. Reprod. **15**: 704–713.
21. CATO, A. C. B., S. GEISSE, M. WENZ, H. M. WESTPHAL & M. BEATO. 1984. The nucleotide sequences recognized by the glucocorticoid receptor in the rabbit uteroglobin gene region are located far upstream from the initiation of transcription. EMBO J. **3**: 2731–2736.
22. JNATZEN, C., H. P. FRITTON, T. IGO-KEMENES, E. ESPEL, S. JANICH, A. C. B. CATO, K. MUGELE & M. BEATO. 1987. Partial overlapping of binding sequences for steroid hormone receptors and DNaseI hypersensitive sites in the rabbit uteroglobin gene region. Nucleic Acids Res. **15**: 4535–4552.
23. SLATER, E. P., G. REDEUIHL, K. THEIS, G. SUSKE & M. BEATO. 1990. The uteroglobin promoter contains a noncanonical estrogen responsive element. Mol. Endocrinol. **4**: 604–610.
24. NISHIDA, M., K. KASAHARA, M. KANEKO & H. IWASAKI. 1985. Establishment of a new human endometrial adenocarcinoma cell line, Ishikawa cells, containing estrogen and progesterone receptors. Acta Obstet. Gynecol. Jpn. **37**: 1103–1111.
25. HAGEN, G., M. WOLF, S. L. KATYAL, G. SINGH, M. BEATO & G. SUSKE. 1990. Tissue-specific expression, hormonal regulation and 5′-flanking gene region of the rat Clara cell 10 kDa protein: Comparison to rabbit uteroglobin. Nucl. Acids Res. in press.
26. WIEHLE, R. D., G. HELFTENBEIN, H. LAND, K. NEUMANN & M. BEATO. 1990. Establishment of rat endometrial cell lines by retroviral mediated transfer of immortalizing and transforming oncogenes. Oncogene **5**. In press.
27. SIMMEN, R. C. M., V. SRINIVAS & R. M. ROBERTS. 1989. cDNA sequence, gene organization, and progesterone induction of mRNA for uteroferrin, a porcine uterine iron transport protein. DNA **8**: 543–554.
28. RENKAWITZ, R., G. SCHÜTZ, D. VON DER AHE & M. BEATO. 1984. Identification of hormone regulatory elements in the promoter region of the chicken lysozyme gene. Cell **37**: 503–510.

Studies on Human Endometrial Cells in Primary Culture

F. SCHATZ,[a] V. HAUSKNECHT,[a] R. E. GORDON,[b]
D. HELLER,[b] L. MARKIEWICZ,[a]
L. DELIGDISCH,[b] AND E. GURPIDE[a]

[a]Department of Obstetrics/Gynecology and Reproductive Science
[b]Department of Pathology
Mount Sinai School of Medicine
New York, New York 10029-6574

INTRODUCTION

In rodents, prostaglandin (PG) $F_{2\alpha}$ stimulates hatching of the preimplantation blastocyst,[1] and appears to mediate two early implantational events, increased endometrial vascular permeability at the sites of implantation, and decidualization of the underlying endometrial stromal cells (see review by Kennedy[2]). During the period of the menstrual cycle corresponding to hatching and implantation of the human blastocyst, concentrations of $PGF_{2\alpha}$ reportedly increase three- to fivefold in endometrial extracts[3] and in jet washes of the uterine lumen.[4] This pattern suggests that endometrial $PGF_{2\alpha}$ is involved in periimplantational events in women.

A role for estrogens in the cyclic production of $PGF_{2\alpha}$ in human endometrium is indicated from observations that estradiol (E_2) elevates $PGF_{2\alpha}$ output in explants of human endometrium taken from secretory,[5-8] but not proliferative phase[5-7] specimens. To eliminate the potential contribution to these *in vitro* results of E_2 acting directly and/or indirectly on blood cells present in human endometrial explants, E_2 effects were studied on the glandular epithelial and stromal cells, the predominant human endometrial cell types, grown conventionally on tissue culture plastic. Through these experiments, the glandular epithelial cells were singled out as estrogen targets leading to enhanced $PGF_{2\alpha}$ production in human endometrium. Paradoxically, despite the unresponsiveness of proliferative endometrium, these results also revealed that E_2 elevated $PGF_{2\alpha}$ levels significantly in epithelial cell cultures derived from proliferative tissue.[6,9] Recently, we were able to culture both cell types under "polarizing" conditions,[10] thereby providing a physiological milieu with the potential for investigating alternative explanations for the paradoxical *in vitro* responsiveness to E_2 of proliferative phase grandular epithelial cells: that the stromal cells inhibit E_2-enhanced production of $PGF_{2\alpha}$ in the glands of intact tissue; that loss of structural polarity of the glandular epithelial cells during conventional culture alters this E_2 response.

METHODS

Tissues

Endometrial specimens were obtained from patients undergoing biopsy for fertility examination or hysterectomy. The tissues were trimmed and minced under a laminar flow hood in Minimum Essential Medium containing 1% of an antibiotic-antimycotic mixture (Grand Island Biological Co., Grand Island, NY). A small portion of each specimen was fixed in formalin and dated histologically by the criteria of Noyes *et al.* [11]

Isolation of Glands and Stromal Cells

The isolation procedure was carried out using Ham's F-10 supplemented with 10 µg/ml porcine insulin (Nordisk-USA, Bethesda MD), 1% antibiotic-antimycotic mixture (Gibco) and 10% charcoal-stripped calf serum (Ham's F-10 + 10% SCS). As detailed elsewhere[10,10a] it involves: 1) digestion of the minced tissue using Type I collagenase; 2) separation of glands and stroma by filtration through a stainless steel sieve; 3) backwashing the glands from the sieve, followed by pelleting by centrifugation; and 4) isolation of the stromal cells from contaminating epithelial and blood cells in the filtrate by taking advantage of the more rapid adhesion of the stromal cells than the contaminants to tissue culture plastic at 37°C.

$PGF_{2\alpha}$ Output by Glandular Epithelial Cells and Stromal Cells Grown on Tissue Culture Plastic

The isolated glands and stroma from each specimen were distributed equally among polystyrene culture dishes in Ham's F-10 + 10% SCS. The dishes were kept in a 37°C incubator for a 24 h "Plating Period" to enable the glands to adhere to the plastic surface, then the medium was removed along with floating glands, and replaced with fresh Ham's F-10 + 10% SCS.

Incubation Protocol 1

As detailed by Schatz *et al.*,[6] it involves daily replacement of the conditioned medium with fresh medium containing 10-8 M E_2, added in 0.1% ethanol, the vehicle control. The cell-conditioned media were centrifuged and the supernatants frozen for later measurement of $PGF_{2\alpha}$. Incubations were terminated by harvesting the cells with trypsin-EDTA. Cell numbers were measured by counting an aliquot in a hemocytometer, and protein content of the cell pellets determined.

Incubation Protocol 2

As detailed by Schatz *et al.*,[12] it involves incubation with fresh control medium, or medium containing 10-8 M E_2, arachidonic acid (AA) at 4 and 20 µg/ml, and combinations of E_2 + AA for a 24–74 h "Monolayer Formation Period." Conditioned media were then replaced with corresponding fresh media, and the cultures incubated for a 64 h "Testing Period." At the end of this period, the collected media were centrifuged, and analyzed for $PGF_{2\alpha}$ content. Cell numbers and cell protein content were determined as described for *Incubation Protocol 1.*

Stromal cells isolated from the same endometrial specimens as the glands, were incubated in parallel with the glandular epithelial cells according to *Protocols 1 and 2.* For those endometrial specimens in which the yield of only the glands or the stroma was judged sufficient to procede with the incubation, experiments were carried out with that cell type alone. Measurements of $PGF_{2\alpha}$ levels in the conditioned media, and determinations of cell numbers and cell protein were performed as described for the glandular epithelial cells.

Measurement of $PGF_{2\alpha}$

Levels of $PGF_{2\alpha}$ in the conditioned medium of glandular epithelial and stromal cells grown on tissue culture plastic were measured by radioimmunoassay as previously described by Schatz and Gurpide.[9]

Statistics

Statistical significance of differences between means were estimated by Student's paired or unpaired t-test, as appropriate for the data.

Incubation of Glandular Epithelial and Stromal Cells under Polarizing Conditions

As described in detail in Schatz *et al.*,[10] the culturing configuration used consists of a cylindrical polystyrene insert (Millicell® CM, Millipore) that sits on small projections in the well of a tissue culture plate. Thus, access of culture medium is provided to the underside of a permeable (Biopore) filter that serves as support for the endometrial cells. In these experiments, 0.2 ml of type I collagen, prepared as an acid extract from rat tails and titrated to neutral pH, was applied to each 12-mm diameter filter. After allowing the collagen to gel at 37°C, and sterilizing with ethanol, the collagen gels were stored in basal medium (BM) (a phenol red-free mixture of Dulbecco's minimum essential medium (Gibco) and Ham's F-12 (Flow Laboratories), 1:1 v/v, supplemented with 100 U/ml penicillin, and 100 μg/ml streptomycin, 0.25 μg/ml fungizone), under sterile conditions. Endometrial glands carrying stromal cells were suspended in BM to which 10% charcoal stripped calf serum (SCS) was added. An aliquot of the cell suspension was transferred to each collagen gel, and the tissue culture plate was placed in a 37°C incubator. After 3 days, the conditioned BM + SCS was replaced with fresh BM supplemented with ITS (+) (Colaborative Research) and 10-8 M E2 + 10-6 M medroxyprogesterone (MPA). The tissue culture plate was returned to the incubator for 4 days.

Fixation and Immunocytochemistry of Cells Cultured under Polarizing Conditions

Incubations were terminated by removing the conditioned medium and rinsing the cultures with PBS. The cultures were fixed for 30 minutes in 3.5% paraformaldehyde dissolved in PBS, and the cultures washed with PBS. The collagen-coated filters containing the endometrial cells were cut out of each Millicell insert, subjected to graded ethanol dehydration, and embedded in paraffin. Parallel sections were examined after staining immunocytochemically, and with hemotoxylin-eosin. Immunocytochemistry was performed by the avidin-biotin-peroxidase complex method using a polyclonal primary antibody to human cytokeratin (Becton Dickinson) that was appropriately diluted. Specificity was determined by substituting for the primary antibody, PBS at pH 7.4, as well as nonimmune serum.

RESULTS

Estradiol-regulated $PGF_{2\alpha}$ Output in Human Endometrial Glandular Epithelial Cells

Estradiol effects on $PGF_{2\alpha}$ output were measured during consecutive days in culture in primary glandular epithelial cells from several specimens of proliferative and secretory phase endometrium. TABLE 1 summarizes the results for the first 24 h of incubation. It indicates that E_2 elicits significant, threefold increases in levels of $PGF_{2\alpha}$ measured in the media of both proliferative ($p < 0.002$ and secretory $p < 0.035$) phase epithelial cells. Estradiol has been shown to elevate levels to a similar extent in epithelial cells from both phases of the menstrual cycle during several days in culture.[6] Moreover, E_2-enhanced $PGF_{2\alpha}$ output apparently reflects an increase in the synthesis of $PGF_{2\alpha}$. Thus, 10^{-8} M E_2 did not affect cell number[9] or total cell protein[6,9] in the cultured epithelial cells, indicating that increased $PGF_{2\alpha}$ output does not reflect altered cell growth, whereas radiolabeled $PGF_{2\alpha}$ was metabolized to a similar, relatively small extent in control and E_2-treated cultures,[6] indicating the E_2 does not inhibit the catabolism of $PGF_{2\alpha}$.

TABLE 1. Prostaglandin $F_{2\alpha}$ Levels in Epithelial Cell Cultures

Source of Epithelial Cells	Number of Specimens	ng $PGF_{2\alpha}$/dish[a]		% of Control[a,b]
		Control	+ E_2 (10^{-8}M)	
Proliferative endometrium	12[c]	3.6 ± 0.72	12.0 ± 2.6	330 ± 32
Secretory endometrium	6[d]	5.0 ± 0.83	11.9 ± 2.4	300 ± 77

[a] Mean ± SE.

[b] % of control = $\dfrac{\text{conc. of } PGF_{2\alpha} \text{ in dishes containing } E_2}{\text{conc. of } PGF_{2\alpha} \text{ in corresponding control}} \times 100$

[c] Three specimens of early, 4 specimens of mid and 2 specimens of late proliferative endometrium.

[d] One specimen of day 15, 1 specimen of day 16, 2 specimens of day 18, and 2 specimens of day 19 endometrium.

TABLE 2. Prostaglandin $F_{2\alpha}$ Levels in Epithelial and Stromal Cell Cultures

Endometrial Cell Type	Number of Specimens	Control[a] ng PGF$_{2\alpha}$/mg prot. × 64h	E$_2$ (10^{-8}M); % of Control[b]
Epithelial[c]	11	12.3 ± 3.1	862 ± 227
Stromal[d]	9	9.4 ± 2.3	146 ± 27

[a] Mean ± SE.
[b] Percentage of control.
[c] Nine specimens of proliferative and 2 specimens of secretory endometrium.
[d] Eight specimens of proliferative and 1 specimen of secretory endometrium.

Effects of Estradiol and Arachidonic Acid on PGF$_{2\alpha}$ Output in Human Endometrial Glandular Epithelial and Stromal Cells

The effects of E$_2$ were studied on PGF$_{2\alpha}$ output by epithelial and stromal cells that were isolated from several specimens of human endometrium and incubated according to Protocol 2 (METHODS). As indicated in TABLE 2, basal production of PGF$_{2\alpha}$ is comparable in the two cell types. However, E$_2$ evoked large, statistically significant increases in the levels of PGF$_{2\alpha}$ in cultures of epithelial cells (8.6-fold ± 2.3, $p <$ 0.01), but not in the stromal cells (1.4-fold ± 2.4, $p < 0.3$).

Since AA is the obligatory substrate for PG synthase-mediated synthesis of PGF$_{2\alpha}$, the similarity in basal PGF$_{2\alpha}$ output evident in TABLE 2 implies the presence of functional PG synthase in both epithelial and stromal cells. Confirmation of this came from adding AA to primary cultures of epithelial and stromal cells within the concentration range shown to produce a linear increase in PGF$_{2\alpha}$ output by the epithelial monolayers.[13]

Accordingly, TABLE 3 indicates that AA added at 4 and 20 μg/ml, increased PGF$_{2\alpha}$ output proportionally in primary cultures of both cell types. In the epithelial cell cultures, moreover, addition of AA together with E$_2$ resulted in PGF$_{2\alpha}$ output that was approximately two and half times the sum of that produced by E$_2$ and AA added separately. In contrast, no E$_2$ effects were produced in the stromal cell cultures whether the estrogen was added alone, or in combination with AA.

Cocultured Glandular Epithelial and Stromal Cells under Polarizing Conditions

Primary mammary epithelial cells lose important structurally and functionally polarized features of the cells *in vivo* when grown on tissue culture plastic that are retained during culture on the stromal cell-derived extracellular matrix component, Type I collagen.[14,15] To determine whether collagen I is similarly suitable for culturing human endometrial cells, glands carrying stromal cells were derived from a specimen of late secretory phase tissue (approximately day 24) and incubated under the polarizing conditions described in METHODS. The cultured cells were then fixed and examined immunocytochemically for the presence of human keratin.

As shown in FIGURE 1, the glands formed an epithelial cell monolayer which was stained strongly with the human cytokeratin antibody. The epithelial cells lie on a cluster of immunocytokeratin negative stromal cells, which appear to have penetrated

TABLE 3. Effects of E_2 and Arachidonic Acid on $PGF_{2\alpha}$ Output by Endometrial Cells[a]

	Basal Output (ng $PGF_{2\alpha}$)		+ E_2 (10^{-8}M)	+ Arachidonic Acid		+ E_2 (10^{-8}M) + Arachidonic Acid	
% Controls							
Cell Type	mg prot. × 64 h			4 μg/ml	20 μg/ml	4 μg/ml	20 μg/ml
Epithelial	Mean[b]	9.4	510	550	1900	2700	6200
	SE	± 3.0	± 130	± 100	± 180	± 830	± 1900
	n	5	5	5	3	5	3
Stromal	Mean[b]	11.0	110	320	1300	330	1300
	SE	± 4.1	± 2.0	± 100	± 280	± 150	± 310
	n	5	5	2	3	2	3

[a] Averages from results of duplicate dishes.

[b] Cultures of epithelial and stromal cells derived from a specimen of early proliferative endometrium, 3 from mid-proliferative endometrium and 1 from late proliferative endometrium, and from additional cultures of stromal cells derived from another specimen of secretory endometrium.

the gel. Examination of parallel sections with an antiserum for vimentin (results not shown) confirmed the differential nature of the two cell types. As expected, the stromal cells were strongly positive for the presence of vimentin, whereas, the epithelial cells were only weakly positive. Use of polarizing culture conditions extends the period of the menstrual cycle in which interactions between epithelial and stromal cells can be studied *in vitro*. Thus, unlike the results shown here for glands from late secretory endometrium, endometrial glands obtained from specimens after day 21 of the menstrual cycle (approximately the time of implantation), do not show appreciable adherence to tissue culture plastic.

DISCUSSION

Extrapolation of results from primary human endometrial glandular epithelial and stromal cells grown on tissue culture plastic to intact tissue indicates that the epithelial cells and not the stroma are sites of estrogen action leading to increased $PGF_{2\alpha}$ production.[6,9,13,16] Thus, although basal $PGF_{2\alpha}$ release is comparable in both cell types, addition of E_2 elevates $PGF_{2\alpha}$ production only in the epithelial cells (TABLE 2). This response appears to be mediated by specific estrogen receptors since 4-OH-tamoxifen is at least an order of magnitude more potent than tamoxifen in inhibiting E_2-enhanced $PGF_{2\alpha}$ output in the epithelial cells and in endometrial fragments.[12] Alternatively, lack of an estrogen response in the stroma cannot be readily attributed to a deficiency in functional estrogen receptors, since E_2 is known to augment progesterone effects on decidualization-related changes in these cells.[17-19] The differential estrogen responsiveness of the epithelial and stromal cell monolayers is accentuated in the presence of exogenous AA, the obligatory substrate for $PGF_{2\alpha}$ synthesis via PG synthase. Both cell types effectively converted added AA to $PGF_{2\alpha}$, showing that each possesses functional PG synthase. For the epithelial cells, incubation with E_2 and AA produced synergistic increases in $PGF_{2\alpha}$ output, an E_2-enhanced utilization of AA that reflects in-

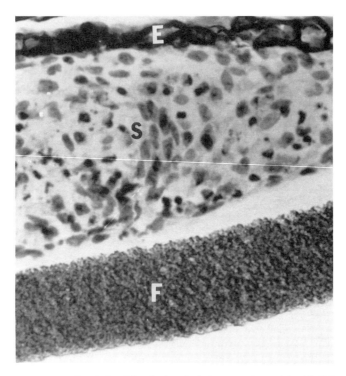

FIGURE 1. Immunocytochemical staining for keratin in human endometrial epithelial and stromal cells derived from a day-24 specimen and cultured on collagen I. A = Epithelial cells; S = Stromal cells; F = (Biopore) filter. *Magnification:* ×740.

creased PG synthase activity. In contrast, the stromal cell monolayers were unresponsive to E_2 even in the face of AA-evoked $PGF_{2\alpha}$ output (TABLE 3).

Reports that E_2 enhances $PGF_{2\alpha}$ production in secretory, but not proliferative phase endometrial explants,[5-7] suggest a regulatory role for E_2 in the higher levels of $PGF_{2\alpha}$, measured in endometrial biopsies[3] and luminal secretions[4] during the secretory than proliferative phases. This *in vitro* refractoriness of proliferative endometrium contrasts with the equivalent effectiveness exhibited by E_2 in elevating $PGF_{2\alpha}$ production in epithelial cell monolayers derived from tissues of both phases (TABLE 1). These results suggest that glands in intact proliferative-phase tissue are under a repressive influence. That the endometrial stromal are a likely source of such repression is indicated by the profound effects that stroma exert on epithelial cell function in several embryonic[20] and adult tissues.[21] However, determining whether endometrial stroma can inhibit E_2-enhanced $PGF_{2\alpha}$ production in the glandular epithelial cells requires controlled co-incubation of both cell types, for which tissue culture plastic is an ill-suited culturing substrate. Furthermore, as noted in several epithelial cell types grown on impermeable surfaces, monolayers of the human endometrial glandular epithelial cells flatten and lose structural polarity on plastic.[14,22,23] Disappearance of structural polarity may alter estrogen effects on $PGF_{2\alpha}$ production in these cells since shape changes are known to disrupt the cytoskeleton and affect epithelial cell function.[24]

Several epithelial cell types retain structural polarity and differentiated function (functional polarity) when grown on extracellular matrix materials, and/or in a culturing configuration that promotes cellular feeding from the basolateral surface,[14,22,23] thereby simulating key aspects of the *in vivo* epithelial cell environment. Rat uterine epithelial cells, for example, exhibit both structural and functional polarity on the surface of the reconstituted basement membrane preparation Matrigel,[25,26] whereas the stromal cells reportedly penetrate it.[27] Seeding of human proliferative phase endometrial glands and stroma on Matrigel in a culturing configuration which provides access of the culture medium to the basal cell surface (see METHODS) resulted in a similar distribution of the two cell types. Thus, the glands formed polarized cuboidal-columnar epithelial cell monolayers on the Matrigel surface, exhibiting such *in situ* ultrastructural features as well-developed microvilli and tight junctional complexes. These were absent from the flattened epithelial cells in parallel cultures on plastic.[10] In contrast, the stromal cells formed clusters within the Matrigel.[10] This culturing configuration promotes epithelial-stromal interactions via cell-derived diffusible paracrine effectors such as growth factors and prostanoids, and insoluble extracellular matrix proteins.

Carrying out appropriately controlled experiments aimed at evaluating the influence of E_2 and stromal cells on $PGF_{2\alpha}$ production in human endometrial glandular epithelial cells would appear difficult when the cells are grown on Matrigel, since significant levels of growth factors and protease activity are associated with its components.[28] Moreover, harvesting primary human endometrial cells from Matrigel has proved difficult, suggesting problems in quantitating cell recoveries following experimental incubations. Alternatively, type I collagen, which like Matrigel retains structural polarity and differentiated function in primary epithelial cells,[14,15] appears to be relatively free of these objections. Accordingly, cells are readily recovered from it following digestion with collagenase I, whereas it has not been shown to contain potential paracrine effectors. Thus, the observation that collagen I can substitute for Matrigel in co-culturing human endometrial glands and stroma (FIG. 1) should prove to be a significant step in developing a relevant *in vitro* model with which to test effects of hormones and stromal cells on $PGF_{2\alpha}$ production by the epithelial cells.

REFERENCES

1. CHIDA, S., S. UEHARA, H. HOSHIAI & A. YAJIMA. 1986. Effects of indomethacin, prostaglandin E_2, prostaglandin $F_{2\alpha}$ and 6-keto-prostaglandin $F_{1\alpha}$ on hatching of mouse blastocysts. Prostaglandins **31:** 337.
2. KENNEDY, T. G. 1987. Interactions of eicosanoids and other factors in blastocyst implantation. *In* Eicosanoids and Reproduction. K. Hillier, Ed.: 3–88. MTP Press. Lancaster, PA
3. DOWNIE, J., N. L. POYSER & M. WUNDERLICH. 1974. Levels of prostaglandins in human endometrium during the normal menstrual cycle. J. Physiol. (Lond.) **236:** 465–472.
4. DEMERS, L. M., D. R. HALBERT, D. E. D. JONES, *et al.* 1975. Prostaglandin F levels in endometrial jet wash specimens during the normal menstrual cycle. Prostaglandins **10:** 1057–1065.
5. ABEL, M. H. & D. T. BAIRD. 1980. The effect of 17b-estradiol and progesterone on prostaglandin production by endometrium maintained in organ culture. Endocrinology **106:** 1599–1606.
6. SCHATZ, F., L. MARKIEWICZ, P. BARG & E. GURPIDE. 1985. In vitro effects of ovarian steroids on prostaglandin $F_{2\alpha}$ output by human endometrium and endometrial epithelial cells. J. Clin. Endocrinol. Metabol. **61:** 361–367.

7. LEAVER, H. A. & D. H. RICHMOND. 1984. Effect of oxytocin, estrogen, calcium ionophore and hydrocortisone on prostaglandin $F_{2\alpha}$ and 6-oxy-prostaglandin $F_{1\alpha}$ production by cultured human endometrial and myometrial explants. Prostaglandins Leukotrienes Med. **13**: 179–196.

8. TSANG, B. K. & T. C. OOI. 1982. Prostaglandin secretion by human endometrium. Am. J. Obstet. Gynecol. **142**: 626–633.

9. SCHATZ, F. & E. GURPIDE. 1983. Effects of estradiol on prostaglandin $F_{2\alpha}$ levels in primary monolayer cultures of epithelial cells from human proliferative endometrium. Endocrinology **113**: 1274–1279.

10. SCHATZ, F., R. E. GORDON, N. LAUFER & E. GURPIDE. 1990. Culture of human endometrial cells under polarizing conditions. Differentiation **42**: 184–190.

10a. SATYASWAROOP, P. G., R. S. BRESSLER, M. M. DE LA PENA & E. GURPIDE. 1979. Isolation and culture of human endometrial glands. J. Clin. Endocrinol. Metab. **48**: 639–641.

11. NOYES, R. W., A. T. HERTIG & J. ROCK. 1950. Dating the endometrial biopsy. Fertil. Steril. **1**: 3–25.

12. SCHATZ, F., L. MARKIEWICZ, P. BARG & E. GURPIDE. 1986. In vitro inhibition with antiestrogens of estradiol effects on prostaglandin $F_{2\alpha}$ production by human endometrium and endometrial epithelial cells. Endocrinology **118**: 408–412.

13. SCHATZ, F., L. MARKIEWICZ & E. GURPIDE. 1987. Differential effects of estradiol, arachidonic acid, A23187 on prostaglandin $F_{2\alpha}$ output by epithelial and stromal cells of human endometrium. Endocrinology **120**: 1465–1471.

14. LI, M. L., J. AGGELER, D. A. FARSON, C. HATIER, J. HASSELL & M. J. BISSELL. 1987. Influence of a reconstituted basement membrane and its components on casein gene expression and secretion in mouse mammary epithelial cells. Proc. Natl. Acad. Sci. USA. **84**: 136–140.

15. STREULI, C. H. & M. J. BISSELL. 1990. Expression of extracellular matrix components is regulated by substratum. J. Cell Biol. **110**: 1405–1415.

16. SMITH, S. K. & R. W. KELLY. 1987. The effect of estradiol-17B and actinomycin D on the release of PGF and PGE from separated cells of human endometrium. Prostaglandins **34**: 553–561.

17. HUANG, J. R., L. TSENG, P. BISCHOFF & O. A. JANNE. 1987. Regulation of prolactin production by progestin, estrogen and relaxin in human endometrial stromal cells. Endocrinology **121**: 2011–2017.

18. IRWIN, J. C., D. KIRK, R. J. B., M. M. QUIGLEY & R. B. L. GWATKIN. 1989. Hormonal regulation of human endometrial stromal cells in culture: An in vitro model for decidualization. Fertil. Steril. **52**: 761–768.

19. BENEDETTO, M. T., S. TABANELLI & E. GURPIDE. 1990. Estrone sulfate sulfatase activity is increased during in vitro decidualization of stromal cells from human endometrium. J. Clin. Endocrinol. Metab. **70**: 342–345.

20. CUNHA, G. R. 1983. Hormone-induced morphogenesis and growth: Role of mesenchymal-epithelial interactions. Rec. Prog. Hor. Res. **39**: 559–598.

21. CUNHA, G. R., H. FUJII, B. L. NEUBAUER, J. M. SHANNON, L. SAWYER & B. A. REESE. 1983. Epithelial-mesenchymal interactions in prostatic development. I Morphological observations of prostatic induction by urogenital sinus mesenchyme in epithelium of the adult rodent urinary bladder. J. Cell Biol. **107**: 1662–1670.

22. SIMONS, K. & S. D. FULLER. 1985. Cell surface polarity in epithelia. Annual Rev. Cell Biol. **1**: 243–288.

23. RODRIGUEZ-BOULAN, E. & W. J. NELSON. 1989. Morphogenesis of the polarized epithelial cell phenotype. Science **245**: 718–725.

24. FOLKMAN, J. & A. MOSCONA. 1978. Role of cell shape in growth control. Nature **273**: 245.

25. GLASSER, S. R., J. JULIAN, G. L. DECKER, J-P. TANG & D. D. CARSON. 1988. Development of morphological and functional polarity in primary cultures of immature rat uterine epithelial cells. J. Cell Biol. **107**: 2409–2423.

26. CARSON, D. D., J-P. TANG, J. JULIAN & S. R. GLASSER. 1988. Vectorial secretion of proteoglycans by polarized rat uterine epithelial cells. J. Cell Biol. **107**: 2425–2434.

27. WELSH, A. O. & A. C. ENDERS. 1989. Comparisons of the ability of cells from rat and mouse blastocysts and rat uterus to alter complex extracellular matrix in vitro. In Blastocyst Implantation—Sorono Symposia USA. K. Yoshinaga, Ed.: 55–74. Adams Publishing Group LTD.

28. MCGUIRE, P. G. & N. W. SEEDS. 1989. The interaction of plasminogen activator with a reconstituted basement membrane matrix and extracellular macromolecules produced by cultured epithelial cells. J. Cell Biochem. **40**: 215–227.

Cytokine Regulation of Human Endometrial Function[a]

S. TABIBZADEH[b]

Department of Pathology
City Hospital Center at Elmhurst
Elmhurst, New York 11373
and
Mount Sinai School of Medicine
New York, New York 10029

INTRODUCTION

Human endometrium is composed of glandular structures that are invested by endometrial stroma. Both components characteristically undergo a predictable series of structural, morphologic, cytochemical, and immunohistochemical changes. These changes are accompanied by sequences of proliferation (proliferative phase), secretion (secretory phase), and menstrual shedding (menstruation). It is thought that these changes are primarily driven by two steroid hormones, estrogen and progesterone. However, it is unclear whether some of the effects of these hormones are directed at target tissue or are indirectly exerted through elaboration of other factors within endometrium. In addition, in view of the complex structure of the endometrial stroma, it is conceivable that many of these cells interact in endometrium via production of factors, collectively called cytokines. We have entertained this possibility and attempted within the last few years to define whether cytokines may be important signals for controlling different aspects of endometrial physiology. In this review the complexity of the endometrial stroma is briefly summarized. In addition, some of the salient features regarding the production, cytokine receptor expression and potential cytokine actions in human endometrium are highlighted. These data enforce the view that cytokines may play important roles in directing certain endometrial functions.

COMPLEXITY OF ENDOMETRIAL STROMA

Human endometrial stroma consists of a heterogeneous population of cells. The presence of aggregates of lymphoid cells, polymorphonuclear leukocytes, mast cells and stromal granulocytes in endometrial stroma has been known for some time.[1] However, with the advent of monoclonal antibodies that react with specific types of cells, the diversity of the constituent cells of endometrial stroma has become more ap-

[a] This work is supported in part by Public Health Research Grant CA6866-01A1.

[b] *Address for reprint requests and correspondence:* S. Tabibzadeh, MD, Department of Pathology, City Hospital Center at Elmhurst, Elmhurst, NY 11373 (Tel: 718-830-1685).

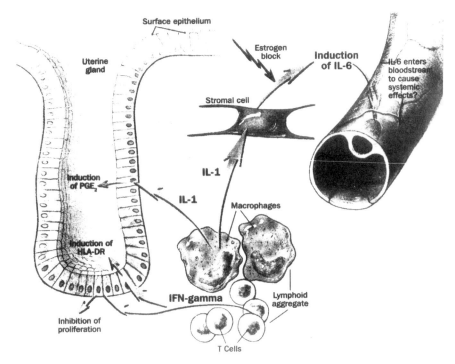

FIGURE 1. Diagrammatic representation of potential cytokine actions in human endometrium.

parent.[2-10] As portrayed by the reactivity with leukocyte common antigen, it is evident that lymphoid cells are a major participant in the formation of endometrial stroma. This group is scattered as single cells in endometrial stroma, or within endometrial glands or as aggregates primarily adjacent to endometrial glands in the basalis (FIG. 1).[2] T lymphocytes both with helper/inducer and cytotoxic/suppressor phenotypes and monocytes/macrophages constitute the majority of the lymphoid cells in human endometria.[2-10] B cells, dendritic cells, and NK cells form a smaller population of lymphoid cells in human endometria.[9-10] Endometrial lymphoid cells including T cells and monocytes/macrophages similar to the endometrial glands and stromal cells exhibit proliferative activity.[6] This proliferative activity which is enhanced in the secretory phase is primarily limited to the lymphoid cells in the latter phase of the menstrual cycle.[6] Endometrial lymphoid cells similar to other lymphoid cells exhibit adhesion molecules.[7] However, a subset of lymphoid cells of endometrium show unique properties such as expression of steroid receptors.[8] Presence of significant number of lymphoid cells in human endometrium suggests that they may serve as key driving forces in endometrial physiology. It is also important to emphasize that in view of the diversity of the cells in endometrial stroma, it is exceedingly important that the term endometrial stromal cell not be loosely used. At present time, however, lack of a specific marker for the stromal cells makes it difficult to identify this group with certainty both *in vitro* and *in vivo*.

CYTOKINE PRODUCTION IN HUMAN ENDOMETRIUM

IFN-Gamma Production

We have isolated endometrial T cells by sheep red blood cell rosetting technique (unpublished results). These cells form colonies reminiscent of those observed after activation of peripheral blood T cells *in vitro*. Direct addition of the endometrial T cells to cultures of autologous endometrial glands induces HLA-DR molecules in epithelial cells which in terms of the intensity of expression and the number of the HLA-DR positive cells correlates with the number of added T cells. In addition, this expression can be induced by the supernatant collected from endometrial T cell cultures. The expression of HLA-DR molecules induced by endometrial T cell supernatant can be inhibited by a neutralizing antiserum to IFN-gamma. Radioimmunoassay has confirmed the presence of IFN-gamma in the supernatant of the endometrial cells. Recently, it was shown that cells attached to intrauterine devices produce IFN-gamma.[11] These findings are consistent with the hypothesis that endometrial T cells represent activated cells secreting IFN-gamma in human endometrium.

IL-1 Production

Our early trials using the D–10 bioassay indicates that supernatant of the heterogeneous population of the endometrial stromal cell culture show significant IL-1 like activity. Further work is required to establish the identity of this factor as IL-1. The contention that IL-1 is produced in endometrium is supported by recent data that indicates of the presence of IL-1 mRNA in endometrium. IL-1 mRNA was shown by *in situ* hybridization in mouse uteri and by northern blotting in human endometria in the secretory phase of the menstrual cycle.[12,13]

IL-6 Production

Multiple species of stromal cell IL-6 in the size range of 23 to 30 kDa are detected using immunoprecipitation and immunoblotting procedures in the supernatant of induced stromal cells. The stromal IL-6 species are phosphorylated and differentially glycosylated similar to the IL-6 secreted by the monocytes from peripheral circulation and fibroblasts.[14]

CYTOKINE RECEPTOR EXPRESSION IN HUMAN ENDOMETRIUM

IFN-Gamma Receptor

Using a monoclonal antibody to IFN-gamma receptor, we have localized the receptor by immunohistochemical method in human endometria throughout the menstrual cycle. IFN-gamma receptor is expressed in endometrial epithelium and scattered cells in endometrial stroma. This expression is invariable throughout the menstrual cycle.[15] In addition to IFN-gamma receptor a factor encoded by chromosome 21 is also required to confer to cells biological sensitivity to IFN-gamma.[16] Thus, for demonstration of response to the IFN-gamma, we tested the sensitivity of endometrial epithelium to this cytokine, *in vitro*. Incubation of these cells *in vitro* with IFN-gamma induced HLA-DR molecules in a time and dose dependent fashion and inhibited their proliferation.[17,18]

IL-1 Receptor

Experiments using radioiodinated rIL-1α reveal that the membranes prepared from human endometrial epithelium possess high affinity receptors for IL-1.[19] Scatchard plot analysis indicates a dissociation constant of approximately 19.7 pmol/L, in close agreement with the dissociation constants found on other cell types.[20] Binding of radio-labeled rIL-1α is inhibited by both rIL-1α and rIL-1β. This is consistent with other reports indicating that both rIL-1α and rIL-1β bind to the same receptor.[21] In similar experiments high affinity receptors for IL-1 are observed in cells cultured from endometrial stroma. In the experiments carried out, a Kd of approximately 10^{-10} M and 690 IL-1 binding sites per cell were found (FIG. 2, S. S. Tabibzadeh and P. L. Kilian, unpublished).

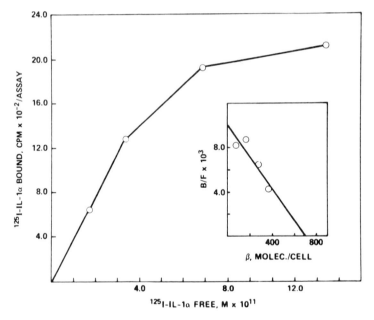

FIGURE 2. Binding of radioiodinated rIL-1α to stromal cells as a function of concentration. Confluent cultures of stromal cells were prepared in twelve-well mutilwell plates. The adherent stromal cells were incubated with concentrations of radioiodinated rIL-1α ranging from 17 to 140 pM in the absence (total binding) or presence of 50 nM unlabeled rIL-1α (nonspecific binding). Scatchard plot analysis (*inset*) indicates a single type of binding site having an apparent dissociation constant of 5×10^{-11} M and the presence of approximately 690 IL-1 binding sites.

REGULATION OF ENDOMETRIAL FUNCTION BY CYTOKINES AND STEROID MODULATION OF CYTOKINE ACTION

IFN-Gamma–Induced Expression of Major Histocompatibility Complex in Endometrial Epithelial Cells

Experiments using endometrial gland cultures reveal that IFN-gamma induces primarily the HLA-DR molecules in epithelial cells of endometrium, and HLA-DP and HLA-DQ determinants are rarely observed after induction. This expression is both time and dose dependent and can be induced in glands isolated from both proliferative and secretory phases of the menstrual cycle.[5]

IFN-Gamma–Mediated Inhibition of Proliferation in Endometrial Epithelial Cells

The proliferation of endometrial epithelial cells as evidenced by incorporation of bromodeoxyuridine, a thymidine analog, is markedly reduced after incubation of epithelial cells with IFN-gamma. Both epithelial cells of proliferative and secretory phases show this sensitivity to IFN-gamma action in regard to inhibition of proliferation.[18]

IL-1–Induced Expression of Major Histocompatibility Complex in Epithelial Cells

IL-1 induces HLA-DR molecules in human endometrial (EnCal01AE) and breast (T47D) carcinoma cell lines in a dose and time dependent manner. ^{35}S-methionine incorporation into IL-1-induced immunoprecipitable HLA-DR molecules demonstrates *de novo* synthesis of both light and heavy chains of HLA-DR molecules. Lipopolysaccharide, IL-2 and IL-6 fail to induce HLA-DR molecules in these epithelial cells.[22] Pretreatment of T47D cells with estradiol 17-β (10^{-7}, 10^{-8}, 10^{-9} M) decreases the IL-1 induced HLA-DR expression. However, using endometrial glands, we have not been able to demonstrate the induction of HLA-DR molecules by IL-1. The failure to induce HLA-DR molecules in endometrial glandular epithelium is not due to lack of expression of IL-1 receptor or lack of response to IL-1. We demonstrated that glands possess IL-1 binding sites and in addition respond to IL-1 by PGE_2 production.[19] The lack of IL-1 mediated induction of HLA-DR is also not due to the inability of the endometrial glands to express HLA-DR, as these cells express HLA-DR *in vivo* and after incubation with IFN-gamma *in vitro*.[2,17] We speculate that this failure of induction of expression of HLA-DR molecules in endometrial glands may be related to the production of a factor that inhibits IL-1 action. In early trials, culture supernatant of epithelial cells inhibited HLA-DR inducing effect of IL-1 in T47D cell line (unpublished results).

IL-1–Induced PGE_2 Production by Endometrial Epithelial Cells

A significant increase in PGE_2 production as determined by radioimmunoassay is observed by incubation of epithelial cells with IL-1. A significant increase is obtained with 17 and 170 ng/L of rIL-1α. A maximal effect is obtained within 24 hour of incubation with IL-1. The maximal increase relative to the basal levels varies from 2- to 10-fold for a given preparation. The IL-1-mediated PGE_2 production is blocked by the addition of a neutralizing antibody to IL-1 or indomethacin.[19]

IL-1-Induced IL-6 Production by Endometrial Stromal Cells

Stromal cells similar to peripheral blood monocytes and fibroblasts produce IL-6 in response to IL-1. However, the stromal cells unlike the peripheral blood monocytes and fibroblasts are insensitive to the IL-6 inducing activity of bacterial lipopolysaccharide. In addition, the secretion of IL-6 by endometrial stromal cells is strongly inhibited by as low as 10^{-9} M of estradiol-17β.[14]

POTENTIAL CYTOKINE ACTIONS IN HUMAN ENDOMETRIUM

The production of IFN-gamma *in vitro* by endometrial T cells is indicative of their activation. Also consistent with the hypothesis of activation of endometrial T cells is the expression of a host of hallmarks of T cell activation on endometrial T cells *in vivo*. Concomitant with the activation of the resting peripheral blood T cells, a group of antigens appear on these cells, including IL-2 receptor, HLA-DR, HLA-DP, HLA-DQ, and VLA-1. Within 24 hours of the activation of T cells *in vitro,* IL-2 receptor is expressed.[23,24] Within 3 to 4 days of activation, HLA-DR, HLA-DP, HLA-DQ of the major histocompatibility complex II appear on the T cells.[25] More recently, molecules have been described on T cells that are maximally expressed 2–4 weeks after *in vitro* activation.[26-28] One of these proteins, VLA-1 which reacts with the monoclonal antibody TS2/7, is not present on the resting T cells and appears on long-term activated T cells.[26] We demonstrated the presence of HLA-DR, HLA-DP, HLA-DQ, and VLA-1 on endometrial T cells.[15] Whereas T cells from peripheral blood express IL-2 receptor and proliferate upon activation, endometrial T cells, despite evidence for their proliferative activity, do not exhibit IL-2 receptor.[6,8,15] Taken together, these findings indicate that endometrial T cells represent a unique group of activated cells that by production of IFN-gamma may influence neighboring cells including epithelial cells. Inhibition of proliferation of epithelial cells and the expression of HLA-DR molecules at the level of basalis may be a consequence of IFN-gamma-mediated effect in human endometrium (FIG. 1). This hypothesis is consistent with the *in vivo* finding of low proliferative activity and enhanced expression of HLA-DR in the basalis glands as compared to high proliferative activity and weak HLA-DR expression in the functionalis glands (FIG. 1).[2,6] From the three classes of the major histocompatibility complex (HLA-DR, HLA-DP and HLA-DQ), only HLA-DR is expressed on endometrial epithelium.[5] We could demonstrate that this differential expression may be simulated *in vitro*. This is shown by induction primarily of HLA-DR molecules by IFN-gamma in epithelial cells grown *in vitro*.[5]

Several lines of evidence suggest that prostaglandins are important factors in the endometrial physiology. Acidic lipid, first described in the menstruum is shown to contain both prostaglandins E_2 and $F_{2\alpha}$.[29,30] Evidence has been accumulating that these products are involved in the menstruation, parturition and in the pathogenesis of the endometrial abnormalities and endometrial bleeding.[30-32] Production of prostaglandins appear to vary with the menstrual cycle. Increased levels of PGE_2 are observed in the endometrial tissue homogenates as well as freshly explanted endometrial tissue fragments from the secretory phase of the menstrual cycle.[33,34] The underlying mechanism for the observed variation of PGE_2 during the secretory phase is not known. Demonstration of the IL-1-mediated increased synthesis of PGE_2 by endometrial epithelium suggests that IL-1 may serve as a mediator regulating the level of PGE_2 production *in vivo* (FIG. 1).

IL-6 is a pleiotropic cytokine that elicits local as well as systemic effects including induction of physiological, immunological and biochemical changes.[35] Local effects of stromal IL-6 may be directed at various endometrial constituents including epithelial and lymphoid cells. On the other hand, potentially, stromal IL-6 may enter peripheral circulation and induce systemic effects. Since pyrogenic activity has recently been attributed to IL-6,[36] it is important to explore in detail the role that the IL-6 in peripheral circulation may play in the observed temperature rise in the secretory phase of the menstrual cycle (FIG. 1).

IN VITRO MODELS FOR STUDYING CYTOKINE ACTIONS

Glandular epithelium is an important constituent of human endometrium. Many of the cytokine effects may be targeted at this tissue. Thus, it is important that in studying the cytokine effects on human endometrium, and their interaction with steroid hormones suitable models of endometrial epithelium be used. Satyaswaroop *et al.* described isolation of endometrial glands in 1979.[37] Since then, cultures of the isolated glands are routinely used for a variety of functional assays. Using the glands has several drawbacks. Glandular epithelium loses its estrogen and progesterone receptors *in vitro* and does not respond to estrogen in regard to E_2-mediated growth and progesterone-mediated down regulation of ER.[38] Inability to obtain endometria in the same phase of the menstrual cycle, variations observed among different individuals, and region-to-region and gland-to-gland variations represent additional difficulties. Fragmented glands obtained by this procedure do not allow obtaining cell counts at the time of initial plating. Finally, these primary cultures have a finite life-span and do not lend themselves to more than merely one passage. These drawbacks necessitate use of alternative cell sources that represent more homogeneous population and express steroid hormone receptors. Satyaswaroop *et al.* have developed two cell lines that express steroid receptors.[39] The EnCal01AE cell line is derived from a well-differentiated adenocarcinoma of human endometrium that after transplantation into nude mice formed tumors indistinguishable from the original tumor.[40] ECC1 cells are cloned from EnCal01AE cells for the expression of progesterone receptors.[39] These cell lines represent alternative cell sources to endometrial gland cultures for testing cytokine effects.[41] We have utilized these cell systems to investigate in detail certain aspects of cytokine action in human endometrium.[18,19,41]

CONCLUSIONS

There is a growing body of evidence that supports the notion that cytokines such as IL-1 and IL-6 are involved in different aspects of inflammation.[35,42] Thus, it is not difficult to understand why endometrium, a tissue where continuous tissue damage and repair is taking place, may be ideally equipped with the cytokine network that their effect may be aimed at limiting tissue damage.[35] It is conceivable that in a backdrop of the systemic effects of steroids, the cytokines in human endometrium regulate endometrial function at an autocrine and paracrine level. The work regarding the expression of cytokine receptors in human endometrium, their production by endometrial constituents and the potential roles that they play in endometrial physiology provide a firm foundation for further exploration of this new area of research.

SUMMARY

Human endometrium undergoes sequences of proliferation, and secretion followed by menstruation in a predictable fashion. The importance of systemic factors, steroid hormones, in driving endometrium through these phases is well known. However, it is becoming increasingly apparent that a group of factors collectively called cytokines may also serve a key role as local modulators of endometrial function. Expression of the receptors for cytokines, production of cytokines and the ability to demonstrate modulation of a host of functions of both endometrial epithelium and stroma indicate that human endometrium is uniquely poised to respond to cytokines.

ACKNOWLEDGMENTS

The author thanks Dr. P. G. Satyaswaroop (Hershey Medical Center, Hershey, PA) for reviewing this manuscript and Terese Winslow for the FIG. 1 artwork (*Journal of NIH Research*).

REFERENCES

1. BLAUSTEIN, A. 1982. Pathology of the female genital tract. Second edition. A. Blaustein, Ed.: 241. Springer-Verlag. New York, NY.
2. TABIBZADEH, S. S., A. BETTICA & M. A. GERBER. 1986. Variable expression of Ia antigens in human endometrium and in chronic endometritis. Am. J. Clin. Pathol. 86: 153–160.
3. TABIBZADEH, S. S. & M. A. GERBER. 1986. Immunohistologic analysis of lymphoid cells by a rapid double immunoenzymatic labeling. J. Immunol. Meth. 91: 169–174.
4. TABIBZADEH, S. S., S. MORTILLO & M. A. GERBER. 1987. Immunoultrastructural localization of Ia antigens in human endometrium. Arch. Pathol. Lab. Med. 111: 32–37.
5. TABIBZADEH, S. S., & P. G. SATYASWAROOP. 1989. Differential expression of HLA-DR, HLA-DP and HLA-DQ antigenic determinants of the major histocompatibility complex in human endometrium. Am. J. Reprod. Immunol. Microbiol. 18: 124–130.
6. TABIBZADEH, S. S. 1990. Proliferative activity of lymphoid cells in human endometrium throughout the menstrual cycle. J. Endocrinol. Metab. 70: 437–443.
7. TABIBZADEH, S. S. & D. POUBOURIDIS. 1990. Expression of leukocyte adhesion molecules in human endometrium. Am. J. Clin. Pathol. 93: 183–189.
8. TABIBZADEH, S. S. & P. G. SATYASWAROOP. 1989. Sex steroid receptors in lymphoid cells of human endometrium. Am. J. Clin. Pathol. 91: 656–663.
9. KAMAT, B.R. & P. G. ISAACSON. 1987. The immunocytochemical distribution of leukocyte subpopulations in human endometrium. Am. J. Pathol. 127: 66–73.
10. MORRIS, H., J. EDWARDS, A. TILTMAN & M. EMMS. 1985. Endometrial Lymphoid tissue: An immunohistological study. J. Clin. Pathol. 38: 644–652.

11. GRASSO, G., M. MUSCETTOLA & V. BOCCI. 1983. The physiologic interferon response. I. Cells attached to intrauterine devices release interferon in vitro. Proc. Soc. Exp. Biol. Med. **173:** 276–280.

12. TAKACS, L., E. J. KOVACS, R. S. SMITH, H. A. YOUNG & S. K. DRUM. 1988. Detection of IL-1α and IL-1β gene expression by in situ hybridization. Tissue localization of IL-1 mRNA in the normal C57BL/6 mouse. J. Immunol. **141:** 3081–3095.

13. KAUMA, S. W. 1989. HLA-DR and interleukin-1β (IL-1β) mRNA expression in human decidua. 36th Meeting of the Society of Gynecologic Investigation. Abstract, March 15–18, 1989.

14. TABIBZADEH, S. S., U. SANTHANAM, P. B. SEHGAL & L. MAY. 1989. Cytokine-induced production of interferon β2/interleukin-6 by freshly explanted human endometrial stromal cells. Modulation by estradiol-17β. J. Immunol. **142:** 3134–3139.

15. TABIBZADEH, S. S. 1990. Evidence of T cell activation and potential cytokine action in human endometrium. J. Endocrinol. Metab. **71:** 645–649.

16. JUNG, V., A. RASHIDBAIGI, C. JONES, J. A. TISCHFIELD, T. B. SHOWS & S. PESTKA. 1987. Human chromosome 6 and 21 are required for sensitivity to human interferon gamma. Proc. Natl. Acad. Sci. USA **84:** 4151–4155.

17. TABIBZADEH, S. S., M. A. GERBER & P. G. SATYASWAROOP. 1986. Induction of HLA-DR antigen expression in human endometrial epithelial cells in vitro by recombinant gamma-interferon. Am. J. Pathol. **125:** 90–96.

18. TABIBZADEH, S. S., P. G. SATYASWAROOP & P. N. RAO. 1988. Antiproliferative effect of interferon gamma in human endometrial epithelial cells in vitro: Potential local growth modulatory role in endometrium. J. Endocrinol. Metab. **67:** 131–138.

19. TABIBZADEH, S. S., K. L. KAFFKA, P. G. SATYASWAROOP & P. L. KILIAN. 1990. IL-1 regulation of human endometrial function: Presence of IL-1 receptor correlates with IL-1 stimulated PGE2 production. J. Endocrinol. Metab. **70:** 1000–1006.

20. DOWER, S. K. & D. L. URDAL. 1987. The interleukin-1 receptor. Immunol. Today **8:** 46–51.

21. DOWER, S. K., S. R. KRONHEIM, T. P. HOPP, M. CANTRELL, M. DEELEY, S. GILLIS, C. S. HENNEY & D. L. URDAL. 1986. The cell surface receptors for interleukin-1α and interleukin-1β are identical. Nature **324:** 266–268.

22. TABIBZADEH, S., A. SIVARAJAH, D. CARPENTER, B. M. OHLSSON-WILHELM & P. G. SATYASWAROOP. 1990. Modulation of HLA-DR expression in epithelial cells by interleukin 1 and estradiol-17β. J. Endocrinol. Metab. **71:** 740–747.

23. CANTRELL, D. A. & K. A. SMITH. 1983. Transient expression of interleukin 2 receptors. Consequences for T cell Growth. J. Exp. Med. **158:** 1895–1911.

24. MEUER, S. C., R. E. HUSSEY, D. A. CANTRELL, J. C. HODGDON, S. F. SCHLOSSMAN, K. A. SMITH & E. L. REINHERZ. 1984. Triggering of the T3-Ti antigen receptor complex results in clonal T-cell proliferation through an interleukin 2-dependent pathway. Proc. Natl. Acad. Sci. USA **81:** 1509–1513.

25. GANSBACHER, B. & K. S. ZIER. 1988. Regulation of HLA-DR, DP and DQ molecules in activated T cells. Cellular Immunol. **117:** 22–34.

26. HELMER, M. E., J. G. JACOBSON, M. B. BRENNER, D. MANN & J. L. STROMINGER. 1985. VLA-1: A T cell surface antigen which defines a novel late stage of human T cell activation. Eur. J. Immunol. **15:** 502–508.

27. HELMER, M. E., F. SANCHEZ-MADRID, T. J. FLOTTE, A. M. KRENSKY, S. J. BURAKOFF, A. K. BHAN, T. A. SPRINGER & J. L. STROMINGER. 1984. Glycoproteins of 210,000 and 130,000 M. W. on activated T cells. Cell distribution and antigenic relation to components on resting cells and T cell lines. J. Immunol. **132:** 3011–3018.

28. HELMER, M. E., J. G. JACOBSON & J. L. STROMINGER. 1985. Biochemical characterization of VLA-1 and VLA-2. Cell surface heterodimers on activated T cells. J. Biol. Chem. **28:** 15246–15252.

29. PICKLES, V. R. 1957. A plain muscle stimulant in the menstruum. Nature **180:** 1198–1202.

30. PICKLES, V. R., W. J. HALL, F. A. BEST & G. N. SMITH. 1965. Prostaglandins in endometrium and menstrual fluid from normal and dysmenorrheic subjects. J. Obstet. Gynaecol. Br. Commonwealth **72:** 185–192.

31. WILLIAM, E. A., W. P. COLLINS & S. G. CLAYTON. 1976. Studies in the involvement of prostaglandins in uterine symptomatology and pathology. Br. J. Obstet. Gynaecol. **83:** 337–341.

32. KARIM, S. M. M., R. C. TRUSSELL, R. C. PATEL & K. HILLIER. 1968. Response of pregnant human uterus to prostaglandin F_2 alpha induction of labour. Br. Med. J. **4**: 621–623.
33. PEEK, M. J., I. S. FRASER, C. A. PHILLIPS, T. M. RESTA, P. M. BLACKWELL & R. MARKHAM. 1985. The measurement of human endometrial prostaglandin production. A comparison of two in vitro methods. Prostaglandins **29**: 3–18.
34. LEVITT, M. J., H. TOBON & J. B. JOSIMOVISH. 1976. Prostaglandin content of human endometrium. Fertil. Steril. **26**: 296–300.
35. SEHGAL, P. B. 1990. Interleukin-6. A regulator of plasma protein gene expression in hepatic and non-hepatic tissues. Mol. Biol. Med. **7**: 117–130.
36. LEMAY, L. G., A. J. VANDER & M. J. KLUGER. 1990. Role of interleukin 6 in fever in rats. Am. J. Physiol. **258**: R798-R803.
37. SATYASWAROOP, P. G., R. S. BRESSLER, M. M. DE LA PENA & E. GURPIDE. 1979. Isolation and culture of human endometrial glands. J. Clin. Endocrinol. Metab. **48**: 639–641.
38. NARDULLI, A. M. & B. S. KATZENELLENBOGEN. 1986. Dynamics of estrogen receptor turnover in uterine cells in vitro and in uteri in vivo. Endocrinology **119**: 2038–2046.
39. SATYASWAROOP, P. G., A. SIVARAJAH, R. J. ZAINO & R. MORTEL. 1988. Hormonal control of growth of human endometrial carcinoma in nude mouse model. In Progress in Cancer Research and Therapy. F. Bresciani, R. G. B. King, M. E. Lippman & J. P. Raynud, Eds.: **35**: 430–435. Raven Press. New York, NY.
40. ZAINO, R. J., P. G. SATYASWAROOP & R. MORTEL. 1984. Morphology of human uterine cancer in nude mice. Effects of hormone and antihormone treatment. Arch. Pathol Lab. Med. **108**: 571–578.
41. TABIBZADEH, S. S., K. L. KAFFKA, P. L. KILIAN & P. G. SATYASWAROOP. 1990. EnCa101AE and ECC1 cell lines, suitable models for studying cytokine actions in human endometrium. In Vitro. In press.
42. DINARELLO, C. A. 1986. Multiple biological properties of recombinant human interleukin 1 (beta). Immunobiology **172**: 301–315.

Responsiveness of Human Endometrial Stromal Cells to Cytokines[a]

DIANE SEMER,[b] KEITH REISLER,[b]
PAUL C. MACDONALD, AND
M. LINETTE CASEY

*The Cecil H. and Ida Green Center for Reproductive Biology Sciences
and the Departments of Biochemistry and Obstetrics-Gynecology
The University of Texas Southwestern Medical Center
Dallas, Texas 75235-9051*

INTRODUCTION

Cytokines are known to act, most commonly in a paracrine manner, to evoke a variety of responses in a number of tissues. In most responsive cell types, cytokines act to stimulate the production of prostaglandins (PGs) and other metabolites of arachidonic acid (*e.g.*, leukotrienes). In addition, cytokines serve in a cell-specific manner to effect modifications in cell replication and to induce the synthesis of specific proteins. Exemplary cytokines include monokines, *i.e.*, protein products of monocytes/macrophages such as interleukin-1 (IL-1) and tumor necrosis factor-α (TNF-α), as well as lymphokines, *i.e.*, protein products of lymphocytes such as interleukin-2. Other cytokines are produced by a variety of cell types and include interleukin-6 (IL-6), colony-stimulating factors, transforming growth factor-β (TGF-β), interferons, and others. Generally, cytokines are produced as a part of the response to inflammation or else as part of the host response to infection or immune challenge; but, it is now believed that the production and actions of cytokines may not be limited to those that occur solely as a consequence of inflammation and infection. It is known, for example, that endometrial stromal cells produce IL-6 in a hormonally responsive manner.[1]

In previous investigations, we obtained evidence that human endometrial stromal cells are responsive to the actions of IL-1. Specifically, we found that IL-1 acts in human endometrial stromal cells maintained in monolayer culture to stimulate the production of PGE_2 and $PGF_{2\alpha}$[2] (FIG. 1). The present study was undertaken to identify other responses of endometrial stromal cells to the action of cytokines and to evaluate the possibility that selected cytokines are biosynthesized in these cells.

We demonstrated that pro-IL-1β mRNA and protein are expressed in endometrial stromal cells and that the levels of expression of these are increased in response to treatment with LPS or IL-1α. Importantly, we could detect little or no IL-1β in the culture medium of endometrial stromal cells even under conditions in which IL-1β

[a] This investigation was supported, in part, by USPHS Grant No. 5-P50-HD11149 and March of Dimes National Foundation Grant No. 5-622.

[b] Drs. Semer and Reisler were postdoctoral trainees, supported in part by USPHS Grant No. 1-T32-HD07190.

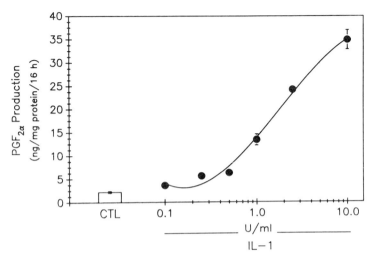

FIGURE 1. Data are taken from reference 2. Stimulation of prostaglandin $F_{2\alpha}$ production in endometrial stromal cells by IL-1. Confluent endometrial stromal cells were treated with IL-1 (naturally occurring) in various concentrations (0.1–10 U/ml; 1 U $\approx$ 80 pg) for 16 h. Thereafter, prostaglandins in the culture media were quantified by radioimmunoassay. (Reprinted with permission from *Australian Journals of Scientific Research*, Melbourne, Victoria, Australia.) Similar findings were obtained when prostaglandin E_2 was evaluated (data not shown).

synthesis was maximal. We found that IL-1 acts to stimulate the expression of IL-6 mRNA in a manner that is consistent with the known increase in IL-6 protein synthesis in the endometrial stromal cells in response to IL-1 treatment.

MATERIALS AND METHODS

Isolation and Culture of Human Endometrial Stromal Cells

Endometrial tissue was collected from the uteri of premenopausal women after hysterectomy that was conducted for reasons other than endometrial disease. Informed consent for the use of tissues was obtained from each woman prior to the surgical procedure. The consent form and protocol used were approved by the Institutional Review Board of this University. Endometrial stromal cells were prepared as described[3] and as modified in our laboratory.[4] Briefly, endometrial tissue was minced into small pieces (~ 1 mm³), and the minced tissue was incubated at 37°C for 20–40 min in Hanks balanced salt solution that contained Hepes (25 mM), penicillin (200 units/ml), streptomycin (200 mg/ml), collagenase (1 mg/ml; 134 units/mg), and DNAse (0.08 mg/ml; 1950 Kunitz units/ml). The dispersed endometrial stromal cells were separated from endometrial glands by filtration through a wire sieve (75 mm). The endometrial stromal cells (in the filtrate) were pelleted by centrifugation (400 $\times$ g, 10 min) and washed twice by centrifugation and suspension in culture medium that did not contain collagenase or DNAse. The cells were suspended finally in Waymouth enriched culture medium [Waymouth MB752/1, minimal essential medium vitamins, minimal essential medium amino acids, nonessential amino acids, antibiotics-antimycotics[4]] that contained fetal bovine serum (10%, by volume). The cells were plated in plastic culture dishes (24-well plates, 16 mm diameter wells) at a density of approximately 200,000 cells/well/ml of culture medium. The endometrial stromal cells were maintained in a tissue culture incubator at 37°C in a humidified atmosphere of CO_2 (5%) in air. Experiments were conducted with endometrial stromal cells in confluent primary monolayer culture or after first or second passage.

Quantification of IL-1β by ELISA

Endometrial stromal cells were scraped from the tissue culture dishes in Dulbecco phosphate buffered saline solution. The cells were pelleted by centrifugation then disrupted by sonication in a solution of Dulbeccos phosphate buffered saline that contained CHAPS (9 mM) and phenylmethylsulfonyl fluoride (PMSF, 1 mM). To ensure extraction of the IL-1β, the disrupted cells were incubated at 4°C in an ice bath for 90 min. The homogenates were centrifuged for 2 min in a microfuge and the supernatant fraction was frozen at $-20°C$ prior to the conduct of the ELISA.

The ELISA for IL-1β was conducted by use of a kit purchased from Cistron Biotechnology (Pine Brook, NJ). The PMSF/CHAPS extraction buffer was used as the diluent for the standard curve (5–600 pg/assay well) and for aliquots (10–100 μl) of the cell extract. Intraassay and interassay coefficients of variation were 10 and 12%, respectively. Parallelism was maintained in assays of cell extracts in various volumes. The amount of IL-1β in the cell extracts is expressed as a function of the amount of protein quantified by the method of Lowry *et al.*[5] with bovine serum albumin as standard.

Alternatively, IL-1β was quantified in culture medium collected from endometrial stromal cell cultures after various treatment paradigms. In the conduct of these assays, Waymouth enriched culture medium that contained fetal bovine serum (10%, v/v) was used as the diluent for the standard curve. The assay was validated in this culture medium by use of authentic human recombinant IL-1β.

Analysis of IL-1β mRNA

Total RNA was prepared by extraction of the tissue with guanidinium thiocyanate as described by Chirgwin *et al.*[6] The RNA was purified by centrifugation through cesium chloride. The RNA was size fractionated on agarose (1%) gels and transferred to nylon membranes.[7] The membranes were baked at 80°C *in vacuo* for 2 h. A cDNA probe for IL-1β (1.7 kb) was isolated from *E. coli* that contained the pIL-1b-47 plasmid (pBR322), provided to us by Michael Tocci (Merck, Sharp, Dohme, Rahway, NJ). Prehybridizations were conducted by incubation of the membranes for 4–24 h at 42°C in prehybridization buffer made up of 5 × SSC, 10 × Denhardt solution, formamide (50%, v/v), dextran sulfate (5%, w/v), NaH_2PO_4 (50 mM), and salmon sperm DNA (0.5 mg/ml). Hybridizations were conducted for 16 h at 42°C in buffer composed of 5 × SSC, 2 × Denhardt solution, formamide (50%, v/v), dextran sulfate (10%, w/v), NaH_2PO_4 (20 mM), salmon sperm DNA (0.1 mg/ml), and cDNA probe (5–15 μCi) radiolabeled with [α-^{32}P]dCTP by the random hexamer priming method. Thereafter, the blots were washed with 2 × SSC and SDS (0.1%, w/v) for 30 min at room temperature, twice with 0.1 × SSC and SDS (0.1%, w/v) for 15 min at room temperature, and 2–4 times with 0.1 × SSC and SDS (0.1%, w/v) for 30 min at 65°C. The membranes were blotted on filter paper, sealed in a plastic bag, and exposed to film for autoradiography at −70°C.

Analysis of IL-6 mRNA

The human IL-6 cDNA clone pCSF309 (ATCC 67153) was obtained from the American Type Culture Collection, Rockville, MD. The 1.16 kb EcoR1 restriction fragment of the IL-6 cDNA insert was subcloned into pGEM-3Zf (Promega, Madison, WI). In this construction (pGEM-IL6gcl), the orientation of the insert, which we evaluated by restriction enzyme mapping, is such that an antisense RNA probe is synthesized from the T7 RNA polymerase promoter. Northern analyses were conducted using total RNA and the IL-6 antisense RNA probe radiolabeled with [α-^{32}P]UTP. The membranes were baked at 80°C *in vacuo* for 2 h. Prehybridization was conducted for 4–24 h at 65°C in hybridization buffer that consists of 5 × SSC, 10 × Denhardt solution, formamide (50%, v/v), SDS (1%, w/v), EDTA (5 mM), sodium pyrophosphate (0.1%, w/v), Tris HCl (50 mM), salmon sperm DNA (150 μg/ml), and yeast tRNA (150 μg/ml). Hybridizations were conducted for 16 h at 65°C in hybridization buffer that contained the radiolabeled riboprobe (2 × 10^6 cpm/RNA sample). After hybridization, the blots were washed 2–3 times in 0.1 × SSC and SDS (0.1%, w/v) for 30 min at 65°C. The membranes were blotted on filter paper, sealed in a plastic bag, and exposed to film for autoradiography at −70°C.

RESULTS

We found that human endometrial stromal cells respond to LPS in a time- and dose-dependent manner by induction of IL-1β synthesis (FIGS. 2 and 3).

In studies conducted to evaluate further the responsiveness of endometrial stromal cells to IL-1, we investigated the effect of IL-1α on IL-1β protein and mRNA synthesis. In FIGURE 4, we present the results of a study in which endometrial stromal cells at confluence were incubated in culture media that contained LPS (1 μg/ml) or IL-1α in various concentrations (8–8000 pg/ml). After incubation for 16 h, the cells were collected and processed for assay of intracellular IL-1β and total protein. IL-1α stimulated IL-1β synthesis in a dose-dependent manner; maximal stimulation was effected by IL-1α at a concentration of 800 pg/ml. The time course of IL-1β protein induction is presented in FIGURE 5. Maximal induction of IL-1β synthesis was demonstrable after 16–14 h of treatment with IL-1α (800 pg/ml).

To investigate the mechanism by which IL-1β synthesis in the endometrial stromal cells was stimulated, we evaluated the effects of IL-1α on IL-1β mRNA synthesis. In cells treated with IL-1α (800 pg/ml) for 2 h, an increase in IL-1β mRNA was found (FIG. 6). The IL-1α-induced increase in IL-1β mRNA was maximal at 4–8 h of treatment. An increase in the level of IL-1β protein in the same endometrial stromal cells was detectable at 2–4 h after commencement of IL-1α treatment (FIG. 6).

In another study, we obtained evidence that endometrial stromal cells respond to TNF-α by way of an increase in the synthesis of IL-1β protein (FIG. 7). The effect

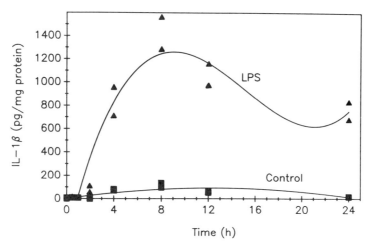

FIGURE 2. Stimulation of IL-1β synthesis in human endometrial stromal cells by lipopolysaccharide (LPS, *E. coli* 055:B5): Time course. Confluent endometrial stromal cells were treated with culture medium that contained LPS (300 ng/ml) for various times. Thereafter, the cells were scraped from the plates and cell sonicates were prepared in CHAPS/PMSF buffer as described in MATERIALS AND METHODS. IL-1β in the cell sonicates was quantified by ELISA. Data were obtained for duplicate dishes of cells and are presented in the figure; individual data points are depicted. IL-1β in the culture medium was undetectable (<50 pg/mg protein).

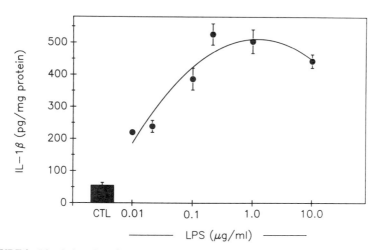

FIGURE 3. Stimulation of IL-1β synthesis in human endometrial stromal cells by lipopolysaccharide (LPS, *E. coli* 055:B5). Confluent endometrial stromal cells were treated with culture medium that contained LPS in various concentrations for 16 h. Thereafter, cell sonicates were prepared as described and IL-1β was quantified by ELISA. Data are mean ±SEM for replicates of four dishes of cells.

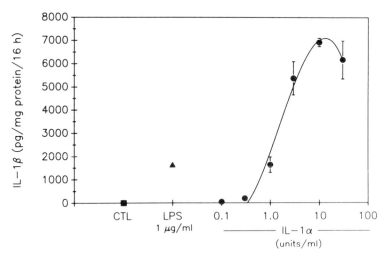

FIGURE 4. IL-1α concentration-dependent induction of IL-1β synthesis in human endometrial stromal cells. Confluent endometrial stromal cells in monolayer culture were incubated for 16 h in Waymouth enriched culture medium that contained fetal bovine serum (10%, v/v) in the absence or presence of lipopolysaccharide (LPS; *E. coli* 05:B55; 1 μg/ml) or IL-1α (0.1–100 U/ml ≈ 8–8000 pg/ml). Thereafter, the culture medium was removed and the cells were collected by scraping; the cells were pelleted and disrupted by sonication in PMSF/CHAPS-containing buffer (as described in MATERIALS AND METHODS). IL-1β in the cell sonicates was quantified by ELISA. Data are mean ±SEM for replicates of 4–6 dishes of cells. IL-1β in the culture medium was undetectable.

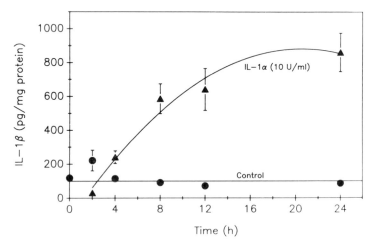

FIGURE 5. Time course of IL-1α induction of IL-1β synthesis in human endometrial stromal cells. Confluent endometrial stromal cells in monolayer culture were incubated for various times (2–24 h) in Waymouth enriched culture medium that contained fetal bovine serum (10%, v/v) in the absence or presence of IL-1α (human recombinant 10 U/ml or ~800 pg/ml). At the end of the incubation period, the culture media were removed and IL-1β was quantified by ELISA. Data are mean ±SEM for replicates of four.

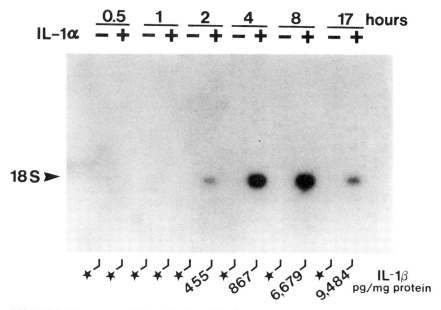

FIGURE 6. Time course of IL-1α induction of IL-1β mRNA and protein synthesis in human endometrial stromal cells. Confluent endometrial stromal cells in monolayer culture were incubated for various times in Waymouth enriched culture medium that contained fetal bovine serum (10%, v/v) in the absence or presence of IL-1α (human recombinant 10 U/ml or ~800 pg/ml). At the end of the incubation period, the culture media were removed and total RNA was prepared from the cells. IL-1β mRNA was detected by northern analysis of total RNA (10 μg per lane) conducted as described in MATERIALS AND METHODS. IL-1β in cell sonicates prepared from replicate dishes of the endometrial stromal cells was quantified by ELISA (data are the average of duplicate determinations).

of TNF-α in increasing the level of IL-1β protein was concentration-dependent and additive with that of LPS (FIG. 7).

Finally, we found that IL-1α and TNF-α act in endometrial stromal cells to stimulate IL-6 transcription. The expression of IL-6 mRNA was maximal after treatment of endometrial stromal cells with IL-1α (800 pg/ml) for 6–12 h (FIG. 8). TNF-α also effected induction of IL-6 mRNA synthesis in these cells; TNF-α, however, was less potent than IL-1α in inducing IL-6 transcription (FIG. 9). Epidermal growth factor (EGF) was ineffective in stimulating the synthesis of IL-6 mRNA in these cells (FIG. 9).

DISCUSSION

There is considerable evidence, obtained in studies of a variety of tissues, that epithelial cell differentiation and function is modulated substantially by interactions with mesenchymal components. The findings of a number of studies are indicative that the differentiation of embryonic tissues [*e.g.*, urogenital sinus,[8] mullerian duct,[8] lung,[9] pancreas,[10] and thyroid[11]] is modulated by interactions between mesenchymal and epithelial (or endothelial) constituents. In addition, interactions between stromal

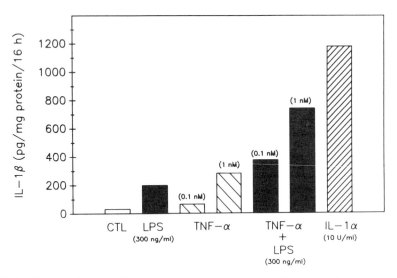

FIGURE 7. Responsiveness of human endometrial stromal cells to TNF-α. Confluent endometrial stromal cells in monolayer culture were treated for 16 h with culture media that contained various test agents, *i.e.*, LPS (300 ng/ml), TNF-α (0.1 or 1 nM) and TNF-α in the presence of LPS (300 ng/ml) or IL-1α (800 pg/ml). At the end of the incubation period, the cells were collected and sonicated for quantification of intracellular IL-1β by ELISA. Data are the average for duplicate dishes of cells.

and epithelial components of the human endometrium is believed to be important in the function of this tissue.[12] The human endometrium is characterized by the well-defined glandular epithelial component and the hormonally responsive stromal component.[13] It is likely that the function of the glandular epithelium is influenced by biochemical signals derived from the contiguous stromal cells. And, it is likely that the contributions of stromal cells to epithelial cell function are regulated hormonally. Thus, the physiological and pathophysiological function of this tissue may be governed by metabolic events that involve interactions between mesenchymal and epithelial components.

One mechanism by which interactions between the cell types of the endometrium may be mediated is by way of the action of cytokines. This is an important issue in defining mesenchymal-epithelial interactions; and in the case of endometrium, it is potentially important in defining the role of decidua in the maintenance of pregnancy and in the initiation of parturition. The decidua constitutes the maternal tissue interface that is contiguous with fetal tissues. The decidua parietalis is contiguous with the chorion laeve and the decidua basalis is infiltrated by extravillous trophoblasts. Many investigators have sought to define the mechanisms by which the fetal allograft is tolerated by the mother; and in the conduct of these studies, many have sought to ascertain whether there were unique features of the decidua that facilitated this apparent exception to the laws of transplantation immunology. In addition, it seems likely that the uterine decidua constitutes a tissue interface that will promote the prevention of infection of the conceptus. Thereby, on two counts, the decidua is a potential target tissue of an inflammatory response, *i.e.*, immunological as well as infectious challenges.

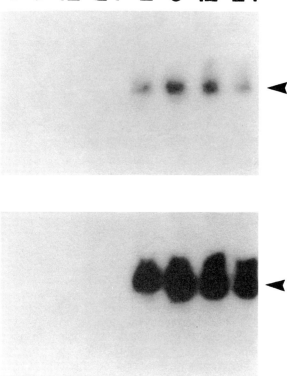

FIGURE 8. IL-6 mRNA expression in human endometrial stromal cells. Confluent endometrial stromal cells in monolayer culture were treated with IL-1α (800 pg/ml) for various times (2–24 h). At the end of the incubation period, total RNA was isolated as described. Northern analysis of total RNA (10 µg/lane) was conducted to evaluate the expression of IL-6. Hybridization to a single species of mRNA (~ 1.4 kb) was detected in cells treated with IL-1α. The data presented in both panels are from the same blot that was exposed to film for different times (*viz.*, top panel, 2 h; bottom panel, 18 h).

The mounting of an inflammatory response as well as the response to mediators of this response in tissues is centered about the formation of cytokines. Accordingly, the formation of cytokines and the response of uterine endometrium and decidua to cytokines is likely important to the function of this tissue in women both before and during pregnancy. Indeed, many investigators take the view that the formation of selected components of the inflammatory response may be important in the initiation of labor and in the puerperal involution of the uterus after delivery of the fetus. To define more clearly the potential role of cytokines in the physiological, and possibly pathophysiological, processes of endometrial and decidual function, we have initiated a systematic study of the formation of cytokines by this tissue and we have begun studies to define the response of these tissues to these bioactive agents. In this study, we used endometrial stromal cells in monolayer culture as a model system.

We find that endometrial stromal cells produce pro-IL-1β and that these cells respond to treatment with LPS or IL-1α by an increase in mRNA for pro-IL-1β and by an increase in pro-IL-1β protein. But even with maximal response to treatment,

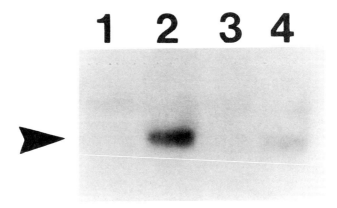

FIGURE 9. Stimulation of IL-6 mRNA expression in human endometrial stromal cells by IL-1 and TNF-α. Confluent endometrial stromal cells in monolayer culture were treated with IL-1α (800 pg/ml), mEGF (15 ng/ml) or TNF-α (10⁻⁸ M) for 24 h. At the end of the incubation period, total RNA was isolated as described. Northern analysis of total RNA (10 μg/lane) was conducted with an IL-6 cDNA probe. Hybridization to a species of mRNA (~ 1.4 kb, denoted by the arrow) was detected in cells treated with IL-1α or TNF-α but not in cells treated with EGF. *Lane 1*, nontreated; *lane 2*, IL-1α (10 U/ml); *lane 3*, EGF (15 ng/ml); and, *lane 4*, TNF-α (10⁻⁸M).

there is little or no mature (*i.e.*, 17 kDa) IL-1β secreted into the medium. This finding is similar to that of a number of other tissues. Namely, a variety of cells seem to synthesize pro-IL-1β, but perhaps only a few, possibly only mononuclear phagocytes, process and secrete the mature, biologically active IL-1β.[14,15] From these findings alone, we cannot deduce the importance of the formation of pro-IL-1β by these cells. Others have suggested that pro-IL-1β may be active in the cells in which it is produced.[14] Alternatively, these cells may be induced in some manner to process pro-IL-1β or else, under selected conditions, may secrete pro-IL-1β, which is processed in a nonspecific manner by proteases in the extracellular environment.[16] In any event, we must tentatively conclude that the formation of mature, 17 kd IL-1β in endometrium or decidua must be attributed to its formation in mononuclear phagocytes in this tissue and not to the endometrial stromal cell.

On the other hand, we find, as have others,[1] that the case for IL-6 is quite different. Namely, the endometrial stromal cells produce IL-6 and it is secreted into the medium. The secretion of IL-6 is preceded by a striking increase in mRNA upon stimulation of these cells with LPS or with IL-1α. We have demonstrated previously that TNF-α mRNA and protein is produced by decidual tissue and that the mRNA and protein are increased appreciably in response to treatment with LPS.[17]

We also have demonstrated that the endometrial stromal cells and decidua respond to treatment with IL-1 and TNF-α by a striking increase in prostaglandin formation.[2] Thus, the endometrial stromal cell in culture and decidual tissue in explant culture are poised to mount an impressive response to immunological or infectious challenge. The hormonal modulation of these responses may serve to regulate further the precise physiological role of cytokine formation and response in endometrial and decidual tissues. It has been demonstrated already, for example, that estrogen treatment of endometrial stromal cells will attenuate the formation of IL-6.[1] This exciting finding may lead to other experimental paradigms that will permit a better understanding of the mechanism(s) by which the sex steroids act, sometimes indirectly, and sometimes by way of actions on contiguous cells, to effect growth, differentiation, and function. It seems reasonable to suspect that cytokines and other growth factor production and action may be modulated by sex steroid hormone action. If this were the case, significant insights will be obtained in deducing the physiological mechanisms of steroid action.

SUMMARY

Cytokines are known to act in a variety of tissues, most commonly in a paracrine manner, to effect a number of biochemical processes. Previously, we found that human endometrial stromal cells respond to the action of interleukin-1 (IL-1) with an increase in the production of prostaglandins. In these investigations, we also found that IL-1 acts in endometrial stromal cells to stimulate the synthesis of IL-1 and IL-6 mRNA and protein. Specifically, in human endometrial stromal cells maintained in monolayer culture, treatment with IL-1α leads to a striking increase in the synthesis of IL-1β mRNA and protein; this increase is IL-1α-dose- and time-dependent. The pro-IL-1β produced, however, is not secreted into the culture medium but is retained within the stromal cell. The failure of secretion of IL-1β is characteristic of non-monocyte/macrophage cell types; this obtains because the enzyme that effects processing of pro-IL-1β (31 kDa) to the mature, secreted form of IL-1β (17 kDa) is believed to be present only in monocytes/macrophages. We also find that IL-1 and tumor necrosis factor-α (TNF-α) act in endometrial stromal cells to stimulate the synthesis of interleukin-6 (IL-6) mRNA and protein; the IL-6 produced by these cells is secreted into the culture medium. In addition, we find that IL-1 acts in endometrial stromal cells to inhibit the expression of mRNA for connexin43, a gap junction protein that is believed to be the principal component of gap junctions in cardiac and smooth muscle. Thus, it is likely that IL-1 action leads to a decrease in gap junction–dependent intercellular communication among endometrial stromal cells. Based on these findings, we conclude that endometrial stromal cells are responsive to the actions of IL-1 and TNF-α. These cells synthesize both IL-1 and IL-6; and, IL-6 is released into the extracellular medium. Thus, the possibility exists that the synthesis and action of cytokines may be involved in the mechanisms that serve to regulate the mesenchymal-epithelial interactions between endometrial stromal and glandular components; and, the formation and action of cytokines in decidua may serve to modulate immunological and infectious challenges encountered by this tissue in pregnancy.

REFERENCES

1. TABIBZADEH, S. S., U. SANTHANAM, P. B. SEHGAL & L. T. MAY. 1989. Cytokine-induced production of IFN-β_2/IL-6 by freshly explanted human endometrial stromal cells. J. Immunol. **142:** 3134–3139.

2. CASEY, M. L., S. M. COX, R. A. WORD & P. C. MACDONALD. 1990. Cytokines and infection-induced preterm labor. Reprod. Fertil. Dev. **2:** 499–509.

3. SATYASWAROOP, P. G., R. S. BRESSLER, M. M. DE LA PENA & E. GURPIDE. 1979. Isolation and culture of human endometrial gland. J. Clin. Endocrinol. Metab. **48:** 639–641.

4. KORTE, K., P. C. MACDONALD, J. M. JOHNSTON, J. R. OKITA & M. L. CASEY. 1983. Metabolism

of arachidonic acid and prostanoids in human endometrial stromal cells in monolayer culture. Biochim. Biophys. Acta 752: 423–433.

5. LOWRY, O. H., N. J. ROSEBROUGH, A. L. FARR & R. J. RANDALL. 1951. Protein measurement with the Folin phenol reagent. J. Biol. Chem. 193: 265–275.

6. CHIRGWIN, J. M., A. E. PRZYBYLA, R. J. MACDONALD & W. J. RUTTER. 1979. Isolation of biologically active ribonucleic acid from sources enriched in ribonuclease. Biochemistry 18: 5294–5299.

7. SAMBROOK, J., E. F. FRITSCH & T. MANIATIS. 1989. Molecular Cloning. A Laboratory Manual, 2nd edit. Cold Spring Harbor Laboratory Press. Cold Spring Harbor, NY.

8. CUNHA, G. A., L. W. K. CHUNG, J. M. SHANNON & B. A. REESE. 1980. Stromal-epithelial interaction in sex differentiation. Biol. Reprod. 22: 19–42.

9. SPOONER, B. S. & N. K. WESSELLS. 1970. Mammalian lung development: Interaction in primordium formation and bronchial morphogenesis. J. Exp. Zool. 175: 445–454.

10. WESSELLS, N. K. & J. H. COHEN. 1967. Early pancreas organogenesis: Morphogenesis, tissue interactions, and mass effects. Develop. Biol. 15: 237–270.

11. HILFER, S. R. 1968. Cellular interactions in the genesis and maintenance of thyroid characteristics. In Epithelial-Mesenchyme Interactions. R. Fleischmayer & R. E. Billingham, Eds. :177–199, the Williams & Wilkins Company. Baltimore, MD.

12. GAL, D., M. L. CASEY, J. M. JOHNSTON & P. C. MACDONALD. 1982. Mesenchyme-epithelial interactions in human endometrium: Prostaglandin synthesis in separated cell types. J. Clin. Invest. 70: 798–805.

13. HUANG, J. R., L. TSENG, P. BISCHOF & O. A. JÄNNE. 1987. Regulation of prolactin production by progestin, estrogen, and relaxin in human endometrial stromal cells. Endocrinology 121: 2011.

14. FENTON, M. J., M. W. VERMEULEN, B. D. CLARK, A. C. WEBB & P. E. AURON. 1988. Human pro-IL-1β gene expression in monocytic cells is regulated by two distinct pathways. J. Immunol. 140: 2267–2273.

15. KOSTURA, M. J., M. J. TOCCI, G. LIMJUCO, J. CHIN, P. CAMERON, A. G. HILLMAN, N. A. CHARTRAIN & J. A. SCHMIDT. 1989. Identification of a monocyte specific pre-interleukin 1β convertase activity. Proc. Natl. Acad. Sci. USA 86: 5227–5231.

16. HAZUDA, D. J., J. STRICKLER, F. KUEPPERS, P. L. SIMON & P. R. YOUNG. 1990. Processing of precursor interleukin 1β and inflammatory disease. J. Biol. Chem. 265: 6318–6322.

17. CASEY, M. L., S. M. COX, B. BEUTLER, L. MILEWICH & P. C. MACDONALD. 1989. Cachectin/tumor necrosis factor-α formation in human decidua. J. Clin. Invest. 83: 430–436.

Autocrine/Paracrine Regulation of Prolactin Release from Human Decidual Cells[a]

STUART HANDWERGER[b] AND RANDALL RICHARDS[b]

Departments of Pediatrics and Cell Biology
Duke University Medical Center
Durham, North Carolina 27710

EDITH MARKOFF

Department of Pediatrics
University of Cincinnati and Children's Hospital Medical Center
Cincinnati, Ohio 45229

Human decidual tissue synthesizes and releases a protein that is identical in its chemical and biological properties to pituitary prolactin.[1,2] The mRNA for prolactin has been isolated from human decidual tissue,[3,4] and the nucleotide sequence of the cDNA for decidual prolactin has been shown to be identical to that of the human pituitary prolactin gene.[5,6]

Prolactin is first detected in decidualized endometrium during the late luteal phase of the menstrual cycle.[7,8] If pregnancy ensues, the decidual content of prolactin increases markedly following implantation.[9] Since prolactin is also detected in endometrial tissues of women receiving progesterone or combined progesterone/estrogen therapy[10] and in endometrial tissue exposed *in vitro* to progesterone,[11,12] the induction of prolactin synthesis appears to be dependent upon the progesterone-induced decidualization of the endometrium.

Although decidual and pituitary prolactin have identical chemical and biological properties, the factors that regulate the synthesis and release of the two hormones are different. For example, thyrotropin-stimulating hormone (TRH), dopamine and bromocriptine, which markedly affect the synthesis and release of pituitary prolactin, have no effects on decidual prolactin.[13] As discussed below, recent studies indicate that the synthesis and release of decidual prolactin is regulated, at least in part, by autocrine/paracrine factors.

The first evidence for paracrine regulation of decidual prolactin release was the demonstration that decidual explants co-incubated with placental explants or exposed to placental conditioned medium (PCM) release three- to fourfold more prolactin than control explants (FIG. 1).[14] The increase in prolactin release in these experiments was not accompanied by a generalized increase in protein release and was not secondary

[a] Supported by National Institutes of Health Grant HD-15201.

[b] *Present address:* Departments of Pediatrics and Anatomy and Cell Biology, University of Cincinnati and Children's Hospital Medical Center, Cincinnati, Ohio 45229.

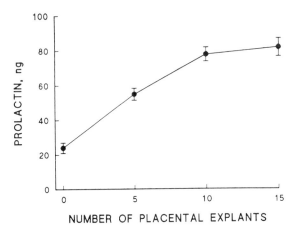

FIGURE 1. The effect of placental explants on the release of decidual prolactin. Fifteen human decidual explants with a total weight of approximately 100 mg were exposed for 0.5 h to control medium or medium containing 5, 10, or 15 human placental explants (average weight approximately 8–10 mg/explant). The amount of prolactin released into the medium is expressed as the total amount of prolactin contained in the medium after the 0.5 h exposure. Each point represents the mean ± SEM of triplicate cultures.

to a toxic effect of the placenta on decidual cells. Exposure of decidual explants to conditioned media from human fibroblasts, hepatocytes and other tissues had no effect on decidual prolactin release. In addition, exposure of pituitary explants to placental explants or PCM had no effect on pituitary prolactin release. Preliminary studies indicated that the prolactin-releasing factor (PRL-RF) in placental extracts and PCM was non-dialyzable (10 kD cut-off) and was not extracted by lipid solvents. The releasing activity, however, was completely destroyed by treatment with proteolytic enzymes, indicating that the activity is due to a protein(s) released by the placenta.

The factor has now been purified to homogeneity from placental extracts and PCM by a scheme consisting of ion exchange, gel exclusion and affinity chromatography.[15] The purified material, which consists of a single band following SDS polyacrylamide gel electrophoresis, has a M_r of 23,500 and stimulates the acute release of prolactin from decidual cells with a half maximal dose of 50 ng/ml (5 pM). More recent investigations with purified PRL-RF indicate that the releasing factor stimulates a biphasic increase in prolactin release (FIG. 2).[16] The initial acute increase in prolactin release is followed approximately 6 h later by a prolonged secondary increase in prolactin release that is secondary to stimulation of prolactin synthesis. The acute stimulation is blocked by somatostatin but not cycloheximide, while the prolonged increase in prolactin release is blocked by cycloheximide but not somatostatin.

The placenta has recently been shown to synthesize and release IGF-I.[17] To determine whether IGF-I affects the synthesis and release of decidual prolactin, we exposed decidual cells to IGF-I for 69 h (FIG. 3A).[18] IGF-I stimulated a dose-dependent increase in prolactin release beginning about 48 h after exposure. Half-maximal stimulation occurred at a physiologic dose of 25–50 ng/ml, and maximal stimulation occurred at doses ⩾100 ng/ml. The stimulation was blocked by cycloheximide and a

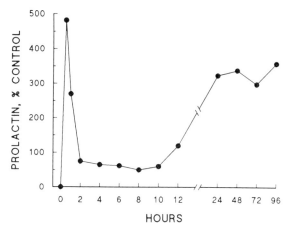

FIGURE 2. The acute and long-term effects of PRL-RF on the release of decidual prolactin. Decidual explants weighing approximately 120 mg were exposed for 96 h to control medium or medium containing PRL-RF (0.6 µg/ml). An aliquot of medium was removed at each of the indicated times during the first 24-h, and the medium was changed at 24-h intervals. The amounts of prolactin released by the cells exposed to PRL-RF are expressed as a percentage of that released by control cells. Each point represents the mean ± SEM for cultures. (Modified from Golander *et al.*[16])

monoclonal antibody (α-IR3) to the IGF-I receptor. This latter observation strongly suggests that the effect of IGF-I is mediated through the IGF-I receptor. Since human decidua does not synthesize IGF-I, these studies suggest a physiologic role for placental IGF-I in the regulation of prolactin synthesis and release.

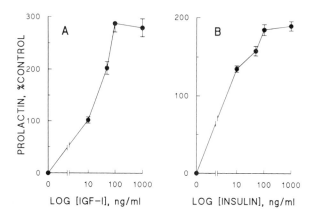

FIGURE 3. The effects of decidual conditioned medium on the release of prolactin from human decidual explants. Decidual explants with a total weight of approximately 120 mg were exposed for 0.5 h to control medium or decidual conditioned medium at concentrations of 50, 100, or 200 µg/ml. The results are expressed as a percent of the prolactin released by the control explants during the 0.5 h interval. Each point represents the mean ± SEM of triplicate cultures. (Modified from Markoff *et al.*[21])

In other studies, insulin was also observed to stimulate a dose dependent increase in prolactin release with a similar time course as IGF-I (FIG. 3B).[19] This affect, however, does not appear to be secondary to the interaction of insulin with the IGF-I receptor since the half maximal stimulation by insulin is also in the range of 25–50 ng/ml and the effect is not blocked by α-IR3. Relaxin, which is synthesized by both placenta and decidua and has structural similarities to IGF-I and insulin, also stimulates decidual prolactin release.[20]

Inhibitory factors also appear to be involved in the regulation of decidual prolactin release. Several years ago, we observed that human decidua releases a factor that inhibits decidual but not pituitary prolactin release.[21] Exposure of human decidual explants or cell cultures to decidual extracts or decidual conditioned medium (DCM) causes a dose-dependent and specific inhibition of prolactin release (FIG. 4). The inhibition is not secondary to feedback inhibition by prolactin since the addition of prolactin to decidual cells fails to inhibit prolactin release, and the M_r of the inhibitory factor is greater than that of prolactin. Chemical characterization of partially purified PRL-IF indicates that the factor is not lipid soluble and is destroyed by treatment with proteolytic enzymes. The active material in DCM and decidual extracts migrates on Sephadex G-150 with an apparent M_r of 40 000–45 000. To date, PRL-IF has been purified to a specific activity of approximately 350. Further purification has been complicated by the lability of the releasing activity on prolonged storage. Recent studies using perifused human decidual cells have shown that PRL-IF also inhibits the stimulation of prolactin release in response to PRL-RF.[22]

The lipocortins are a family of calcium-dependent, phospholipid-binding proteins that are induced by glucocorticoids and inhibit phospholipase A2 activity.[23] At least

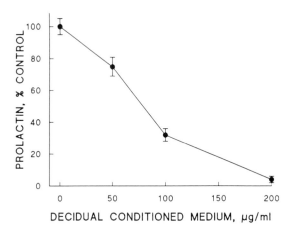

FIGURE 4. The effects of insulin-like growth factor I (IGF-I) (**A**) and insulin (**B**) on prolactin release from decidual cells. Human decidual cells (approximately 1.2×10^6 cells/well) were exposed for 72 h to IGF-I or insulin at the indicated doses. The medium was changed at 24-h intervals. The results are expressed as the percentage of the amount of prolactin released by the treated cells during the third day of culture relative to that released by control cells during the same time interval. Each point represents the mean ± SEM of triplicate cultures. (Modified from Thraillkill *et al.*[18] and Thrailkill *et al.*[19])

6 members of the lipocortin family have been shown to be present in the placenta.[24] However, little is known about the role of the lipocortins during pregnancy. Since inhibition of phospholipase A2 results in a decrease in the production of prostaglandins and other arachidonic acid metabolites, the lipocortins might play a role in the initiation of parturition and other biological actions that may be influenced by arachidonic acid metabolites. In recent experiments from our laboratories, we demonstrated that recombinant lipocortin I, one of the major lipocortins synthesized by the placenta, causes a dose-dependent inhibition of basal prolactin release from human decidual cells.[25] In addition, lipocortin I inhibited prolactin release in response to PRL-RF. The action of lipocortin I, however, does not appear to be glucocorticoid dependent since neither hydrocortisone nor dexamethasone inhibits prolactin release. Furthermore, the effect of the action of lipocortin does not appear to be dependent upon activation of phospholipase A2 since, as discussed below, activation of phospholipase A2 inhibits prolactin release. If the effect of lipocortin were due to inhibition of phospholipase A2 activity, one would anticipate that lipocortin would stimulate rather than inhibit prolactin release. Northern blot analysis of human decidual mRNA indicated that the mRNA hybridized with high stringency to a synthetic oligonucleotide specific for lipocortin I. Western blot analysis of human decidual cell homogenates and conditioned medium with a monclonal antibody to lipocortin I indicated the presence of lipocortin I in both decidual cells and medium. Taken together, these studies strongly suggest that decidual cells synthesize and release lipocortin I. Thus the effect of lipocortin on decidual prolactin may result from an autocrine as well as paracrine effect.

In other studies, human chorionic gonadotrophin (hCG) has been reported to stimulate the release of prolactin from decidual explants,[26] and a significant correlation has been observed between prolactin concentrations in human decidual tissue and decidual progesterone and androgen receptors.[27] In addition, incubation of decidual explants in hyperosmolar medium of greater than 350 mosm/L has been reported to decrease prolactin release.[28] However, prolactin release is unaffected when decidual explants are incubated in medium containing 240–340 mosm/L.[29] In one study, decidual tissues obtained after spontaneous vaginal deliveries were found to release more prolactin than decidual tissues obtained after elective caesarian delivery.[30] We, however, have not observed a difference.

At present, the second messengers involved in the regulation of decidual prolactin release are unknown. However, studies from our laboratory strongly suggest roles for cAMP, protein kinase C and arachidonic acid. In the experiments implicating a role for cAMP in prolactin release, the cAMP analogue dibutyryl cAMP, the phosphodiesterase inhibitors IBMX and theophylline and the adenylate cyclase activators cholera toxin and forskolin all cause dose-dependent inhibition of prolactin release (FIG. 5A).[31] Inhibition occurs within the first few minutes of exposure and quickly returns to basal levels despite continued exposure to the various agents. In the experiments implicating protein kinase C, the synthetic diacylglycerol sn-1,2-dioctanylglycerol (diC8), which stimulates decidual protein kinase C, caused a dose-dependent rapid inhibition of prolactin release (FIG. 5B).[32] Acylglycerols that did not affect protein kinase C were without effect. In addition, PMA and other phorbol esters that stimulate decidual protein kinase C, inhibits prolactin release, while 4-β PMA and other phorbol esters that do not activate protein kinase C are without effect. Since the major source of cellular diacylglycerols results from the breakdown of membrane phosphoinosotides by phospholipase C, these studies also implicate phospholipase C-mediated PI hydrolysis in the regulation of prolactin release. In experiments im-

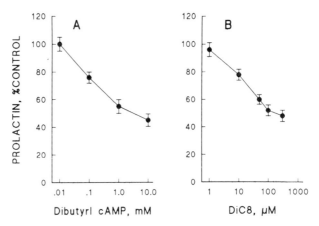

FIGURE 5. The effects of dibutyrl cAMP (A) and SN-1,2-dioctanoylglycerol (diC$_8$) (B) on the release of prolactin from human decidual cells. Decidual cells (approximate weight 1×10^6 cells/well) were exposed for 0.5 h to either dibutyrl cAMP or diC$_8$ at the indicated concentrations. The results are expressed as a percent of the amount of prolactin released by cells exposed to control medium alone. Each point represents the mean $\pm$ SEM of triplicate cultures. (Modified from Handwerger et al.[31] and Harman et al.[32])

plicating arachidonic acid in prolactin release, both phospholipase A2 and arachidonic acid caused dose-dependent inhibition of prolactin release.[33] The inhibition by arachidonic acid, however, was not prevented by cyclo-oxygenase or lipoxygenase inhibitors, indicating that the inhibition is due to either arachidonic acid itself or a non-cyclo-oxygenase, non-lipoxygenase product. Since plasma arachidonic acid concentrations increase during pregnancy, the decrease in the prolactin content of decidual tissue and amniotic fluid prolactin concentrations during the second half of pregnancy may result, at least in part, from the increase in plasma arachidonic acid concentrations. Thus arachidonic acid may function as both a primary and secondary messenger in the regulation of prolactin release. Like PRL-IF, arachidonic acid and the pharmacologic agents that increase intracellular cAMP levels or stimulate protein kinase C also inhibit prolactin release in response to PRL-RF.[22]

In summary, the release of prolactin from human decidual cells is regulated by both stimulatory and inhibitory factors (FIG. 6). Release is stimulated by PRL-RF, IGF-I, insulin and relaxin and is inhibited by PRL-IF and lipocortin I. Since the placenta has been shown to release PRL-RF, IGF-I, relaxin and lipocortin and decidual tissue releases PRL-IF, relaxin and lipocortin, these findings implicate a role for paracrine/autocrine factors in the regulation of decidual prolactin release.

SUMMARY

Studies from this laboratory indicate that the synthesis and release of prolactin from human decidual cells are regulated by factors released by the placenta, decidua and fetal membranes. A 23.5 kD protein (decidual prolactin-releasing factor, PRL-RF) has been purified to homogeneity from human placental tissue and placental con-

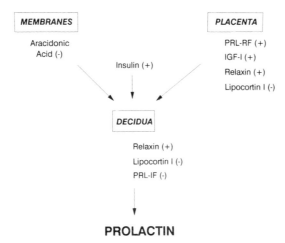

PROLACTIN

FIGURE 6. A schematic representation of the factors regulating the release of prolactin from human decidua.

ditioned medium. The releasing factor stimulates an acute release of prolactin that occurs within the first few minutes of exposure and a prolonged release, secondary to new hormone synthesis, that begins about 6–8 hours later. In addition, the synthesis and release of decidual prolactin are stimulated by IGF-I, insulin and relaxin, each acting through distinct plasma membrane receptors. In contrast, the synthesis and release of decidual prolactin are inhibited by arachidonic acid, lipocortin I and a 35–45 kD decidual protein (prolactin-releasing inhibitory factor) that has been partially purified from decidual conditioned medium. Studies of the second messengers involved in the regulation of decidual prolactin release strongly suggest that decidual prolactin release may be mediated, at least in part, by activation of phosphoinositide metabolism and stimulation of adenylate cyclase. The demonstration that the synthesis and release of decidual prolactin are regulated by PRL-RF, IGF-I, insulin, relaxin, arachidonic acid, PRL-IF and lipocortin I strongly suggests that there is novel autocrine/paracrine feedback regulation between the placenta, fetal membranes, and decidua in the regulation of decidual prolactin.

REFERENCES

1. GOLANDER, A., T. HURLEY, J. BARRETT, A. HIZI & S. HANDWERGER. 1978. Prolactin synthesis by human chorion-decidual tissue: A possible source of amniotic fluid prolactin. Science **202:** 311–313.
2. RIDDICK, D. H., A. A. LUCIANO, W. F. KUSMIK & I. A. MASLAR. 1978. De novo synthesis of prolactin by human decidua. Life Sci. **23:** 1913–1919.
3. ROCKET, R., J. MARTIAL & J. L. PASTEELS. 1982. Detection and characterization of human prolactin messenger RNA in chorion-decidua. DNA **1:** 193–198.
4. TAII, S., Y. IHARA & T. MORI. 1984. Identification of the mRNA coding for prolactin in the human decidua. Biochem. Biophys. Res. Commun. **124:** 530–537.
5. CLEMENTS, J., P. WHITFELD, N. COOKE, D. HEALY, B. MATHESON, J. SHINE & J. FUNDE. 1983. Expression of the prolactin gene in human decidua-chorion. Endocrinology **112:** 1133–1134.

6. TAKAHASHI, H., Y. NABESHIMA, Y-I. NABESHIMA, K. OGATA & S. TAKEUCHI. 1984. Molecular cloning and nucleotide sequence of DNA complementary to human decidual prolactin mRNA. J. Biochem. **95:** 1491–1499.

7. MASLAR, I. A. & D. H. RIDDICK. 1979. Prolactin production by human endometrium during the normal menstrual cycle. Am. J. Obstet. Gynecol. **135:** 751–754.

8. DALY, D. C., I. A. MASLAR, S. M. ROSENBERG, N. TOHAN & D. H. RIDDICK. 1981. Prolactin production by luteal phase defect endometrium. Am. J. Obstet. Gynecol. **140:** 587–591.

9. MASLAR, I. A., B. M. KAPLAN, A. A. LUCIANA & D. H. RIDDICK. 1980. Prolactin production by the endometrium of early human pregnancy. J. Clin. Endocrinol. Metab. **51:** 1288–1295.

10. MEURIS, S., G. SOUMENKOFF, A. MALENGREAU & C. ROBYN. 1980. Immunoenzymatic localization of prolactin-like immunoreactivity in decidual cells of the endometrium from pregnant and nonpregnant women. J. Histochem. Cytochem. **28:** 1347–1350.

11. DALY, D., I. MASLAR & D. RIDDICK. 1983. Term decidua response to estradiol and progesterone. Am. J. Obstet. Gynecol. **145:** 679–683.

12. MASLAR, I. A. & R. AUSBACHER. 1986. Effects of progesterone on decidual prolactin production by organ cultures of human endometrium. Endocrinology **118:** 2102–2108.

13. GOLANDER, A., J. BARRETT, T. HURLEY, S. BARRY & S. HANDWERGER. 1979. Failure of bromocriptine, dopamine and thyrotropin-releasing hormone to affect prolactin secretion by decidual tissue *in vitro.* J. Clin. Endocrinol. Metab. **49:** 787–789.

14. HANDWERGER, S., S. BARRY, E. MARKOFF, J. BARRETT & P. M. CONN. 1983. Stimulation of the synthesis and release of decidual prolactin by a placental polypeptide. Endocrinology **112:** 1370–1374.

15. HANDWERGER, S., D. CAPEL, G. KORNER & R. RICHARDS. 1987. Purification of decidual prolactin-releasing factor, a placental protein that stimulates prolactin release from human decidual tissue. Biochem. Biophys. Res. Commun. **147:** 452–459.

16. GOLANDER, A., R. RICHARDS, K. THRAILKILL, D. CAPEL, D. ROGERS & S. HANDWERGER. 1988. Decidual prolactin-releasing factor stimulates the synthesis of prolactin from human decidual cells. Endocrinology **123:** 335–339.

17. MILLS, N. C., A. J. D'ERCOLE, L. E. UNDERWOOD & J. ILAN. 1986. Synthesis of somatomedin C/insulin-like growth factor I by human placenta. Mol. Biol. Rep. **11:** 231–236.

18. THRAILKILL, K. M., A. GOLANDER, L. E. UNDERWOOD & S. HANDWERGER. 1988. Insulin-like growth factor I (IGF-I) stimulates the synthesis and release of prolactin from human decidual cells. Endocrinology **123:** 2930–2934.

19. THRAILKILL, K. M., A. GOLANDER, L. E. UNDERWOOD, R. G. RICHARDS & S. HANDWERGER. 1989. Insulin stimulates the synthesis and release of prolactin from human decidual cells. Endocrinology **124:** 3010–3014.

20. HUANG, J. R., L. TSENG, P. BISCHOF & O. A. JANNE. 1987. Regulation of prolactin production by progestin, estrogen, and relaxin in human endometrial stromal cells. Endocrinology **121:** 2011–2017.

21. MARKOFF, E., S. HOWELL & S. HANDWERGER. 1983. Inhibition of decidual prolactin by a decidual peptide. J. Clin. Endocrinol. Metab. **57:** 1282–1286.

22. HANDWERGER, S., I. HARMAN, D. A. HANDWERGER & A. GOLANDER. Dynamics of prolactin release from perifused decidual explants. Submitted for publication.

23. HIRATA, F. & W. FUSAO. 1989. The role of lipocortins in cellular function as a second messenger of glucocorticoids. *In* Anti-inflammatory Steroid Action: Basic and Clinical Aspects. Academic Press, Inc.

24. PEPINSKY, R. B., R. TIZARD, R. J. MATTALIANO, *et al.* 1988. Five distinct calcium and phospholipid binding proteins share homology with lipocortin I. J. Biol. Chem. **263:** 10799–10811.

25. PIHOKER, C., R. PHEENEY & S. HANDWERGER. Lipocortin I inhibits the synthesis and release of prolactin from human decidual cells. Endocrinology. In press.

26. ROSENBERG, S. M. & A. S. BHATNAGAR. 1984. Sex steroid and human chorionic gonadotropin modulation of *in vitro* prolactin production by human term decidua. Am. J. Obstet. Gynecol. **148:** 461–465.

27. TAMAYA, T., K. ARBORI & H. OKADA. 1985. Relation between steroid receptor levels and prolactin level in the decidua of early human pregnancy. Fertil. Steril. **43:** 761–765.

28. ANDERSEN, J., B. BORGGAARD, E. SCHROEDER, E. OLSEN, H. STIMPEL & H. NYHOLM. 1984.

The dependence of human decidual prolactin production and secretion on the osmotic environment *in vitro*. Acta Endocrinol. **106:** 405–410.

29. MARKOFF, E., S. BARRY & S. HANDWERGER. 1982. Influence of osmolality and ionic environment on the secretion of prolactin by human decidua *in vitro*. J. Endocrinol. **92:** 103–110.

30. KRUG, E. C., A. D. ROGOL, W. D. JARVIS, S. THIAGARAJAH & C. A. SINGHAS. 1983. Prolactin secretion by human chorion-decidua *in vitro*: Influence of mode of delivery and agents that modify prostaglandin synthesis. Am. J. Obstet. Gynecol. **147:** 38–42.

·31. HANDWERGER, S., I. HARMAN, A. COSTELLO & E. MARKOFF. 1987. Cyclic AMP inhibits the synthesis and release of prolactin from human decidual cells. Mol. Cell. Endocrinol. **50:** 99–106.

32. HARMAN, I., A. COSTELLO, B. GANONG, R. M. BELL & S. HANDWERGER. 1986. Activation of protein kinase C inhibits the synthesis and release of decidual prolactin. Am. J. Physiol. **251:** E172–E177.

33. HANDWERGER, S., S. BARRY, J. BARRETT, E. MARKOFF, P. ZEITLER, B. CWIKEL & M. SIEGEL. 1981. Inhibition of the synthesis and secretion of decidual prolactin by arachidonic acid. Endocrinology **109:** 2016–2021.

The Insulin-like Growth Factor Binding Proteins—The Endometrium and Decidua[a]

STEPHEN C. BELL

Departments of Obstetrics & Gynaecology and Biochemistry
The Medical School, University of Leicester
Leicester, LE1 7RH, England

INTRODUCTION

The insulin-like growth factors (IGFs), IGF-I and IGF-II, are mitogenic peptides structurally related to insulin, and are synthesized by a variety of embryonic, fetal, post-natal and adult mammalian tissues.[1-6] The serum levels of IGFs alter during development and in general terms IGF-II is involved in fetal development whilst IGF-I is characteristic of post-natal growth and development. Assessment of mRNA expression for these growth factors has confirmed their differential developmental and tissue restricted pattern of expression. An N-terminal truncated variant of IGF-I, des-1,3-IGF-I, has been identified in the brain.[5] IGFs as well as acting in an endocrine manner, act via autocrine or paracrine mechanisms to stimulate growth and differentiation and to maintain differentiated cell function. IGFs may interact with two classes of cell surface receptors.[7-9] Type I IGF receptors (IGF-I receptor), structurally homologous to insulin receptors, are heterotetramers comprising two α (M_r 135K) and β subunits (M_r 95K). The Type II IGF receptor (IGF-II receptor) is a 260K monomeric multifunctional protein which shares identity with the cation-independent mannose-6-phosphate receptor. Although the insulin and IGF receptors do not exhibit absolute specificity, for example IGF-I interacts with 2–10% lower affinity than IGF-II with the IGF-II receptor and 1% lower affinity than insulin with the insulin receptor, the IGFs exert their mitogenic actions through the Type I receptor. The role of IGFs within cells of tissue will therefore depend upon exogenous availability and endogenous production of IGFs, the pattern of receptors present and their relative ligand affinities. To this complex equation must be added the influence of members of the specific high-affinity IGF binding proteins which exhibit developmental and tissue specific patterns of expression, and to which virtually all the IGFs are complexed in plasma and other biological fluids.

IGF BINDING PROTEINS (IGFBPs)

IGFs circulate in the blood bound to binding proteins in the form of two complexes, a growth hormone-dependent saturated 150K "large" complex in which the bulk of

[a] The author acknowledges financial support from the Wellcome Trust and the Medical Research Council.

IGFs are detected, and a 40K "small" complex which is unsaturated.[10] Studies on these complexes in human serum revealed microheterogeneity in terms of binding protein species of differing molecular weight, pI and ligand specificity.[11,12] Similar observations have been made on other physiological fluids and cell and tissue culture medium.[13] In particular the techniques of affinity labeling and ligand blotting revealed the presence of at least five IGF binding protein species whose relative preponderance varied according to source. In the human three distinct IGFBP species have been characterized and amino acid-nucleotide sequences determined[16-21] validating studies which indicated the existence of at least three groups of IGFBP,[14,15] and their homologues in the rat have now been described.[22-24] A nomenclature for these characterized IGFBPs has recently been proposed.[25] Although specific reagents to assay levels of these individual BPs are not yet widely available it is probable that binding species of equivalent molecular weight detected by ligand blotting in different fluids represent identical BP species.

IGFBP Structure

The primary structure of the three human IGFBPs, hIGFBP-1, -2 and -3 are shown in FIGURE 1 with the detailed nucleotide sequence of IGFBP-1 in FIGURE 2. The three BPs are 234, 289, and 264 amino acids in length with the major discrepancy between predicted and observed molecular weight being for IGFBP-3. However IGFBP-3 (previously termed BP53) is a glycoprotein isolated in two forms of M_r of 53K and 43K. These two forms represent the 41.5 and 38.5K BP species identified by ligand blotting and predominant in the "large" serum complex. It has been demonstrated that the IGFBP-3 complexed with IGF binds to an acid-labile component of 80–85K to form the 150K "large" complex detected in serum.[15,26,27] IGFBP-1 and -2 are not glycosylated, no N-glycosylation sites are present, and do not appear to associate with other units. A characteristic feature of these sequences is the sequence homology detected in the N and C terminus particularly with respect to number and spacing of cysteine residues. In the N terminus region the spacing of the 12 cysteines is identical for IGFBP-1 and -3 and can be matched with IGFBP-2 if a gap is inserted in the former BPs. In the C terminus region the spacing of 5 cysteines is identical in all three. Cysteine-rich regions appear to define ligand specificity in the binding domain of a number of receptors and both the N and C terminus regions could represent separate binding domains since both N terminal and C terminal containing fragments bind IGFs.[28,29] The C terminus of IGFBP-1 and -2 are also characterized by a peptapeptide IRGDP sequence containing the RGD tripeptide, a consensus sequence for proteins binding to cell surfaces via integrins.[30] The central region of the BPs share the least homology, with the IGFBP-1 sequence possessing a PEST sequence, a sequence which is associated with proteins with short intracellular half-lives.[31] Although certain regions of the proteins also exhibit higher homologies there is no indication as to the structural basis for their differential ligand specificity, i.e., IGFBP-1 and -3 exhibit approximately equal affinity for IGF-I and -II, with IGFBP-3 exhibiting higher affinity, whereas IGFBP-2 exhibits higher relative affinity for IGF-II. Competitive binding assays also indicate that IGFBP-1 and -2 do not bind des-(1-3)-IGF-I in contrast to IGFBP-3.[32] Only single gene copies and single mRNA species appear to exist for IGFBP-1 and for -2; therefore, other related low molecular weight BP species (with shared immunoreactivity and sequence) probably reflect cleavage of these BPs. However the

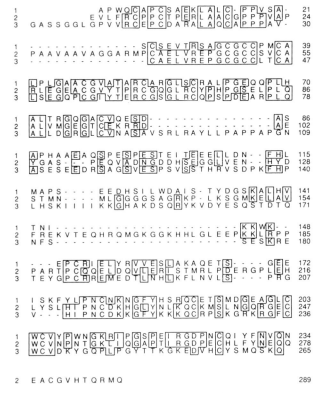

FIGURE 1. Amino acid sequences of hIGFBP-1, -2[20] and −3[21] with gaps included to maximize sequence alignments. Numbers on right refer to amino acid residue.

24K BP detected in ligand blots and predominant in certain cell conditioned media may represent a fourth distinct BP since no antibody cross-reactivity has been noted with this form.

Tissue and Developmental Distribution and Regulation

The employment of specific antibodies and specific cDNAs, and studies involving the rat have indicated that the IGFBPs exhibit dramatic differences in expression and regulation and presumably function. IGFBP-3, the predominant BP of the "large" complex of adult plasma, is strongly dependent upon GH. In adult serum for example IGFBP-3 levels are 100 fold those of IGFBP-1. The appearance of the large complex is developmentally controlled with a switch from IGF containing "small" to "large" complexes in human fetal serum occurring at 30 weeks gestation. In rats this switch corresponds to the developmental switch from IGF-II to IGF-I during early post-natal life.[7] Altered levels of IGFBP-3 have been reported in a variety of clinical conditions as well as in situations of altered GH levels.[15] IGFBP-3 and BPs of similar molecular weight

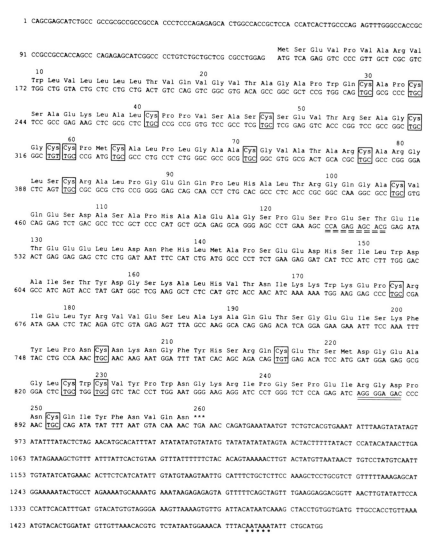

```
  1 CAGCGAGCATCTGCC GCCGCGCCGCCGCCA CCCTCCCAGAGAGCA CTGGCCACCGCTCCA CCATCACTTGCCCAG AGTTTGGGCCACCGC

                                                                       Met Ser Glu Val Pro Val Ala Arg Val
 91 CCGCCGCCACCAGCC CAGAGAGCATCGGCC CCTGTCTGCTGCTCG CGCCTGGAG        ATG TCA GAG GTC CCC GTT GCT CGC GTC

       10                                       20                                       30
    Trp Leu Val Leu Leu Leu Leu Thr Val Gln Val Gly Val Thr Ala Gly Ala Pro Trp Gln Cys Ala Pro Cys
172 TGG CTG GTA CTG CTC CTG CTG ACT GTC CAG GTC GGC GTG ACA GCC GGC GCT CCG TGG CAG TGC GCG CCC TGC

                              40                                       50
    Ser Ala Glu Lys Leu Ala Leu Cys Pro Pro Val Ser Ala Ser Cys Ser Glu Val Thr Arg Ser Ala Gly Cys
244 TCC GCC GAG AAG CTC GCG CTC TGC CCG CCG GTG TCC GCC TCG TGC TCG GAG GTC ACC CGG TCC GCC GGC TGC

              60                                       70                                       80
    Gly Cys Cys Pro Met Cys Ala Leu Pro Leu Gly Ala Ala Cys Gly Val Ala Thr Ala Arg Cys Ala Arg Gly
316 GGC TGT TGC CCG ATG TGC GCC CTG CCT TCG GGC GCC GCG TGC GGC GTG GCG ACT GCA CGC TGC GCC CGG GGA

                      90                                      100
    Leu Ser Cys Arg Ala Leu Pro Gly Glu Gln Gln Pro Leu His Ala Leu Thr Arg Gly Gln Gly Ala Cys Val
388 CTC AGT TGC CGC GCG CTG CCG GGG GAG CAG CAA CCT CTG CAC GCC CTC ACC CGC GGC CAA GGC GCC TGC GTG

                             110                                     120
    Gln Glu Ser Asp Ala Ser Ala Pro His Ala Ala Glu Ala Gly Ser Pro Glu Ser Pro Glu Ser Thr Glu Ile
460 CAG GAG TCT GAC GCC TCC GCT CCC CAT GCT GCA GAG GCA GGG AGC CCT GAA AGC CCA GAG AGC ACG GAG ATA
                                                                         ========

    130                                     140                                     150
    Thr Glu Glu Glu Leu Leu Asp Asn Phe His Leu Met Ala Pro Ser Glu Glu Asp His Ser Ile Leu Trp Asp
532 ACT GAG GAG GAG CTC CTG GAT AAT TTC CAT CTG ATG GCC CCT TCT GAA GAG GAT CAT TCC ATC CTT TGG GAC

                             160                                     170
    Ala Ile Ser Thr Tyr Asp Gly Ser Lys Ala Leu His Val Thr Asn Ile Lys Lys Trp Lys Glu Pro Cys Arg
604 GCC ATC AGT ACC TAT GAT GGC TCG AAG GCT CTC CAT GTC ACC AAC ATC AAA AAA TGG AAG GAG CCC TGC CGA

                     180                                     190                                     200
    Ile Glu Leu Tyr Arg Val Val Glu Ser Leu Ala Lys Ala Gln Glu Thr Ser Gly Glu Glu Ile Ser Lys Phe
676 ATA GAA CTC TAC AGA GTC GTA GAG AGT TTA GCC AAG GCA CAG GAG ACA TCA GGA GAA GAA ATT TCC AAA TTT

                             210                                     220
    Tyr Leu Pro Asn Cys Asn Lys Asn Gly Phe Tyr His Ser Arg Gln Cys Glu Thr Ser Met Asp Gly Glu Ala
748 TAC CTG CCA AAC TGC AAC AAG AAT GGA TTT TAT CAC AGC AGA CAG TGT GAG ACA TCC ATG GAT GGA GAG GCG

                     230                                     240
    Gly Leu Cys Trp Cys Val Tyr Pro Trp Asn Gly Lys Arg Ile Pro Gly Ser Pro Glu Ile Arg Gly Asp Pro
820 GGA CTC TGC TGG TGC GTC TAC CCT TGG AAT GGG AAG AGG ATC CCT GGG TCT CCA GAG ATC AGG GGA GAC CCC
                                                                                  ___ ___ ___

    250                                     260
    Asn Cys Gln Ile Tyr Phe Asn Val Gln Asn ***
892 AAC TGC CAG ATA TAT TTT AAT GTA CAA AAC TGA AAC CAGATGAAATAATGT TCTGTCACGTGAAAT ATTTAAGTATATAGT

973 ATATTTATACTCTAG AACATGCACATTTAT ATATATATGTATATG TATATATATATAGTA ACTACTTTTTATACT CCATACATAACTTGA

1063 TATAGAAAGCTGTTT ATTTATTCACTGTAA GTTTATTTTTTCTAC ACAGTAAAAACTTGT ACTATGTTAATAACT TGTCCTATGTCAATT

1153 TGTATATCATGAAAC ACTTCTCATCATATT GTATGTAAGTAATTG CATTTCTGCTCTTCC AAAGCTCCTGCGTCT GTTTTTAAAGAGCAT

1243 GGAAAAAATACTGCCT AGAAAATGCAAAATG AAATAAGAGAGAGTA GTTTTTCAGCTAGTT TGAAGGAGGACGGTT AACTTGTATATTCCA

1333 CCATTCACATTTGAT GTACATGTGTAGGGA AAGTTAAAAGTGTTG ATTACATAATCAAAG CTACCTGTGGTGATG TTGCCACCTGTTAAA

1423 ATGTACACTGGATAT GTTGTTAAACACGTG TCTATAATGGAAACA TTTACAATAAATATT CTGCATGG
                                                      •••••
```

FIGURE 2. Nucleotide and deduced amino acid sequences of IGFBP-1 cDNA obtained from a human first trimester gestational endometrial library (J. Garde, I. C. Eperon & S. C. Bell, unpublished observations).

have been demonstrated by a number of cells in culture including neonatal skin fibroblasts,[33] astrocyte cells[34] and cell lines derived from carcinomas.[35] Both r and h IGFBP-1 and -2 are developmentally regulated in that for both highest mRNA levels are detected in the fetal liver, compared to other fetal tissues, and levels are dramatically reduced in adult liver.[17,36] In certain fetal rat tissues IGFBP-2 mRNA was more abundant than IGFBP-1 mRNA, e.g., 8-fold more abundant in kidney and 25-fold in the brain, and this has suggested a specific role in these tissues.[36] The predominance of the liver as the source of human fetal IGFBP-1 is supported by Mab based immunocytochemistry.[37] During the neonatal period mRNA levels for both proteins in the rat liver fall dramatically by 3 weeks and a 50% fall for IGFBP-2 mRNA has been produced in neonatal rats by glucocorticosteroid administration.[36,38] In contrast to the neonatal decline in hepatic IGFBP-2, in the choroid plexus of the adult brain expression persists and possibly accounts for the predominance of IGFBP-2 in cerebrospinal fluid.[39]

In the adult other tissues and physiological conditions are associated with differential expression of IGFBP-1 and -2. In the human serum levels of immunoreactive IGFBP-1 exhibit a diurnal variation and this has been related to ambient glucose concentrations and hormonal environment.[40] Hypoglycemia increased, and high glucose intake suppressed,[41] serum levels whereas insulin infusion during a euglycemia clamp suppressed levels.[42] These effects of substrate availability and insulin have been replicated, and inhibition by a glucocorticosteroid and stimulation by agents which raise cAMP have been demonstrated, in human fetal liver explants.[43] Employing reagents which block glucose uptake and effect cAMP levels it has been suggested that a common pathway may be involved whereby regulation of IGFBP-1 production would be positively linked with cAMP levels.[44] In the HEPG2 hepatoma cell line although a glucocorticosteroid was without effect, insulin suppressed and progesterone induced production.[45] Whether IGFBP-2 levels are altered and regulated by similar mechanisms in the human is unknown. In the rat both hepatic IGFBP-1 and -2 expression are affected by metabolic alterations however rIGFBP-1 appears to respond differently to the protein in the human. Whereas in the human serum levels of IGFBP-1 increase 4- to 12-fold after fasting no effects on hepatic mRNA expression or serum levels are observed in the rat, whereas IGFBP-2 mRNA and serum levels increase 10–20 fold.[36] Streptozotocin-induced diabetes however preferentially induces over 100-fold increase in hepatic IGFBP-1 mRNA levels and serum levels.[36] The reason for this differential response in these BPs in the human and rat is not known although they suggest differential regulation and functions of IGFBP-1 and -2 during catabolic states. Examination of a number of tumor-derived cell lines and primary cultures of carcinomas suggest, that apart from hepatomas, IGFBP-2 or BPs of similar molecular weight production is more commonly associated with these cells.[34,35] The other adult tissue associated with reactivation of high levels of IGFBP expression is the endometrium during pregnancy (see next section). Evidence suggests that the 24K BP detected on ligand blots may represent a fourth distinct IGFBP and in conditioned medium from human fibroblasts, where it represented the major form, production was suppressed by a glucocorticoid and stimulated by GH.[35]

IGFBPs AND THE ENDOMETRIUM

The ultimate function of the endometrium is to support implantation of the embryo and subsequent pregnancy, however the involvement of individual endometrial cell populations reflects the species-specific nature of implantation and placentation. In epithelialchorial placental species the role of the luminal and glandular epithelium is predominant whereas in hemochorial species, where trophoblast invasion is extensive, differentiation of the stromal compartment is marked with the formation in the human of the decidual cell of the decidualized gestational endometrium or decidua. The endometrium also undergoes periodic bursts of proliferative activity, most marked in species where in the absence of pregnancy a portion of the endometrium is shed. Within the endometrium, embryo and placenta, where IGF expression and IGF receptors have been detected, given the alterations in the cellular juxtaposition that occur during implantation and placental development the potential IGF-receptor-BP relationships are likely to reach a high degree of complexity.

IGFBP-1 and the Menstrual Cycle

Of the two phases of the cycle it may be anticipated that the proliferative activity in the endometrium during the follicular phase may be associated with the dramatic alterations in growth factor activity. Estrogens which dominate this phase have been implicated in regulation of EGF and IGF-I in the rodent uterus.[46,47] However only very low levels of endometrial IGFBP-1 synthesis was detected during this phase in the human[48] and was undetectable by Mab-based immunohistochemical techniques in both the human and baboon.[49,50] During the luteal phase histological alterations in the early and mid-secretory endometrium occur primarily in the luminal and glandular epithelial populations, whereas stromal alterations dominate the late-secretory endometrium and presumably subserve functions in implantation. An elevation in IGFBP-1 synthesis and secretion by late secretory endometrial explants has been reported[48] and this has been supported by western blotting where immunoreactive protein was detected in cytosolic extracts of only late secretory endometrium.

This was confirmed by Mab-based immunocytochemical techniques. IGFBP-1 was first detected in the glandular epithelium of mid-secretory endometrium, however staining was weak and was restricted to a few cells and glands in contrast to the consistent staining detected in late secretory endometrium. In this latter tissue intense staining was detected in the cytoplasm of specific stromal fibroblastic populations in the sub-luminal region and surrounding spiral arteries. Outside these regions the stroma was negative.[49] These populations of stromal cells are those which initially undergo decidual differentiation during the menstrual cycle. Mature predecidual cells possessed lower intensity of staining or were often negative. These results contrasted with reports employing polyclonal antisera where immunoreactivity was solely detected at high intensity in the glandular epithelium of the mid-secretory endometrium.[51] However paradoxically employing the same antisera substantial IGFBP-1 levels were detected in cytosols of late secretory endometrium in contrast to being undetectable in endometrium prior to this stage.[52] IGF-I receptors have been detected in endometrial membrane preparations throughout the menstrual cycle suggesting that the fluctuation in IGFBP-1 levels could have an effect upon IGF availability. Serum levels of immunoreactive IGFBP-1 did not fluctuate during the menstrual cycle. IGFBP-1 production is also increased in the late secretory endometrium in the baboon as demonstrated at the mRNA and protein level.[50] However, in direct contrast to the human, immunocytochemical techniques have demonstrated its restriction to the glandular epithelium. Within these cells localization to vesicles in the apical cytoplasm suggested that the protein is destined for luminal secretion. In these studies no histological alterations were observed in the stroma consistent with the absence of predecidualization within the menstrual cycle in this species.

IGFBP-1, Decidualization and Pregnancy

Pregnancy appears to represent a unique physiological state with respect to the production of tissue selectively expressing high levels of IGFBP-1. Historically in pregnancy IGFBP-1 was originally described as an amniotic fluid IGFBP,[53] a placental protein (PP12),[54] and the major *in vitro* secretory protein product of the decidualized first trimester gestational endometrium (endometrial protein 14 or pregnancy-associated α_1-globulin).[25,26] In medium from decidualized endometrial explants the protein is secreted as two pI isoforms of identical molecular weight. During the first trimester of pregnancy rates of *in vitro* synthesis and secretion, on a tissue wet weight basis, increased and in the earliest specimens another protein, a human glycosylated homologue of β-lactoglobulin (endometrial protein 15, pregnancy-associated endometrial α_2-globulin, placental protein 14, progestagen-associated endometrial protein), represents the major secretory soluble protein product with IGFBP-1 a minor product.[57] During the late first trimester IGFBP-1 represents the major product and in some species >95% of radioactive precursors are incorporated into this single protein. During the first trimester in the gestational endometrium, the decidua parietalis or non-implanted region of the uterus obtained in these studies, two histologically distinguishable zones of tissue are observed. The upper decidua compacta is made up of relatively non-secretory or attenuated glands in a stroma in which the stromal fibroblastic cells are differentiated into decidual cells. The lower zone, the decidua spongiosa, is comprised of secretory glands supported by a non-differentiated stroma. During the first trimester the decidua spongiosa zone undergoes involution such that a greater proportion of gestational endometrium is represented by decidua compacta. Immunohistochemical techniques employing monoclonal antibodies to IGFBP-1 have principally localized the protein to decidual cells of the compacta zone[58] and β-lactoglobulin to the secretory glandular-epithelium of the spongiosa.[59] The increasing production of IGFBP-1 during the first trimester therefore probably does not reflect increased production per decidual cell but progressive decidualization of the endometrium. In the decidua a variety of staining patterns have been observed supporting secretion and localization to the extracellular matrix (FIG. 3). At other intra-uterine sites during the first trimester, decidua capsularis and basalis, and third trimester, the basal plate and fetal membranes, IGFBP-1 was localized to decidual cells.[38] These studies suggest that the decidual cell represents a unique normal cell with respect to its selective production of IGFBP-1, and the protein representing its major soluble protein product. Highest levels of IGFBP-1 mRNA have been detected in decidual tissue[19] and in an immunohistochemical study of a range of normal and pathological tissues this tissue exhibited the highest staining intensity.[7]

The decidual cell at the light and ultrastructural level exhibits features such as abundant intracellular filaments and an encapsulating basement membrane, and other biochemical features suggested to reflect the decidual cell phenotype include synthesis of prolactin and aromatase.[30] However, immunohistological evidence suggests IGFBP-1 production is not always tightly linked with histologically defined decidual cell differentiation since ectopic decidual tissue has been detected devoid of IGFBP-1 (unpublished observations). These studies on human gestational endometrium have been extended to other primate species, the baboon and rhesus monkey. In both these species explants of gestational endometrium synthesize and secrete a protein detected as 2 pI isoforms, immunochemically and biochemically indistinguishable from human IGFBP-1, as their quantitatively major soluble protein (I. A. Maslar & S. C. Bell, unpublished observations).[61] The *in vitro* rates of production are higher in these species than in the human with highest rates detected in the rhesus monkey. Histologically the gestational-associated changes in endometrial stromal cells in these latter species have not been considered to represent decidual cell differentiation and have been referred to as "stromal hypertrophy." However at the ultrastructural level these hypertrophied cells do exhibit features of decidual cells and immunohistochemical studies employing the Mab's to the hIGFBP-1 localize the BP to these cells and suggests that these cells represent the functional analogue of decidual cells.[61,62] It remains to be determined whether this feature is found for gestational endometrium of other species exhibiting haemochorial placentation and represents an evolutionary conserved property of the decidual cell.[63]

The examination of the cellular distribution of IGFBP-1 in an early pregnancy specimen from the rhesus monkey may provide insight into the relationship between the differential expression in the primates during the menstrual cycle (FIG. 4). In this specimen IGFBP-1 was localized to the glandular epithelium, reflecting a continuation of expression observed in the menstrual cycle of non-human primates. However staining was also detected in stromal fibroblastic cells surrounding spiral arteries, analogous to those observed within the human menstrual cycle, and at high intensity in large cells associated with the implantation site. If these cells are confirmed to represent decidual cells this would suggest that the trophoblast may be involved in inducing IGFBP-1 production in decidual cells.

During the mid-trimester of pregnancy high levels of IGFBP-1 are detected in amniotic fluid which fall dramatically during the third trimester.[64-66] Amniotic fluid BP could arise from the fetus particularly during early pregnancy when amniotic fluid composition reflects fetal serum rather than maternal serum composition. High levels of IGFBP-1 mRNA have been detected in fetal liver[17] and immunoreactive protein detected in the fetal liver[7] and fetal serum. However, it is more likely that amniotic fluid IGFBP-1 is derived from the decidualized endometrium since similar phenomena of amniotic fluid directed transport of endometrial products have been implicated for h-β-lactoglobulin and prolactin. Levels of immunoreactive IGFBP-1 in maternal serum increase 9-fold from non-pregnant values to a maximum at weeks 22–23 after which levels are relatively constant.[64] Although this increase has been considered to represent decidual-derived protein, this has not been unequivocally established and since factors involved in regulation of the decidual source could act upon the maternal liver, the latter tissue could contribute to this increase.

Regulation

In the primate endometrium IGFBP-1 production is associated with both the epithelial and stromal cell populations; however, in the human and baboon markedly different patterns of expression occur. These observations are compatible with similar mechanisms of regulation if, as has been proposed, IGFBP-1 expression in the stroma is principally associated with the process of decidual cell differentiation,[63] which is not observed within the menstrual cycle of the baboon, and the species differences in glandular epithelial production are quantitative rather than qualitative. In the baboon, employing ovariectomized animals, progesterone administration to estradiol-primed animals induced production of endometrial IGFBP-1 which was localized to the glandular epithelium.[50] The pattern of ovarian steroids would account for the epi-

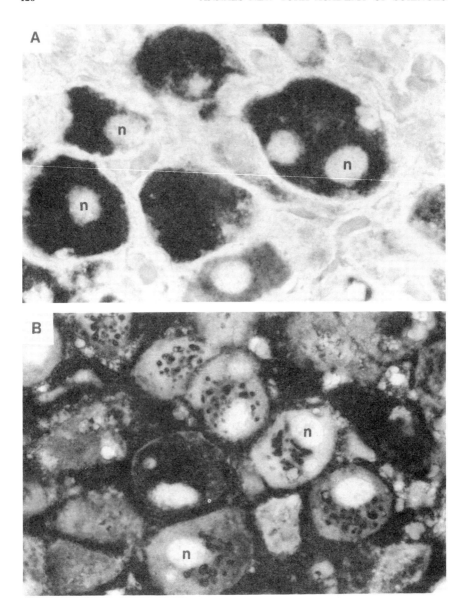

thelial appearance in the secretory endometrium of the baboon and human, albeit at very low levels in the latter species, presumably mediated via a progesterone receptor-mediated mechanism. That IGFBP-1 synthesis and secretion, albeit at low levels, is detected initially in stromal fibroblastic populations during the late luteal phase destined to undergo histologically defined differentiation to predecidual cells, suggests

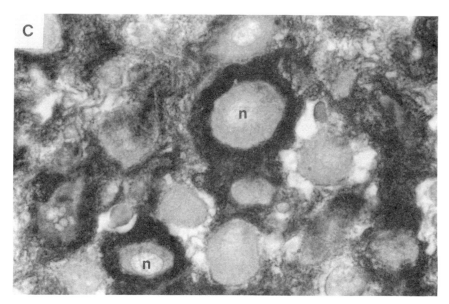

FIGURE 3. Patterns of immunocytochemical localization of hIGFBP-1 associated with decidual cells in the decidua compacta of human first trimester gestational endometrium (decidua parietalis) employing monoclonal antibody code B2H10. Staining patterns detected include A) uniform cytoplasmic staining, B) intracellular peri-nuclear vesicular structures with extracellular staining and C) essentially extracellular staining where it appears to be of highest intensity in the pericellular region and is also associated with fibrillar material. Nuclei of selected cells are indicated by n.

an association with decidual cell differentiation. Thus production could be dependent upon the same hormonal stimuli which control stromal cell differentiation and represent another marker of the decidual cell phenotype.

In primary cultures of endometrial stromal cells progestagen-induced morphological alterations, production of prolactin and aromatase have been reported, consistent with *in vitro* decidualization. Relaxin exerts a potent effect upon aromatase and PRL synthesis in stromal cell cultures, and it has been proposed that aromatase induction is mediated by a cAMP independent mechanism but for PRL a cAMP-dependent pathway may be involved. In decidual cell cultures obtained at term many regulatory factors have been reported to affect PRL production including IGF-I, insulin, decidual and placental proteins. In these cells activation of protein kinase C inhibits synthesis and secretion of PRL (see S. Handwerger, this volume). In endometrial stromal cell cultures IGFBP-1 production is also induced by progestin, but under the conditions employed PRL is produced at 17–33% the levels of IGFBP-1 and ligand blotting has revealed that IGFBP-1 represented a minor BP product. During culture after the initial appearance of a BP of molecular weight 34K, consistent with its identity as IGFBP-2, BPs of 25, 40 and 44 are also apparent (FIG. 5).

The relevance of studies on regulation of IGFBP-1 and -2 in the liver to the endometrium is uncertain; however, progesterone stimulated production by HEP G2 cells[45] and this feature may also reflect a property of the normal hepatocyte. In the human

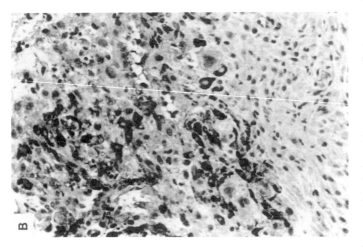

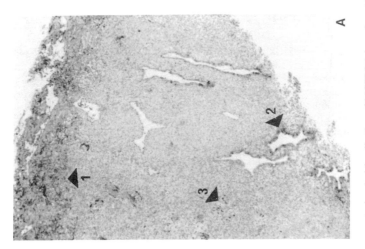

FIGURE 4. Immunocytochemical localization of hIGFBP-1 in endometrium of the rhesus monkey during early pregnancy employing monoclonal antibody code B2H10. Examination of whole endometrial specimen containing implantation site revealed three regions containing positive cells. Stroma was only positive in the implantation site (A1 and B at higher power) where numerous intensely staining cells were detected. Glandular cells of deep glands were positive (A2 and C at higher power) and positive cells were detected surrounding spiral arteries (A3 and D at higher power).

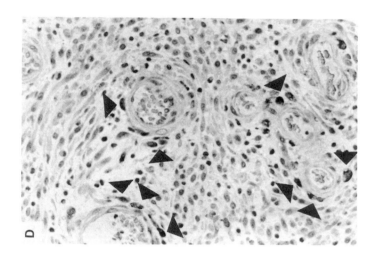

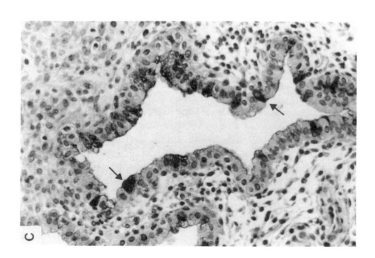

KDa

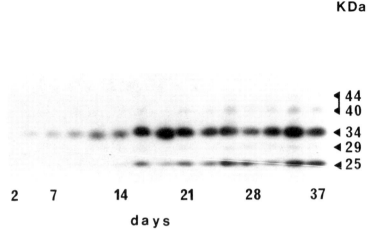

FIGURE 5. IGFBP species in medium of endometrial stromal cells obtained during the menstrual cycle and cultured in presence of medroxyprogesterone acetate for days indicated. Medium was subjected to SDS-polyacrylamide gel electrophoresis and [^{125}I]-IGF-I ligand blotting. Molecular weight of IGF-I binding components indicated. (S. C. Bell and L. Tseng, unpublished observations.)

fetal liver a common cAMP-dependent pathway has been implicated in the regulation of IGFBP-1 production, and studies in the rat would suggest that IGFBP-2 may also be regulated by similar regulators. To induce stromal cell cultures to produce IGFBP-1 as their major secretory product, at levels analogous to decidualized endometrial explants, the cultures also required the inclusion of RLX. Under these conditions IGFBP-1 was preferentially produced, *i.e.*, 5- to 60-fold the levels of PRL, and represented the major BP present and major soluble secretory product (S. C. Bell & L. Tseng, unpublished observations; FIG. 6). Whether RLX is involved *in vivo*, either as an endocrine[67] or autocrine[68] inducer, or is acting as an analogue for another factor involved *in vivo* is unknown. That paracrine inducers are involved is supported by the detection of decidual cells without associated high levels of IGFBP-1, *i.e.*, predecidual cells of the human menstrual cycle and ectopic decidual tissue and the observations of early pregnancy specimens in the rhesus monkey. However, these observations together with the possibility that the autocrine and placentally derived protein implicated in the regulation of decidual PRL are involved suggests that PRL and IGFBP-1 may be independently regulated by complex endocrine, paracrine, and autocrine mechanisms.

Function

Certain features of IGFBPs indicate that they potentially fulfill a determinant role in IGF action, and the cell-specific and IGFBP type-specific expression as observed in the endometrium indicate that they may subserve important effects upon IGF action in implantation and pregnancy. The most important feature has been the report that IGFBP-1 exists in two forms which either inhibit or enhance IGF-1 action upon cells

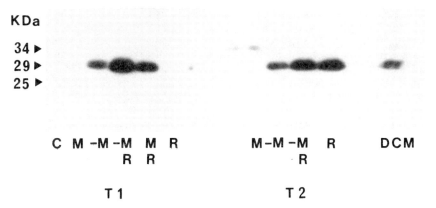

FIGURE 6. IGFBP-1 and other IGF-BP species in medium of endometrial stromal cells obtained during the menstrual cycle and cultured in presence of medroxyprogesterone acetate, MPA (M) or relaxin (R) for 26 days, MPA then subsequently with no hormone ($-$M), relaxin ($-$M, R), or MPA plus relaxin (M,R). Medium from explants of first trimester gestational endometrium (DCM) is also shown. Medium was subjected to SDS-polyacrylamide gel electrophoresis and [^{125}I]-IGF-I ligand blotting. Note appearance of IGFBP species of 34KDa in MPA treated cultures from tissue 2 (T2) which is replaced by IGFBP-1 (29KDa) after MPA withdrawal. Molecular weight of IGF-I binding components indicated. (S. C. Bell and L. Tseng, unpublished observations.)

in vitro.[69,70] These pI isoforms differ in their ability to bind to the cells tested, with the stimulatory form exhibiting cell adherence which also enhanced cellular IGF-1 binding.[70] The stimulatory effect has been reported to be dependent upon the inclusion of human plasma which implies the possibility of extracellular conversion of the inhibitory to stimulatory form.[71] The non-glycosylated IGFBPs, including IGFBP-1, possess the RGD consensus sequence for "integrin" binding and it has been proposed that this may reflect a function in cell surface binding; however, the former studies indicate that other alterations in IGFBP-1 structure may also be required for binding. Also for this stimulatory effect to be apparent a cell may also have to possess an appropriate cell membrane-associated receptor or matrix. If all these conditions are not present the IGFBP-1 may be inhibitory and explain why in most *in vitro* studies the protein has been reported to be inhibitory for IGF-I action.[71-74] However, the situation remains to be clarified since IGFBP-3, which does not contain the RGD sequence, has been demonstrated to enhance IGF-I action under appropriate conditions,[75] and soluble IGFBP-1/IGF complexes to be more stimulatory than IGF-I.[76] A second feature which has profound implications is the differential ligand specificity of the IGFBPs. The IGFBP-2 induced by progestin in endometrial stromal cells exhibits higher affinity for IGF-II than for IGF-I, and IGFBP-1 and -2 in contrast to IGFBP-3 does not exhibit substantial affinity with des-1-3-IGF-I, a form isolated from the uterus.[32] This would suggest that local production of mitogenic des-1,3-IGF-I unlike exogenous IGFs would not be subject to the regulatory effects of local IGFBPs. The high potency of this form of IGF has been suggested to be due to its release from the inhibitory effects of IGFBPs.

Within the context of these considerations it is obvious that the function of uterine

IGFBP production, particularly decidual IGFBP-1, whether systemic, autocrine or paracrine, remains essentially one of speculation. Given the strong evidence for a role of serum IGFBP-1 alterations in glucose homeostasis in the non-pregnant adult and the increased levels of IGFBP-1 in the second half of pregnancy it must be considered that if decidual tissue represents its source this also represents a principal function of decidual IGFBP-1. In the non-pregnant adult levels reflect feeding-fasting cycles with low levels during high glucose uptake or intracellular substrate availability suggested to allow insulin-like activity to be expressed and the converse during hypoglycemia. A decidual source not subject to the same regulatory influences as the liver would disrupt this link and produce high levels independent of these maternal factors which would prevent maternal insulin-like activity of IGFs under all conditions. It could be hypothesized that this would enhance insulin resistance of maternal tissues and contribute to the alteration of glucose homeostasis in pregnancy. This may be of importance since IGF levels are elevated during pregnancy. The production of IGFBP-1 by the glandular epithelium, more pronounced in the baboon, and its intracellular localization suggests the protein is destined for intraluminal secretion during the peri-implantation period. The function of this source of BP may live in a paracrine relationship with the implanting embryo and it may be involved in IGF transport. The more superficial implantation exhibited in the baboon may be reflected by a greater dependence upon a glandular contribution.

The common feature of high IGFBP-1 production by decidual tissue in these species exhibiting hemochorial placentation suggests an important function associated with pregnancy in these species. However, this could reflect an autocrine or paracrine function involved with the decidualization process itself, a complex process of growth differentiation and regression, or a systemic or paracrine function of decidual tissue.[77] Decidual differentiation is associated with prior cell proliferation and the initial appearance of IGFBP-1 in regions destined to decidualize could localize mitogenic effects of endogenous IGFs. This effect may be associated with decidual tissue since IGFBP-1 appears to be localized in the extracellular matrix and this may provide a local reservoir of IGF-I. Decidual cell production of PRL has been demonstrated to be stimulated by IGF-I,[78] therefore, decidual IGFBP-1 production may be anticipated to affect this regulator. The local high concentrations of IGFBP-1 soluble or extracellular matrix-bound may potentially affect other cell types found in this tissue whether maternal (*i.e.*, macrophages or large endometrial granulocytes) or embryonic (*i.e.*, invading interstitial trophoblast populations). The effects will depend upon the previously mentioned factors such as whether IGFBP-1 is inhibitory or stimulatory, whether the extracellular BP is a reservoir of IGF, and distribution of IGF receptors. IGF receptors have been detected upon placental membranes and trophoblast cell lines and IGFBP-1 is inhibitory for IGF-I binding to these receptors[56] and IGF-I action upon these cells[72] and a possibility exists that decidual IGFBP-I may regulate trophoblast activity. However the demonstration that trophoblast-derived factors may regulate decidual cell activity, the detection of regions of decidual tissue without IGFBP-1 expression, and extracellular modulation of the biological activity of IGFBP-1, suggests a potentially complex dynamic situation.

To determine the full implications of these features together with the changing cellular patterns of IGFBP expression for function, future efforts must now be directed towards the elucidation of the expression and cellular distribution of the IGFs and their receptors during implantation and pregnancy, since the IGFBPs are only one element in the complex picture of IGF physiology.

REFERENCES

1. SUSSENBACH, J. S. 1989. Prog. Growth Factor Res. **1**: 33–48.
2. DAUGHADAY, W. H. & P. ROTWEIN. 1989. Endocrinol. Rev. **10**: 68–91.
3. FROESCH, E. R., C. SCHMID, J. SCHWANDER & J. ZAPF. 1985. Ann. Rev. Physiol. **47**: 443–467.
4. D'ERCOLE, A. J. 1987. J. Develop. Physiol. **9**: 481.
5. SARA, V. R. & C. CARLSSON-SKWIRUT. 1988. Prog. Brain Res. **73**: 87–99.
6. RECHLER, M. M., Y. W-H. YANG, R. L. BROWN, J. A. ROMANUS, S. O. ADAMS, W. KIESS & S. P. NISSLEY. 1988. Insulin-like growth factors in fetal growth. *In* Basic and Clinical Aspects of Growth Hormone. B. B. Bercu, Ed.: 233. Plenum Press, New York.
7. NISSLEY, S. P. & M. M. RECHLER. 1984. Insulin-like growth factors: Biosynthesis, receptors and carrier proteins. *In* Hormonal Proteins and Peptides. C. Hoa Li, Ed. **12**: 127–203. Academic Press, Inc., New York.
8. ULLRICH, A., A. GRAY, A. W. TAM, T. YANG-FENG, M. TSUBOKAWA, C. COLLINS, W. HENZEL, T. LEBON, S. KALHURIA, E. CHEN, S. JACOBS & U. FRANKE. 1986. EMBO J. **5**: 2503.
9. MORGAN, D. O., J. C. EDMAN, D. N. STANDRING, V. A. FRIED, M. C. SMITH, R. A. ROTH & W. J. RUTTER. 1987. Nature **329**: 301–307.
10. ZAPF, J., M. WALDVOGEL & E. R. FROESCH. 1975. Arch. Biochem. Biophys. **168**: 638–645.
11. WILKINS, J. R. & A. J. D'ERCOLE. 1985. J. Clin. Invest. **75**: 1350–1358.
12. HARDOUIN, S., P. HOSSENLOPP, B. SEGOVIA, D. SEURIN, G. PORTOLAN, C. LASSARRE & M. BINOUX. 1987. Eur. J. Biochem. **170**: 121–132.
13. BINOUX, M., P. HOSSENLOPP, S. HARDOUIN, D. SEURIN, C. LASSARRE & M. GOURMELEN. 1986. Horm. Res. **24**: 141–151.
14. OOI, G. T. & A. C. HERINGTON. 1988. J. Endocrinol. **118**: 7–18.
15. BAXTER, R. C. & J. L. MARTIN. 1989. Prog. Growth Factor Res. **1**: 49–68.
16. LEE, Y-L., R. L. HINTZ, P. M. JAMES, P. D. K. LEE, J. E. SNIVELY & D. R. POWELL. 1988. Mol. Endocrinol. **2**: 404–411.
17. BRINKMAN, A. C. GROFFEN, D. J. KORTLEVE, A. GEURTS VAN KESSLL & S. L. S. DROP. 1988. EMBO J. **7**: 2417–2423.
18. BREWER, M. T., G. L. STETLER, C. H. SQUIRES, R. C. THOMPSON, W. H. BUSBY & D. R. CLEMMONS. 1988. Biochem. Biophys. Res. Commun. **152**: 1289–1297.
19. JULKUNEN, M., R. KOISTINEN, K. AALTO-SETALA, M. SEPPALA, O. A. JANNE & K. KONTULA. 1988. FEBS Lett. **236**: 295–302.
20. BINKERT, C., J. LANDWEHR, J-L. MARY, J. SCHWANDER & G. HEINRICH. 1989. EMBO J. **8**: 2497–2502.
21. WOOD, W. I., G. CACHIANES, W. J. HENZEL, G. A. WINSLOW, S. A. SPENCER, R. HELLMISS, J. L. MARTIN & R. C. BAXTER. 1988. Mol. Endocrinol. **2**: 1176–1185.
22. BROWN, A. L., L. CHIARIOTTI, C. C. ORLOWSKI, T. MEHLMAN, W. H. BURGESS, E. J. ACKERMAN, C. B. BRUNI & M. M. RECHLER. 1989. J. Biol. Chem. **264**: 5148–5154.
23. MARGOT, J. B., C. BINKERT, J-L. MARY, J. LANDWEHR, G. HEINRICH & J. SCHWANDER. 1989. Mol. Endocrinol. **3**: 1053–1080.
24. YANG, V. W-H., A. L. BROWN, C. C. ORIOWSKI, D. E. GRAHAM, L. Y-H. TSENG, J. A. ROMANUS & M. M. RECHLER. 1990. Mol. Endocrinol. **4**: 29–38.
25. BALLARD, F. J., R. C. BAXTER, M. BINOUX, D. R. CLEMMONS, S. L. S. DROP, K. HALL, R. L. HINTZ, M. M. RECHLER, E. M. RUTANEN & J. C. SCHWANDER. 1990. J. Clin. Endocrinol. Metab. **70**: 817–818.
26. BAXTER, R. C. 1988. J. Clin. Endocrinol. Metab. **67**: 265–272.
27. BAXTER, R. C., J. L. MARTIN & V. A. BENIAC. 1989. J. Biol. Chem. **264**: 11843–11848.
28. WANG, J-F., B. HAMPTON, T. MEHLMAN, W. H. BURGESS & M. M. RECHLER. 1988. Biochem. Biophys. Res. Commun. **157**: 718–726.
29. HUHTALA, M. L., R. KOISTINEN, P. PALOMAKI, P. PARTANEN, H. BOHN & M. SEPPALA. 1986. Biochem. Biophys. Res. Commun. **141**: 263–270.
30. RUOSLAHTI, E. & M. D. PIERSCHBACHER. 1987. Science **238**: 491–497.
31. ROGERS, S., R. WELLS & M. RECHSTEINER. 1986. Science **234**: 364–368.
32. FORBES, B., L. SZABO, R. C. BAXTER, F. J. BALLARD & J. C. WALLACE. 1988. Biochem. Biophys. Res. Commun. **157**: 196–202.
33. MARTIN, J. L. & R. C. BAXTER. 1988. Endocrinology **123**: 1907–1915.

34. OCRANT, I., H. PHAM, Y. OH & R. G. ROSENFELD. 1989. Biochem. Biophys. Res. Commun. **159:** 1316–1322.
35. DE LEON, D. D., D. M. WILSON, B. BAKKER, G. LAMSON, R. L. HINTZ & R. G. ROSENFELD. 1989. Mol. Endocrinol. **3:** 567–574.
36. OOI, G. T., C. C. ORIOWSKI, A. L. BROWN, R. E. BECKER, T. G. UNTERMAN & M. M. RECHLER. 1990. Mol. Endocrinol. **4:** 321–328.
37. WAITES, G. T., R. F. L. JAMES, R. A. WALKER & S. C. BELL. 1990. J. Endocrinol. **124:** 333–339.
38. ORLOWSKI, C. C., A. L. BROWN, G. T. OOI, Y. W. H. YANG, L. Y. H. TSENG & M. M. RECHLER. 1990. Endocrinology **126:** 644–652.
39. TSENG, L. Y-H., A. L. BROWN, Y. W-H. YANG, J. A. ROMANUS, C. C. ORLOWSKI, T. TAYLOR & M. M. RECHLER. 1989. Mol. Endocrinol. **3:** 1559–1569.
40. BAXTER, R. C. & C. T. COWELL. 1987. J. Clin. Endocrinol. Metab. **65:** 432–440.
41. SUIKKARI, A-M., V. A. KOIVISTO, E-M. RUTANEN, H. YKI-JARVINEN, S-L. KARONEN & M. SEPPALA. 1987. J. Clin. Endocrinol. Metab. **66:** 266–272.
42. YEOH, S-I. & R. C. BAXTER. 1988. Acta Endocrinol. **119:** 465–473.
43. LEWITT, M. S. & R. C. BAXTER. 1989. J. Clin. Endocrinol. Metab. **69:** 246.
44. LEWITT, M. S. & R. C. BAXTER. 1990. Endocrinology **126:** 1527–1533.
45. CONOVER, C. A., F. LIU, D. POWELL, R. G. ROSENFELD & R. L. HINTZ. 1989. J. Clin. Invest. **83:** 852–859.
46. DIAUGUSTINE, R. P., P. PETRUSZ, G. I. BELL, C. F. BROWN, K. S. KORACH, J. A. MCLACHLAN & C. T. TENG. 1988. Endocrinology **122:** 2355–2363.
47. MURPHY, L. J., L. C. MURPHY & H. G. FRIESEN. 1987. Mol. Endocrinol. **1:** 445–450.
48. BELL, S. C., S. R. PATEL, P. H. KIRWAN & J. O. DRIFE. 1986. J. Reprod. Fertil. **77:** 221–231.
49. WAITES, G. T., R. F. L. JAMES & S. C. BELL. 1988. J. Clin. Endocrinol. Metab. **67:** 1100–1104.
50. FAZLEABAS, A. T., R. C. JAFFE, H. G. VERHAGE, G. WAITES & S. C. BELL. 1989. Endocrinology **124:** 2321–2329.
51. WAHLSTROM, T. & M. SEPPALA. 1984. Fertil. Steril. **41:** 781–784.
52. RUTANEN, E-M., F. PEKONEN & T. MAKINEN. 1988. J. Clin. Endocrinol. Metab. **66:** 173–180.
53. CHOCHINOV, R. H., I. K. MARIZ, A. S. HAJEK & W. H. DAUGHADAY. 1977. J. Clin. Endocrinol. Metab. **44:** 902–908.
54. KOISTINEN, R., N. KALKKINEN, M-L. HUHTALA, M. SEPPALA, H. BOHN & E-M. RUTANEN. 1986. Endocrinology **118:** 1375–1378.
55. BELL, S. C., M. W. HALES, S. PATEL, P. H. KIRWAN & J. O. DRIFE. 1985. Br. J. Obstet. Gynaecol. **92:** 793–803.
56. BELL, S. C., S. R. PATEL, J. A. JACKSON & G. T. WAITES. 1988. J. Endocrinol. **118:** 317–328.
57. BELL, S. C. 1988. J. Reprod. Fertil., Suppl. **36:** 109–125.
58. WAITES, G. T., R. F. L. JAMES & S. C. BELL. 1989. J. Endocrinol. **120:** 351–357.
59. WAITES, G. T. & S. C. BELL. 1989. J. Reprod. Fertil. **87:** 291–300.
60. BELL, S. C. 1989. Decidualization and relevance to menstruation. *In* Contraception and Mechanisms of Endometrial Bleeding. C. D'Arcangues, I. S. Fraser, J. R. Newton & V. Odlind Eds. :187–209. Cambridge University Press. Cambridge, England.
61. FAZLEABAS, A. T., H. G. VERHAGE, G. WAITES & S. C. BELL. 1989. Biol. Reprod. **40:** 973–985.
62. FAZLEABAS, A. T., H. G. VERHAGE & S. C. BELL. 1990. Insulin-like growth factor binding protein and pregnancy: regulation and function in the primate. *In* Proceedings of the UCLA Symposium on Early Embryo Development and Paracrine Relationships. S. Hayner and L. Wiley, Eds.: 137–152. Alan R. Liss Inc. New York.
63. BELL, S. C. 1989. Hum. Reprod. **4:** 125–130.
64. RUTANEN, E-M., H. BOHN & M. SEPPALA. 1982. Am. J. Obstet. Gynecol. **144:** 460–463.
65. BELL, S. C., M. W. HALES, S. R. PATEL, P. H. KIRWAN, J. O. DRIFE & A. MILFORD-WARD. 1986. Br. J. Obstet. Gynaecol. **93:** 909–915.
66. BAXTER, R. C., J. L. MARTIN & M. H. WOOD. 1987. J. Clin. Endocrinol. Metab. **65:** 423–431.
67. BELL, R. J., L. W. EDDIE, A. R. LESTER, E. C. WOOD, P. D. JOHNSON & H. D. NIALL. 1987. Obstet. Gynecol. **69:** 585–589.
68. SAKBUN, V., S. M. ALI, R. C. GREENWOOD & G. D. BRYANT-GREENWOOD. 1990. J. Clin. Endocrinol. Metab. **70:** 508–514.
69. ELGIN, R. G., W. H. BUSBY & D. R. CLEMMONS. 1987. Proc. Natl. Acad. Sci. USA **84:** 3254–3258.
70. BUSBY, W. H., D. G. KLAPPER & D. R. CLEMMONS. 1988. J. Biol. Chem. **263:** 14203–14210.

71. CLEMMONS, D. R. 1989. Meeting of Endocrine Soc. (US) Abs. 2.
72. RITVOS, O., T. RANTA, J. JALKANEN, A-M. SUIKKARI, R. VOUTILAINEN, E-M. BOHN & E-M. RUTANEN. 1988. Endocrinology 122: 2150–2157.
73. FRAUMAN, A. G., S. TSUZAKI & A. C. MOSES. 1989. Endocrinology 124: 2289–2296.
74. HAN, V. K. M., J. M. LAUDER & A. J. D'ERCOLE. 1988. J. Neurosci. 8: 3135–3143.
75. DE MELLOW, J. S. M. & R. C. BAXTER. 1988. Biochem. Biophys. Res. Commun. 156: 199–204.
76. BLUM, W. F., E. W. JENNE, F. REPPIN, K. KIETZMANN, M. B. RANKE & J. R. BIERICH. 1989. Endocrinology 125: 766–772.
77. BELL, S. C. 1985. Comparative aspects of decidualization in rodents and human: Cell types, secreted products and associated function. *In* Implantation of the Human Embryo. R. G. Edwards, J. Purdy & P. C. Steptoe, Eds.: 71–122. Academic Press, London.
78. THRAILKILL, K. M., A. GOLANDER, L. E. UNDERWOOD & S. HANDWERGER. 1988. Endocrinology 123: 2930–2934.

Relative Potency of Relaxin, Insulin-like Growth Factors, and Insulin on the Prolactin Production in Progestin-primed Human Endometrial Stromal Cells in Long-term Culture[a]

MIRIAM ROSENBERG,[b] JAMES MAZELLA,
AND LINDA TSENG[c]

Department of Obstetrics and Gynecology
State University of New York at Stony Brook
Stony Brook, New York, 11794

INTRODUCTION

Previous studies have shown that prolactin (PRL) is synthesized and secreted from human endometrium and decidua.[1-4] Progesterone and medroxyprogesterone acetate (MPA) stimulate PRL production in a dose- and time-dependent manner in endometrial tissue explants and isolated stromal cells.[5] In addition, a peptide hormone, relaxin (RLX), was found to stimulate the production of PRL in progestin primed endometrial stromal cells in long-term culture.[5] Relaxin is a member of a family of structurally related polypeptide hormones which also includes insulin and insulin-like growth factors (IGFs). Because of the similarity in their tertiary structures and amino acid sequence homology (25–35%), it was expected that IGFs and insulin would also stimulate the PRL production in endometrial stromal cells. The present study was undertaken to investigate if IGF-1 and insulin are able to stimulate PRL production and to compare the relative potency of RLX, IGF-1 and insulin on the induction of PRL secretion by progestin-primed endometrial stromal cells.

[a] This work was supported by USPHS grant HD–19247 from the National Institutes of Health.
[b] On sabbatical leave from December 1989 to November 1990 at OB/GYN, SUNY at Stony Brook. Permanent address: Agricultural Research Organization, Institute of Animal Sciences, Bet Degan, Israel.
[c] Address correspondence to L. Tseng, Dept. of OB/GYN, School of Medicine, State University of New York at Stony Brook, Stony Brook, New York 11794.

MATERIALS AND METHODS

Isolation and Culture of Human Endometrial Stromal Cells and PRL RIA

One proliferative and five secretory endometrial specimens were obtained from premenopausal and cycling women who had undergone hysterectomies for medical reasons: three specimens of fibroid uterus, two specimens of uterine prolapse, and one adenocarcinoma of the cervix. Endometrial stromal cells were separated from epithelial glands by digesting the tissue fragments with 0.02 to 0.05% collagenase as previously described.[6] Stromal cells were suspended in medium A[RPMI-1640 and antibiotics (GIBCO, Grand Island, NY)], containing 0.1 U/ml insulin, and 10% fetal calf serum (FCS, Hyclone, Logan, UT) and plated in culture dishes (~ 0.5 to 1×10^6 cells/10 cm^2 well). The purity of each preparation was estimated by gross examination of the morphology of stromal cells in culture (flat spindle monolayer) distinctly different from glandular epithelial cells (tadpole-shaped curl around monolayer).[6] Stromal cell preparations with purity greater than 95% were used in this study. Relaxin was not detectable in culture medium containing 10% FCS (Hyclone, Lot #1102490).[7] MPA (a gift from Upjohn, Inc., Kalamazoo, MI) porcine RLX (1 mg RLX = 3,000 units by the mouse pubic symphysis bioassay, NIDDK, Bethesda, MD), recombinant hIGF-1 (Amgen Biologicals) and human insulin (Lilly, Inc.) were used in this study.

The relative potency of RLX, IGF-1 and insulin in stimulating the production of PRL was studied in long-term culture. Endometrial stromal cells were cultured in medium A with FCS reduced to 2% which minimized the production of PRL to an undetectable level in the control samples. The relative potency of RLX, IGF-1 and insulin was examined at a concentration of 20 ng/ml. This dose was selected because it had been found to elicit maximal response in a dose response study on the effect of RLX (0.1 to 100 ng/ml) on PRL production shown in FIGURE 3.[4] Endometrial stromal cells were initially cultured with 0.2 μM MPA for 8–14 days and subsequently cultured in the following conditions: no hormone, addition of 20 ng/ml RLX, IGF-1 or insulin. During the long-term culture, medium was changed every day. Stromal cells were all viable during the culture period based on the trypan blue dye exclusion test.

Immunoreactive PRL was identified using Anti-hPRL-IC-2 (AFP-C11580, NIDDK). Results of RIA were previously verified by another RIA kit.[4] The limit of detection was 0.25 ng/assay tube.[4] The inter-assay coefficient of variation was maintained at less than 8%. Any batch of iodinated PRL which did not meet this requirement was discarded. Medium (not exposed to cells) was used as the assay blank (~ 1 ng/ml). The production rate was calculated and expressed as μg PRL/0.1 mg total DNA in cells/day. The DNA content at various incubation times was determined in each experiment by the method of Giles and Myers.[8]

RESULTS

FIGURE 1A shows the magnitude of stimulation of the PRL production in stromal cells treated with MPA continuously in comparison to cells treated with MPA for 8 days and subsequently cultured with no hormone added. MPA increased the PRL production steadily from an undetectable level to ~ 5.5 μg/0.1 mg cell DNA/day on Day

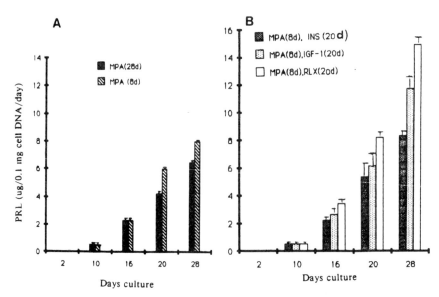

FIGURE 1. Production rate of immunoreactive PRL in endometrial stromal cells from a secretory endometrium. A) shows the production rate in stromal cells treated with 0.2 µM MPA continuously and with MPA for 8 days and subsequently cultured with no hormone. B) shows the production of PRL in stromal cells primed with MPA for 8 days and subsequently cultured with 20 ng/ml each of RLX, IGF-1 or insulin. Each point represents the mean value of duplicate determinations from two separate dishes (mean ± range).

28 of culture. Additional stimulation was observed after MPA withdrawal similar to the results observed previously.[5]

The relative potency of RLX, IGF-1 and insulin on the production of prolactin in progestin primed stromal cells is shown in FIGURE 1B. Stromal cells were primed with MPA for 8 days and these cells were subsequently cultured with RLX, IGF-1 or insulin for 22 days. The production rate of PRL remained the same after 2 days of incubation of the stromal cells with these polypeptides as shown on Day 10 of culture. On the following days, the production rate in cells treated with RLX or IGF-1 gradually increased to higher levels than in MPA withdrawn samples. The potency of different treatments to stimulate PRL production was determined using data combined from four specimens on Days 14, 16, 18, 20 and 22 of culture. Analysis of variance revealed a significant difference ($p < 0.01$) on the effects of MPA withdrawal, insulin, IGF-1 and RLX (1 ± 0.2, 0.8 ± 0.2, 1.1 ± 0.2, and 1.3 ± 0.4, respectively, mean ± SD).

The relative potency of IGF-1 and RLX increased further as the culture continued. On Day 28 of culture, the PRL production in cells incubated with IGF-1 and with RLX was 1.5- and 2.0-fold that of MPA withdrawal, respectively (FIG. 1B). The PRL production was consistently higher in RLX treated cells than that in IGF-1 treated cells which was confirmed in three other specimens. The potency to stimulate PRL production by different hormonal treatments in MPA-primed stromal cells was also determined from different specimens (n=2-12) on Day 28 of culture. The relative potency of MPA withdrawal (n=12), insulin (n=2), IGF-1 (n=4) and RLX (n=7)

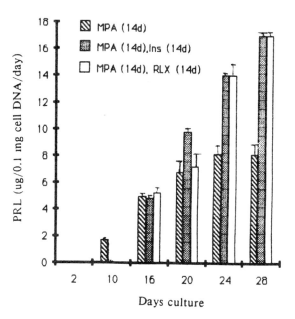

FIGURE 2. Production of PRL in endometrial stromal cells (secretory phase) treated with MPA for 14 days and subsequently treated with no hormone, 8 μg/ml insulin and 20 ng/ml RLX. Data represent triplicate determinations from three separate dishes (mean ± SD).

was 1, 1, 1.4, and 2.4, respectively. This estimation includes previously published data on the effects of MPA withdrawal and of RLX.[5] In cells which had not been pretreated with MPA, IGF-1 and insulin had no effect on the PRL production.

Although 20 ng/ml insulin did not increase the PRL production in progestin-primed stromal cells (FIG. 1B), 8 μg/ml insulin increased the PRL production to the same extent as 20 ng/ml RLX (2.3-fold higher than in cells of MPA withdrawn, FIG. 2). This result indicates that insulin is able to stimulate the PRL production, but that the potency of insulin is much less than that of IGF-1 and RLX, 8 μg/ml insulin alone without MPA treatment had no effect on the PRL production.

DISCUSSION

Increased production of endometrial PRL is essential for the development of the oocyte and the endometrial cells, and for the maintenance of pregnancy.[9,10] Recently, Yoshimura *et al.*[9] have shown that PRL promotes the maturation of rabbit oocyte *in vitro* indicating that PRL may be an important constituent in the process of oocyte maturation. Also, PRL controls uteroglobin gene expression in rabbit endometrium[11] and regulates estrogen receptor and cell proliferation in a human endometrial adeno-carcinoma cell line.[12] These observations suggest that *de novo* synthesized PRL is important for the differentiation of endometrial stromal cells. The relation between the production of PRL and the degree of decidualization requires special attention. In human endometrium, stromal cells undergo profound morphological changes to transform the fibroblastic elements to decidual cells from the mid stage to the late luteal phase of the menstrual cycle. Daly *et al.* first demonstrated that the PRL production correlated with the degree of decidualization of the endometrial stroma.[13] Thus the PRL production can be considered as a biochemical marker to indicate the extent of decidualization. It is interesting to mention that a PRL-like protein has been identified in rat decidual cells.[14] On the other hand, our recent finding indicates that bovine endometrial stromal cells cultured under the same hormonal milieu as human endometrial stromal cells did not produce PRL. Indeed, it is known that the bovine endometrium does not decidualize throughout the reproductive cycle. It appears that endometrial PRL production is a biochemical characteristic of those species in which decidualization of the endometrium is a prerequisite for implantation. Thus, it is important to analyze factors, (both exogenous and endogenous hormones) which regulate the production of PRL during the differentiation of endometrial cells as well as the maintenance of the high rate of production during pregnancy.

We have shown previously that RLX has a dose- and time-dependent effect on PRL production by endometrial stromal cells in the presence of MPA, or MPA plus estradiol (E_2) (FIG. 3). Estradiol alone did not stimulate but it potentiated the MPA to increase the PRL production.[4] It should be pointed out that the combination of MPA plus E_2 potentiates the effect of RLX more at higher RLX concentrations (*i.e.*, >10 ng/ml) than MPA alone (FIG. 3). The maximal response to MPA, E_2 and RLX was ~54 ng PRL/0.1 mg cell DNA/day while MPA and RLX increased the production rate up to ~30 ng PRL/0.1 mg cell DNA/day. Relaxin alone, stimulated the PRL production in short term culture (~2-fold increase over the control).[4] In long-term culture, a cyclic variation of the production of PRL in response to RLX was observed in stromal cells obtained from the mid-secretory phase.[5]

Our present results demonstrate that IGF-1, at concentrations below the physiological plasma level (100–180 ng/ml, 15), stimulates the PRL production of cultured MPA-primed human endometrial stromal cells. IGF-1 and insulin have been reported to stimulate PRL production by decidual cells from term pregnancy.[16,17] However, the decidual cells from term pregnancy are fully differentiated and are therefore different

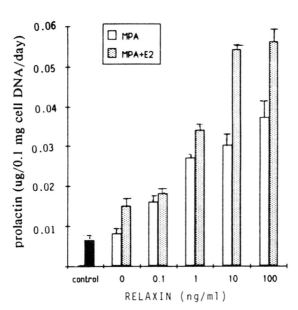

FIGURE 3. Dose-response of RLX on the production rate of immunoreactive PRL in the presence of 0.2 μM MPA alone or MPA plus 0.03 μM estradiol (E_2) in stromal cells isolated from a proliferative endometrium. PRL production rates at various concentrations of RLX on Day 5 of culture were measured by RIA. Results were adapted from reference 4, Table 1, exp. 6. Data represent mean value (± range) of duplicate determination from two separate dishes.

from the undifferentiated endometrial stromal cells. Contrary to endometrial stromal cells, decidual cells do not require progestin priming for the effect of IGF-1 and insulin on PRL production.[16,17]

The present study indicates that the time course of the effect of IGF-1 is similar to the RLX-mediated stimulation. However, the magnitude of the stimulation is less than that of RLX. One of the factors which may explain the lower potency of IGF-1 is the secretion of IGFBP-1 by endometrial stromal cells. We and others have found that IGFBP-1 is the major secretory protein in hormone-stimulated endometrial stromal cells.[18,19] Although IGFBP-1 stabilizes IGFs in body fluids,[20] it may also compete with the binding of IGF-1 to its receptor.[21] Whether RLX and IGF-1 are mediated through the same second messenger system is not known, since little information is available on RLX receptor status in endometrial cell. We have shown that RLX increased the accumulation of intracellular cAMP in endometrial glands[22] and in MPA-stimulated stromal cells suggesting that the effect of RLX may be mediated through the adenylate cyclase system.

Contrary to the RLX receptor, IGF type I receptor has been identified in the secretory endometrium.[21] Whether the effect of IGF-1 is mediated directly through the activation of tyrosine kinase on the IGF type I receptor or through the interaction of the IGF-1 receptor with the other second messengers remains to be studied. The present study shows that a high concentration of insulin is required to stimulate the PRL production in endometrial stromal cells. This suggests that the effect of insulin may be mediated through the IGF-1 receptor.

IGF-1 has been shown to regulate the production of various types of hormones via autocrine/paracrine control by diverse tissues, including the placenta, gonads and pituitary.[23,24] Preliminary studies indicate that the IGF-I mRNA is present in the endometrium, in cultured endometrial stromal cells and in decidua of the first trimester. This suggests autocrine control of endometrial/decidual PRL production. In addition, several studies have shown that the human placenta synthesizes and secretes IGF-1, predominantly during the first trimester[23] suggesting a paracrine mechanism of decidual PRL production during pregnancy. We conclude that stimulation of PRL production by IGF-1 is physiologically important.

ACKNOWLEDGMENTS

We thank the clinical staff of the Departments of Obstetrics and Gynecology and Pathology at State University of New York at Stony Brook; and physicians and pathologists at St. Charles Hospital (Port Jefferson, NY) for providing us with viable endometrial specimens and histological diagnosis of the specimens.

REFERENCES

1. RIDDICK, D. H., A. A. LUCIANO, W. F. KUSMIK & I. A. MASLAR. 1978. De novo synthesis of prolactin in human decidua. Life Sci. **23:** 1913–1921.
2. DALY, D. C., I. A. MASLAR & D. H. RIDDICK. 1982. Prolactin production during in vitro decidualization of proliferative endometrium. Am. J. Obstet. Gynecol. **145:** 672–678.
3. ROSENBERG, S. M., I. MASLAR & D. H. RIDDICK. 1980. Decidual production of prolactin in late gestation. Am. J. Obstet. Gynecol. **138:** 681–755.
4. HUANG, J. R., L. TSENG, P. BISCHOF & O. A. JANNE. 1987. Regulation of prolactin production by progestin, estrogen, and relaxin in human endometrial stromal cells. Endocrinology **121:** 2011–2017.

5. ZHU, H. H., J. R. HUANG, J. MAZELLA, M. ROSENBERG & L. TSENG. 1990. Synergistic effects of progesterone and relaxin on the synthesis of prolactin in long term culture of human endometrial stromal cells. J. Clin. Endocrinol. Metab. **71:** 889–899.

6. LIU, H. C. & L. TSENG. 1979. Estradiol metabolism in isolated human endometrial epithelial glands and stromal cells. Endocrinology **104:** 1674–1680.

7. TSENG, L., J. MAZELLA & G. A. CHEN. 1979. Effect of relaxin on aromatase activity in human endometrial epithelial glands and stromal cells. Endocrinology **120:** 2220–2226.

8. GILES, K. W. & A. MYERS. 1965. An improved diphenylamine method for the estimation of deoxyribonucleic acid. Nature **206:** 931–932.

9. YOSHIMURA, T., Y. HOSOI, A. IRITANI, Y. NAKAMURA, S. J. ATALAS & E. E. WALLACH. 1989. Developmental potential of rabbit oocyte matured in vitro: The possible contribution of prolactin. Biol. Reprod. **40:** 26–33.

10. RIDDICK, D. H. 1985. Secretory products of the human uterus. In Mechanism of Menstrual Bleeding. D. T. Baird & E. A. Michie, Eds. Serono Symposia Publications, Raven Press. **25:** 57–81.

11. CHILTON, B. S. & J. C. DANIEL. 1985. Influence of PRL on DNA synthesis and glandular differentiation in rabbit uterine endometrium. In PRL Basic and Clinical Correlation. R. M. MacLeod, M. O. Thorner & U. Scapagnini, Eds., Section V: 351–359. Liviana Press.

12. KIMURA, J., Y. KATO, T. HIROSE & H. OKADA. 1986. Growth promotion of human endometrial adenocarcinoma cell line HHUA by prolactin. Acta Obst. Gynaecol. Jap. **38:** 1779–1780.

13. DALY, D. C., I. A. MASLAR, S. M. ROSENBERG, N. TOHAN & D. H. RIDDICK. 1981. Prolactin production by luteal phase defect endometrium. Am. J. Obstet. Gynecol. **140:** 587.

14. JAYATILAK, P. G., T. K. PURYEAR, Z. HERZ, A. FAZLEABAS & G. GIBORI. 1989. Protein secretion by mesometrial and antimesometrial rat decidual tissue: Evidence for differential gene expression. Endocrinology **125:** 659–666.

15. UNDERWOOD, L. E., A. J. D'ERCOLE, D. R. CLEMMONS & J. J. VAN WYK. 1986. Paracrine functions of somatomedins. Clin. Endocrinol. Metab. **15:** 59.

16. THRAILKILL, K. M., A. GOLANDER, L. E. UNDERWOOD & S. HANDWERGER. 1988. IGF-I stimulates the synthesis and release of prolactin from human decidual cells. Endocrinology **123:** 2930–2934.

17. THRAILKILL, K. M., A. GOLANDER, L. E. UNDERWOOD, R. G. RICHARDS & S. HANDWERGER. 1989. Insulin stimulates the synthesis release of prolactin from human decidual cells. Endocrinology **124:** 3010–3014.

18. BELL, S. C., J. A. JACKSON, J. ATIKINS, H. H. ZHU & L. TSENG. 1991. Regulation of 28–32 Kd IGFBP-1 production by progestin and relaxin in human endometrial stromal cells. JCEM. In press.

19. RUTANEN, E. M., R. KOISTINEN, J. SJOBERG, M. JUKUNEN, T. WAHLSTROM, H. BOHN & M. SEPPALA. 1986. Synthesis of placental protein 12 by human endometrium. Endocrinology **118:** 1067–1071.

20. COHEN, K. L. & S. P. NISSLEY. 1976. The serum half-life of somatomedin activity: Evidence for growth hormone dependence. Acta Endocrinol. **83:** 243.

21. RUTANEN, E. M., F. PEKONEN & T. MAKINEN. 1987. Soluble 34K binding protein inhibits the binding of Insulin-like Growth Factor I to its cell receptors in human secretory phase endometrium: Evidence for autocrine/paracrine regulation of growth factor action. J. Clin. Endocrinol. Metab. **66:** 173.

22. CHEN, G. A., J. R. HUANG & L. TSENG. 1988. The effect of relaxin on cAMP concentration in human endometrial glandular epithelial cells. Biol. Reprod. **39:** 515–519.

23. BHAUMICK, B., E. P. DAWSON & R. M. BALA. 1987. The effects of insulin-like Growth Factor-I and insulin on placental lactogen production by human term placental explants. Biochem. Biophys. Res. Commun. **144:** 674.

24. LIN, T., J. HASKELL, N. VINSON & L. TERRACIO. 1986. Direct stimulatory effects of insulin-like growth factor-I on Leydig cell steriodogenesis in primary culture. Biochem. Biophys. Res. Commun. **137:** 950.

25. CEDA, G. P., R. G. DAVIS, R. G. ROSENFELD & A. R. HOFFMAN. 1987. The growth hormone (GH)-releasing hormone GHRH-GH-somatomedin axis: Evidence for rapid inhibition of GHRH-elicited GH release by insulin-like growth factors I and II. Endocrinology **120:** 1658.

Autocrine and Paracrine Effects in the Endometrium

ROBIN LEAKE, LOUISE CARR,
AND FRANK RINALDI

Department of Biochemistry
University of Glasgow
Glasgow G12 8QQ, Scotland

INTRODUCTION

For many years, the simple view of the regulation of growth of endometrial epithelial cells was that estradiol stimulated cell growth in the proliferative phase of the cycle, then progesterone inhibited estrogen-induced DNA synthesis, promoting instead differentiation and secretory activity throughout the secretory phase. About 10 years ago, evidence began to accumulate that induction of endometrial DNA synthesis by estrogens was, in fact, achieved by some indirect mechanism(s). For example, Gorski's group[1] showed that injection of estradiol into the blood stream of an immature rat led to a 15-fold increase in uterine DNA synthesis whereas direct application of the equivalent amount of estradiol directly onto the luminal surface of the cells resulted in only minimal DNA synthesis. In our laboratory, we showed[2,3] that primary cultures of human endometrial epithelial cells responded to estradiol in various metabolic ways but did not show significant increases in DNA synthesis. On the other hand, epidermal growth factor (EGF) could double the number of cells, relative to control. This could be increased to fourfold if EGF was given in combination with insulin.

EGF AND TGF-α CONTENT OF ENDOMETRIAL CANCER

The effects of EGF in culture could, of course, be artefactual. In order to investigate whether EGF could be a physiological regulator of endometrial growth, we established a study of EGF content in normal and malignant endometrium. As evidence had been presented by others that transforming growth factor-α (TGF-α) also acts through the EGF receptor (EGFR),[4] we also assayed for content of TGF-α. Our radioimmunoassays use rabbit polyclonal antibodies (kindly supplied by Dr. Harry Gregory of ICI Pharmaceuticals), the sensitivity of both the assays for EGF and TGF-α is down to 10 pg/g tissue. The cross-reactivity is such that 20 ng of either growth factor remains undetected (*i.e.* records as < 10 pg/g) in the assay for the other factor. Results for the first 50 endometrial cancer biopsies showed that TGF-α is detected in over 90% of tumors (range 377–15,177 pg/g wet weight; median value = 1,259). However, EGF is detected in just under 50% of biopsies (range 172–1,204 pg/g; median value = 759 pg/g). This might suggest that TGF-α is the natural ligand for the EGF receptor in endometrial cancer. However, as the EGFR is only detected in 55% of biopsies, it is also possible that the TGF-α may act on surrounding tissues.

Because TGF-α has strong angiogenic and colony-forming activities,[5,5a] one can argue the case for TGF-α content being of potential prognostic value. Median follow-up in our study is too short for meaningful analysis. However, it is interesting that those patients who have died within 18 months of biopsy had tumors which contained a mean of 5,200 pg/g TGF-α, whereas those remaining alive had a mean value of 950 pg/g. Concentration of TGF-α was also observed to be higher in those tumors which showed the greater degrees of myometrial invasion.

An important role for TGF-α, as the mediator of estrogen-induced growth, has been shown in breast cancer by Lippmann's group.[6] However, elegant work from Artega *et al.*[7] has warned against any assumption that TGF-α is the only factor involved. The latter group showed that estrogen-induced growth was preceeded by TGF-α secretion, as expected. However, if the EGF receptor is blocked with an appropriate antibody, the direct action of TGF-α is blocked. Unfortunately, cells can still be stimulated to grow by estradiol suggesting that, at least, cells have an alternative pathway to TGF-α mediation of estrogen-induced growth.

TRANSFORMING GROWTH FACTOR-β

In contrast to the growth stimulation shown in response to TGF-α, transforming growth factor-β (TGF-β) will effectively inhibit growth of reproductive epithelial cells. This has been shown in detail for breast cancer epithelial cells[8,9] and the growth inhibition was further shown to be due to increased production of TGF-β mRNA followed by synthesis and release of the growth factor. TGF-β is released in an inactive precursor form and has to be activated prior to its autocrine effect on the epithelial cell.[10] This information has been used[10] to develop a model for regulation of reproductive epithelial cells *in vitro* in which growth is stimulated by TGF-α but down-regulated by TGF-β. However, there is no reason to suppose that, in the intact endometrium, secreted and activated TGF-β might not act, in a paracrine manner, on the surrounding stroma. The affects of TGF-β on stromal cells is to promote growth and increase blood supply. As the source of the TGF-α found in endometrium has not yet been established, it would be wrong to use the *in vitro* model as a guide to the potential effects of TGF-β *in vivo*.

EPIDERMAL GROWTH FACTOR RECEPTOR

In view of the potential importance of TGF-α as a regulator of endometrial epithelial cell growth, a study was initiated on the distribution of its receptor. Since TGF-α is thought to act solely through the EGFR, we assayed EGFR in all adequate biopsies of endometrial carcinoma using a micro-assay involving 15 different concentrations of EGF over the range $0.045-12.5 \times 10^{-9}$ M. Non-specific binding was determined at each point using 100-fold unlabeled EGF. The EGF was iodine-labeled "in-house" using the iodogen method. EGFR was detected in 55% of tumors (36/66). All 36 tumors showed a high affinity binding site for EGF (range $0.01-7.1 \times 10^{-9}$ M). A lower affinity binding site (range $1.8-62 \times 10^{-9}$ M) was also detected in 31 of the tumors. No clinical significance of two binding sites, as opposed to one, has yet been established. In breast cancer, it is clear that there is an inverse relationship between EGFR status and estrogen receptor (ER) status.[11] However, in this study there was no correlation of EGFR with either ER status or ER concentration. The prognostic value of EGFR status is potentially interesting in that, in breast cancer,[11] EGFR is a positive index of poor prognosis, whereas in ovarian cancer[12] EGFR is an index of good prognosis. Although our own data on EGFR in endometrial cancer are too immature for analysis, it is interesting to note that the concentration of EGFR in the tumors of patients still alive is almost twice that found in the tumors of patients now dead. This is true for both the high and low affinity binding sites.

Interest in paracrine and autocrine effects in the endometrium lies in the fact that both stromal and epithelial cells of the endometrium respond to steroid hormones and, further, gonadotrophin effects on ovarian stromal cells may be a precursor to endometrial cancer.[13] Thus, exogenous hormones may well be the prime regulators of growth factor release in the intact endometrium. If hormone-induced growth is, in fact, mediated by paracrine growth factor action, then it is possible to explain both why some hormone-dependent tumors fail to respond to hormone therapy and also why 10% of endometrial tumors[14] which are estrogen and progesterone receptor negative, nevertheless, respond to endocrine therapy. In the first case, the hormone acts on the growth factor-releasing cell but fails to release the growth factor (or the growth factor receptor is missing from the tumor cell) despite the fact that the tumor cell contains ER and PR. In the second case the tumor cell is ER and PR negative but the hormone is acting on stroma which retains hormone sensitivity, releases growth factors and these bind to functional growth factor receptor on the tumor cells. Thus the endocrine therapy inactivates growth factor release from the endometrial stroma and hence the tumor regresses.

CONCLUSIONS

Stromal-epithelial interaction is critical to both the development of normal endometrium and to the initial development of endometrial cancers. Many of these stromal-epithelial interactions may be achieved by growth factors. Endometrial epithelial cells in culture can be stimulated to grow by both EGF and TGF-α. In endometrial cancer biopsies, TGF-α is found in over 90% and is often present at high concentration. However, the EGFR, the sole known receptor for TGF-α, is only detected in 55% of endometrial cancers. This might imply that the target tissue for the TGF-α is, in fact, the surrounding stroma. However, there is not yet any evidence to support such a view. Although our study is too immature to permit statistical analysis, two facts have emerged so far: (a) high concentrations of TGF-α in the biopsy are associated with clinical indices of poor prognosis and, correspondingly, with short survival; (b) high concentrations of EGFR do not, at this stage, predict short survival. Future work will be concentrated on the regulation of EGFR and the interaction of TGFs-α and -β.

ACKNOWLEDGMENTS

We are most grateful to Harry Gregory for supply of antibodies against EGF and TGF-α and are particularly pleased to thank ICI Pharmaceuticals for their generous support.

REFERENCES

1. STACK, G. & J. GORSKI. 1984. Direct mitogenic effect of estrogen on the prepuberal rat uterus: Studies on isolated nuclei. Endocrinology 115: 1141–1145.
2. MUNIR, I. & R. E. LEAKE. 1984. Growth potential of endometrial cells in primary culture. Biochem. Soc. Trans. 12: 259–260.
3. LEAKE, R. E., R. I. FRESHNEY & M. I. MUNIR. 1987. *In vitro* assay of responses to steroid hormones. *In* Steroid Hormones: A Practical Approach. B. Green & R. E. Leake, Eds.: 205–218. IRL Press. Oxford, UK.
4. SCHLESSINGER, J. 1988. The epidermal growth factor receptor as a multifunctional allosteric protein. Biochemistry 27: 3119–3123.
5. SCHREIBER, A. B., M. F. WINKLER & R. DERYNCK. 1988. Transforming growth factor-α—a more potent angiogenic mediator than epidermal growth factor. Science 232: 1250–1254.
5a. HANAUSKE, A. R., C. L. ARTEGA, G. M. CLARK, C. K. OSBORNE, P. HAZARIKA, R. L. PARDUE, R. E. PAQUE & D. D. VON-HOFF. 1987. α-Transforming growth factor activity (αTGF) in ovarian cancer effusions correlates with *in vivo* tumor colony formation, cytologic findings, tumor burden and patient survival. Proc. Ann. Meet. Am. Assoc. Cancer Res. 28: 178–179.
6. DICKSON, R. B. & M. E. LIPPMANN. 1987. Estogenic regulation of growth and polypeptide growth factor secretion in human breast carcinoma. Endocrine Rev. 8: 29–45.
7. ARTEGA, C. L., E. CORONADO & C. K. OSBORNE. 1988. Blockade of the epidermal growth factor receptor inhibits transforming growth factor α-induced but not estrogen-induced growth of hormone-dependent breast cancer. Mol. Endocrinol. 2: 1064–1075.
8. KERR, D. J., I. B. PRAGNELL, A. SPROUL, S. COWAN, T. MURRAY, D. GEORGE & R. LEAKE. 1989. The cytostatic effects of α-interferon may be mediated by transforming growth factor-β. J. Mol. Endocrinol. 2: 131–136.
9. KNABBE, C., M. E. LIPPMAN, L. M. WAKEFIELD, K. C. FLANDERS, A. KASID, R. DERYNCK & R. B. DICKSON. 1987. Evidence that TGF-β is a hormonally-regulated negative growth factor in breast cancer. Cell 48: 417–428.
10. LEAKE, R. E., D. KERR & F. RINALDI. 1990. Steroid hormones and growth factors in breast cancer. Ann. NY Acad. Sci. 595: 236–241.
11. SAINSBURY, J. R. C., G. K. NEEDHAM, A. MALCOLM, J. R. FARNDON & A. L. HARRIS. 1987. Epidermal growth factor receptor status as predictor of early recurrence and death from breast cancer. Lancet i: 1398–1401.
12. BAUKNECHT, T., M. RUNGE, M. SCHWALL & A. PFLEIDERER. 1988. Occurrence of epidermal growth factor receptors in human adnexal tumours and their prognostic value in advanced ovarian carcinomas. Gynecol. Oncol. 29: 147–157.
13. SNOWDEN, J. A., P. J. R. HARKIN, J. G. THORNTON & M. WELLS. 1989. Morphometric assessment of ovarian stromal proliferation—a clinicopathological study. Histopathology 14: 369–379.
14. SOUTTER, W. P. & R. E. LEAKE. 1987. Steroid hormone receptors in gynaecological cancer. Recent Advances in Obstetrics and Gynaecology 15: 175–194.

Estrogen and Progestin Receptors in the Macaque Endometrium[a]

ROBERT M. BRENNER,[b] MARYANNE C. McCLELLAN,[c]
NEAL B. WEST,[b] MILES J. NOVY,[b]
GEORGE J. HALUSKA,[b] AND MARK D. STERNFELD[d]

[b]Division of Reproductive Biology and Behavior
Oregon Regional Primate Research Center
Beaverton, Oregon 97006

[c]Department of Biology
Reed College
Portland, Oregon 97202

[d]School of Medicine
Oregon Health Sciences University
Portland, Oregon 97201

INTRODUCTION

In the past few years we and others have conducted biochemical and immunocyto-chemical studies of steroid receptors in the female reproductive tract to analyze receptor regulation and to localize steroid receptors within specific cell types. In the course of this work we have found convincing evidence that stromal-epithelial interactions play important roles in regulating the growth and differentiation of the primate endometrium. In this overview, we will discuss our work on the normal endometrium, the decidual tissue of pregnancy and the endometriotic lesions of macaques, and we will summarize our conclusions on receptor regulation and cell interactions in these tissues.

THE NORMAL ENDOMETRIUM

Animals

We used rhesus (*Macaca mulatta*), cynomolgus (*Macaca fascicularis*), and pig-tail (*Macaca nemestrina*) monkeys. Some animals were laparotomized at different times during the menstrual cycle and the reproductive tract was removed. In other experiments, animals were spayed and then treated by implanting Silastic capsules filled with crystalline steroids in subcutaneous sites.[1] Thin cross-sectional slices of the whole uterine wall were cut at the point where the endometrium was the thickest.

[a] This work, ORPRC Publication No. 1740, was supported by NIH Grants HD-19182, HD-18185, HD-06159 and RR-00163.

149

These slices were frozen for immunocytochemistry (ICC) or fixed for histology,[2] and the remainder of the endometrium and myometrium were homogenized for estrogen (E) and progestin (P) receptor (R) assays.

Antibodies

The monoclonal antibody H222 was originally prepared against purified ER obtained from a human breast cancer cell line (MCF-7) by Greene *et al.*[3] The antiPR antibody (B39) had been prepared against human PR.[4] These antibodies cross-react strongly with the rhesus monkey ER and PR.[5] A monoclonal antibody of the same immunoglobulin subclass (IgG_{2a}), anti-Timothy grass pollen (AT) was used as an irrelevant control antibody, courtesy of Dr. Arthur Malley, Oregon Regional Primate Research Center (Beaverton, OR).

Estrogen Receptor (ER) Assays

Nuclear and cytosolic ER were analyzed with binding assays as previously described.[6] We have also developed a quantitative gradient shift assay for activated nuclear ER which uses ^{3}H-estradiol (E_2) and the anti-ER monoclonal antibody H222 to effect a physical separation on a high salt sucrose gradient of the ^{3}H-E_2-ER:anti-ER complex from nonspecific binders. The specificity and quantitative characteristics of the gradient shift assay have been reported.[7,8]

Immunocytochemistry (ICC)

Receptors were localized with the immunocytochemical method previously described[1] and subsequently modified.[9] Frozen tissue was sectioned (5 µm) on a cryostat, sections were mounted on gelatin-coated glass slides then freeze-substituted for 48 h in absolute acetone at $-80°C$ (which improves cell morphology), lightly fixed, washed, and incubated overnight at $4°C$ with either H222 (10 µg/ml), B39 (1 µg/ml), or AT (10 µg/ml) as a control for nonspecific staining. The primary antibodies were detected with an avidin-biotin peroxidase kit from Vector Laboratories.

Results of Hormonal Variations

Spayed vs. Estrogen vs. Sequential Progestin

In one of our studies,[10] spayed cynomolgus macaques were either untreated, treated with a 2 cm E_2 implant for two weeks, or treated first with E_2 for 2 weeks and then E_2 plus progesterone (P) for 2 additional weeks (sequential P). The binding assays showed that in untreated spayed animals most of the receptor was cytosolic, but the ICC studies indicated that all of the specific staining was nuclear (Fig. 1A). After E_2 treatment more ER was found in both the cytosolic and nuclear fractions and there was an increase in both the intensity of nuclear staining and the number of positively stained cells (Fig. 1B). Sequential P treatment lowered cytosolic and nuclear ER in

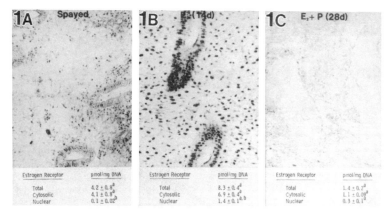

FIGURE 1. This figure is a composite that compares immunocytochemistry of ER in the functionalis zone of the endometrium with a tabulation of binding assays of ER in the whole endometrium from spayed animals that were either untreated (A), treated for 14 days with E_2 (B), or treated for 14 days with E_2 then 14 days with E_2 and P (C). ICC shows that ER is low but detectable in the nuclei of spayed untreated animals, that E_2 treatment increases the number of cells positive for ER and that sequential P treatment suppresses ER below detectable levels in the functionalis. In the tabulation, treatment groups with the same superscript letter were significantly different (Students t-test, $p < 0.01$). *Original magnification: ×250.*

the oviduct and endometrium significantly below the amount present in these tissues in E_2-treated animals, and lowered the cytosolic, but not the nuclear levels significantly below the levels found in spayed animals. After such sequential P treatment, nuclear staining was undetectable, well below the amount seen in spayed animals (FIG. 1C). Thus the nuclear staining for ER detected by ICC paralleled the total cellular ER (cytosolic plus nuclear) measured by binding assays and was increased by treatment with E_2 and decreased by sequential P treatment. These findings support the current view[11] that the ER is a nuclear protein which is synthesized in the cytoplasm and rapidly enters the nucleus in spayed as well as in hormone-treated animals. In this view, under physiological conditions, most of the ER in target cells is not occupied by ligand and therefore has low affinity for chromatin. Consequently, large amounts enter the cytosolic fractions when cells are ruptured in dilute buffers and smaller amounts remain in nuclei. However, ER is always detected in cell nuclei by ICC regardless of the hormonal state of the animal.

Immunocytochemistry also showed that in the E_2-treated animals, there was an increase in the intensity of nuclear staining of the progestin receptor (PR) in the stromal fibroblasts and the glandular epithelium of all endometrial zones (FIG. 2) compared to spayed untreated animals. The induction of PR by E_2 treatment has also been shown in rhesus monkey endometrium by Okulicz *et al.*[12] After 14 days of E_2 plus P treatment, PR staining was suppressed in most of the glandular epithelium, except for those epithelial cells in the glands of zone IV of the basalis which retained their PR (FIG. 3). However, stromal PR remained easily detectable in all zones (FIG. 4). This latter observation suggests that P suppresses its own receptor much more in the glandular epithelium than in the stroma and that the sustained effects of P on the glands of the functionalis in the late luteal phase may be mediated through the stroma, as

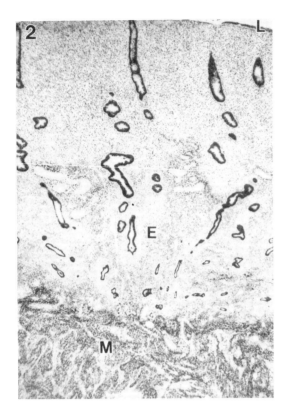

FIGURE 2. ICC of PR in animals treated for 14 days with E_2. Positive staining is evident in the stroma and glandular epithelium throughout the entire thickness of the endometrium. L = lumen, E = endometrium, M = myometrium. *Original magnification:* ×45.

the stromal cell population was the only one with detectable PR in the functionalis during most of the luteal phase. During sequential P treatment, however, ER became undetectable in most stromal cells in all regions, though like PR, ER remained detectable in the glands of the deeper basalis. In addition, ER remained detectable in the perivascular stroma and smooth muscles of the spiral arteries. The great reduction of ER in the stroma and glandular epithelium throughout the functionalis argues against any significant direct role for estrogen on these cells during progestational development of this endometrial zone, but the retention of ER in the perivascular regions of the spiral arteries indicates that E_2 could directly affect blood vessels during the luteal phase.

Menstrual Repair and the Luteal-Follicular Transition

As noted above, P suppresses endometrial ER in hormone-treated spayed animals. A similar suppression occurs during the luteal phase of the natural menstrual cycle.[13] During the luteal-follicular transition (LFT) between cycles in macaques, serum P declines while serum E_2 remains relatively constant. Consequently, P antagonism of ER is diminished and ER levels rise. To examine this increase in detail, we created

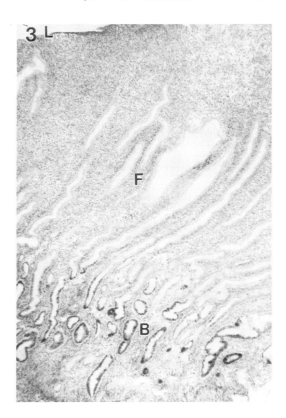

FIGURE 3. ICC of PR in animals treated with 14 days of E_2 followed by 14 days of E_2 plus P. PR staining is greatly reduced in the glandular epithelium of all zones except the deeper portions of the basalis. Stromal cells retain PR staining throughout all zones. This is more clearly seen in FIGURE 4. L = lumen, F = functionalis, B = basalis. *Original magnification:* ×45.

artificial menstrual cycles in 27 spayed macaques through the use of E_2 and P-filled Silastic capsules, and sampled the endometrium during the LFT between the end of one cycle and the first few days of the next.[1,14] We measured ER levels with binding assays and used ICC to evaluate changes in the distribution of ER and PR among the various uterine cell types.

Binding assays showed that endometrial ER concentrations increased linearly during the artificially induced follicular phase in the primate endometrium.[1] However, immunocytochemistry revealed that up to and including the time when epithelial mitotic activity began, most of the ER (FIG. 5, A–D) and PR (FIGS. 6 & 7) were specifically localized in the stromal fibroblasts, not in the epithelial cells that were mitotically active. Compaction of the stroma resulted in close associations between stromal fibroblasts and epithelial cells. These results suggested that estrogen-dependent mitotic renewal began in ER/PR-negative glandular epithelial cells that were in close association with ER/PR-positive stromal cells.

In a further test of this hypothesis, we combined steroid receptor immunocytochemistry with ^{3}H-thymidine autoradiography on the same tissue sections to determine whether the specific cells making DNA during the LFT contained ER or PR.[14] In addition, we retreated animals with progesterone (P) during the LFT to determine whether P could antagonize the effects of E_2 on epithelial mitosis when PR was only

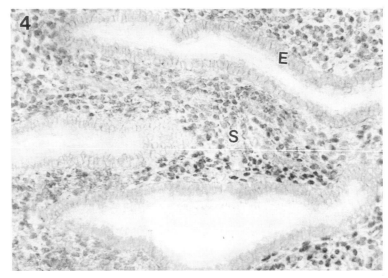

FIGURE 4. ICC of PR in the functionalis of E_2 and P treated animals. After P treatment, PR staining becomes undetectable in the glandular epithelium but remains detectable in the stromal cells. E = glandular epithelium, S = stroma. *Original magnification:* ×400.

present in stromal cells. To simplify the analysis, we confined our studies to that region of the functionalis (zone II/III) that remains after menstrual sloughing, because this is the region that undergoes estrogen-dependent proliferation after serum P declines. At 4 days after P withdrawal, there was little ^{3}H-thymidine uptake (FIG. 8). At 4.5 days after P withdrawal there was a burst of DNA synthesis in the epithelium, but the great majority of epithelial cells that were autoradiographically positive for ^{3}H-thymidine uptake were immunocytochemically negative for both ER and PR (FIG. 9). By day 5 of P withdrawal most of the ^{3}H-thymidine positive cells were still PR-negative and many were still ER-negative, though ER had become detectable in many ^{3}H-thymidine positive cells (FIG. 10). Retreatment with P on days 3–4 of the LFT (when PR was only present in the stroma) significantly inhibited DNA synthesis in epithelial cells, as measured by a decrease in the number of ^{3}H-thymidine labeled cells (FIG. 11). P retreatment also significantly lowered the amount of total endometrial ER measured biochemically, but ICC showed that this suppressive effect of P on ER occurred only in the stroma.[14] Taken together these data indicated that E_2 treatment could stimulate DNA synthesis in epithelial cells that lacked ER, and P treatment could suppress DNA synthesis in epithelial cells that lacked PR. These findings support our hypothesis that the effects of E_2 on epithelial DNA synthesis in endometrial zone II/III during the very early proliferative phase of the menstrual cycle in non-human primates may be mediated indirectly through factors released from the stroma. Whether stromal cells continue to mediate the effects of E_2 on epithelial mitosis as the cycle progresses remains to be determined.

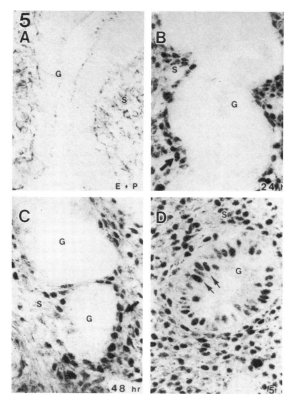

FIGURE 5. ICC of ER in the functionalis during the luteal-follicular transition (LFT). ER staining is negative in stroma and glands after 28 days of sequential E_2 plus P administration (**A**), is positive only in the stroma 24 (**B**), and 48 (**C**) hours after P withdrawal and does not become positive in large numbers of glandular epithelial cells until 5 days (**D**) after P withdrawal. G = glands, S = stroma. *Original magnification:* ×400.

Naturally Cycling Animals

In naturally cycling animals, the pattern of ER and PR staining in the endometrium throughout the cycle and during the transition between cycles is essentially as described above for the hormonally treated ones. Other laboratories have reported similar findings in women.[15,16] By midcycle, the majority of stromal fibroblasts and glandular epithelial cells are positively stained for ER and PR. After ovulation there is a decline in the intensity of ER staining in both stromal and epithelial cells that is evident first in the outer zones (I and II) and later in zone III. The stromal cells in zone IV are also suppressed, but the glandular epithelium of zone IV retains its ER staining. After ovulation the endometrial glands showed a loss of PR staining in the glandular epithelium, first in the outer zones and later in the inner zones. The glands in the deepest

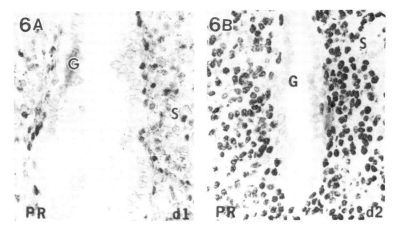

FIGURE 6. ICC of PR in the functionalis during days 1 and 2 of the LFT. PR staining is only detectable in the stroma, not the glandular epithelium on days 1 (A) and 2 (B) of P withdrawal. *Original magnification:* ×400.

region of the basalis (zone IV) retained their PR staining longer than the other zones. Stromal cells retained PR staining throughout the entire endometrium.

DECIDUAL STEROID RECEPTORS AND THE EFFECTS OF RU 486

In preliminary work, we noted that in pregnant monkeys the P-induced suppression of endometrial ER and PR which began in the luteal phase was maintained

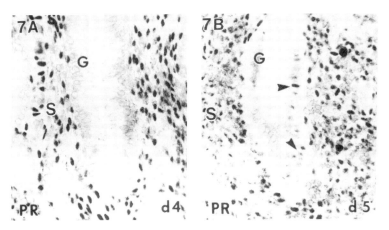

FIGURE 7. ICC of PR in the functionalis during days 4 (A) and 5 (B) of the LFT. PR is detectable in the stroma throughout this period, but does not appear in the glandular epithelium until day 5. Arrowheads point to PR positive nuclei in the glandular epithelium on day 5. *Original magnification:* ×400.

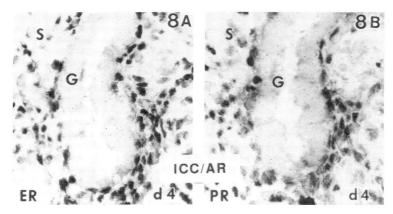

FIGURE 8. Combined immunocytochemical/autoradiographic (ICC/AR) preparations on day 4 of the LFT showing ER on the left (A) and PR on the right (B) in sections labeled with ³H-thymidine. ER and PR are only detectable in the stroma and there are no cells making DNA. *Original magnification:* ×400.

throughout pregnancy. Immunocytochemical studies of the decidua and the myometrium showed that while ER remained suppressed in both the epithelium and the stroma, and PR remained suppressed in the epithelium, PR continued to be detectable in the endometrial stroma just as in the late luteal phase.

To further study these relationships we examined the effects of the progestin antagonist RU 486[17] whose contragestational effects are due to an effective P withdrawal.[18] To date we have studied the changes in ER levels during midgestation, during

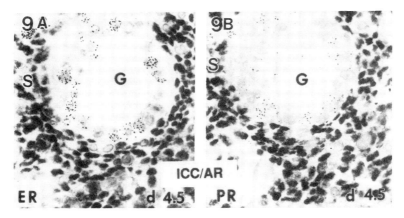

FIGURE 9. Combined immunocytochemical/autoradiographic (ICC/AR) preparations on day 4.5 of the LFT showing ER on the left (A) and PR on the right (B) in sections labeled with ³H-thymidine. On day 4.5, DNA synthesis is evident in many glandular epithelial cells, most of which are negative for ER (A) and PR (B). In both A and B, the slight nuclear staining evident is due to hematoxylin staining of chromatin. Only the stroma contains detectable levels of ER and PR. *Original magnification:* ×400.

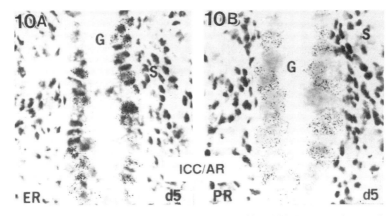

FIGURE 10. Combined immunocytochemical/autoradiographic (ICC/AR) preparations on day 5 of the LFT. As above, ER is on the left (A) and PR on the right (B) in sections labeled with ^{3}H-thymidine. About half the cells making DNA have become ER positive by day 5 (A), but almost none are PR positive. *Original magnification:* ×400.

and after spontaneous term labor and after RU 486 treatment of midpregnant animals. We have also obtained preliminary data concerning changes in PR in similar animals.[19]

Animals

Timed pregnant rhesus macaques (*Macaca mulatta*) were obtained from the breeding colony. At approximately day 110 of pregnancy, the animals were conditioned to a jacket and tether system.[20] Animals were surgically instrumented with maternal femoral arterial and venous catheters, intra-amniotic pressure catheters, myometrial bipolar electromyographic electrodes and fetal electrocardiographic electrodes as previously described.[21] Surgical instrumentation occurred on days 119–124 of pregnancy for RU 486–treated animals (n = 6). Six to nine days after surgery, some animals received RU 486 at a dose of 20 mg/kg/d for 3 days at 10:00 h each day. The fetuses were delivered by cesarean section 72 hours after the last dose. Uterine wall biopsies were collected from 7 control animals (vehicle only) on days 121–136 of pregnancy.

Two pregnant animals that had been instrumented received no treatment except for control vehicle. When they were in labor the fetuses were delivered by cesarean section. Biopsies of tissues were also collected from a third animal 2.5 hours postpartum (parturient controls). Full thickness sections of the uterine wall, including amnion, chorion, decidua and myometrium, were collected in Hepes buffered Hanks solution, separated under a dissecting microscope and prepared for gradient shift assay of ER levels and immunocytochemical detection of ER and PR.

RESULTS

Immunocytochemistry revealed a great increase in staining for ER in the decidual stromal cells in RU 486-treated rhesus macaques when compared to pregnant control

11

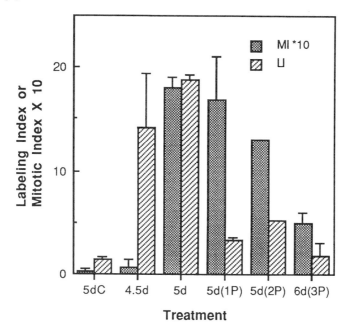

FIGURE 11. Labeling index (LI) and mitotic index (MI) in endometrial zone II/III under different hormonal conditions associated with the LFT. In each case, animals had been treated with the sequential P regimen for 28 days before the procedures below were initiated. The treatments indicated by the code under each pair of bars are as follows:

Code	Treatment
5C	Controls, sampled on day 5 after withdrawal of both E_2 and P capsules.
4.5	Sampled on day 4.5 of LFT.
5	Sampled on day 5 of LFT.
5(1P)	Sampled on day 5 of LFT but with P reinserted 1 day previously.
5(2P)	Sampled on day 5 of LFT but with P reinserted 2 days previously.
6(3P)	Sampled on day 6 of LFT but with P reinserted 3 days previously.
	n = 3 except for group 5(2P), where n = 2.

animals (FIG. 12). This increase did not occur in any other decidual cell type; the luminal epithelium was immunocytochemically negative. However, there was no similar increase in ER staining in the decidual stromal cells obtained from animals in or shortly after labor. The gradient shift assay, which measures the amount of receptor shifted by antibody to the 8S peak (expressed as femtomoles of E_2 bound per mg DNA) showed that RU 486 treatment greatly increased the amount of nuclear ER in decidual tissues (52.3 $\pm$ 16.8) compared to pregnant controls (7.3 $\pm$ 2.4; $p < 0.05$). In tissues obtained during or immediately after natural labor, the nuclear ER (7.7 $\pm$ 3.1) remained unchanged compared to the levels found earlier in pregnancy. Cytosolic ER levels showed similar patterns: levels were higher in RU 486-treated than pregnant

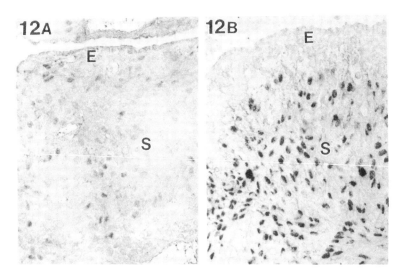

FIGURE 12. ICC of ER in decidua of control (A) and RU 486 treated (B) pregnant rhesus monkeys. In controls, ER is barely detectable in the decidual stromal cells and nondetectable in the maternal epithelium. After RU 486 treatment, ER becomes easily detectable in the stromal cells but remains undetectable in the maternal epithelium. *Original magnification:* ×400.

controls (240.5 $\pm$ 145.3 vs. 17.1 $\pm$ 6.4 fmol/mg DNA respectively) and there was no increase during labor (16.4 $\pm$ 8.8 fmol/mg DNA).

Analysis of fetal membranes by immunocytochemistry and the gradient shift assay revealed no ER in either amnion or chorion from pregnant control or parturient animals. Despite RU 486 treatment, there was no appearance of ER in any of the specimens of fetal membranes.

In preliminary work[19] we have found that PR was also absent from the amnion, chorion and the luminal epithelial cells of the decidua. PR was present throughout pregnancy in decidual stromal and myometrial smooth muscle cells, but showed little change during spontaneous or RU 486–induced labor.

In summary, the data clearly indicate that RU 486 treatment greatly increased ER levels in both the decidua and myometrium of rhesus macaques in late pregnancy compared to age-matched, vehicle-treated pregnant controls. Previous studies in rhesus macaques have shown that 3 to 4 days of actual P withdrawal is sufficient time for a significant increase in endometrial ER to occur.[1] Presumably, RU 486 blocks the suppressive effect of P on ER by causing an effective P withdrawal at the cellular level. RU 486 can have a similar effect on P-suppressed ER levels in uteri of rats.[22] ER was not detected either before or after RU 486 treatment in amnion or chorion of our animals. ER was also absent from human fetal membranes collected at normal delivery.[23,24] Evidently, the reason RU 486 had no effect on ER levels in amnion, chorion and the luminal epithelium of the decidua is that PR was not present in these cell types.[19]

It remains to be shown whether the RU 486–induced increase in decidual/myometrial ER contributes to any biological effect of E_2 in the pregnant uterus. The high level of uterine contractility and the atypical contraction pattern generated by RU 486[21] may be related to the increase in ER levels. Data from our laboratory indicates that myometrial gap junctions are increased by RU 486 treatment in pregnant rhesus macaques.[25,26] In pregnant rats, because RU 486 treatment led to increased numbers of myometrial gap junctions, Garfield *et al.*[27] concluded that estrogens favor and progestins suppress gap junction formation. However, we found no increase in ER in decidual or myometrial cells during spontaneous labor, and serum P does not decline during normal parturition. Consequently, we have concluded that although labor can be induced by an experimentally imposed P withdrawal, the natural trigger for the onset of labor in primates remains to be elucidated.

RECEPTOR REGULATION IN ENDOMETRIOSIS

We studied changes in ER by biochemical and immunocytochemical techniques in a group of rhesus monkeys diagnosed with endometriosis in order to examine the distribution of ER in the stromal and glandular epithelial cells of endometriotic lesions.[28]

Spontaneous endometriosis has been described in rhesus macaques[29] cynomolgus macaques[30] and baboons.[31] Endometriosis generally occurs in middle-aged or older monkeys, as in women, and symptoms include menstrual irregularities, infertility, and dysmenorrhea. Comparative histological observations indicate close similarities between human and monkey forms of the disease.

Although Roddick *et al.*[32] have reported that endometriotic lesions differentiate synchronously with endometrium during the menstrual cycle, other biochemical, ultrastructural, and autoradiographic studies of endometriotic lesions suggest that endometriotic lesions can exhibit incomplete progestational responses.[33-35] Several investigators have reported that ER and PR levels in endometriotic lesions differ significantly from levels found in normal endometria.[36,37] In our studies, we selected normally cycling animals with endometriosis and compared changes in the lesions with those in the endometrium of the same monkeys during the menstrual cycle.

Animals

Rhesus macaques (*Macaca mulatta*) with confirmed endometriosis were identified in the breeding colony at the Oregon Regional Primate Research Center. These animals were serially bled over 60 days, and E_2 and P levels were determined by radioimmunoassay (RIA), as previously described.[6] Hormone levels in the selected animals at the time of tissue sampling were as follows: follicular phase, n = 7 (E_2 = 120.8 $\pm$ 42.4 pg/ml, P = 0.5 $\pm$ 0.2 ng/ml); luteal phase, n = 8 (E_2 = 61.2 $\pm$ 12.0 pg/ml, P = 3.0 $\pm$ 0.7 ng/ml).

Tissue Handling

Although most animals were laparotomized, others were euthanized because recovery from surgery was precluded due to the severity of the disease. Wherever possible, endometriotic lesions and endometrium were removed from the same animal (n = 9). Endometrium could not be obtained from some animals where the endometriosis had caused severe physical distortion of the uterus. The endometrium was dissected from myometrium, and the mucosa of endometriotic cysts was separated from the underlying fibrous tissue. Fresh tissues were then apportioned for analysis by immunocytochemistry of ER, receptor binding assays, and light microscopy. The percentages of ER positive cells in both the stromal and the epithelial compartments were determined by counting 300 to 400 cells per tissue compartment per tissue sample. Epithelial counts included only cells in the glands of zones II and III (functionalis) of the endometrium[38] and in the glands of the endometriotic lesions. In endometrium, stromal counts included only stromal fibroblasts; lymphocytes, neutrophils, macrophages, endothelia, and vascular smooth muscle cells were excluded. In lesions, only stromal fibroblasts that resembled eutopic endometrial stromal cells were counted. Very slender, spindle shaped fibroblasts that had apparently invaded the lesion from neighboring connective tissues were not counted.

Comparisons of Endometria and Lesions in the Follicular and Luteal Phases

Eutopic Endometria

During the follicular phase, the mean percentage of ER positive epithelial and stromal cells was 95% $\pm$ 1.7 and 86% $\pm$ 11.6, respectively. During the luteal phase, the mean percentages of ER positive epithelial and stromal cells fell to 27.8% $\pm$ 13.0 and 32% $\pm$ 11.0, respectively (FIG. 1A). Hence, the percentage of ER positive cells was significantly less during the luteal than the follicular phase in both epithelial ($p < .05$), and stromal ($p < .025$) compartments of the functionalis (endometrial zones II and III). Staining intensity was also greatly diminished during the luteal phase.

Endometriotic Lesions

In the lesions there were no significant differences between the follicular and luteal phases in the mean percent of ER positive epithelial or stromal cells. The number of ER positive stromal cells was significantly lower in lesions than in eutopic endometria during the follicular phase. The lack of change in the mean percent of ER positive stromal cells in the lesions during the cycle, and their lower number during the follicular phase indicates an important difference in the mode of ER regulation between lesions and endometria.

Biochemical analysis of ER in endometriotic lesions indicated that the levels of receptor did not significantly change throughout the menstrual cycle. Receptor levels (fmol/mg DNA $\pm$ standard error of mean) in lesion biopsies from 3 follicular animals (cytosolic, 403 $\pm$ 447; nuclear, 492 $\pm$ 527) were statistically indistinguishable from values obtained from 6 luteal animals (cytosolic, 561 $\pm$ 512; nuclear, 539 $\pm$ 174). Too few eutopic endometria were obtained for biochemical analysis to test for significant differences during the cycle, but the normally suppressive effect of elevated serum P on endometrial ER levels has been well established by ourselves and others.[6]

Histological evaluation revealed that the eutopic endometria were similar to those taken from normal monkeys during the menstrual cycle.[38] In the lesions however, the characteristic zonation typical of eutopic endometrium was never observed. Some endometriotic lesions were primarily composed of glandular elements, but it was more common for stromal fibroblasts to predominate. In most lesions both proliferative and secretory features were present simultaneously, such as the presence of highly sinuous, secretory glands (progestational) with extensive mitotic activity (proliferative). Glands of the lesions were usually surrounded by a dense, compact stroma much denser than normally seen in eutopic endometria.

Our study demonstrated that in a group of regularly cycling animals with endometriosis, the endometriotic lesions exhibited several features distinct from the endometrium. The lesions were histologically out of phase with the endometrium from the same animal. Most lesions had low numbers of ER-positive stromal cells and exhibited great variation in the percentage of ER-positive epithelial cells during the menstrual cycle. Stromal and epithelial cells both showed an insensitivity to the normally suppressive effect of P[6,39] on levels of endometrial ER. The low percentage of ER-positive cells in stroma of all lesions (and the epithelia of some lesions) during the follicular phase also suggested a loss in the capacity of these cells to increase ER in response to both the decline in serum P during the LFT and the increase in serum E_2 that occurs during the mid and late follicular phase.

Although we have not yet evaluated PR in endometriotic lesions, it appears that P does not suppress ER in either stromal or epithelial cells, and the usual progestational effects of P are not expressed uniformly in either cell type. Studies on cellular localization of PR in macaque endometriotic lesions are needed to evaluate more fully the mechanisms underlying the aberrant behavior patterns exhibited by stromal and epithelial cells in these tissues.

OVERALL CONCLUSIONS

Our major conclusion is that paracrine interactions between the cells of the normal macaque endometrium are more important than previously appreciated. During the natural cycle, PR is retained in the stromal cells but disappears from most of the glandular epithelium early in the luteal phase. Yet, the progestational effects of P on glandular differentiation continue throughout the luteal phase. During the LFT, ER and PR are only present in the stromal cells, yet E_2-dependent DNA synthesis occurs in the glandular epithelial cells, and such E_2-dependent epithelial cell DNA synthesis can be blocked by P administration.

In the decidua during pregnancy, ER is nondetectable in epithelial cells and barely detectable in stromal cells because of the suppressive effects of P on ER that begin during the luteal phase of the cycle. Although PR is also lacking from epithelial cells during pregnancy, it is retained in decidual stromal cells. RU 486 can act to relieve the suppression of ER in stromal cells, which have PR, but not in epithelial cells, which lack PR. These data suggest that receptors are regulated differently within different cell types, and that the direct genomic effects of E_2 and P are only expressed in cells that contain ER and PR respectively. This was also evident when we retreated animals with P during the LFT; ER was only suppressed in cells that had PR. Therefore, another conclusion we have drawn is that steroid receptor regulation appears to be an intracellular event directly influenced by the relevant steroids and not by intercellular factors.

In endometriotic lesions, ER regulation in stromal and epithelial cells is abnormal, and the typical effects of E_2 and P on histological differentiation are aberrant as well. Endometriosis thus appears to be a disease associated with derangements in both receptor regulation and cell-cell interaction. A fuller understanding of receptor regulation and stromal-epithelial communication in the female reproductive tract should lead to improved therapy for this and other endometrial diseases.

ACKNOWLEDGMENTS

We thank Angela Adler for word processing and Kunie Mah for technical assistance.

REFERENCES

1. McClellan, M., N. B. West & R. M. Brenner. 1986. Immunocytochemical localization of estrogen receptors in the macaque endometrium during the luteal-follicular transition. Endocrinology 119: 2467–2475.
2. Sandow, B. A., N. B. West, R. L. Norman & R. M. Brenner. 1979. Hormonal control of apoptosis in hamster uterine luminal epithelium. Am. J. Anat. 156: 15–36.
3. Greene, G. L., C. Nolan, J. P. Engler & E. V. Jensen. 1980. Monoclonal antibodies to human estrogen receptor. Proc. Natl. Acad. Sci. USA 77: 5115–5119.
4. Press, M. F. & G. L. Greene. 1988. Localization of progesterone receptor with monoclonal antibodies to the human progestin receptor. Endocrinology 122: 1165–1175.
5. Brenner, R. M. & N. B. West. 1987. Immunocytochemistry of the progestin receptor in the reproductive tract of female macaques. Program of the 69th Annual Meeting of the Endocrine Society, Indianapolis, IN, p. 79 (Abstract).
6. West, N. B. & R. M. Brenner. 1985. Progesterone-mediated suppression of estradiol receptors in cynomolgus macaque cervix, endometrium and oviduct during sequential estradiol-progesterone treatment. J. Steroid Biochem. 22: 29–37.
7. West, N. B., C. E. Roselli, J. A. Resko, G. L. Greene & R. M. Brenner. 1988. Estrogen and progestin receptors and aromatase activity in rhesus monkey prostate. Endocrinology 123: 2312–2322.
8. West, N. B., K. S. Carlisle & R. M. Brenner. 1990. Progesterone treatment suppresses estrogen receptor in the sex skin of *Macaca nemestrina*. J. Steroid Biochem. 35: 481–485.
9. Brenner, R. M., K. Mah, N. B. West & M. C. McClellan. 1988. An improved immunocytochemical technique for localization of estrogen and progestin receptors in cryostat sections. *In* Program of the 8th International Congress of Histochemistry and Cytochemistry, Washington, DC, p. 924 (Abstract).
10. West, N. B., M. C. McClellan, M. D. Sternfeld & R. M. Brenner. 1987. Immunocytochemistry versus binding assays of the estrogen receptor in the reproductive tract of spayed and hormone treated macaques. Endocrinology 121: 1789–1800.
11. Gorski, J., W. V. Welshons, D. Sakai, J. Hansen, J. Walent, J. Kassis, J. Shull, G. Stack & C. Campen. 1986. Evolution of a model of estrogen action. *In* Recent Progress in Hormone Research. R. O. Greep, Ed.: 297–329. Academic Press, NY.
12. Okulicz, W. C., A. M. Savassta, L. M. Hoberg & C. Longcope. 1989. Immunofluorescent analysis of estrogen induction of progesterone receptor in the rhesus uterus. Endocrinology 125: 930–934.
13. West, N. B. & R. M. Brenner. 1983. Estrogen receptor levels in the oviducts and endometria of cynomolgus macaques during the menstrual cycle. Biol. Reprod. 29: 1303–1312.
14. McClellan, M. C., S. Rankin, N. B. West & R. M. Brenner. 1990. Estrogen receptors, progestin receptors and DNA synthesis in the macaque endometrium during the luteal-follicular transition. J. Steroid Biochem. & Mol. Biol. In press.
15. Garcia, E., P. Bouchard, J. De Brux, J. Berdah, R. Frydman, G. Schaison, E. Milgrom

& M. PERROT-APPLANAT. 1988. Use of immunocytochemistry of progesterone and estrogen receptors for endometrial dating. J. Clin. Endocrinol. Metab. **67:** 80–87.

16. BERGERON, C., A. FERENCZY, D. O. TOFT, W. SCHNEIDER & G. SHYAMALA. 1988. Immunocytochemical study of progesterone receptors in the human endometrium during the menstrual cycle. Lab. Invest. **59:** 862–869.

17. HALUSKA, G. J., N. B. WEST, M. J. NOVY & R. M. BRENNER. 1990. Uterine estrogen receptors are increased by RU486 in late pregnant rhesus macaques but not after spontaneous labor. J. Clin. Endocrinol. Metab. **70:** 181–186.

18. GERMAIN, G., D. PHILIBERT, J. POTTIER, M. MOUREN, E. E. BAULIEU & C. SUREAU. 1985. Effects of the antiprogesterone agent RU 486 on the natural cycle and gestation in the intact cynomolgus monkeys. *In* The Antiprogesterone Steroid RU 486 and Human Fertility Control. E. E. Baulieu & S. J. Segal, Eds.: 155–168. Plenum Press, NY.

19. HIRST, J. J., N. B. WEST, R. M. BRENNER & M. J. NOVY. Myometrial and decidual progesterone receptors during gestation, in spontaneous labor and after RU486 treatment in rhesus monkeys. *In* Abstracts of Serono Symposia, USA Symposium, Uterine Contractility: Mechanisms of Control (St. Louis, MO, 3/17–20/90), p. 41, abstract 17.

20. DUCSAY, C. A., M. J. COOK & M. J. NOVY. 1988. Simplified vest and tether system for maintenance of chronically catheterized pregnant rhesus monkeys. Lab. Anim. Sci. **38:** 343–344.

21. HALUSKA, G. J., STANCZYK, F. Z., M. J. COOK & M. J. NOVY. 1987. Temporal changes in uterine activity and prostaglandin response to RU486 in late gestation rhesus macaques. Am. J. Obstet. Gynecol. **157:** 1487–1495.

22. OKULICZ, W. C. 1987. Effect of the antiprogestin RU-486 on progesterone inhibition of occupied nuclear estrogen receptor in the uterus. J. Steroid. Biochem. **28:** 117–122.

23. KHAN-DAWOOD, F. S. & M. D. DAWOOD. 1984. Estrogen and progesterone receptor and hormone levels in human myometrium and placenta in term pregnancy. Am. J. Obstet. Gynecol. **150:** 501–505.

24. PADAYACHI, T., R. J. PEGORARO, J. HOFMEYR, S. M. JOUBERT & R. J. NORMAN. 1987. Decreased concentrations and affinities of oestrogen and progesterone receptors of intrauterine tissue in human pregnancy. J. Steroid Biochem. **26:** 473–479.

25. HALUSKA, G. J., I. C. JAY & M. J. NOVY. Gap junctions in the primate myometrium: Effect of RU 486. Biol. Reprod. **40** (Suppl. 1): 131 (abst. 250).

26. SAITO, Y., H. SAKAMOTO, N. J. MACLUSKY & F. NAFTOLIN. 1985. Gap junctions and myometrial steroid hormone receptors in pregnant and postpartum rats: A possible cellular basis for the progesterone withdrawal hypothesis. Am. J. Obstet. Gynecol. **151:** 805–812.

27. GARFIELD, R. E., J. M. GASC & E.-E. BAULIEU. 1987. Effects of the antiprogesterone RU 486 on preterm birth in the rat. Am. J. Obstet. Gynecol. **157:** 1281–1285.

28. STERNFELD, M.D., N. B. WEST & R. M. BRENNER. 1988. Immunocytochemistry of the estrogen receptor in spontaneous endometriosis in rhesus macaques. Fertil. Steril. **49:** 342–348.

29. KLUVER, H. & G. W. BARTELMEZ. 1951. Endometriosis in a rhesus monkey. Surg. Gynecol. Obstet. **92:** 650–660.

30. FANTON, J. W. & G. B. HUBBARD. 1983. Spontaneous endometriosis in a cynomolgus monkey (*Macaca fascicularis*). Lab. Anim. Sci. **33:** 597–599.

31. FOLSE, D. S. & L. C. STOUT. 1978. Endometriosis in a baboon (*Papio doguera*). Lab. Anim. Sci. **28:** 217–219.

32. RODDICK, J. W., JR., G. CONKEY & E. J. JACOBS. 1960. The hormonal response of endometrium in endometriotic implants and its relationship to symptomatology. Am. J. Obstet. Gynecol. **79:** 1173–1177.

33. VIERIKKO, P., A. KAUPPILA, L. RONNBERG & R. VIHKO. 1985. Steroidal regulation of endometriosis tissue: Lack of induction of 17 beta-hydroxysteroid dehydrogenase activity by progesterone, medroxyprogesterone acetate, or danazol. Fertil. Steril. **43:** 218–224.

34. SCHWEPPE, K. W., R. M. WYNN & F. K. BELLER. 1984. Ultrastructural comparison of endometriotic implants and eutopic endometrium. Am. J. Obstet. Gynecol. **148:** 1024–1039.

35. GOULD, S. F., J. M. SHANNON & G. R. CUNHA. 1983. Nuclear estrogen binding sites in human endometriosis. Fertil. Steril. **39:** 520–524.

36. TAMAYA, T., T. MOTOYAMA, Y. OHONO, N. IDE, T. TSURUSAKI & H. OKADA. 1979. Steroid receptor levels and histology of endometriosis and adenomyosis. Fertil. Steril. **31:** 396–400.

37. JANNE, O., A. KAUPPILA, E. KOKKO, T. LANTTO, L. RONNBERG & R. VIHKO. 1981. Estrogen and progestin receptors in endometriosis lesions: Comparison with endometrial tissue. Am. J. Obstet. Gynecol. **141:** 562–566.
38. BARTELMEZ, G. W. 1951. Cyclic changes in the endometrium of the rhesus monkey (*Macaca mulatta*). Contrib. Embryol. **34:** 99–144.
39. BRENNER, R. M., N. B. WEST, R. L. NORMAN, B. A. SANDOW & H. G. VERHAGE. 1979. Progesterone suppression of the estradiol receptor in the reproductive tract of macaques, cats and hamsters. Adv. Exp. Med. Biol. **117:** 173–196.

Plasminogen Activators in Endometrial Physiology and Embryo Implantation: A Review

BRUCE A. LITTLEFIELD[a]

Section of Biology
Eisai Research Institute
Andover, Massachusetts 01810

INTRODUCTION

Plasminogen activators (PAs) are highly specific serine proteases which cleave the inactive zymogen plasminogen to the potent general protease plasmin. In its classical role, the PA/plasmin system constitutes the body's fibrinolytic system. However, it is now clear that this system also plays a critical role in cell attachment, migration, and invasiveness by providing a source of localized extracellular proteolysis. Interest in the role of the PA/plasmin system in endometrial physiology accelerated markedly in the late 1970s after it was found that uterine PAs were regulated throughout the endometrial cycle of proliferation, maturation, decidualization, and menstruation. Other studies at the same time implicated embryo-derived PAs as mediators of trophoblast implantation and early embryonic differentiation. In the last decade, most of the key components of the PA/plasmin system have been identified, purified, characterized, and cloned: uPA, tPA, plasminogen/plasmin, the two PA inhibitors PAI-1 and PAI-2, and cell surface uPA receptors. These advances have led to new levels of sophistication in studies of the PA/plasmin system in the endometrium. This paper will present an historical perspective of investigations in this area and summarize our current knowledge of the PA/plasmin system in endometrial physiology and embryo implantation.

THE PA/PLASMIN SYSTEM

In its role as the primary mediator of fibrinolysis (blood clot dissolution) the PA/plasmin system is the functional counterpart of the blood clotting cascade. In fact, the two systems share many similarities: both consist of a series of inactive and active proteases and inhibitors, each active protease specifically activating the next inactive protease in the cascade. The clotting cascade culminates in cleavage of prothrombin to thrombin, which initiates blood clot formation by cleaving fibrinogen to fibrin, polymerization of the latter leading to blood clot formation. In contrast, the PA/plasmin system culminates in cleavage of plasminogen to plasmin, a broad spectrum serine

[a] *Direct all correspondence to*: Bruce A. Littlefield, Ph.D., Section of Biology, Eisai Research Institute, 4 Corporate Drive, Andover, MA 01810; (508) 794-1117.

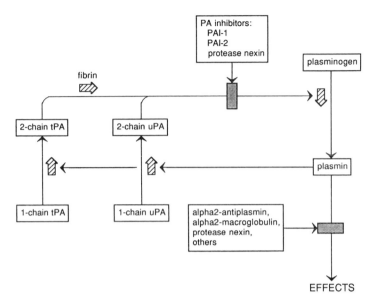

FIGURE 1. Essential components of the PA/plasmin system. *Striped arrows* indicate stimulation; *cross-hatched boxes* indicate inhibition. (See text and refs. 1–6 for details.)

protease which, among other things, can lyse clots by degrading fibrin to soluble degradation products.

The essential components of the PA/plasmin system are shown in FIGURE 1. Since the details of this complex system have been presented in several recent reviews,[1-6] only the most salient points will be discussed here. The central feature of the system is conversion of plasminogen to plasmin by either of the two PAs urokinase (uPA) or tissue-type PA (tPA). While uPA and tPA share a common specificity for a single arginine-valine bond in plasminogen (Arg[560]-Val[561]), an important difference between the two is that tPA's enzymatic activity is highly dependent on binding to fibrin, consistent with the greater importance of tPA in fibrinolysis relative to cellular migration and invasiveness (see below). Both PAs are produced in single chain forms with low (tPA) or no (uPA) enzymatic activity; cleavage of either by trace amounts of plasmin generates the fully active two-chain forms of both enzymes. Local activity of the PA/plasmin system is controlled by regulated cellular production of uPA and tPA as well as two specific PA inhibitors (PAIs) PAI-1 and PAI-2 and a more general protease inhibitor, protease nexin. The action of plasmin itself is confined to locations where local concentrations are high enough to overcome inhibition by ubiquitous plasmin inhibitors such as α_2-antiplasmin and α_2-macroglobulin. For more detailed discussions of the PA/plasmin system, the reader is again referred to several excellent reviews on the topic.[1-6]

In addition to its importance in fibrinolysis, the PA/plasmin system is also involved in or associated with other biological processes which depend on regulated, localized, extracellular proteolysis. Several of these processes are listed in TABLE 1. A common denominator of most of these processes is cellular degradation of extracellular barriers

TABLE 1. Involvement of the PA/Plasmin System in Non-Fibrinolytic Processes

Process	Reference(s)
Ovulation	38,56–58
Embryo implantation	33–43
Mammary gland involution	59
Prostate gland involution	60,61
Angiogenesis	62
Bone resorption, remodeling	63,64
Cellular differentiation	33,34,65–69
Embryonic nerve cell growth	70
Tumor metastasis and invasion	1,2,5,71–74

such as extracellular matrix (ECM) or basement membrane (BM). In this capacity, the PA/plasmin system provides localized extracellular proteolysis for ECM and BM degradation and subsequent cellular migration or invasiveness. PA/plasmin-dependent ECM and BM degradation involves not only direct degradation of non-collagenous components by plasmin, but also degradation of collagen via activation of latent collagenases by plasmin. The relationships between these processes are shown in FIGURE 2; greater details are presented in the review articles mentioned above.[1-6]

Of the two PAs, uPA plays the most important role in generating extracellular proteolysis for ECM and BM degradation, cellular migration, and invasiveness.[1-6] The importance of uPA in these processes is consistent with the fibrin-independent nature of its activity as well as its binding to high affinity uPA receptors on the surfaces of invasive cells.[1-6] In contrast, the primary physiological action of tPA appears to be fibrinolysis, consistent with the fibrin-dependent nature of its activity.[1-6]

PAs AND THE ENDOMETRIUM

Studies of the PA/plasmin system in the human endometrium essentially began about seventy-five years ago when Whitehouse,[7] and then Kross,[8] attributed the inability of human menstrual blood to clot to the presence of fibrinolytic agents in uterine secretions. Thirty years later the fluidity of menstrual blood was attributed to the release from the endometrium of specific fibrinolytic proteases during menstruation.[9-11] In 1956, Albrechtsen demonstrated that the human uterus is a rich source of PA.[12]

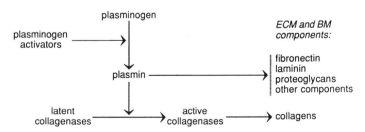

FIGURE 2. Involvement of the PA/plasmin system in ECM and BM degradation. (See text and refs. 1–6 for details.)

Later studies by others indicated that tPA is probably the dominant PA type in the myometrium,[13-16] while both uPA and tPA are found in the endometrium.[17-20] PA activity in both human endometrium and myometrium varies throughout the menstrual cycle, increasing during the proliferative phase, reaching maximal levels at mid-cycle, decreasing during the luteal phase, and increasing again prior to menstruation.[12,20-23] In 1981, PA activity was found in non-menstrual human uterine luminal fluid.[17,24-26] Similar to findings in uterine tissues, uterine luminal fluid PA activity increases during the proliferative phase, reaches maximal levels at mid-cycle, decreases during the luteal phase, and increases again prior to menstruation.[17,24-26] Finally, in addition to being regulated during the menstrual cycle, alterations in endometrial and uterine luminal fluid PA activities are seen with the use of both oral contraceptives and intrauterine contraceptive devices.[17,18,20,23,25,26]

Such observations suggested to several investigators that endometrial PA expression was hormonally regulated. In the 1950s and 1960s, Albrechtsen[27] and Kwann and Albrechtsen[28] observed that estradiol altered the fibrinolytic activity of extracts from rat uterus. This concept was further explored by Kneifel et al.[29] who used immature female rats to show steroid-specific stimulation of uterine PA activity by estrogens, an effect which was suppressible by triphenylethylene antiestrogens. These investigators then showed that estrogen stimulation of PA activity was observed in both stromal/myometrial and epithelial fractions of the rat uterus.[30] Importantly, the highest PA activity levels on a per milligram protein basis were observed not in the uterine tissues themselves but in uterine luminal fluid from estradiol-stimulated rats.[30] In the same year, Finlay et al.[31] demonstrated estradiol-stimulated uptake of plasminogen into mouse uterine luminal fluid. Taken together, these observations in animal models provided strong evidence that estrogen regulation of PA activity played an important role in uterine physiology.

Hormonal regulation of PA activity in the human endometrium was addressed by Casslen et al.,[19] who used explants of proliferative phase human endometrium in organ culture to assess effects of estradiol and progesterone on PA secretion. While both uPA and tPA were secreted by the explant cultures, the amount of uPA secreted was two to threefold greater than that of tPA. Estradiol greatly increased uPA secretion but had little if any effect on tPA. In contrast, progesterone markedly inhibited both uPA and tPA secretion.[19] These patterns of hormonal regulation of endometrial PA secretion in vitro parallel earlier observations made in uterine tissue extracts[12,20-23] and uterine luminal fluid[17,24-26] (see above). Thus, it appears that high levels of circulating estrogen during the proliferative and mid-cycle phases result in the high uterine and luminal PA activity levels observed, whereas high progesterone levels during the luteal phase result in PA activity decreases. It is worth noting that uPA, the PA type associated with differentiation, cellular migration, and invasiveness (see previous section), is the endometrial PA most responsive to regulation by female sex steroids.

PAs AND TROPHOBLAST IMPLANTATION

The concept that embryo implantation involves proteolytic degradation of the endometrium has existed for over a century (reviewed in refs. 25, 32). In 1976, studies by Strickland et al.[33] and Sherman et al.[34] focused attention on the PA/plasmin system as an important source of embryo-derived proteolysis participating in embryo implantation. These authors demonstrated production of PAs by mouse blastocysts in vitro, the temporal characteristics of such production corresponding precisely with the initial differentiation of trophoblast during the period of maximal embryonic invasiveness.[33,34] In 1981, Kubo et al.[35] showed that blockage of PAs and trypsin-like proteases (including plasmin) with nitrophenol-p-guanidino benzoate, ε-aminocaproic acid, and soybean trypsin inhibitor inhibits mouse blastocyst attachment to decidual cell monolayers and subsequent trophoblast outgrowth. The same group then showed temporal correlations between mouse blastocyst PA secretion and the period of trophoblast outgrowth on decidual cells in vitro.[36] More support for a role of PAs in embryo implantation came from studies by Axelrod,[37] who demonstrated that mouse embryos homozygous for the t[w73] implantation-defect mutation showed decreased invasiveness when implanted into mouse testes as well as decreased secretion of PA activity. Care was taken in this study to show that such effects were not secondary to reduced embryonic proliferative capacity or reduced trophoblastic differentiation.[37] Most recently, Sappino et al.[38] used in situ hybridization with uPA and tPA cRNA probes to demonstrate that uPA, and not tPA, is the PA type expressed by invasive trophoblast cells of implanting mouse embryos. This finding is consistent with the known association of uPA with invasive processes (see above).

Although most studies addressing the role of PAs in embryo implantation have been done in the mouse, PA production by porcine[39,40] and bovine[41] embryos has also been reported. Unfortunately, little is known regarding the role of PAs in human embryo implantation, owing primarily to the complex legal and ethical considerations associated with performing studies in this area. Nevertheless, some information on the participation of PAs in trophoblast-endometrium-myometrium interactions in the human has been obtained by studying PA production in early pregnancy and term human trophoblast cultures in vitro. In 1982, Martin and Arias[42] showed that cultured human trophoblasts from 8–12 week gestations secreted PA activity, although the specific PA type involved was not identified. Interestingly, such PA activity was not found to be regulated by estradiol or progesterone, although the synthetic glucocorticoid dexamethasone caused significant PA inhibition.[42] A later report by Queenan et al.[43] showed that uPA was secreted by human trophoblast cultures obtained from term placentas, and that such secretion was stimulated markedly, albeit transiently, by 8-bromo-3′,5′-cyclic adenosine monophosphate (8-bromo-cAMP), suggesting that trophoblast uPA expression is under hormonal or growth factor control.

UTERINE INHIBITORS OF PAs AND PLASMIN

While many studies have addressed PA production by human uterine tissues, including myometrium and the epithelial and stromal fractions of endometrium (see above), fewer have addressed the presence of PA/plasmin inhibitors in these tissues. In part, this undoubtedly reflects the fact that identification, characterization, and cloning of the two specific PAIs, PAI-1 and PAI-2 (see above), have only recently been achieved.[3,4,6] Nevertheless, several reports suggest that PA/plasmin inhibitors may play a role in endometrial physiology. In 1943, Huggins et al.[11] suggested the possibility that menstrual blood may contain inhibitors of fibrinolysis in addition to active fibrinolytic enzymes. Twenty-six years later, the presence of a uPA-inhibiting substance in myometrium obtained from term pregnancies at caesarean section was reported.[44] Liedholm and Astedt[45] showed in 1976 that human decidual tissue in organ culture produced fibrinolytic and uPA inhibitors. Also during the 1970s, several investigators presented evidence for the presence of α_2-antiplasmin, α_2-macroglobulin, α_1-antitrypsin, α_1-antichymotrypsin, and other unidentified PA/plasmin inhibitors in nonmenstrual human uterine fluid (reviewed in ref. 25). However, Soszka and Olszewski[46] found little if any evidence for the presence of acid-sensitive fibrinolytic inhibitors in homogenates from normal human endometrium, although they did find evidence for such inhibitors in hyperplastic and cancerous endometrium. In contrast, Casslen et al.[19] showed that normal human endometrium cultured in vitro releases a PA inhibitor with a molecular weight of about 50,000 daltons, similar in size to both PAI-1 and PAI-2.[3,4,6] Recently, Jonasson et al.[47,48] presented enzymatic and enzyme immunoassay data in support of the presence of PAI-1 and PAI-2, respectively, in human decidual tissue homogenates from first trimester pregnancies. On the other hand, Feinberg et al.[49] found no evidence for the expression of these two PAIs in proliferative, secretory, or decidualized human endometrium using immunohistochemical staining procedures. Thus, the question of whether PAI-1 and PAI-2 are produced by the human endometrium is still controversial and needs to be investigated further.

Several interesting studies point to a role of PA/plasmin inhibitors in uterine or endometrial physiology in non-human species. In the pig, progesterone induces uterine secretion of a low molecular weight (14,600 dalton) plasmin inhibitor which appears to differ from other known porcine plasma protease inhibitors.[39,40,50] It was suggested that this inhibitor may play a role in the unique, non-invasive relationship between trophoblastic tissue and endometrium in this species.[39,40,50] Another interesting study was undertaken to assess whether uterine PA inhibitors might be involved in the obligate 200–220 day period of delayed blastocyst implantation in the Western spotted skunk (Spilogale putorius latifrons).[51] These authors found a 70,000 dalton PA inhibitor in uterine flushings which was present at highest specific activity during the 20–70 days prior to blastocyst implantation. Moreover, this inhibitor was produced by explant cultures of skunk endometrium in vitro. However, the authors concluded that a role of this PA inhibitor in delayed implantation could not be clearly established because the total amount of inhibitor (as opposed to specific activity) increased throughout pre-implantation embryonic activation and the ensuing post-implantation period.[51] Nevertheless, further studies of PA/plasmin inhibitor involvement in regulating embryo implantation in this interesting species should be pursued.

PAI PRODUCTION BY PLACENTAL AND TROPHOBLASTIC TISSUES

As discussed above, current evidence suggests that PAs, particularly uPA, are involved in trophoblast invasion and embryo implantation into maternal tissues. In 1968, Kawano et al.[52] demonstrated the presence of an inhibitor of uPA in human placental tissue, now known to be PAI-2.[3,4,6,47,53] PAI-1 has also been reported in placenta,[54] although PAI-2 appears to be the dominant PAI in this tissue. Analyzing term placental tissue by immunohistochemical staining techniques, Astedt et al.[55] localized PAI-2 expression to villous trophoblastic epithelium, but observed no PAI-2 staining in stromal cells of the chorionic villi. Using similar techniques, Feinberg et al.[49] then further localized PAI-2 expression to the syncytiotrophoblasts, as opposed to cytotrophoblasts, of placental villous tissue from term as well as first and second trimester pregnancies. In the same studies, faint but detectable staining for PAI-1 was also observed in villous syncytiotrophoblasts. In contrast, the opposite situation was observed in extravillous invading trophoblasts, where PAI-1 staining was dominant and PAI-2 staining was weak. These data suggest that expression of PAI-1 and PAI-2 by trophoblasts is dependent on the location and type of trophoblastic tissue being considered. Indeed, Feinberg et al.[49] showed that cytotrophoblasts cultured in vitro expressed both PAI-1 and PAI-2 antigen and mRNA. Interestingly, PAI-1 antigen staining was primarily on the cell surface whereas PAI-2 staining was observed mostly in the cytoplasm.[49] This suggests the presence of control mechanisms which determine the extent and cellular localization of PAI-1 and PAI-2 expression by trophoblast cells in vivo. The nature of such controlling mechanisms is unknown at this time.

SUMMARY AND FURTHER QUESTIONS

Much evidence now supports a role for the PA/plasmin system in endometrial physiology, embryo implantation, and uterine-placental relationships. The identification, characterization, and cloning of PA/plasmin system components have fostered more sophisticated investigations of this area. Nevertheless, several important questions still await resolution. For instance, what are the precise roles of endometrial uPA and tPA, and do they perform different functions in different phases of menstrual cycle? Are PAI-1 and PAI-2 produced by the endometrium, and if so, what are their functions? What is the importance of PAs in implantation relative to other proteases? What roles do PAI-1 and PAI-2 play in villous and invading trophoblasts, and why are they differently regulated in these tissues? What factors govern the regulation of PA and PAI expression in the endometrium and embryonic tissues? Do species differences exist in the roles of the PA/plasmin system in endometrial and implantation physiology? Finally, what are the clinical ramifications of our increased understanding of this area, particularly with respect to infertility, pregnancy complications, and contraception? These and other important questions should guide further investigations into this interesting and complex area of reproductive physiology.

REFERENCES

1. DANO, K., P. A. ANDREASEN, J. GRONDAHL-HANSEN, P. KRISTENSEN, L. S. NIELSEN & L. SKRIVER. 1985. Adv. Cancer Res. **44:** 139–266.
2. SAKSELA, O. 1985. Biochim. Biophys. Acta **823:** 35–65.
3. BLASI, F., J.-D. VASSALLI & K. DANO. 1987. J. Cell Biol. **104:** 801–804.
4. KRUITHOF, E. K. O. 1988. Enzyme **40:** 113–121.
5. MARKUS, G. 1988. Enzyme **40:** 158–172.
6. ANDREASEN, P. A., B. GEORG, L. R. LUND, A. RICCIO & S. N. STACEY. 1990. Mol. Cell. Endocrinol. **68:** 1–19.
7. WHITEHOUSE, H. B. 1914. Lancet **1:** 877–885, 951–957.
8. KROSS, I. 1924. Am. J. Obstet. Gynecol. **7:** 310–313.
9. GLUECK, H. I. & I. A. MIRSKY. 1941. Am. J. Obstet. Gynecol. **42:** 267–271.
10. LOZNER, E. L., Z. E. TAYLOR & F. H. L. TAYLOR. 1942. N. Eng. J. Med. **226:** 481–483.
11. HUGGINS, C., V. C. VAIL & M. E. DAVIS. 1943. Am. J. Obstet. Gynecol. **46:** 78–84.
12. ALBRECHTSEN, O. K. 1956. Acta Endocrin. **23:** 207–218.
13. SOSZKA, T. 1977. Thromb. Res. **10:** 823–832.
14. RIJKEN, D. C., G. WIJNGAARDS, M. ZAAL-DE JONG & J. WELBERGEN. 1979. Biochim. Biophys. Acta **580:** 140–153.
15. KOK, P. 1979. Thromb. Haemost. **41:** 718–733.
16. MATSUO, O., H. FUKAO, S. IZAKI, C. MATSUO & S. UESHIMA. 1989. Cell Struct. Funct. **14:** 45–60.

17. CASSLEN, B., J. THORELL & B. ASTEDT. 1981. Contraception 23: 435–445.
18. CASSLEN, B. & B. ASTEDT. 1983. Contraception 28: 553–564.
19. CASSLEN, B., A. ANDERSSON, I. M. NILSSON & B. ASTEDT. 1986. Proc. Soc. Exp. Biol. Med. 182: 419–424.
20. CASSLEN, B. & B. ASTEDT. 1983. Contraception 28: 181–188.
21. RYBO, G. 1966. Acta Obstet. Gynecol. Scand. 45: 429–450.
22. SHAW, S. T., JR., L. K. MACAULAY, M. S. TANAKA, JR., W. R. HOHMON, D. L. MOYER & N. C. SUN. 1980. Biochem. Med. 24: 170–178.
23. SHAW, S. T., JR., L. K. MACAULAY, N. C. SUN, M. S. TANAKA, JR. & P. C. ROCHE. 1983. Contraception 27: 131–140.
24. CASSLEN, B. & B. ASTEDT. 1981. Acta Obstet. Gynecol. Scand. 60: 55–58.
25. CASSLEN, B. 1981. Acta Obstet. Gynecol. Scand. Suppl 98: 1–38.
26. CASSLEN, B. & K. OHLSSON. 1981. Acta Obstet. Gynecol. Scand. 60: 97–101.
27. ALBRECHTSEN, O. K. 1957. Proc. Soc. Exp. Biol. Med. 94: 700–702.
28. KWAAN, H. C. & O. K. ALBRECHTSEN. 1966. Am. J. Obstet. Gynecol. 95: 468–473.
29. KNEIFEL, M. A., S. P. LEYTUS, E. FLETCHER, T. WEBER, W. F. MANGEL & B. S. KATZENEL-LENBOGEN. 1982. Endocrinology 111: 493–499.
30. PELTZ, S. W., B. S. KATZENELLENBOGEN, M. A. KNEIFEL & W. F. MANGEL. 1983. Endocrinology 112: 890–897.
31. FINLAY, T. H., J. KATZ, L. KIRSCH, M. LEVITZ, S. A. NATHOO & S. SEILER. 1983. Endocrinology 112: 856–861.
32. DENKER, H. W. 1983. Obstet. Gynecol. Annu. 12: 15–42.
33. STRICKLAND, S., E. REICH & M. I. SHERMAN. 1976. Cell 9: 231–240.
34. SHERMAN, M. I., S. STRICKLAND & E. REICH. 1976. Cancer Res. 36: 4208–4216.
35. KUBO, H., A. SPINDLE & R. A. PEDERSEN. 1981. J. Exp. Zool. 216: 445–451.
36. KUBO, H., S. KATAYAMA, H. AMANO & A. I. SPINDLE. 1982. Acta Obstet. Gynecol. Jpn. 34: 801–808.
37. AXELROD, H. R. 1985. Dev. Biol. 108: 185–190.
38. SAPPINO, A.-P., J. HUARTE, D. BELIN & J.-D. VASSALLI. 1989. J. Cell Biol. 109: 2471–2479.
39. MULLINS, D. E., F. W. BAZER & R. M. ROBERTS. 1980. Cell 20: 865–872.
40. FAZLEABAS, A. T., R. D. GEISERT, F. W. BAZER & R. M. ROBERTS. 1983. Biol. Reprod. 29: 225–238.
41. MENINO, A. R., JR. & J. S. WILLIAMS. 1987. Biol. Reprod. 36: 1289–1295.
42. MARTIN, O. & F. ARIAS. 1982. Am. J. Obstet. Gynecol. 142: 402–409.
43. QUEENAN, J. T., JR., L.-C. KAO, C. E. ARBOLETA, A. ULLOA-AGUIRRE, T. G. GOLOS, D. B. CINES & J. F. STRAUSS, III. 1987. J. Biol. Chem. 262: 10903–10906.
44. USZYNSKI, M. & R. USZYNSKI-FOLEJEWSKA. 1969. Am. J. Obstet. Gynecol. 105: 1041–1043.
45. LIEDHOLM, P., & B. ASTEDT. 1976. Acta Obstet. Gynecol. Scand. 55: 217–219.
46. SOSZKA, T. & K. OLSZEWSKI. 1986. Thromb. Res. 42: 835–846.
47. JONASSON, A., B. LARSSON, I. LECANDER & B. ASTEDT. 1989. Thromb. Res. 53: 91–97.
48. JONASSON, A., B. LARSSON, I. LECANDER & B. ASTEDT. 1989. Int. J. Gynecol. Obstet. 29: 73–77.
49. FEINBERG, R. F., L.-C. KAO, J. E. HAIMOWITZ, J. T. QUEENAN, JR., T.-C. WUN, J. F. STRAUSS, III & H. J. KLIMAN. 1989. Lab. Invest. 61: 20–26.
50. FAZLEABAS, A. T., F. W. BAZER & R. M. ROBERTS. 1982. J. Biol. Chem. 257: 6886–6897.
51. FAZLEABAS, A. T., R. A. MEAD, A. W. ROURKE & R. M. ROBERTS. 1984. Biol. Reprod. 30: 311–322.
52. KAWANO, T., K. MORIMOTO & Y. UEMURA. 1968. Nature (London) 217: 253–254.
53. ASTEDT, B., I. LECANDER, T. BRODIN, A. LUNDBLAD & K. LOW. 1985. Thromb. Haemost. 53: 122–125.
54. PHILIPS, M., A.-G. JUUL, S. THORSEN, J. SELMER & J. ZEUTHEN. 1986. Thromb. Haemost. 55: 213–217.
55. ASTEDT, B., I. HAGERSTRAND & I. LECANDER. 1986. Thromb. Haemost. 56: 63–65.
56. BEERS, W. H. 1975. Cell 6: 379–386.
57. BEERS, W. H., S. STRICKLAND & E. REICH. 1975. Cell 6: 387–394.
58. STRICKLAND, S. & W. H. BEERS. 1976. J. Biol. Chem. 251: 5694–5702.
59. OSSOWSKI, L., D. BIEGEL & E. REICH. 1979. Cell 16: 929–940.
60. RENNIE, P. S., R. BOUFFARD, N. BRUCHOVSKY & H. CHENG. 1984. Biochem. J. 221: 171–178.
61. RENNIE, P. S., J. F. BOWDEN, N. BRUCHOVSKY & H. CHENG. 1988. Biochem. J. 252: 759–764.
62. GROSS, J. L., D. MOSCATELLI & D. B. RIFKIN. 1983. Proc. Natl. Acad. Sci. USA 80: 2623–2627.

63. HAMILTON, J. A., S. R. LINGELBACH, N. C. PARTRIDGE & T. J. MARTIN. 1984. Biochem. Biophys. Res. Commun. **122:** 230–236.
64. HAMILTON, J. A., S. LINGELBACH, N. C. PARTRIDGE & T. J. MARTIN. 1985. Endocrinology **116:** 2186–2191.
65. STRICKLAND, S. & V. MAHDAVI. 1978. Cell **15:** 393–403.
66. STRICKLAND, S., K. K. SMITH & K. R. MAROTTI. 1980. Cell **21:** 347–355.
67. SAKSELA, O. & H. HOLTHOFER. 1987. Differentiation **34:** 131–138.
68. AMICI, C., A. BENEDETTO, O. SAKSELA, E. M. SALONEN & A. VAHERI. 1989. Int. J. Cancer **43:** 171–176.
69. ISSEROFF, R. R., N. E. FUSENIG & D. B. RIFKIN. 1983. J. Invest. Dermatol. **80:** 217–222.
70. PITTMAN, R. N. & H. M. BUETTNER. 1989. Dev. Neurosci. **11:** 361–375.
71. WANG, B. S., G. A. MCLOUGHLIN, J. P. RICHIE & J. A. MANNICK. 1980. Cancer Res. **40:** 288–292.
72. OSSOWSKI, L. & E. REICH. 1983. Cell **35:** 611–619.
73. CARLSEN, S. A., I. A. RAMSHAW & R. C. WARRINGTON. 1984. Cancer Res. **44:** 3012–3016.
74. OSSOWSKI, L. 1988. Cell **52:** 321–328.

Factors Regulating Interaction between Trophoblast and Human Endometrium

C. FLAMIGNI,[a,b] C. BULLETTI, V. POLLI,
P. M. CIOTTI, R. A. PREFETTO,
A. GALASSI,[c] AND E. DI COSMO

[a] Reproductive Medicine Unit
Department of Obstetrics and Gynecology
University of Bologna
40138 Bologna, Italy

[c] Department of Pathology
Bassano del Grappa General Hospital
Viale delle Fosse, 43
36062 Bassano del Grappa (VI), Italy

After the extensive study of ovulation and fertilization that has taken place in the last two decades, a series of cooperative biochemical and physical events (involving both conceptus and maternal tissues) called implantation, became the focus of scientific research because it is seen as the basic feature of human reproduction.

It has been estimated that only about 30% of all conceptions survive to birth, 15% end in recognizable miscarriage, and the other 55% are lost in the early stages of pregnancy.[1] A total of 61.9% of conceptuses are lost prior to 12 weeks. Most of these losses (91.7%) occur subclinically, without the mother's knowledge.[2] Roberts and Loewe, using a mathematical estimation, suggested that 78% of fertilizations fail to result in a live birth.[3] Implantation of the embryo rather than fertilization, is the crucial event which differentiates fertile and non-fertile ovulatory cycles.[4,5]

The interactive steps of the event begin with adhesion of the blastocyst to the endometrium and end with formation of a placenta (FIG. 1). Although various facets of this process have been described in much detail, relatively little is known at the molecular or cellular level about the actual mechanisms responsible for implantation of the human embryo.

Implantation involves communication between embryonic and maternal tissues and it is difficult to attribute whether failure to establish an ongoing pregnancy is due to inappropriate morphophysiologic/biochemical conditions in the uterus or to an embryonic inability to grow or to both. The importance of endometrial adequacy is evident from results of *in vitro* fertilization and embryo transfer (IVF/ET) which report high fertilization frequencies (70% to 90%) whereas the pregnancy rate after embryo transfer ranges from 15% to 25%.[6,7] Only 3 to 5 out of 100 embryos transferred after

[b] Address for correspondence: Carlo Flamigni, MD, Reproductive Medicine Unit, Dept. Ob/Gyn, University of Bologna, Via Massarenti, 13, 40138 Bologna, Italy (tel. (51)-343934; FAX (51)-342820).

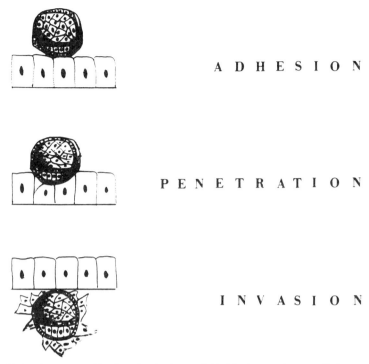

A D H E S I O N

P E N E T R A T I O N

I N V A S I O N

FIGURE 1. The process of implantation is shown divided in three main steps. Each step may be regulated by different factors.

in vitro fertilization usually complete implantation and begin pregnancy. Embryo loss before recognition of pregnancy seems to be the major loss rate, but it is impossible to quantify.

In vivo or *in vitro* fertilization and embryo transfer fails to produce a pregnancy because of pre- and post-implantation embryo loss. Embryo mortality is largely concentrated in the early months with only 1% of stillbirths after the 28th week.[8]

The incidence of chromosomal abnormalities in spontaneous abortion after pregnancy recognition and before 12 weeks of gestation is high (30 to 60%), but it can still be estimated that 40% to 70% of embryo mortality is not related to grossly abnormal karyotype.[8]

Even the extent of early embryonic mortality, prior to both implantation and recognition of pregnancy, is obviously under-represented; it has been estimated at around 40–60%,[2,8] and the most important question that arises from analytical studies[8,9] is whether the abortion of 40% of chromosomally "normal" abortuses (plus part of "silent abortuses" that occur before implantation) is brought about by physiological defects in the mother or in the maternal-embryonic interaction. It might be possible to save these embryos by improving our knowledge of factors influencing human embryo implantation.

Furthermore, statistical analysis gives us an indirect measurement of events occurring during implantation and it indicates that the uterus and not the ovary or the embryos themselves is the cause of the drop in pregnancies of women over 40 years of age, as reported by R. G. Edwards.[6] In fact there appears to be no difference between the hormone profiles of luteal phases in young and older patients and the embryos do not display any evidence of cleavage impairment *in vitro*, as assessed by their growth to blastocysts. Furthermore, lack of ovaries or ovarian function is no longer an absolute impediment to having a baby if the endometrial cycle is adequately obtained with estrogen/progesterone administration.[7] We know that embryos and uterus must be synchronized: the period of uterine receptivity is limited and the transition from nonsensitivity to receptivity is associated with many changes in the endometrium ending with the so called "predecidualization" (FIG. 2). The endometrium provides the embryo with a unique substrate to attach, penetrate and grow on. Details of these steps vary in different species and, although data obtained from non-primates or non-human primates are helpful for comparison (TABLE 1), only data obtained from human embryos and human endometrium are useful for final conclusions.

Early human embryonic conceptus migrate through the predecidualized endometrium and penetrate the basement membrane (BM) underlying the luminal uterine epithelium to tap the maternal blood supply; during this histotrophic phase, but not later, the embryo displays both highly invasive and proliferative properties without an embryonic blood circulation.

The highly proliferative phase of cytotrophoblasts during early human embryogenesis may be due to the endogenous production of growth factors that may establish an autocrine/short range paracrine stimulator loops which explain the tumor-like properties of this tissue.[10] Penetration of endometrial BM and invasion of stroma may be due to the proteolytic capability of the human embryo. Collagenase and urokinase-like plasminogen activators are candidates for this activity.[11-13]

During its penetration into the decidua, the human embryo elicits a response from the maternal immunity system as a result of its paternal antigens.[14] Despite this, the embryo is capable of surviving in a host that is immunologically hostile due to the presence of non-specific suppressor cells in the decidua[15] or because of the presence of an embryo-associated immunosuppressor factor.[16]

It is evident that the blastocyst can influence endometrial protein synthesis and secretion before implantation;[17] it is not known whether synthesis is due to stromal or epithelial cells, but cooperation of these cells is an established biological phenomenon.[18]

To clarify the molecular mechanisms involved in human embryo implantation several models are suggested: blastocyst culture,[17] endometrial cell culture,[19] endometrial explant co-culture,[20] endometrial organic culture[4] (FIG. 3), endometrial monolayer co-culture,[21] and endometrial trophoblast suspension on co-culture.[22] With these models it may be possible to differentiate between facets of embryo implantation in human endometrium.

ESTROGEN AND PROGESTERONE RECEPTORS

Estrogen and progesterone receptors (ER, PR) are present in the endometrium in relatively large concentrations which change throughout the menstrual cycle and can be modified by hormonal and metabolic factors.[23]

The cyclic nature of these changes in ER and PR in the endometrium has been

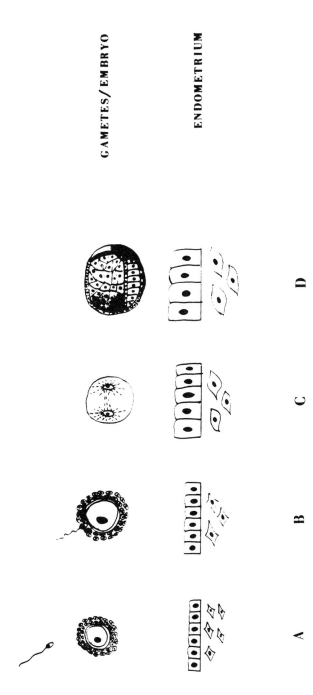

FIGURE 2. Endometrium and embryos undergo growth and differentiation and these steps must be synchronized to complete implantation successfully. After ovulation the oocyte is fertilized (A) and the corresponding endometrium is modified by differentiation to a predecidualized endometrium. During these steps (B, C, D) stromal cells change their biochemical and physical features, the luminal epithelium grows, glycogen content increases, and embryo grows and penetrates the luminal epithelium without blood connection.

TABLE 1. The Stages of Pregnancy (Approximate Days after Ovulation) and the Embryo Development Stages at the Time of Implantation (Definite Attachment)

Mammalians	Day of Implantation	Embryo Development Stage
Human	6–7	
Chimpanzee	6–7	
Rhesus monkey	8–9	Blastocyst
Baboon	8–9	
Marmoset	11–12	

determined by many workers. In general, the tissue concentration of ER and PR is maximal during the proliferative phase and minimal during the secretory phase. Progesterone (P) and progestins induce a decline in ER levels.[23] The changes in PR levels coincide with the patterns of estradiol concentrations in the endometrium during the cycle.

The PR are under estrogen (E) control.[23] ER and PR in decidual cells are also under hormonal control and there is a significant loss of ER during the first four days

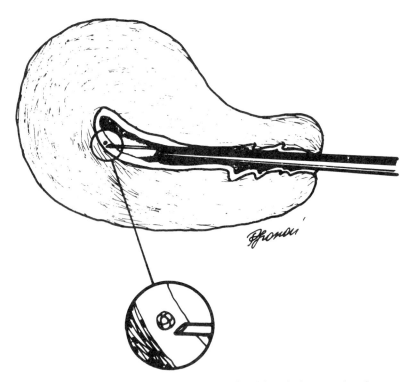

FIGURE 3. Human blastocyst can be injected or transferred into the lumen cavity of an extracorporeally perfused human uterus. The uterus, obtained at +5th, +6th day after LH ovulatory peak, can be preserved for 52 hours, a time sufficient to complete the implantation.

of decidualization of non-primates that could not be attributed to changes in serum steroid levels.[24]

ENDOMETRIAL MATURATION

The temporal window of human endometrial receptivity is restricted to days 16–19 of a 28-day cycle[25] and it is important to synchronize embryo development stage with the endometrial maturation of the recipient. The endometrium must undergo specific proliferative and differentiative events including secretion,[13] edema formation, vascular proliferation, and decidualization of the stroma. Decidualization is an important step in endometrial maturation and it may modulate embryo implantation.

Decidualization is common to many species and obviously plays an essential role in implantation and pregnancy maintenance. Decidual cells are large, rich in glycogen and lipids.[13,26] They derive from stromal cells and P seems to be involved in the transformation.[27] In many species the uterine stroma undergoes a change, known as decidualization, after its initial reaction with the embryo (but physical stimulation of the endometrium may also induce reactive endometrial decidualization), whereas in the human uterus the stromal cells display a similar type of modification during the menstrual cycle at around day 21[27] which resembles predecidualization.

Biochemically, stromal cells at this step of differentiation produce prolactin and laminin,[28] secrete prostaglandins,[29] and are provided with ER and PR.[30,31] Stromal cells turn into decidual cells containing prolactin (PRL),[32] regulating trophoblast invasion,[33] and protecting the embryo against rejection by the maternal immune response.[34,35] They may also serve in the nutrition or protection of the embryo or they may protect the mother by limiting the invasiveness of the embryonic trophoblast.

Furthermore, the endometrium may provide secretory products which help the embryo to maintain its high degree of proliferative and differentiative activity since the embryo enters the uterine cavity about 3 days before implantation and it grows without blood supply. The biochemical characteristics of the luminal epithelium seem to be important for embryo adhesion and for the beginning of implantation.[36]

ENDOMETRIAL SECRETIONS

Most of the endometrial secretions in the uterine lumen are considered to be important for implantation and they appear to play this role through autocrine and paracrine effects. Since E and P are so closely involved in the control of production of many of the secretory substances in the uterus, the enzymes that enable their biological action are of particular importance.

The most important enzyme controlling estrogen metabolism is estradiol-17β hydroxy steroid dehydrogenase (17β E_2-HSD). The activity of this enzyme in the secretory endometrium is markedly increased under the influence of P and is highest shortly following ovulation. 17β E_2-HSD catalyzes the conversion of estradiol to estrone, a reaction that markedly reduces the biological effect of E. The stimulation of this enzyme by progestins, both during the normal menstrual cycle and when administered pharmacologically, is one of the two primary mechanisms by which progesterone is anti-estrogenic (the other is the reduction of available receptors for estradiol).

P also stimulates the production of nicotinamide adenine dinucleotide-dependent

15-hydroxyprogesterone dehydrogenase (NAD-15-HPD). This enzyme catalyzes the metabolism of estradiol and PGF2α as well.[37] The third enzyme of importance in E metabolism is sulfotransferase. This enzyme converts estrone to estrone sulfate which does not bind ER and thus prevents the recycling of estradiol.[38,39] However since sulfatase activity is also present in the endometrium the activity of these enzymes influences the bioavailability of E in the endometrium itself. P controls its own biological activity by inhibiting the biological activity of estradiol, resulting in a diminution of PR and induction of 20 α-hydroxysteroid dehydrogenase (20 α-HSD) that reduces the biological action of P by altering its capacity to bind PR.[37]

The last enzyme to be considered is 11β-hydroxysteroid dehydrogenase, present at high concentrations in decidua and which converts cortisone to the much more biologically active cortisol and corticosterone. Its importance is more linked to labor and fetal maturation than implantation.

EICOSANOIDS

The importance of prostaglandins in the development of endometrial vascular permeability and subsequent decidual transformation is well known[40,41] and the use of indomethacin during the first days of pregnancy inhibits or delays implantation in several non-primates.[42-45] *In vitro* E stimulate and progestins diminish prostaglandin output. This effect is evident in epithelial but not in stromal cells. Other endogenous agents such as interleukin 1 (IL_1) and colony-stimulating factor 1 (CSF_1) may be physiologic stimulators.

Cytokines[46] and growth factors[47] can be produced by endometrial cells and serve as local intrauterine regulators of prostaglandin production. Other arachidonic acid metabolites formed by the action of lipogenoses, such as leukotrienes, have been identified as endometrial products of potential importance in the regulation of vasomotor activity.

PROGESTIN-ASSOCIATED ENDOMETRIAL PROTEIN

Progestin-associated endometrial protein (PEP) is a glycoprotein with a molecular weight of about 47 000 which can be reductively dissociated into two subunits each having molecular weights of approximately 27 000. It is also known by a variety of other names such as placental protein 14 (PP14), $α_2$-microglobulin, α-uterine protein, pregnancy associated $α_2$-globulin or EE 15 β-lactoglobulin.

PEP is synthesized from human decidua[48] and is only present in progestin-dominated endometrium (*e.g.* mid- and late-secretory phase endometria and decidua), but not in estrogen-dominated proliferative endometrium or in pregnancy or non-pregnancy sera.[49]

The endometrium is the major, if not the only, source of PEP. In women PEP is synthesized within the endometrium and is not sequestered from peripheral blood;[49] it is confined to the glands.

PEP serum levels are positively correlated with the degree of the secretory change intensity within the endometrium and not with serum E_2 or P levels; its patterns during the menstrual cycle may provide quantitative information about short or inadequate luteal phases or insensitivity to P.[49] The biological function of PEP is completely unknown.

24K PROTEIN

24k Protein (or stress responsive protein 27 as it is now called) can be detected in normal human endometrium and endometrial carcinoma as well as in the MCF-7 human breast cancer cell line where it is stimulated by E and heat shock.[50] The protein has been localized immunohistochemically in both glandular and surface epithelium as well as on decidual cells.[51]

Immunostaining for 24k protein in the glandular epithelium peaks at ovulation time, declines sharply thereafter, whereas staining in surface epithelium peaks later, at about the time of the cycle corresponding to implantation (FIG. 4). Immunostaining shifts later to decidual cells during the luteal phase. *In vitro* predecidualized stromal cells show immunostaining for 24k protein of deciduate endometrium.

CARBOHYDRATE, GLYCOCONJUGATE, AND GLYCOPROTEIN

The potential importance of 24k as a preparatory marker of the surface epithelium for blastocyst attachment is evident and implies the search for marker-focusing studies for the identification of glycoproteins and microvilli of surface epithelial cells. Some of the lectins seem to bind the apical border of the luminal epithelium during the implantation window.[52,53] Glysoaminoglycan may play an important role in promoting embryo implantation.[54] Hyaluronate facilitates attachment and outgrowth of embryos.[54] Like other cancer cells[55] embryo trophoblastic cells also seem to be able to utilize hyaluronate for in tissue invasion. Other extracellular matrix molecules, such as laminin and fibronectin, also support embryo attachment and outgrowth.[56]

The increased expression of hyaluronate seems to be one aspect of a complex but coordinated response of the uterus designed to provide a favorable medium for embryonic migration and growth after the initial stages of embryo attachment. Other molecules expressed by epithelial cells may mediate initial embryo adhesion to the uterus (*e.g.*, laminin).[57] Laminin, the major noncollagenous glycoprotein of basement membranes, is important for cell attachment, cell spreading, cell migration and binding to other matrix components.

BASEMENT MEMBRANES AND PROTEOLYTIC ENZYMES

The blastocyst has to penetrate the endometrial basement membrane underlying the luminal epithelium and the thick decidual wall during implantation (FIG. 5). Penetration of the BM is a crucial step in implantation[4] and requires BM degradation. In the rabbit, protease activity of trophoblast has been demonstrated and is under control of stromal regulation with the possible involvement of uterine protease inhibitors in the hormonal regulation.[58]

After human embryo attachment to the luminal epithelium, the trophoblast laminin interaction may provide the initial anchorage which facilitates trophoblast migration in the same way as postulated for tumor cell. Human embryos produce type IV collagen-degrading enzyme and the secretion of this enzyme increases with time in culture, while unfertilized oocytes secrete low, stable amounts of this enzyme *in vitro*.[11]

Urokinase-type plasminogen activator (uPA) is involved in invasive and destructive phenomena that occur both in physiological as well as in pathological conditions.[59] Its activity is involved in the implantation of embryonic trophoblast cells in the endo-

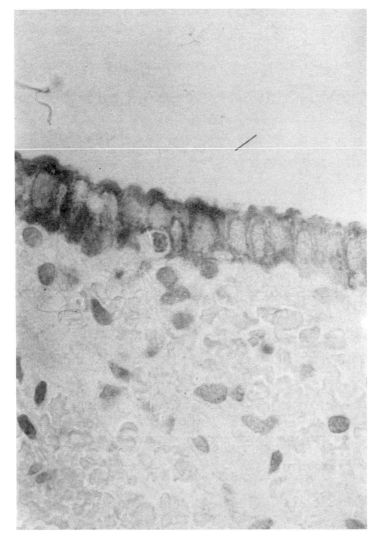

FIGURE 4. Immunostaining for 24k protein in the luminal epithelium. The positive immunoreaction is clearly detectable at the time of the cycle corresponding to implantation.

metrium[60] and its production has been demonstrated in trophoblastic and parietal endoderm[60] as well as its activity regulators, *e.g.* plasminogen activator inhibitors.[61]

PROLACTIN

The production of PRL by the human endometrium has been shown to correlate with the degree of histological decidualization.[28] Stromal cells produce PRL when

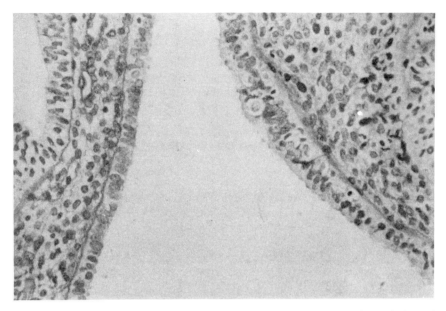

FIGURE 5. Laminin, one of the most important components of basement membrane, is detected by immunohistochemistry under the epithelial cells of luminal epithelium. Embryos should penetrate this barrier to invade the stroma and to tap maternal blood supply beginning the pregnancy.

stimulated by P in a dose-dependent manner and this production is higher when cells are stimulated with MPA and Norethindrone than with those receiving P.[62]

Decidual PRL is a protein synthesized and secreted by predecidualized and decidualized cells which has clinical and biological properties identical to pituitary PRL. The physiological role of decidual PRL is unclear, but numerous studies suggest its role in water and mineral metabolism in amniotic fluid, synthesis of pulmonary surfactant, inhibition of uterine contractility, suppression of the immunoresponse,[63] and possibly in stromal cell differentiation into decidual cells.

PRL production *in vitro* reflects the histologic maturity of the endometrium rather than the cycle date. P has been reported to stimulate decidua PRL production and a role for PRL in the early implantation events has been suggested. Studies on this aspect are hampered by the fact that PRL appears to be produced by decidualized endometrial stroma only in primates and human beings. The effect of PRL on implantation and early embryonic development might be involved in regulating cellular responses in early gestation. On this point PRL is known to function as a growth factor in a variety of lower animals.[37]

GROWTH FACTORS

The existence of growth factor activity in human endometrium and embryos should be postulated because of their intense proliferative and differentiative activity. Many growth factors have been identified in the endometrium while the possibility of performing similar studies on human embryos at an early stage remains unexplored due to the ethical problems of using human embryonic cells at an early stage of development.

However the endometrium membrane has receptors for insulin growth-factor-I (IGF-I) and synthesizes and secretes a 34k IGF-binding protein.[47,64]

Colony-stimulating factor I is a glycosylated polypeptide, originally characterized as a microphase-specific hematopoietic growth factor.[65] It may act as an endometrial growth factor stimulating proliferation and/or secretion in epithelial cells as it is capable of stimulating proliferation in Ishikawa cells.[66]

Transforming growth factor α (TGF-α) is a 50 aminoacid glycoprotein[67] that is synthesized by day 7 decidua in rats. We recently identified it in human endometrium with immunohistochemistry, but it is not known if epithelial cells express TGF-α and whether it promotes proliferation and angiogenesis;[69] it is likely to be intimately involved in repair.

Epidermal growth factor (EGF) is a 53 aminoacid peptide[70] that may be involved in the regulation of human endometrium proliferation. Mouse and rabbit endometrial cells proliferate in response to EGF.[71,72] Epithelial but not stromal cells proliferate in response to estradiol and EGF.

Fibroblast growth factor is an important mediator of angiogenesis but it has still not been demonstrated to be synthesized by human endometrium.

IMPLANTATION AND MATERNAL IMMUNORESPONSE

In human pregnancy the embryo needs to invade the maternal decidua and vessels for successful implantation and development of a normal blood supply to the feto-placental unit. One may view this process as a type of allograft that is capable of survival in a host that is immunologically hostile.[73,74]

The fetus itself has paternal antigens which can and often do elicit a response from the maternal immunity system. Certain trophoblast populations also express class I antigens of the major histocompatibility complex and paternal minor histocompatibility antigens that may serve as a target for sensitized maternal effector cells.[75] Non-specific suppressor cells can be isolated from the human decidua[76] and a local immunologic suppression of T-cell responses that may protect the early embryo conceptus from maternal rejection has been demonstrated.[15]

Suppressor cell deficiency may explain very early occult embryonic loss[77,78] as well as some unexplained infertility and habitual abortion. Suppressive activity has been found in humans during the secretory phase of the normal menstrual cycle when implantation would normally occur. This suggests that hormone preparation of the endometrium for successful implantation induces a suppressive activity that prevents the immune response to antigens expressed in the embryo.

It is possible that local suppressive activity may be an important mechanism in the reproductive process. Furthermore, failing IVF embryos are infiltrated by maternal lymphocytes[79] and thus support the hypothesis of human fetal allograft rejection by maternal immunity.

The possibility of manipulating suppression activity cells makes it possible to provide treatment for women with unexplained infertility and unexplained habitual abortion as well as preventing the loss of embryos transferred after IVF.[15]

Perhaps decidual leukocytes exert a cytostatic influence rather than cytolysis. They may also inhibit the response of lymphocytes to immunogenic stimuli, acting as local natural suppressor cells which are known to be large granular lymphocytes both phenotypically and morphologically.[80] It has even been suggested that these decidual cells may actually enhance trophoblast growth by production of appropriate cytokines.[80] However, human embryo-associated immunosuppressor factors were also demonstrated and may play a role in suppressing maternal immune response thereby preventing maternal rejection of the embryo.[16] Recent data suggest that PGF2 secretion by first trimester human decidual cells blocks activation of maternal leukocytes in the decidua, with a potential antitrophoblast killer function, by inhibiting interleukin-2 receptor generation and interleukin-2 production *in situ*.[81]

SUMMARY

Implantation is a crucial step in human reproduction. Disturbances of this process are responsible for pregnancy failure after both *in vivo* and *in vitro* fertilization. The endometrium provides the implanting embryo with a unique substratum where the embryo communicates with biochemical signals, attaches itself, penetrates and grows without blood circulation. The highly proliferative phase of the cytotrophoblast, during early human embryogenesis, may be due to endogenous production of growth factors that may establish autocrine/short range paracrine stimulator loops which explain the tumor-like properties of these tissues. Endometrial BM penetration and stroma invasion may be due to the proteolytic capability of the human embryo. It is suggested that collagenase and the urokinase-like plasminogen activator are responsible for this activity. To clarify the molecular mechanisms involved in human embryo implantation several models are suggested: culture of blastocysts, culture of endometrial cells, and endometrial explant co-culture. Human blastocysts cultured with whole perfused human uteri make it possible to recognize some aspects of the entire implantation process and give us the possibility of improving the benefits provided by new technologies in reproductive medicine and reducing embryonic loss at an early stage.

REFERENCES

1. LINDLEY, M. 1979. Life and death before birth. *Editorial*. Nature **280:** 635–637.
2. EDMONDS, D. K., K. S. LINDSAY, J. F. MILLER, E. WILLIAMSON & P. J. WOOD. 1982. Early embryonic mortality in women. Fertil. Steril. **38:** 447–453.
3. ROBERTS, S. C. J. & D. B. LOEWE. 1975. Where have all the conceptus gone? Lancet **1:** 498–501.
4. BULLETTI, C., V. M. JASONNI, S. TABANELLI, L. GIANAROLI, P. M. CIOTTI, A. P. FERRARETTI & C. FLAMIGNI. 1988. Early human pregnancy in vitro utilizing an artificially perfused uterus. Fertil. Steril. **49:** 991–996.
5. NAVOT, D., T. D. ANDERSON, K. DROESH, R. T. SCOTT, D. KREINER & Z. ROSENWAKS. 1989. Hormonal manipulation of endometrial maturation. J. Clin. Endocrinol. Metab. **68:** 801–807.
6. EDWARDS, R. G. 1985. Normal and abnormal implantation in the human uterus. *In* Implantation of the Human Embryo. **1:** 303–312. Academic Press, Inc. London.
7. NAVOT, D., N. LAUFER & J. KOPOLOVIC. 1986. Artificially induced endometrial cycles and establishment of pregnancies in the absence of ovaries. N. Engl. J. Med. **314:** 806–810.
8. SHORT, R. V. 1979. When a conception fails to become a pregnancy. *In* Maternal Recognition of Pregnancy. Ciba Foundation Series 64 (new series). **1:** 377–394. Excerpta Medica.
9. PHYCHOYOS, A. 1973. Hormonal control of ovum implantation. Vitam. Horm. **31:** 201–256.
10. OHLSSON, R., E. LARSSON, O. NILSSON, T. WAHLSTROM & P. SUNDSTROM. 1989. Blastocyst implantation precedes induction of insulin like growth factor II gene expressive in human trophoblast. Development **106:** 555–559.

11. PUISTOLA, V., L. RONNBERG, H. MARTIKAINEN & T. TURPEENNIEMI-HUJANEN. 1989. The human embryo produces basement membrane collagen (type IV collagen) degrading protease activity. Hum. Reprod. **4**(3): 309–311.

12. MULLINS, D. E. & S. T. ROHRLICH. 1983. The role of proteinases in cellular invasiveness. Biochem. Biophys. Acta **695**: 177–214.

13. NOYES, R. W., A. T. HERTIG & J. ROCK. 1950. Dating the endometrial biopsy. Fertil. Steril. **1**: 3–15.

14. KING, A., C. BIRKBY & Y. W. LOKE. 1989. Early human decidua cells exhibit NK activity against the 562 cell line but not against first trimester trophoblast. Cell. Immunol. **118**: 337–344.

15. DAYA, S., D. A. S. CLARK, C. DEVLIN & J. JARRELL. 1985. Preliminary characterization of the two types of suppressor cells in the human uterus. Fertil. Steril. **44**: 778–783.

16. BOSE, R. 1989. Human embryo associated immunosuppressor factor(s) from pre- and post-implantation stages show some similarities. Immunol. Lett **20**(4): 261–267.

17. SALMONSEN, L. A., B. W. DOUGHTON & J. F. FINDLAY. 1986. The effect of the preimplantation blastocyst in vivo and in vitro on proterin synthesis and secretion by cultured epithelial cells from sheep endometrium. Endocrinology **119**: 622–628.

18. GAL, D., L. CASEY, J. M. JOHNSTON & P. C. MACDONALD. 1982. Mesenchyme-epithelial interactions in human endometrium. J. Clin. Invest. **70**: 798–805.

19. CARSON, D. D., J. P. TANG & S. GAY. 1988. Collagens support embryo attachment and outgrowth in vitro: Effect of the Arg-Gly Asp sequence. Dev. Biol. **127**: 368–375.

20. GLENISTER, T. W. 1961. Organ culture as a new method for studying the implantation of mammalian blastocysts. Proc. Royal Soc. B **154**: 428–431.

21. LINDERBERG, S., P. HYTTEL, S. LENZ & P. V. HOLMES. 1986. Ultrastructure of the early human implantation in vitro. Human Reprod. **1**: 533–538.

22. KLIMAN, H. J., C. COUTIFARIS, R. F. FEINBERG, J. F. STRAUSS III & J. E. HAIMOWTZ. 1988. Interactions between human term trophoblasts and endometrium in vitro. 11th Roch. Troph. Conf., Rochester.

23. GURPIDE, E., R. BLUMENTHAL & H. FLEMMY. 1985. Regulation of steroid receptors in human endometrium. *In* Mechanism of Menstrual Bleeding. D. T. Baird & E. A. Michie, Eds. Vol. **1**: 47–55. Raven Press, New York.

24. LEAVITT, W. W. & A. TAKEDA. 1986. Hormonal regulation of estrogen and progestin receptors in decidual cells. Biol. Reprod. **35**: 475–484.

25. ROSENWAKS, Z. 1987. Donor eggs: Their application in modern reproductive technologies. Fertil. Steril. **47**: 895–900.

26. WEVER, V. M., M. FABER, L. A. LIOTTA & R. ALBRECHTSEN. 1985. Immunochemical and ultrastructural assessment of the nature of pericellular basement membrane of human decidual cells. Lab. Invest. **53**: 624–630.

27. BULLETTI, C., A. GALASSI, V. M. JASONNI, G. MARTINELLI, S. TABANELLI & C. FLAMIGNI. 1988. Basement membrane components in normal hyperplastic and neoplastic endometrium. Cancer **62**: 142–149.

28. MASLAR, I. A. & D. H. RIDDICK. 1979. Prolactin production by human endometrium during the normal menstrual cycle. Am. J. Obstet. Gynecol. **135**: 751–756.

29. RIDDICK, D. H., D. C. DALAY & C. A. WALTER. 1983. The uterus as an endocrine compartment. Clin. Perinatal **10**: 627–631.

30. MARTIN, P. M., P. H. ROLLAND, M. GAMMERRE, H. SERMENT & M. TOGA. 1979. Estradiol and progesterone receptors in normal and neoplastic endometrium correlation between receptors histological examination and clinical response under progestin therapy. Int. J. Cancer **23**: 321–325.

31. PRESS, M. F., N. NOUSER-GOEGL, W. J. KING, A. L. HERBST & G. L. GREENE. 1984. Immunohystochemical assessment of estrogen receptor distribution in the human endometrium throughout the menstrual cycle. Lab. Invest. **51**: 495–501.

32. FRAME, L. T., L. AWILEY & A. D. ROYAL. 1979. Indirect immunofluorescent localization of prolactin to the cytoplasm of decidua and trophoblast cells in human placental membranes at term. Clin. Endocrinol. Metab. **49**: 435–438.

33. PIJENENBORG, F., G. DIXON, W. B. ROBERTSON & I. BROSENS. 1980. Trophoblastic invasion of human decidua from 8 to 18 weeks of pregnancy. Placenta **1**: 3–9.

34. DODD, M., T. A. ANDREW & J. S. COLES. 1980. Functional behaviour of skin allograft transplanted to rabbit deciduomata. J. Anat. **130**: 381–386.

35. GALANDER, A., V. ZAKUTH, Y. SCHECTER & Z. SPIRER. 1981. Suppression of lymphocyte reactivity "in vitro" by a soluble factor secreted by explants of human decidua. Eur. J. Immunol. **11:** 849–853.

36. MARTIN, L. 1980. What roles are fulfilled by uterine epithelial components in implantation? Prog. Reprod. Biol. **7:** 54–57.

37. RIDDICK, D. H. 1985. Secretory products of the human uterus. *In* Mechanism of Menstrual Bleeding. D. T. Baird & E. A. Michie, Eds. Vol. **1:** 57–81. Raven Press. New York.

38. HOLINKA, C. F. & E. GURPIDE. 1980. In vivo uptake of estrone sulphate by rabbit uterus. Endocrinology **60:** 1193–1197.

39. JASONNI, V. M., C. BULLETTI, F. FRANCESCHETTI, M. BONAVIA, G. F. BOLELLI, P. M. CIOTTI & C. FLAMIGNI. 1974. Estrone sulphate plasma levels in postmenopausal women with and without endometrial cancer. Cancer **53:** 2698–2700.

40. KENNEDY, T. G. 1983. Embryonic signals and the initiation of blastocyst implantation. Aust. J. Biol. Sci. **36:** 531–543.

41. KENNEDY, T. G. & D. T. ARMSTRONG. 1981. The role of prostaglandins in endometrial vascular changes at implantation. *In* Cellular Molecular Aspects of Implantation. S. R. Glasser & D. W. Bullock, Eds. Vol. **1:** 349–363. Plenum Press. New York.

42. HOLMES, P. V. & B. J. GORDASKO. 1980. Evidence of prostaglandin involvement in blastocyst implantation. J. Embryol. Exp. Morphol. **55:** 109–122.

43. PHILLIPS, C. A. & N. L. PPYSER. 1981. Studies on the involvement of prostaglandin in implantation in the rat. J. Reprod. Fertil. **62:** 73–81.

44. EVANS, C. A. & T. G. KENNEDY. 1978. The importance of prostaglandin synthesis for the initiation of blastocyst implantation in the hamster. J. Reprod. Fertil. **54:** 255–261.

45. HOFFMAN, L. H. 1978. Antifertility effects of indomethacin during early pregnancy in the rabbit. Biol. Reprod. **18:** 148–153.

46. TABIBZADEH, S. S., P. G. SATYASWAROOP & P. M. RAO. 1988. Antiproliferative effect of interferon-Γ in human endometrial epithelial cells in vitro: Potential local growth modulatory role in endometrium. J. Clin. Endocrinol. Metab. **67:** 131–136.

47. RUTANEN, E. M., F. PEKONEN & T. MAKINEN. 1988. Soluble 34K protein inhibits the binding of Insulin-like growth factor I to its cell receptors in human secretory phase endometrium: Evidence for autocrine/paracrine regulation of growth action. J. Clin. Endocrinol. Metab. **66:** 173–180.

48. JULKUNEN, M. 1986. Human decidua synthesises placenta protein 14 (PP14) in vitro. Acta Endocrinol. **112:** 271–277.

49. JOSHI, S. G. 1985. Progestin-dependent proteins of the human endometrium. *In* Mechanism of Menstrual Bleeding. D. T. Baird & E. A. Michie, Eds. Vol. **1:** 83–95. Raven Press. New York.

50. CIOCCA, D. R., D. J. ADAMS, D. P. EDWARD, R. J. BJERCKE & W. L. McGUIRE. 1984. Estrogen induced 24K protein in MCF7 breast cancer cells is localized in granules. Breast Cancer Res. Treat. **4:** 261–268.

51. CIOCCA, D. R., R. H. ASCH, D. J. ADAMS & W. L. McGUIRE. 1983. Evidence for modulation of a 24K protein in human endometrium during the menstrual cycle. J. Clin. Endocrinol. Metab. **57**(3): 496–499.

52. SCHALFKE, S. & A. C. ENDERS. 1975. Cellular basis of interaction between trophoblast and uterus at implantation. Biol. Reprod. **12:** 41–65.

53. SHERMAN, M. I. & L. R. WUDL. 1976. The implanting mouse blastocyst. *In* The Cell Surface in Animal Embryogenesis and Development. G. Poste & G. L. Nicolson, Eds. Vol. **1:** 81–125. Elsevier/North Holland Biomedical Press. Amsterdam, NL.

54. CARSON, D., A. DUTT & J. P. TANG. 1987. Glyconjugate synthesis during early pregnancy: Hyaluronate synthesis and function. Develop. Biol. **120:** 228–235.

55. TOLE, B. P., C. BISWAS & J. GROSS. 1979. Hyaluronate and invasiveness of the rabbit V2 carcinoma. Proc. Natl. Acad. Sci. USA **26:** 6299–6303.

56. ARMANT, D. R., H. A. KAPLAN & W. J. LENNARZ. 1986. Fibronectin and laminin promote in vitro attachment and outgrowth of mouse blastocysts. Dev. Biol. **116:** 519–523.

57. WEWER, U., G. TARABOLETTI, M. E. SOBEL, R. ALBRECHTSEN & L. A. LIOTTA. 1987. Role of laminin receptor in tumor cell migration. Cancer Res. **47:** 5691–5698.

58. DENKER, H. W. 1972. Blastocyst protease and implantation effect of ovariectomy and progesterone substitution in the rabbit. Acta Endocrinol. **70:** 591–602.

59. BLASI, F. & M. P. STOPPELLI. 1989. *In* Growth regulation and carcinogenesis. W. Penkowits, Eds. CRC Uniscience.
60. STRICKLAND, S., E. REICH & M. I. SHERMAN. 1976. Plasminogen activator in early embryogenesis: Enzyme production by trophoblast and parietal endoderm. Cell 9: 231–240.
61. FEINBERG, R. F., L. C. KAO, J. E. HAIMOWITZ, J. T. QUEENAN, JR., T. C. WUN, J. F. STRAUSS III & H. J. KLIMA. 1989. Plasminogen activator inhibitor 1 and 2 in human trophoblasts. PAI-1 is an immunocytochemical marker of invading trophoblasts. Lab. Invest. 61(1): 20–26.
62. IRWIN, J. C., D. KIRK, R. J. B. KING, M. M. QUINGLEY & R. B. GWATKIN. 1989. Hormonal regulation of human endometrial stromal cells in culture: An in vitro model for decidualization. Fertil. Steril. 52: 761–768.
63. HANDWERGER, S. & M. FREEMARK. 1987. Role of placental lactogen and prolactin in human pregnancy. *In* Regulation of Ovarian and Testicular Function. V. B. Mahesh, D. S. Dhindsa, E. Anderson, S. P. Kalra, Eds. Vol. 1: 399–418, Plenum Publishing Corp. New York.
64. RUTANEN, E. M., R. KOISTINEN, J. SJOBERG, W. JULKUNEN, T. WALSTROM, H. BOHM & M. SEPPALA. 1986. Synthesis of placental protein 12 by human endometrium. Endocrinology 118: 1067–1072.
65. SHEN, C. J. & E. R. STALEY. 1988. Colony stimulating factor-1. *In* Peptide Growth Factors and Their Receptors. M. B. Sporn & A. B. Roberts, Eds. Springer Verlag-Heidelberg. In press.
66. CROXTALL, J. D., M. G. ELDER & J. O. WHITE. 1989. Steroid regulation of lipocortin II in endometrial cancer. J. Endocrinol. 121(suppl.): 176–182.
67. DERYNCK, R., A. B. ROBERTS, M. E. WINKLER, E. Y. CHEN & D. V. GOEDDEL. 1984. Human transforming growth factor-α: Precursor structure and expression in E. Coli. Cell 38: 287–297.
68. HAN, V. K. M., E. S. HUNTER, R. M. PRATT, J. G. ZENDEGUI & D. C. LEE. 1987. Expression of rat transforming factor α mRNA during development occurs predominantly in maternal decidua. Mol. Cell. Biol. 7: 2335–2343.
69. FOLKMAN, J. & M. KLAGSBRUN. 1987. Angiogenic factors. Science 235: 442–447.
70. GRAY, A., J. DULLT & A. ULRICH. 1983. Nucleotide sequence of epidermal growth factor cDNA predicts a 128.000 molecular protein precursor. Nature 303: 722–725.
71. CARPENTER, G. & S. COHEN. 1979. Epidermal growth factor. Ann. Rev. Biochem. 48: 193–216.
72. TOMOOKA, Y., R. P. DI AUGUSTINE & J. A. MACLLACHLAN. 1986. Proliferation of mouse epithelial cells in vitro. Endocrinology 118: 1011–1018.
73. CLARK, D. A., R. SLAPSYS, B. A. CROY, J. KRECK & J. ROSSANT. 1984. Local active suppression by suppressor cells in the decidua: A review. Am. J. Reprod. Immunol. 6: 78–83.
74. CLARK, D. A., R. M. SLAPSYS, B. A. CROY & J. ROSSANT. 1984. Immunoregulation of host versus graft reaction in the uterus. Immunol. Today 5: 111–119.
75. BILLINGTON, W. D. & S. C. BELL. 1989. Immunobiology of murine trophoblast. *In* Biology of Trophoblast. Y. W. Lake, A. Whyte, Eds. Elsevier/North Holland Biomedical Press. Amsterdam, NL.
76. DAYA, S., D. A. CLARK, C. DEVLIN, J. JARRELL & A. CHAPUT. 1985. Suppressor cells in human decidua. Am. J. Obstet. Gynecol. 151: 267–273.
77. SMART, Y. S., I. S. FRASER, T. K. ROBERTS, R. L. CLANCY & H. W. CRIPPS. 1982. Fertilization and early pregnancy loss in healthy women attempting conception. Clin. Reprod. Fertil. 1: 177–182.
78. ROLFER, B. E. 1982. Detection of fetal wastage. Fertil. Steril. 37: 655–660.
79. NEBEL, L. 1984. Malimplantation a cause of failure after IVf and ET. Am. J. Reprod. Immunol. 6: 56–64.
80. KING, A., C. BIRKBY & Y. W. LOKE. 1989. Early human decidual cells exhibit NK activity against first trimester trophoblast. Cell. Immunol. 118: 337–344.
81. PARHAR, R., S. YAGEL & P. K. LALA. 1989. PGE$_2$-mediated immunosuppression by first trimester human decidual cells blocks activation of maternal leukocytes in the decidua with potential antitrophoblast activity. Cell. Immunol. 120: 61–74.

In Vitro Systems for the Study of Human Trophoblast Implantation

C. COUTIFARIS,[a,c] G. O. BABALOLA,[a]
A. O. ABISOGUN,[a] L-C. KAO,[a] U. CHIN,[a]
F. VADILLO-ORTEGA,[a] J. OSHEROFF,[a]
H. J. KLIMAN,[b] AND J. F. STRAUSS, III[a,b]

[a]Department of Obstetrics & Gynecology
[b]Department of Pathology & Laboratory Medicine
University of Pennsylvania School of Medicine
Philadelphia, Pennsylvania 19104

INTRODUCTION

The process of implantation can be viewed as a series of distinct events involving trophoblast-endometrial interactions. Soon after hatching of the blastocyst, there is apposition of the trophectoderm to the endometrial epithelial cell followed by attachment of these two cell types. In the human, the trophoblast cells subsequently intrude in between endometrial epithelial cells and come in contact with the basement membrane. Degradation of this barrier subsequently occurs, thus allowing the frank invasion of the trophoblast into the endometrial stroma. This process of migration through the stroma continues until invasion of the maternal vessels is achieved, establishing hemochorial placentation. The cellular and molecular mechanisms involved in these series of events are virtually unknown. It is postulated that specific signals involving cell adhesion molecules, substrate adhesion molecules, as well as paracrine and autocrine interactions are delicately orchestrated so that successful establishment of pregnancy is achieved. It is hypothesized that well-synchronized activation of cellular processes are involved in attachment and invasion, while reciprocal events are needed to arrest this process once placentation has been completed.

The progress in our understanding of the process of human embryo implantation has been extremely slow. This is principally due to the fact that the process of nidation is morphologically different in humans than in experimental and domestic animals.[1,2] Presumably, these morphologic variations have their basis on fundamental differences at the cellular and molecular levels. *In vivo* human experimentation for the study of implantation is not feasible, and *in vitro* systems would require the use of human embryos which are not available. Given the impressive advances in assisted reproductive technologies that have occurred over the last decade, as well as the increasing needs for establishment of methods for both contraception and contragestion, elucidation of the mechanisms of human implantation is imperative. The recent development of

[c] *Address all correspondence to:* Christos Coutifaris, M.D., Ph.D., Department of Obstetrics and Gynecology, 106 Dulles Building, Hospital of the University of Pennsylvania, 3400 Spruce Street, Philadelphia, PA 19104.

techniques for isolation of purified placental cytotrophoblasts have allowed characterization of their structural, morphologic and functional differentiation at the cellular and molecular levels (ref. 3; for review see 4). The accumulating evidence suggests that these cells possess many of the characteristics of the implanting trophoblasts of the blastocyst and thus can be used as surrogates in *in vitro* models of human implantation.[5-7] In the present report, our current understanding of the morphologic and functional differentiation of isolated human trophoblasts will be reviewed, and some preliminary observations of the behavior of these cells in several *in vitro* model systems will be described. We believe that understanding the behavior of these cells at the molecular level will shed light on the fundamental processes involved in nidation of the human blastocyst.

HUMAN TROPHOBLASTS IN CULTURE

Mononuclear cytotrophoblasts can be isolated from human placentae by a process of mincing, trypsin-DNase digestion of placental villi, and subsequent centrifugation of the digest through a discontinuous percoll gradient. A population of 96 to 98% pure mononuclear cells can be obtained at a density of 1.048–1.065. The isolated cells have been well-characterized and possess the morphologic and functional characteristics of cytotrophoblasts.[3] These cells can be viewed as the trophoblastic precursor cell, which upon differentiation through a process of aggregation and fusion can produce the terminally differentiated syncytial trophoblast. The cytotrophoblast is the mitotically active cell whose behavior with respect to both morphology and function depends upon its environment. The process of morphologic differentiation of the trophoblast from mononuclear cytotrophoblast to multinucleated syncytial trophoblast can be observed *in vitro* using purified cytotrophoblast preparations from human placentae. Using standard culture conditions and serum-containing media, the cells can be seen to migrate towards each other, form aggregates, and finally fuse to form syncytia over a period of 72 to 96 hours.[3] This process of morphologic differentiation can also be achieved in serum-free conditions if the culture surface has been precoated with extracellular matrix components such as fibronectin, laminin, and different types of collagen.[8] It appears that extracellular matrix components provide the lattice for movement of these cells. The presence, though, of extracellular matrix proteins is not obligatory for the process of morphologic differentiation since both aggregation and fusion of the cells can be achieved if the cells are cultured in serum-free media in *suspension*.[9] This culture system allows for random collision of these cells, which allows their aggregation and subsequent fusion. Morphologically, the cellular aggregates form cystic structures which upon subsequent plating on matrix components form outgrowths resembling villi. Under these conditions, scanning electron microscopic studies have indicated these aggregates to be covered with microvilli (FIG. 1). It has been clearly shown that this process of aggregation is protein synthesis dependent, and requires the presence of calcium ions.[9] Preliminary observations have indicated that the calcium-dependent cell adhesion molecule (CAM) E-cadherin is intimately involved in this process.[10,11] In addition, transmission electron microscopic studies have shown the establishment of desmosomes between the aggregating cells[9] and desmoplakins I and II (which are integral components of the desmosomal complex) have been demonstrated to be present at points of cell contact through immunohistochemistry.[11] This organization of the cell adhesion system is transient since the

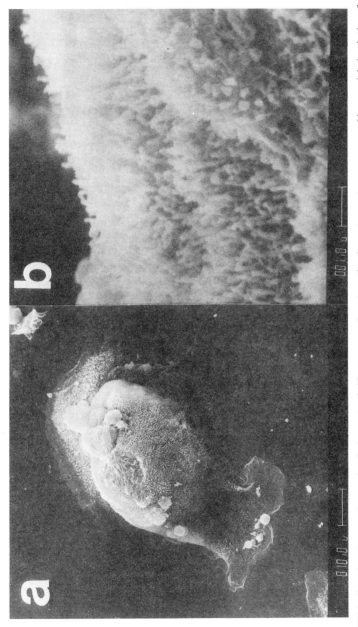

FIGURE 1. Scanning electron micrographs of a human trophoblast aggregate in outgrowth culture. Aggregates were prepared by overnight incubation of purified human cytotrophoblasts in a shaking suspension culture (see ref. 9). The aggregates were subsequently allowed to attach to glass coverslips in serum containing media and fixed and prepared for scanning EM after 24 h of incubation. The aggregates project from the culture surface (**a**) and are covered by microvilli (**b**).

trophoblast cells subsequently fuse and the cell surface expression of E-cadherin and desmoplakins disappears.[10,11]

In parallel to this process of morphological differentiation functional differentiation of the cells with respect to endocrine activity also occurs. The freshly isolated mononuclear cytotrophoblasts do not synthesize or secrete the hormones characteristic of the placenta (*e.g.*, chorionic gonadotropin, placental lactogen, progesterone, and estrogen) while the resultant multinucleated syncytial structures do.[3] This process mimics the *in vivo* situation where the mononuclear cytotrophoblasts do not exhibit this characteristic endocrine function while the syncytial trophoblasts do. Interestingly, the processes of morphologic and endocrine differentiation of the cells can be uncoupled by the addition of cyclic AMP analogues to the culture media or of agents which increase intracellular cyclic AMP.[12] The involvement of this classic "second messenger system" in the functional differentiation of these cells may suggest a role for paracrine or autocrine factors in the function of these cells *in vivo.*

TROPHOBLAST–EXTRACELLULAR MATRIX INTERACTIONS

As described above, morphologic differentiation of the trophoblast cells under standard culture conditions requires extracellular matrix components which presumably provide the lattice for movement of the cells. The intruding/invading trophoblast *in vivo* comes in contact with various extracellular matrix components through its journey from the endometrial epithelium to the maternal vessels. Initially, binding and subsequent degradation of basement membrane needs to be accomplished. This involves interactions of the trophoblast with type IV collagen as well as laminin and proteoglycans. In the *in vitro* system described, precoating of the culture surface with type IV collagen or laminin, allows for binding and movement of these cells.[8] In addition, preliminary immunohistochemical observations using monoclonal antibodies against various integrins have indicated the presence of the α^6-β_1 heterodimer, which corresponds to a laminin receptor (Coutifaris, unpublished observations). Recent studies have indicated that plating of these cells on a critical thickness of matrigel not only allows for the morphologic differentiation of these cells through aggregation and fusion, but also promotes the elaboration of enzyme(s) which degrade the laminin component of this basement membrane construct.[13] This process may involve the elaboration of urokinase-type plasminogen activator and its inhibitors, which have been shown to be secreted by these cells under the described culture conditions.[14,15] It is of interest to note that *in vivo*, urokinase has been implicated to be of importance in the process of implantation.[16] Further, recent evidence suggests the elaboration by these trophoblastic cells of metalloproteinases, which can degrade gelatin and specifically ones with collagenolytic activity (ref. 17; Abisogun & Coutifaris, unpublished observations). Therefore, these trophoblastic cells isolated from placentae not only have the capacity and molecular mechanism to attach to the basement membrane through specific cell-substratum adhesion molecules, but also possess the cellular mechanism for degradation of this structural component which separates the epithelium from the stroma.

Another extracellular matrix protein which the trophoblast encounters is fibronectin. The α^5-β_1 integrin has been demonstrated to be present on the surface of the purified cytotrophoblasts and shows specific distribution along adhesion plaques between the substrate and the cell (Coutifaris, unpublished observations). Normal motility of these cells with subsequent aggregation and fusion has been demonstrated if the culture

surface has been precoated with fibronectin,[8] and placement of aggregates onto millicell filters precoated with fibronectin shows a prompt attachment with subsequent
degradation of the fibronectin surrounding the trophoblast aggregates (FIG. 2). This
is a time-dependent phenomenon, which terminates in the detachment of the trophoblast aggregate from the culture surface once the extacellular matrix has been completely degraded, since the millicell filter cannot support attachment. It appears, that
although addition of cyclic AMP inibits the degradation of laminin by these cells,[13]
the degradation of fibronectin is further enhanced, thus suggesting a possible differential regulation of proteolytic processes by the stage of differentiation of these cells.

HETEROLOGOUS CO-CULTURE SYSTEMS

The first interaction between trophoblast and endometrium involves the adhesion
of trophoblast to the endometrial epithelial cell, followed by intrusion of the trophoblast in between these cells. Characterization of both a two- and a three-dimensional
co-culture system have provided the tools for study of these processes at the cellular
and molecular level.[5-7]

Endometrial epithelial cells can be isolated from human endometrium using a procedure developed by Satyaswaroop *et al.*[18] The endometrial epithelial cells plated
under usual culture conditions on glass or plastic, form islands of cells, which have
been characterized to be epithelial in nature by their characteristic cytokeratin immunostaining. After establishment of these cells in culture, their interaction with trophoblastic cells can be studied by the addition of purified human cytotrophoblasts. When
this is done, the trophoblasts are observed to aggregate around the islands of endometrial epithelial cells, intrude in between them and penetrate deep into these cell
islands.[5] This process appears to be gentle rather than destructive and allows the
gradual separation of the junctions between the epithelial cells by the intruding trophoblasts. The endometrial epithelial cells subsequently remodel themselves around the
trophoblasts, eventually completely encasing them. This process, which occurs in
this two-dimensional co-cuture system, is reminiscent of the early intrusive process
of trophoblasts *in vivo*, during which the trophoblast intrudes between endometrial
cells rather then destroying them. Once the *in vivo* process of intrusion through the
epithelium is complete, the implanting embryo is completely imbedded in the endometrium and covered by epithelium at the original implantation site. As is the case
in vivo, the described *in vitro* system requires the transient dissolution of the adhesion
system between the endometrial epithelial cells. Preliminary immunohistochemical
observations show the disappearance of desmoplakins I and II from the cell surface
at the points of endometrial epithelial cell contact as the intruding trophoblast is allowed to penetrate the epithelial cell islands. The mechanism by which this cellular
dissociation is achieved with no apparent destruction of the epithelial cells is unknown
at the present time.

The process of implantation *in vivo* is a three-dimensional event. Thus, the establishment of a three-dimensional system is imperative in order to have the capability
of studying the regulation of attachment of the trophoblast to the endometrium. If
human endometrial epithelial cells are isolated and placed onto extracellular matrix
coated platforms (type IV collagen, laminin, matrigel) a confluent cell layer can be
established, which shows distinct polarization of the epithelial cells with a basal region adjacent to the matrix-coated platform and an apical region equivalent to the

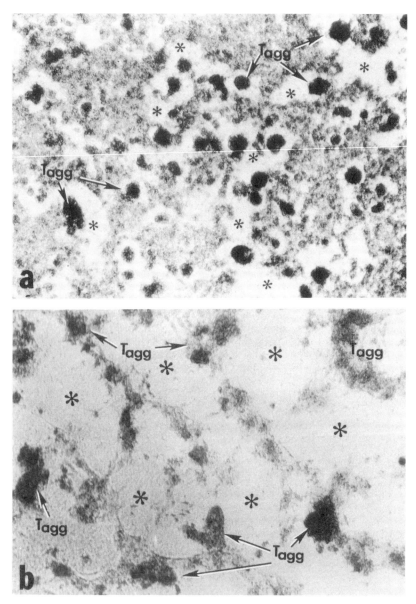

FIGURE 2. Culture of trophoblast aggregates (Tagg) on fibronectin-coated millicell-CM filters. Aggregates were prepared as described in ref. 9, placed onto fibronectin precoated millicell-CM filters, incubated in serum-free media in humidified 95% air–5% CO_2, and observed under an inverted microscope at time intervals up to 96 h (*magnification:* ×100). **a.** At 48 h of incubation, note areas of clearing of the granular fibronectin layer (*) around trophoblast aggregates. **b.** At 96 h, extensive areas of clearing of fibronectin (*) are evident and trophoblast aggregates have detached from the culture surface.

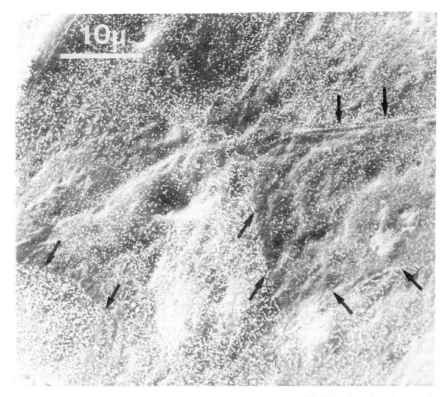

FIGURE 3. Scanning electron micrograph of human endometrial epithelial cells cultured on a collagen membrane (Cellagen,™ ICN Biochemicals). Note the extensive surface microvilli. Individual cell borders in this confluent cell culture are also discernible (*arrows*).

endometrial luminal compartment. In contrast to the epithelial cells cultured on plastic or glass, the polarized cells show a luminal surface rich in microvilli (FIG. 3) and a functional polarity showing transport of labeled amino acids from the basal compartment with preferential secretion into the luminal compartment. Transmission electron microscopy indicates the presence of desmosomes near the apical region between adjacent epithelial cells as well as other elements characteristic of polarized epithelium. Of interest, is the observation that trophoblast aggregates prepared as described earlier and placed onto these polarized epithelia show prompt attachment (FIG. 4), which transmission electron microscopic studies have shown to be mediated by desmosomes (FIG. 5). It is reasonable to conclude that this attachment is specific and is mediated by a cell adhesion molecule. This hypothesis as well as the regulation of the described process awaits confirmation and further elucidation.

CONCLUSIONS

The process of human implantation involves a well-orchestrated series of complex events culminating in successful hemochorial placentation and establishment of preg-

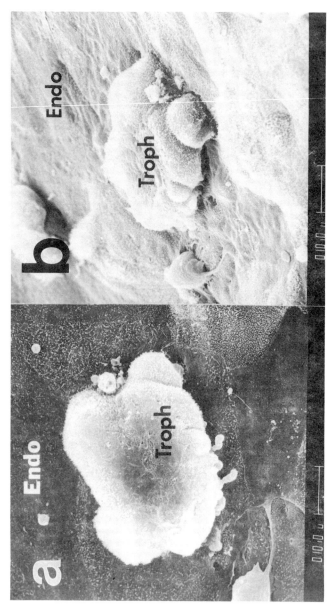

FIGURE 4. Scanning electron micrographs of a trophoblast aggregate (troph) adherent on a confluent layer of endometrial epithelial cells (endo) cultured on a collagen membrane. Both micrographs represent the same aggregate (a. top view; b. 45 degree angle view from the right). Note the microvilli on both the trophoblast and endometrial cell surface.

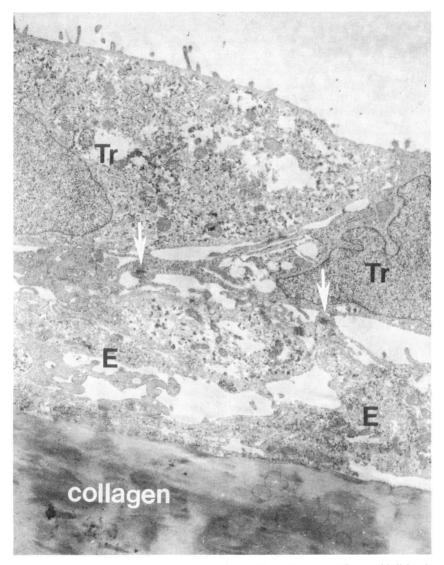

FIGURE 5. Transmission electron micrograph of trophoblasts (Tr) on a confluent epithelial endometrial cell layer (E) cultured on a collagen membrane (×10,140). Note the presence of desmosomes at points of contact of trophoblasts with the endometrial cells (*arrows*).

nancy. Since its study cannot be achieved *in vivo*, *in vitro* systems designed to study each individual step at its cellular and molecular level is necessary. Is it justified to use the purified mononuclear cytotrophoblasts from human placentae as a surrogate for the implanting trophoblast? Our data to date suggests: (1) that these cells can differentiate *in vitro* to form syncytial trophoblasts through a process of aggregation and fusion; (2) aggregates in suspension form cystic structures with evidence of functional and morphologic polarity; (3) these cystic structures form outgrowths in culture reminiscent of chorionic villi; (4) the differentiated syncytial structures secrete the characteristic hormones of the syncytial trophoblast, chorionic gonadotropin, placental lactogen, estrogens and progesterone. Thus, these cells undergo the morphologic differentiation seen in cytotrophoblasts *in vivo*. Most importantly though, the behavior of these cells in the described *in vitro* systems is also remarkably reminiscent of the behavior of the implanting human trophoblast *in vivo*: 1) they attach to polarized endometrial epithelial cells; 2) they are capable of intrusive behavior, insinuating themselves in between endometrial epithelial cells in culture by gently separating the cells without destroying them, and finally, 3) they have the capacity to attach, degrade and remodel extracellular matrix elements which are integral components of the endometrial basement membrane and stroma. We believe that the use of the described *in vitro* models in the study of human trophoblasts, may generate fundamental information at the cellular and molecular levels on the regulation of the processes which result in normal and abnormal human implantation.

REFERENCES

1. WEITLAUF, H. M. 1988. Biology of implantation. *In* The Physiology of Reproduction. E. Knobil & J. Neill, Eds.: 231–262. Raven Press, New York.

2. SCHLAFKE, S. & A. C. ENDERS. 1975. Cellular basis of interaction between trophoblast and uterus at implantation. Biol. Reprod. **12**: 41–52.

3. KLIMAN, H. J., J. E. NESTLER, E. SERMASI, J. M. SANGER & J. F. STRAUSS, III. 1986. Purification, characterization and *in vitro* differentiation of cytotrophoblasts from human term placentae. Endocrinology **118**: 1567–1582.

4. RINGLER, G. E. & J. F. STRAUSS, III. 1990. *In vitro* systems for the study of human placental endocrine function. Endo. Rev. **11**: 105–123.

5. COUTIFARIS, C., H. J. KLIMAN, P. WU & J. F. STRAUSS, III. 1989. Specificity of trophoblast-endometrial interactions in a human *in vitro* implantation model system. 36th Annual Meeting of the Society for Gynecologic Investigation, San Diego, CA. Abstract 489.

6. COUTIFARIS, C., L-C. KAO, H. J. KLIMAN, P. WU & J. F. STRAUSS, III. 1989. Implantation of the human trophoblast: Cell-cell and cell-substratum interactions in an *in vitro* model system. 45th Annual Meeting of the American Fertility Society, San Francisco, CA. Abstract 003.

7. KLIMAN, H. J., C. COUTIFARIS, R. F. FEINBERG, J. F. STRAUSS, III & J. E. HAIMOWITZ. 1989. Implantation: *In vitro* models utilizing human tissues. *In* Blastocyst Implantation. K. Yoshinaga, Ed.: 83. Adams Publishing Group, Ltd., Boston.

8. KAO, L-C., S. CALTABIANO, S. WU, J. F. STRAUSS, III & H. J. KLIMAN. 1988. The human villous cytotrophoblast: Interactions with extracellular matrix proteins, endocrine function and cytoplasmic differentiation in the absence of syncytium formation. Dev. Biol. **130**: 693–702.

9. BABALOLA, G. O., C. COUTIFARIS, E. A. SOTO, H. J. KLIMAN, H. SHUMAN & J. F. STRAUSS, III. 1990. Aggregation of dispersed human cytotrophoblastic cells: Lessons relevant to the morphogenesis of the placenta. Develop. Biol. **137**: 100–108.

10. COUTIFARIS, C., G. O. BABALOLA, U. CHIN, C. A. BUCK & J. F. STRAUSS, III. 1990. Contact induced expression of the cell adhesion molecule E-cadherin during the morphologic differentiation of human trophoblasts. 37th Annual Meeting of the Society for Gynecologic Investigation, St. Louis, MO. Abstract 1.

11. BABALOLA, G. O., C. COUTIFARIS, U. CHIN, W. J. NELSON, C. A. BUCK & J. F. STRAUSS, III. 1990. Differential expression of cell adhesion proteins in human trophoblastic cells. Biol. Reprod. **42**(Suppl. I): 80 (abst. 119).

12. FEINMAN, M. A., H. J. KLIMAN, S. CALTABIANO & J. F. STRAUSS, III. 1986. 8-Bromo-3′5′-adenosine monophosphate stimulates the endocrine activity of human cytotrophoblasts in culture. J. Clin. Endocrinol. Metab. **63**: 1211–1217.

13. KLIMAN, H. J. & R. F. FEINBERG. 1990. Human trophoblast-extracellular matrix (ECM) interactions *in vitro*: ECM thickness modulates morphology and proteolytic activity. Proc. Natl. Acad. Sci. USA **87**: 3057–3061.

14. FEINBERG, R. F., L-C. KAO, J. E. HAIMOWITZ, J. T. QUEENAN, T-C WUN, J. F. STRAUSS III & H. J. KLIMAN. 1989. Plasminogen activator inhibitors 1 and 2 in human trophoblasts. PAI-1 is an immunohistochemical marker of invading trophoblasts. Lab. Invest. **61**: 20–26.

15. QUEENAN, J. T., JR., L-C. KAO, C. E. ARBOLEDA, A. ULLOA-AGUIRRE, T. G. GOLOS, D. B. CINES & J. F. STRAUSS. 1987. Regulation of urokinase type plasminogen activator production by culture human cytotrophoblasts. J. Biol. Chem. **262**: 10903–10906.

16. STRICKLAND, S., E. REICH & M. I. SHERMAN. 1976. Plasminogen activator in early embryogenesis: Enzyme production by trophoblast and parietal endoderm cell. Cell **9**: 231–240.

17. FISHER, S. J., M. S. LEITCH, M. S. KANTOR, C. B. BASBNAUM & R. H. KRAMER. 1985. Degradation of extracellular matrix by trophoblastic cells of first-trimester human placentas. J. Cell. Biochem. **27**: 31–41.

18. SATYASWAROOP, P. G., R. S. BRESSLER, M. M. DE LA PENA & E. GURPIDE. 1979. Isolation and culture of human endometrial glands. J. Clin. Endocrinol. Metab. **48**: 639–641.

Comparative Aspects of Conceptus Signals for Maternal Recognition of Pregnancy[a]

FULLER W. BAZER, ROSALIA C. M. SIMMEN,
AND FRANK A. SIMMEN[b]

Departments of Animal Science and [b]Dairy Science
University of Florida
Gainesville, Florida 32611

INTRODUCTION

Pregnancy is established and maintained in response to interactions between the conceptus (embryo/fetus and associated membranes and fluids) and endometrium. This chapter describes events associated with establishment of intimate contact between the conceptus and uterine endometrium and the conceptus signals affecting the maternal system which allow establishment of pregnancy and maintenance of an intrauterine environment supportive of pregnancy.

ANTILUTEOLYTIC FACTORS FROM CONCEPTUSES OF PIGS AND SHEEP

Conceptus "signals" must be produced at precise times and in adequate amounts for maintenance of morphological and functional integrity of the corpus luteum (CL) and continued production of progesterone by CL, *i.e.*, maternal recognition of pregnancy.[1] Maintenance of an intrauterine environment that will support conceptus development is dependent on progesterone. Endometria of nonpregnant sheep and pigs secrete Prostaglandin $F_{2\alpha}$ (PGF), the uterine luteolytic factor, in a pattern necessary to induce regression of CL (luteolysis). Subprimate species have a uterine-dependent ovarian cycle; therefore, conceptuses of sheep and pigs produce proteins, steroids and/or prostaglandins which inhibit uterine production of luteolytic amounts of PGF. Primates, however, have a uterine-independent ovarian cycle. Luteolysis appears to be dependent on intra-ovarian mechanisms which are inhibited by a luteotrophic signal, *i.e.*, human chorionic gonadotropin (hCG).

Sheep conceptuses secrete an antiluteolytic protein called ovine trophoblast protein-1 (oTP-1) between Days 10 and 21 of pregnancy. oTP-1 secreted by mononuclear cells of the trophectoderm, has a molecular weight of about 19 000 and pI values of 5.3 to 5.7.[2] oTP-1 has high amino acid sequence homology with interferons of the alpha-II ($IFN\alpha_{II}$) class;[3] potent antiviral activity,[4] antiproliferative activity (C. Pontzer, F. W. Bazer, and H. M. Johnson, unpublished results), and immunosuppressive activity.[5]

[a] This paper is published as University of Florida Experiment Station Journal Series No. R-00760.

oTP-1 is the only antiluteolytic protein secreted by sheep conceptuses. oTP-1 inhibits endometrial secretion of luteolytic pulses of PGF.[2]

Endometrium of cyclic ewes releases PGF in a pulsatile manner between Days 14 and 17 of the cycle, which results in luteolysis.[2] In a progesterone-dominated uterus, progesterone and estradiol from ovarian follicles interact to induce endometrial receptors for oxytocin. Oxytocin from CL and/or posterior pituitary stimulates uterine secretion of luteolytic pulses of PGF.[2] The pattern of oxytocin release is not different between cyclic and pregnant ewes; however, endometrial oxytocin receptor numbers are few or absent in pregnant ewes.[6]

In the total array of ovine conceptus secretory proteins (oCSP), oTP-1 alone has antiluteolytic activity.[2] oTP-1 does not interfere with binding of oxytocin to its receptor, oxytocin stimulation of its second messenger system, or oxytocin stimulation of endometrial secretion of PGF when endometrial oxytocin receptors are present.[2] Therefore, synthesis of endometrial oxytocin receptors and oxytocin-induced PI turnover and PGF secretion are inhibited when endometrium of cyclic ewes is exposed to oTP-1 on Days 12 through 14.[7]

Concentrations of prostaglandin E_2 (PGE) in utero-ovarian vein blood of pregnant ewes increase markedly on Days 13 and 14 and PGE may play a luteal protective role.[2] The PGE may interfere with the luteolytic activity of PGF through a competitive mechanism or alternatively, PGE may accelerate depletion of luteal oxytocin prior to formation of endometrial oxytocin receptors on Days 14 to 16.

The theory of maternal recognition of pregnancy in pigs has been reviewed extensively.[2] This theory states that PGF is secreted in an endocrine direction (toward the uterine vasculature) in cyclic pigs and transported to the CL to exert its luteolytic effect. However, in pregnant pigs, the direction of secretion of PGF is exocrine (into the uterine lumen) where it is sequestered to exert its biological effects *in utero*. Available results suggest that estradiol induces endometrial receptors for prolactin in pigs,[2] which may allow prolactin to induce calcium cycling across the epithelium and redirect secretion of PGF into the uterine lumen.

Pig conceptuses secrete two major classes of proteins (pCSP) between Days 10.5 and 18 of gestation[8] which include a protein(s) with antiviral activity.[9] However, available results indicate that pCSP are not antiluteolytic.[10]

RETINOID BINDING PROTEINS

Retinol binding protein(s), a major component of pCSP and oCSP, is secreted by pig conceptuses from Day 10 of pregnancy and by endometrial epithelium of pigs in response to progesterone.[11] Retinoids affect gene transcription, cellular differentiation and proliferation, epithelial cell integrity and function, steroidogenesis, hematopoiesis and immune cell function, and interferon production.[11] Each of these functions is related to the establishment and maintenance of pregnancy.

PLASMINOGEN ACTIVATOR AND PLASMIN/TRYPSIN INHIBITOR

Plasminogen activators of both the tissue (tPA) and urokinase (uPA) type are present in uterine secretions of pigs and may be involved in tissue remodeling, *e.g.*, trophoblast outgrowth, implantation and uterine development, including angiogenesis.[12] Progesterone-induced inhibitors of plasmin and possibly tPA and uPA are present in uterine secretions of pigs and prevent invasive implantation of pig blastocysts, as is the case for PA from trophectoderm of rodent blastocysts. Pig blastocysts are invasive when transferred to ectopic sites, but not in the uterine lumen where protease inhibitors secreted by the endometrial surface epithelium are adsorbed to the trophectoderm. This may restrict effects of PA to remodeling of conceptus tissues. Protease inhibitors may also protect secreted proteins from degradation in the uterine lumen or during transplacental transport into the fetal-placental circulation.

ENDOMETRIAL SECRETIONS IN PIGS AND SHEEP

Conceptuses of pigs and sheep exhibit noninvasive implantation and depend upon secretions of endometrial epithelium for most, if not all of pregnancy.[12]. Peptides and proteins which serve as nutrients, enzymes, regulatory factors, and transport molecules are present in uterine secretions. Enzymes include lysozyme, cathepsins B, D and E, aminoacylpeptidase, plasminogen activator, glucose phosphate isomerase, β-N-acetylglucosaminidase, hyaluronidase, oxytocinase, acid phosphatase (uteroferrin), and a number of glycosidases in pig uterine secretions.[12] Glucose, fructose, riboflavin, ascorbic acid, sodium, potassium, calcium, amino acids, retinol, retinoic acid, prostaglandins, and an array of free and conjugated steroids are also found in uterine luminal fluid.[13] Uterine secretory activity is greatest when the uterus is under the influence of progesterone. However, estrogens stimulate release of progesterone-induced proteins from secretory granules, as well as synthesis and secretion of a number of other proteins.

Estrogens and catecholestrogens secreted by pig blastocysts beginning on Days 10.5–11 act directly or indirectly to cause vasodilation of arterioles, increase uterine blood flow, stimulate uterine growth and endometrial secretory activity, stimulate uterine production of prostaglandins, increase endometrial receptors for prolactin, and possibly alter effects of cholinergic and adrenergic agents on the uterine endometrium and myometrium.[14] In pregnant gilts, there is an increase in calcium on Days 11–12 followed by an increase in total protein, PGF, PGE, sodium, potassium, and selected amino acids between Days 12 and 14. Alanine, glycine, serine, tyrosine, arginine, histidine, isoleucine, leucine, lysine, methionine, phenylalanine, tryptophan, and valine are higher in uterine flushings from pregnant than cyclic gilts.[15] Glucose accumulates in the uterine lumen after Day 12, but only in pregnant pigs. Androgens and progestins increase in uterine flushing of pregnant, but not cyclic gilts between Days 9 and 15 after onset of estrus and can be converted to free estrogens by pig conceptuses.[16]

Pig endometrium and uterine secretions also contain β-endorphin[17] and methionine-enkephalin;[18] however, their function(s) is not known. There is also an increase in the turnover of norepinephrine and dopamine, as well as an increase in cAMP and cGMP in endometrium of pigs in early pregnancy.[19] These results suggest that interactions between the conceptus and endometrium alter uterine and conceptus functions during pregnancy. Proteins secreted by endometrial epithelium of sheep during early gestation have received little attention. Total protein and activities of the enzymes succinic dehydrogenase, glutamic-oxaloacetic transaminase, acid phosphatase, alkaline phosphatase, glucose-6-phosphatase, β-glucuronidase and glycogen phosphorylase are highest in uterine flushings from diestrus ewes and ovariectomized ewes treated with progesterone.[20]

Endometrial secretory proteins have regulatory roles, *e.g.*, regulation of the maternal immune system to allow survival of the conceptus allograft. Uterine secretions of the cow, sheep and pig contain proteins that inhibit *in vitro* proliferation of lymphocytes in response to mitogens. In addition, skin allografts placed into the uterine lumen are protected from rejection in ewes injected with progesterone for 30 days, the time required to stimulate secretion of two major proteins (Mr = 57 and 59k) which are referred to as ovine uterine milk proteins (oUTMP).[21] Endometria and conceptuses of sheep, cows and pigs also secrete high molecular weight glycoproteins which have immunosuppressive activity *in vitro*.[22] The mechanism by which these immunosuppressive proteins block a maternal cytotoxic attack on the conceptus is not known. Lack of expression of polymorphic transplantation antigens by trophoblast/chorion may also be critical to survival of the conceptus allograft.[23]

In pigs, uterine secretory activity is greatest between Days 12 and 16 and Days 35 and 75 of gestation when the progesterone:estrogen ratio in plasma is greatest. Numbers of endometrial receptors for prolactin are highest (Days 35 to 75) when uterine secretory activity and transport of nutrients into the fetal fluids are greatest.[24] In sheep, induction of secretion of oUTMP by progesterone requires about 30 days.[25] In pregnant ewes, the major increase in uterine secretory activity occurs after 90 days of gestation and is temporally associated with increased production of ovine placental lactogen (oPL) and increasing concentrations of progesterone in maternal plasma. It has been suggested that oPL and/or prolactin, as well as estrogen, are necessary for induction of progesterone receptors and, in turn, induction of uterine secretory activity by progesterone in ewes.[25]

UTEROFERRIN, A HEMATOPOIETIC GROWTH FACTOR

Uteroferrin (UF) is a progesterone-induced glycoprotein secreted by the glandular epithelium of pig endometrium. UF has a Mr of about 35 000, a pI of about 9.7, acid phosphatase enzymatic activity and 2 molecules of iron per molecule of UF. The major role of UF has been presumed to be transport of iron from uterine endometrium to conceptus;[26] however, UF has recently been shown to have hematopoietic growth factor activity as well.[27] Localization of UF is in fetal liver, the major hematopoietic organ of fetal pigs, and in yolk sac during early pregnancy.[26] Iron from UF may be released to ferritin and transferred to erythroblasts by a process called ropheocytosis for synthesis of hemoglobin.

Transcriptional activity of the UF gene is low, but distinct between Days 10 and 15 of pregnancy, declines to undetectable levels between Days 16 and 30 and then increases to maximal levels between Days 45 and term (115 days).[28] However, translation of mRNA for UF decreases after Day 60 of pregnancy in pigs, but factors inhibiting translation of UF mRNA are not known.

UF exists as a purple Mr 35 000 monomer and a rose-colored heterodimer (Rose) when bound to one of three UF-associated proteins.[29] The UF-associated proteins have high amino acid sequence homology with serine protease inhibitors; however, the UF-associated proteins are not known to inhibit proteases.[30] Both UF and Rose have colony forming unit (CFU) and burst forming unit (BFU) activities for erythroid (CFU-

E) cells, as well as CFU-granulocyte-monocyte/macrophage (CFU-GM) activities for myeloid cells.[27] Human placenta contains a UF-like protein, the tartrate-resistant Type 5 acid phosphatase, which also has hematopoietic growth factor activity (F. W. Bazer, D. Worthington-White, M. A. Davis, and S. Gross, unpublished results) and 82% amino acid sequence homology with porcine UF.[31,32]

GROWTH FACTORS OF PREGNANCY

Growth factors exhibit diverse modes of action with respect to uterine growth, differentiation and function. At various stages of uterine development, uterine-derived growth factors may, through paracrine and autocrine mechanisms stimulate cellular DNA synthesis, mediate epithelial-stromal interactions, facilitate blastocyst implantation, increase placental vascular circulation, accelerate fetal growth and development and induce extracellular matrix remodeling.[33,34] Recent studies to elucidate the roles of endometrial growth factors in maternal-fetal interactions have derived from use of immunological and molecular probes to monitor the expression levels of mRNAs and corresponding protein(s) in uterine and fetal (placental) tissues. Understandably, studies have been more extensive with rodent models, but sufficient data have emerged to indicate possible involvement of peptide growth factors in maternal-fetal communication in primates and other mammals.

The most extensively characterized peptide growth factors in primate reproduction are epidermal growth factor (EGF) and the insulin-like growth factors (IGFs). EGF actions are targeted to all layers of human uterus including stroma, glandular epithelium and myometrium, based upon detection of specific high affinity EGF receptors in each of these tissues.[35] EGF mRNAs are synthesized primarily in uterine epithelia in the mouse;[36] however, no studies to date have localized production of EGF in any human uterine cell types. The role(s) of EGF in the uterus may be related to creating a favorable environment for the developing conceptuses, as well as a mitogen for endometrial epithelial cells. The role of EGF in myometrium is less clear, although results of recent studies indicated that it stimulates uterine contractions *in vitro*.[37]

Components of the IGF pathway have been elucidated in both the human and baboon. In humans, the placenta is a major site of IGF-I and -II production during pregnancy.[38] Highest expression of placental IGF-I mRNAs occur during the first trimester, whereas IGF-II mRNA levels peak during the second trimester of pregnancy.[39] These developmental changes correspond closely to uterine endometrial steady-state levels of IGF mRNAs in pregnant pigs, in which highest expression of IGF-I and -II mRNAs are detected during the preimplantation period and mid-pregnancy, respectively.[40,41] Similar results have now been demonstrated in sheep endometrium where expression of IGF-I and -II are temporally correlated with the peri-implantation period.[42] The autocrine/paracrine mechanism of IGF action in the placenta likely mediates aspects of placental metabolism, growth, and development. Placental IGFs may also stimulate growth and development of the conceptus, since these tissues contain IGF receptors and respond physiologically to IGFs.[43] IGF binding proteins (IGFBPs) are synthesized in endometrial and decidual tissues and may mediate the biological actions of IGFs.[44] In humans and baboons, IGFBP-1 is the predominant secretory component during gestation and has been localized in decidual stromal cells,[45] amniotic fluid,[46] and endometrial glandular epithelium.[47] It has been shown that IGFBP-1 inhibits binding of IGF-I to its receptor in human endometrial membranes *in vitro*.[48] A role for IGFBP-1 has been postulated in implantation of baboon and human conceptuses.[47,48]

Human placenta also contains factor(s) which stimulate endothelial cell proliferation, migration and angiogenesis *in vivo* and *in vitro*.[49] This factor was found to be homologous to basic fibroblast growth factor (bFGF), which was also localized in conditioned media and homogenates of human fetal membranes and cotyledons from term placentae.[49] FGFs (both acidic and basic forms) have been isolated from uterine tissues of early pregnant gilts,[50] and recent data suggest the presence of these growth factors in sheep uteri also.[42]

Are specific growth factors responsible for initiation of morphological development of conceptuses from spherical to tubular to filamentous forms and initiation of events leading to the secretion of steroids and/or proteins responsible for maternal recognition of pregnancy? Just prior to initiation of estrogen secretion and morphological transition from spherical to tubular to filamentous forms, there is mesodermal outgrowth from the embryonic disc of pig conceptuses, *i.e.*, Days 10 to 12 of pregnancy, which coincides with peak values for IGF-I in uterine secretions of both cyclic and pregnant pigs. Furthermore, conceptuses of prolific Chinese Meishan pigs develop more rapidly, secrete more estrogens and are exposed to higher amounts of IGF-I in uterine secretions than conceptuses of less prolific Large White pigs.[51] Secretion of significant amounts of IFNα-like proteins by pig conceptuses does not begin until Days 13 to 14 or well after mesodermal outgrowth is established.[9]

The growth factor associated with inducing mesoderm in amphibians is βFGF[52] and both αFGF and βFGF stimulate proliferation of mesoderm-derived cells. Fibroblast growth factors are present in pig endometrium and uterine secretions,[34] but temporal associations between secretion of FGFs, morphological changes in conceptuses and initiation of secretion of estrogens by pig conceptuses have not been established.

The most dramatic increase in rate of secretion of oTP-1 by sheep conceptuses occurs on Day 13.[53] Both IGF-I and IGF-II are present in Day 13 uterine secretions of sheep;[42] however, their effects on conceptus development and secretion of oTP-1 are not known. Co-culture of sheep endometrium and conceptuses from Day 16 of pregnancy results in a two- to threefold increase in secretion of oTP-1 which suggests that endometrial factors can influence secretion of oTP-1.[2]

Rates of development of bovine conceptuses are accelerated by injecting cows with exogenous progesterone (100 mg/day) on Days 1–4 after estrus.[54] Bovine trophoblast protein-1 (bTP-1), an IFNα$_{II}$, responsible for maternal recognition of pregnancy in cattle was secreted by conceptuses with accelerated development, but not by conceptuses from control cows.

Platelet-derived growth factor (PDGF) mRNA and protein are expressed in human placenta throughout pregnancy, but highest levels are at midtrimester.[55] This period coincides with maximum proliferation of cytotrophoblast cells, peak levels of IGF-II and accelerated fetal growth. An autocrine mechanism of control is involved in PDGF action in placenta since coordinate expression of mRNAs (and corresponding protein) for PDGF receptor occur at this time. Human and murine decidua and placenta also synthesize colony-stimulating factor-1 (CSF-1),[56,57] coincident with expression of its specific receptor (c-fms) in placenta.[58] Elevated levels of CSF are also found in amniotic fluid throughout gestation, suggesting a role in placental growth regulation. The presence of the transforming growth factor (TGF) family of peptides has not been examined extensively in human uterine tissues. Expression of three forms of murine

TGF-β (β_1, β_2 and β_3) is predominant in the placenta and developing embryos,[59,60] although the relative levels in tissues vary. The TGF-βs may influence mesoderm induction. In frog embryos, a protein called Vg1 exhibits sequence relatedness to TGF-β and is localized in the vegetal hemisphere where it may influence mesoderm formation.[61,62] Uterine production of TGF-β has not been demonstrated in primates and domestic animals, but potential functions are predicted. In sheep, TGF-β may mediate maternal signaling by inducing trophoblast outgrowth and influencing secretion of oTP-1. In pigs, estrogens produced by the conceptus may induce uterine production of TGF-β, which could then facilitate conceptus development. Conceptus estrogens have been shown to induce endometrial secretion of IGF-I in the pig (unpublished observations from our laboratories); and, similarly estrogen increased levels of three isoforms of TGF-β in rat uterus.[63]

Within the uterine microenvironment during pregnancy, the developing conceptus is also a source of growth factors. Using the highly sensitive method of polymerase chain reaction (PCR), synthesis of TGFs, IGF-II, PDGF, FGF and interleukin-6 (IL-6) by developing mouse embryos have been demonstrated.[64,65] Sheep conceptuses also secrete IGF-I and IGF-II,[42] and preimplantation pig conceptuses exhibit low, but detectable levels of IGF-I mRNAs.[40] Although studies on fetal production of growth factors in primates have not been extensive, existing data from studies of rodents and domestic animals suggest similar responses.

SUMMARY

Maintenance of corpus luteum (CL) function is essential for establishment of pregnancy in mammals. Estrogens from pig conceptuses (embryo and associated membranes) initiate events that, with prolactin, redirect secretion of the uterine luteolytic hormone prostaglandin $F_{2\alpha}$ (PGF) from an endocrine (to uterine veins) to an exocrine (to uterine lumen) direction to prevent luteolysis. Ovine conceptuses secrete ovine trophoblast protein-1 (oTP-1), which exhibits high amino acid sequence relatedness with alpha II interferons (IFNα_{II}) and inhibits synthesis of endometrial receptors for oxytocin and uterine production of luteolytic pulses of PGF. Estrogens and oTP-1 are local antiluteolytic signals to endometrium, whereas human chorionic gonadotrophin (hCG) appears to have a direct luteotrophic effect on CL. A progestational endometrium secretes proteins that serve as growth factors, transport proteins, regulatory proteins and enzymes, as well as transporting nutrients into the uterine lumen to support conceptus development.

REFERENCES

1. SHORT, R. V. 1969. Implantation and the maternal recognition of pregnancy. *In* Foetal Autonomy. Ciba Foundation Symposium. Churchill, London.
2. BAZER, F. W., J. L. VALLET, J. P. HARNEY, T. S. GROSS & W. W. THATCHER. 1989. Comparative aspects of maternal recognition of pregnancy between sheep and pigs. J. Reprod. Fertil. (Suppl.) **37:** 85–89.
3. IMAKAWA, K., R. V. ANTHONY, M. KAZEMI, K. R. MAROTTI, H. G. POLITES & R. M. ROBERTS. 1987. Interferon-like sequence of ovine trophoblast protein secreted by embryonic trophectoderm. Nature (Lond.) **330:** 377–379.
4. PONTZER, C. H., B. Z. TORRES, J. L. VALLET, F. W. BAZER & H. M. JOHNSON. 1988. Antiviral

activity of the pregnancy recognition hormone ovine trophoblast protein-1. Biochem. Biophys. Res. Commun. **152:** 801–807.

5. NEWTON, G. R., J. L. VALLET, P. J. HANSEN & F. W. BAZER. 1989. Inhibition of lymphocyte proliferation by ovine trophoblast protein-1 and a high molecular weight glycoprotein produced by preimplantation sheep conceptuses. Am. J. Reprod. Immunol. Microbiol. **19:** 99–107.

6. FLINT, A. P. F. & E. L. SHELDRICK. 1986. Ovarian oxytocin and maternal recognition of pregnancy. J. Reprod. Fertil. **76:** 831–839.

7. MIRANDO, M. A., T. L. OTT, J. L. VALLET, M. A. DAVIS & F. W. BAZER. 1990. Oxytocin-stimulated inositol phosphate turnover in endometrium of ewes is influenced by stage of the estrous cycle, pregnancy and intrauterine infusion of ovine conceptus secretory proteins. Biol. Reprod. **42:** 98–105.

8. GODKIN, J. D., F. W. BAZER, G. S. LEWIS, R. D. GEISERT & R. M. ROBERTS. 1982. Synthesis and release of polypeptides by pig conceptuses during the period of blastocyst elongation and attachment. Biol. Reprod. **27:** 977–987.

9. MIRANDO, M. A., J. P. HARNEY, S. BEERS, C. H. PONTZER, B. A. TORRES, H. M. JOHNSON & F. W. BAZER. 1990. Onset of secretion of proteins with antiviral activity by pig conceptuses. J. Reprod. Fertil. **88:** 197–203.

10. HARNEY, J. P. & F. W. BAZER. 1989. Effect of porcine conceptus secretory proteins on interestrous interval and uterine secretion of prostaglandins. Biol. Reprod. **41:** 277–284.

11. HARNEY, J. P., M. A. MIRANDO, L. G. SMITH, & F. W. BAZER. 1990. Retinol-binding protein: A major secretory product of the pig conceptus. Biol. Reprod. **42:** 523–532.

12. ROBERTS, R. M. & F. W. BAZER. 1988. The functions of uterine secretions. J. Reprod. Fertil. **82:** 875–892.

13. BAZER, F. W. & R. M. ROBERTS. 1983. Biochemical aspects of conceptus-endometrial interactions. J. Exp. Zool. **228:** 373–383.

14. FORD, S. P. 1989. Factors controlling uterine blood flow during estrus and early pregnancy. *In* The Uterine Circulation. C. Rosenfeld, Ed. Perinatology Press, Ithaca, NY.

15. STONE, B. A. 1985. Biochemical Aspects of Early Pregnancy. Doctoral Dissertation, University of Adelaide, Adelaide, S. Australia.

16. STONE, B. A. & R. F. SEAMARK. 1985. Steroid hormones in uterine washings and in plasma of gilts between Days 9 and 15 after oestrus and between Days 9 and 15 after coitus. J. Reprod. Fertil. **75:** 209–221.

17. LI, W. I., C. L. CHEN, P. J. HANSEN & F. W. BAZER. 1987. β-Endorphin in uterine secretions of pseudopregnant and ovariectomized, ovarian steroid-treated gilts. Endocrinology **121:** 1111–1115.

18. LI, W. I. & L. S. SUNG. 1989. Immunoreactive methionine-enkephalin in porcine reproductive tissues. Biol. Reprod. **40** (Suppl. 1): 78 (abstr.).

19. YOUNG, K. H., F. W. BAZER, J. W. SIMPKINS & R. M. ROBERTS. 1987. Effects of early pregnancy and acute 17β-estradiol administration on porcine uterine secretion, cyclic nucleotides and catecholamines. Endocrinology **120:** 254–263.

20. MURDOCH, B. E. & T. O'SHEA. 1978. Activity of enzymes in the mucosal tissues and rinsings of the reproductive tract of the naturally cyclic ewe. Aust. J. Biol. Sci. **31:** 345–354.

21. HANSEN, P. J., F. W. BAZER & E. C. SEGERSON. 1986. Skin graft survival in the uterine lumen of ewes treated with progesterone. Am. J. Reprod. Immunol. Microbiol. **12:** 48–54.

22. MURRAY, M. K., E. C. SEGERSON, P. J. HANSEN, F. W. BAZER & R. M. ROBERTS. 1987. Suppression of lymphocyte activation by a high molecular weight glycoprotein released from preimplantation ovine and porcine conceptuses. Am. J. Reprod. Immunol. Microbiol. **14:** 38–44.

23. KOVATS, S., E. K. MAIN, C. LIBRACH, M. STUBBLEBINE, S. J. FISHER & R. DEMARE. 1990. A class I antigen, HLA-G, expressed in human trophoblast. Science **248:** 220–223.

24. YOUNG, K. H., R. R. KRAELING & F. W. BAZER. 1989. Effects of prolactin on conceptus survival and uterine secretory activity in pigs. J. Reprod. Fertil. **86:** 713–722.

25. MOFFATT, R. J., F. W. BAZER, P. J. HANSEN, P. W. CHUN & R. M. ROBERTS. 1987. Purification and immunocytochemical localization of the uterine milk proteins, the major progesterone-induced proteins in uterine secretions of sheep. Biol. Reprod. **36:** 419–430.

26. ROBERTS, R. M., T. J. RAUB & F. W. BAZER. 1986. Role of uteroferrin in transplacental iron transport in the pig. Fed. Proc. **45:** 2513–2518.

27. FLISS, M. F. V., E. WORTHINGTON-WHITE, S. GROSS & F. W. BAZER. 1989. Uteroferrin and

rose proteins from pig endometrium are hematopoietic growth factors. Biol. Reprod. **40** (Suppl. 1): 112 (Abstr.).

28. SIMMEN, R. C. M., G. BAUMBACH & R. M. ROBERTS. 1988. Molecular cloning and temporal expression during pregnancy of the messenger ribonucleic acid encoding uteroferrin, a progesterone-induced uterine secretory protein. Mol. Endocrinol. **2**: 253–262.

29. MURRAY, M. K., P. V. MALATHY, F. W. BAZER & R. M. ROBERTS. 1989. Structural relationship, biosynthesis, and immunocytochemical localization of uteroferrin-associated basic glycoproteins. J. Biol. Chem. **264**: 4143–4150.

30. MALATHY, P. V. & K. IMAKAWA. 1989. Uteroferrin-associated basic protein, a major progesterone-induced secretory protein of the porcine uterus, is a member of the serpin superfamily of protease inhibitors. Biol. Reprod. **40** (Suppl. 1): 114 (Abstr.).

31. KETCHAM, C. M., R. M. ROBERTS, R. C. M. SIMMEN & H. S. NICK, 1989. Molecular cloning of the type 5, iron-containing, tartrate-resistant acid phosphatase from human placenta. J. Biol. Chem. **264**: 557–563.

32. SIMMEN, R. C. M., V. SRINIVAS & R. M. ROBERTS. 1989. cDNA sequence, gene organization and progesterone induction of mRNA for uteroferrin, a porcine uterine iron transport protein. DNA **8**: 543–554.

33. MERCOLA, M. & C. D. STILES 1988. Growth factor superfamilies and mammalian embryogenesis. Development **102**: 451–460.

34. BRIGSTOCK, D. R., R. B. HEAP & K. D. BROWN. 1989. Polypeptide growth factors in uterine tissues and secretions. J. Reprod. Fertil. **85**: 747–758.

35. HOFMANN, G. E., C. V. RAO, G. H. BARROWS, G. S. SCHULTZ & J. S. SANFILIPPO. 1984. Binding sites for epidermal growth factor in human uterine tissues and leiomyomas. J. Clin. Endocrinol. Metab. **58**: 880–884.

36. HUET-HUDSON, Y. M., C. CHAKRABORTY, S. K. DE, Y. SUZUKI, G. K. ANDREWS & S. K. DEY. 1990. Estrogen regulates the synthesis of epidermal growth factor in mouse uterine epithelial cells. Mol. Endocrinol **4**: 510–523.

37. GARDNER, R. M., R. B. LINGHAM & G. M. STANCEL. 1987. Contractions of the isolated uterus stimulated by epidermal growth factor. FASEB J. **1**: 224–228.

38. FANT, M., H. MUNRO & A. C. MOSES. 1986. An autocrine/paracrine role for insulin-like growth factors in the regulation of human placental growth. J. Clin. Endocrinol. Metab. **63**: 499–505.

39. WANG, C-Y., M. DAIMON, S-J. SHEN, G. L. ENGELMANN & J. ILAN. 1988. Insulin-like growth factor-I messenger ribonucleic acid in the developing human placenta and in term placenta of diabetics. Mol. Endocrinol. **2**: 217–229.

40. LETCHER, R., R. C. M. SIMMEN, F. W. BAZER, & F. A. SIMMEN. 1989. Insulin-like growth factor-I expression during early conceptus development in the pig. Biol. Reprod. **41**: 1143–1151.

41. SIMMEN, R. C. M. & F. A. SIMMEN. 1990. Regulation of uterine and conceptus secretory activity. *In* Control of Pig Reproduction. III. D. J. A. Cole, G. R. Foxcroft & B. J. Weir, Eds.: 279–292. Henry Ling, Ltd, Great Britian.

42. KO, Y., C. Y. LEE, T. L. OTT, M. A. DAVIS, R. C. M. SIMMEN, F. W. BAZER & F. A. SIMMEN. 1990. Identification of insulin-like growth factors and other mitogens in uterine fluids of early pregnant sheep. J. Anim. Sci. **68** (Suppl. 1): 281 (Abstr.).

43. GRIZZARD, J. D., A. J. D'ERCOLE, J. R. WILKINS, B. M. MOATS-STAATS & R. W. WILLIAMS. 1984. Affinity-labeled somatomedin-C receptors and binding proteins from the human fetus. J. Clin. Endocrinol. Metab. **58**: 535–542.

44. CLEMMONS, D. R., V. K. HAN, R. G. ELGIN & A. J. D'ERCOLE. 1987. Alterations in the synthesis of a fibroblast surface associated 35K protein modulates the binding of somatomedin-C/insulin-like growth factor I. Mol. Endocrinol. **1**: 339–347.

45. FAZLEABAS, A. T., H. G. VERHAGE, G. WAITES & S. C. BELL. 1989. Characterization of an insulin-like growth factor binding protein, analogous to human pregnancy-associated secreted endometrial α_1-globulin, in decidua of the baboon (*Papio anubis*) placenta. Biol. Reprod. **40**: 873–885.

46. KOISTINEN, R., M-L. HUHTALA, U. H. STENMAN & M. SEPPALA. 1987. Purification of placental protein PP12 from human amniotic fluid and its comparison with PP12 from placenta by immunological, physicochemical and somatomedin-binding properties. Clin. Chim. Acta **164**: 293–298.

47. FAZLEABAS, A. T., R. C. JAFFE, H. G. VERHAGE, G. WAITES & S. C. BELL. 1989. An insulin-like

growth factor binding protein (IGF-BP) in the baboon (*Papio anubis*) endometrium: Synthesis, immunocytochemical localization and hormonal regulation. Endocrinology **124**: 2321–2329.

48. RUTANEN, E-M., F. PEKONEN & T. MAKINEN. 1988. Soluble 34K binding protein inhibits the binding of insulin-like growth factor-I to its cell receptors in human secretory phase endometrium: Evidence for autocrine/paracrine regulation of growth factor action. J. Clin. Endocrinol. Metab. **66**: 173–180.

49. MOSCATELLI, D., M. PRESTA & D. B. RIFKIN. 1986. Purification of a factor from human placenta that stimulates capillary endothelial cell protease production, DNA synthesis and migration. Proc. Natl. Acad. Sci. USA **83**: 2091–2095.

50. BRIGSTOCK, D. R., R. B. HEAP, P. J. BARKER & K. D. BROWN. 1990. Purification and characterization of heparin-binding growth factors from porcine uterus. Biochem. J. **266**: 273–282.

51. SIMMEN, R. C. M., F. A. SIMMEN, Y. KO & F. W. BAZER. 1989. Differential growth factor content of uterine luminal fluids from Large White and prolific Meishan pigs during the estrous cycle and early pregnancy. J. Anim. Sci. **67**: 1538–1545.

52. KIMELMAN, D., J. A. ABRAHAM, T. HAAPARANTA, T. M. PALISI & M. W. KIRSCHNER. 1988. The presence of fibroblast growth factor in the frog egg: Its role as a natural mesoderm inducer. Science **242**: 1053–1056.

53. NEPHEW, K. P., K. E. McCLURE, T. L. OTT, F. W. BAZER & W. F. POPE. 1989. Cumulative recognition of pregnancy by embryonic production of ovine trophoblastic protein-one. J. Anim. Sci. **67** (Suppl. 1): 404 (Abstr.).

54. GARRETT, J. E., R. D. GEISERT, M. T. ZAVY & G. L. MORGAN. 1988. Evidence for maternal regulation of early conceptus growth and development in the bovine. J. Reprod. Fertil. **84**: 437–446.

55. TAYLOR, R. N. & L. T. WILLIAMS. 1988. Developmental expression of platelet-derived growth factor and its receptor in the human placenta. Mol. Endocrinol. **2**: 627–632.

56. POLLARD, J. W., A. BARTOCCI, R. ARCECI, A. ORLOFSKY, M. B. LADNER & E. R. STANLEY. 1987. Apparent role of the macrophage growth factor, CSF-1 in placental development. Nature (Lond.) **330**: 484–486.

57. POLLARD, J. W., S. PAMPFER, E. DAITER, D. BARAD, E. R. STANLEY & R. J. ARCECI. 1990. Expression of colony stimulating factor-1 (CSF-1) in the uteroplacental unit. *In* Growth Factors in Reproduction, Proceedings of the Serono Symposium (abstr.), 20.

58. MULLER, R., D. J. SLAMON, E. D. ADAMSON, J. M. TREMBLAY, D. MULLER, M. J. CLINE & I. M. VERMA. 1983. Transcription of c-onc genes, c-ras and c-fms during mouse development. Mol. Cell. Biol. **3**: 1062–1069.

59. MILLER, D. A., A. LEE, Y. MATSUI, E. Y. CHEN, H. L. MOSES & R. DERYNCK. 1989. Complementary DNA cloning of the murine transforming growth factor-β_3 (TGFβ3) precursor and the comparative expression of TGFβ3 and TGFβ1 messenger RNA in murine embryos and adult tissues. Mol. Endocrinol. **3**: 1926–1934.

60. MILLER, D. A., A. LEE, R. W. PELTON, E. Y. CHEN, H. L. MOSES & R. DERYNCK. 1989. Murine transforming growth factor-β2 cDNA sequence and expression in adult tissues and embryos. Mol. Endocrinol. **3**: 1108–1114.

61. DALE, L., G. L. MATTHEWS, L. TABE & A. COLMAN. 1989. Developmental expression of the protein product of Vg1, a localized maternal RNA in the frog Xenopus laevis. EMBO J. **8**: 1057–1065.

62. KIMELMAN, D., & M. KIRSCHNER. 1987. Synergistic induction of mesoderm by FGF and TGF-β and the identification of an mRNA coding for FGF in the early Xenopus embryo. Cell **51**: 869–877.

63. MARASCALCO, B. A., K. C. FLANDERS, J. A. SIMON, A. B. ROBERTS & M. B. SPORN. 1990. Immunodetection of 3 isoforms of transforming growth factor beta in the rat uterus in response to steroids. *In* Growth Factors in Reproduction, Proceedings of the Serono Symposium (abstr.), 34.

64. RAPPOLEE, D. A., C. A. BRENNER, R. SCHULTZ, D. MARK & Z. WERB. 1988. Developmental expression of PDGF, TGF-α and TGF-β in preimplantation mouse embryos. Science **241**: 1823–1825.

65. RAPPOLEE, D. A. & Z. WERB. 1990. The expression and function of growth factor ligands and receptors during early development of mouse embryos. *In* Growth Factors in Reproduction, Proceedings of the Serono Symposium (abstr.), 19.

Preparation of the Human Endometrium for Implantation

DANIEL NAVOT[a] AND PAUL BERGH

Mount Sinai Medical Center
Department of Obstetrics, Gynecology and Reproductive Science
New York, New York 10029

The human endometrium is under strict hormonal control throughout women's reproductive life-span. The cyclic morphological changes of the endometrium have been well defined and extensively studied.[1-3] It appears that the main function of the endometrium is to create a suitable environment for embryo implantation and pregnancy sustenance. Nevertheless, the human endometrium, and specifically the decidua may be viewed as an endocrine organ with complex synthetic and secretory capacities.[4,5] This communication summarizes the current knowledge on artificial preparation of the human endometrium for implantation. Morphological as well as functional parameters will be reviewed.

MIMICKING THE NATURAL CYCLE

In the normal ovulatory cycle, the endometrium proliferates under increasing levels of estradiol (E_2). Endometrial regeneration and proliferation are on-going by the time that menstrual sloughing is completed (days 5–6) and continues until day 14–15 of a normalized 28-day cycle. Endometrial secretory transformation begins with a shift from mainly E_2 to preferential progesterone (P_4) production by the dominant ovarian follicle. The first rist in serum P_4 starts in conjunction with the onset of the luteinizing hormone (LH) surge (day 14) and is appreciable by day 15 of the cycle.[6] Day 16 is the earliest day on which secretory changes are consistently observed.[1]

Lutjen *et al.*[7] were the first to devise artificial endometrial cycles that painstakingly minmicked a natural cycle. Navot *et al.*[8] have further refined exogenous hormonal stimulation (FIG. 1). Utilizing the model of ovum donation, in women without ovaries, Navot *et al.* proved the following:

1. Sequential E_2 and P_4 supplementation is capable of producing physiological serum E_2 and P_4 levels (FIG. 1).
2. Sequential administration of E_2 and P_4 is sufficient to produce normal endometrial maturation, as judged by both light and electron microscopy.
3. The normal morphological changes are accompanied by appropriate functional capacity. Namely the ability to promote and sustain embryo implantation.[8]
4. Only sequential E_2 and P_4 and no other ovarian secretagogues are essential for embryo implantation and pregnancy maintenance.

[a] *Address all correspondence to:* Daniel Navot, M.D., Associate Professor, Department of Obstetrics, Gynecology and Reproductive Science, One Gustave L. Levy Place, Box 1175, New York, NY 10029.

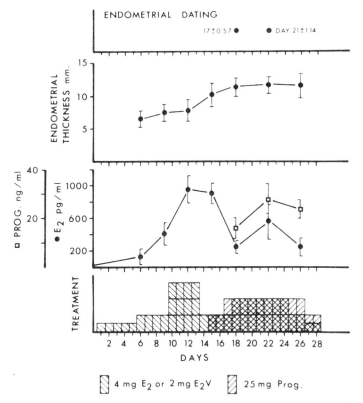

FIGURE 1. Sequential E_2 and P_4 regimen, which closely mimicks the natural cycle. The pattern of serum E_2 and P_4 as well as absolute values are similar to those of a natural cycle. The upper panel depicts histological dating of endometrial biopsies. (From ref. 8.)

DIFFERENT ROUTES FOR E_2 AND P_4 ADMINISTRATION

The pioneering formula of Lutjen et al.[7] was comprised of oral estradiol valerate (E_2V) and natural P_4 in oily base via an intramuscular (IM) route. Navot et al.[8,9] have added oral micronized E_2 into the armamentarium of endometrial stimulatory regimens. Others have suggested transdermal and transvaginal administration.[10,11] Two E_2 regimens merit detailed description:

1. Oral micronized E_2 (Estrace Mead Johnson, Evansville, IN)
2. Transdermal E_2 (Estraderm, CIBA Pharmaceutical Co., Summit, NJ).

The oral E_2 (estrace) regimen[9] has several advantages; it has been extensively and successfully used[9,10] over the last 3 years. The regimen can produce consistent serum values, well within the normal physiological E_2 range.[9] Estrace is relatively inexpensive and has virtually no side effects when given in the physiological E_2 range. However, oral E_2 has a negative effect on overall lipoprotein distribution.[12] The major disadvantage of oral E_2 is the inordinately high serum estrone (E_1) that is invariably produced secondary to E_2 metabolism in the liver.[10] An average E_2 to E_1 ratio of 1/10 is achieved by micronized E_2 administration, while the transdermal regimen is producing a 1:1 E_2:E_1 ratio which is much more physiologic.[10] The excess estrone may in turn compete with E_2 for target organ estrogen receptors.

Transdermal E_2 has become the treatment of choice for the creation of artificial endometrial cycles.[10] It is simple, requires biweekly application, and the transdermally absorbed E_2 reaches the endometrium prior to its passage through the liver. FIGURE 2 illustrates transdermal estraderm regimens with the appropriate E_2 levels in the peripheral circulation.

Although P_4 may be administered through vaginal suppositories, IM injections[8] or as oral micronized P_4,[13] no consistent advantage has been demonstrated by any of the regimens. Adequate P_4 absorption and physiological or higher than physiological serum levels are expected to yield structurally and functionally normal endometrium.[9]

SIMPLIFIED E_2 AND P_4 REGIMENS

Serhal and Craft[14] were the first to suggest a simplified approach for endometrial stimulation. Their regimen is based on a constant dose of E_2V (2 mg orally TID) for an average of 2 weeks prior to the addition of P_4 (either IM or orally 100–300 mg/day). Unfortunately no hormonal evidence or data pertaining to endometrial struc-

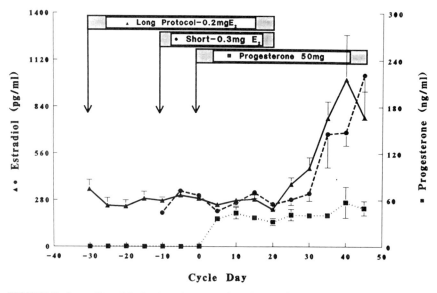

FIGURE 2. Serum E_2 and P_4 levels and patterns throughout endometrial cycles induced by transdermal estrogen and IM P_4. The E_2 values correspond to short vs. long follicular phases (see text). The late luteal rise in E_2 values is due to endogenous hormone production by the implanted embryos. The probable rise in P_4 is masked by the supraphysiological level attained through IM P_4 administration. (© D. Navot)

ture were forwarded to support this regimen. Nevertheless, a high rate of success was reported by Craft's group.[13] proving that the artificially induced endometrium was functionally normal.

TESTING THE LIMITS OF ENDOMETRIAL COMPLIANCE

Three different protocols were devised for the induction of endometrial maturation; each was to serve a dual purpose: to resolve a specific clinical situation and to answer a fundamental question related to endometrial physiology. The pertinent questions regarding the physiology of the endometrium were the following:

1. Can a normal secretory endometrium be achieved subsequent to a short period of estrogen (E) priming?
2. Can secretory transformation be accelerated by very high doses of P_4?
3. Will prolonged unopposed E hyperstimulation modify the integrity of the secretory endometrium?

The adequacy of the induced endometrial cycles was evaluated by hormonal, morphological, and histochemical criteria relevant to endometrial normalcy and receptivity.

A short follicular phase protocol consisted of 5–10 days of transdermal E_2 administration (0.2–0.4 mg every 3 days). A long follicular phase protocol consisted of 21–35 days of unopposed E_2 stimulation prior to P_4 initiation (FIG. 3). An accelerated secretory transformation protocol consisted of 100–150 mg/day of P_4 IM, as opposed to 50 mg/day for the other protocols. Initiation of P_4 administration was normalized to day 15, or luteal day +1 irrespective of the actual length of the preceding artificial follicular phase.

It has previously been shown that in biopsies performed during the peri-implantation period (days 19–22) in artificial cycles, a marked glandular-stromal asynchrony exists.[9] The stroma is typically advanced by 1–2 days, whild glandular maturation lags by about 1 day compared to chronological day at time of biopsy.[9] However, if glandular and stromal maturational stages are averaged (TABLE 1) the chronological and morphological dates correspond to within 1 day. Furthermore, if initiation of P_4 administration would have been normalized to cycle day 14, this one day discrepancy could have been eliminated.

To further evaluate endometrial normalcy after these hormonal manipulations, histochemical studies were performed on biopsies from each treatment group. The results are summarized in TABLE 2. Glycocalyx material was present on the surface of luminal epithelial cells of all biopsies examined. The absence of cationic ferritin (CF) binding and the weak alcian blue (AB) staining indicated minimal, if any, surface electronegativity; no differences in this staining pattern were detected between biopsies obtained during the peri-implantation vs. late luteal cycle intervals. However, alterations in both glycocalyx intensity (periodic acid schiff) and composition (ricinus communis-I agglutinin) were evident between these two sample populations, with a decrease in intensity and presence of galactose-containing glycoconjugates in the latter, corresponding with a presumed loss of uterine receptivity.

There are three components of the endometrium that act in concert throughout the process of implantation: 1) the secretory component, which provides the nourishing milieu to maintain the rapidly dividing embryo that entered the uterine cavity 2–3 days earlier, 2) the luminal epithelium appears to be important in the development

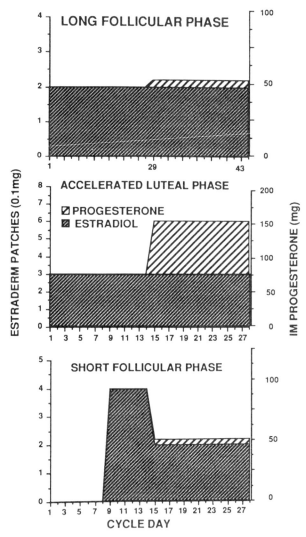

FIGURE 3. Simplified protocols for the induction of artificial endometrial cycles. Sequential transdermal E_2 for variable length and P_4 at variable doses are used to produce the short and long follicular phases and the accelerated luteal transformation, respectively. (© D. Navot)

of uterine receptivity, and 3) the stroma, whose adequacy is the *sine qua non* for sustained implantation. All three components are dependent upon the prevailing steroidal milieu throughout the menstrual cycle.

This study was an attempt to evaluate the integrity of the endometrium and its compliance under drastically manipulated steroidal milieus. The morphology of the glandular and stromal components and the specific biochemical alterations in the uterine

TABLE 1. Morphological Dating of Endometrial Biopsies in the Different Stimulation Protocols (M ± SD)

Protocol	Endometrial Biopsies	
	Chronological Date	Morphological Date
Short follicular phase	19.4 ± 1.0	18.1 ± .9
	25.7 ± .4	24.5 ± .8
Accelerated secretory transformation	18.3 ± 1.5	18.6 ± 2.1
	24.0 ± 0	25.3 ± .4
Long follicular phase	20.0 ± 0	19.1 ± 1.3
	25.5 ± .7	24.3 ± 1.0

luminal surface that are potentially related to the acquisition of ovum receptivity were evaluated.

Prolonged, unopposed E stimulation had no apparent adverse effect on endometrial morphology. The glandular delay in secretory transformation was similar to that of the control protocol, while the stroma seemed to be in phase with the chronological age of the endometrium. It is of special interest that despite the prolonged high dose E exposure, the known mitogenic and proliferative effects of E were not apparent on histological examination. Similarly, a relatively short (5-day) exposure to moderate E_2 levels appeared to be adequate for the introduction of endometrial P_4 receptors and allowed for normal secretory transformation. Very high nonincremental P_4 levels abolished the glandular/stromal disparity in the early biopsy. By cycle day 24, stromal changes characteristic of days 25–26 were attained. This last observation implies that high dose P4 may not only correct the retarded endometrium of P_4-deficient cycles (luteal phase defect), but also may hasten pseudo-decidualization during cycles with adequate P_4 exposure.

Histochemical evaluation of biopsies during the early implantation and late luteal intervals revealed little or no surface negativity, although weak AB staining indicated the presence of carboxyl groups in the glycocalyx; these observations are similar to reports in a variety of other species.[15] The biological significance of luminal negativity reduction at the time of implantation is made apparent by the polymer exclusion theory of cell-cell interactions,[16] which asserts that events such as adhesion are enhanced as repulsive charges on the involved cells are decreased. This is an attractive view in light of the cellular interactions that must occur during the initial stages of blastocyst attachment and invasion.

Glycocalyx intensity (PAS) and galactose residue contact (RCA-I) of the luminal glycocalyx were greatest during the anticipated time of uterine receptivity to implantation, comparing favorably with similar histochemical analyses of endometrial bi-

TABLE 2. Histochemical Properties of Luminal Epithelium during the Peri-implantation and Late Luteal Phases

Timing of Biopsy	PAS	AB	CF	RCA
Peri-implantation phase (Day 20)	+ + +	+	−	+ + +
Late luteal phase (Day 26)	+ +	+	−	+ +

opsies obtained from normal cycling women of proven fertility.[17,18] Increased binding of RCA-I to the uterine luminal surface during the peri-implantation period suggests an embryo recognition and/or adhesion system involving D-galactose. Furthermore, similar endogenous lectins have been identified in several tissues and have been postulated as mediators of both fertilization[19] and embryo-uterine interactions[20] in the mouse.

MORPHOLOGICAL-FUNCTIONAL CORRELATES

In Lutjen's pioneering study,[7] (E_2V and IM P_4) successful implantation occurred in 1 of 7 trials (14.3%). In Navot's series, with a similar regimen,[8] 2 of 8 attempts (25%) have yielded sustained implantation. Asch et al.[21] with a 26-day estrace regimen achieved a 75% implantation rate. Similarly a high rate of success (50%) was reported with the utilization of transdermal E_2 in a 28-day regimen.[10]

Recently in an extensive clinical trial, we tested the suitability of the endometrium for implantation under drastically different hormonal stimulations. Twenty-one women, aged 35 to 46, received donated oocytes from 9 IVF and 6 GIFT patients. From the 15 donors, 295 oocytes were recovered (median 18, range 11–30). One hundred and sixty-four were retained for the donors (median 12, range 6–18) and 131 were donated to the recipients (median 6, range 4–11). Overall fertilization rate was 78.1% (200/256). An average of 4 embryos were transferred to the donors (range 2–7) and 4 to the recipients (range 1–7). In the 15 donation cycles, 35 attempts at conception resulted in 17 pregnancies (48.5%); 7/14 (50.0%) donors and 10/21 (47.6%) recipients conceived. Of the 10 pregnancies in the recipient group 5/9 (55.6%) has *short follicular phases* (5–9 days of E exposure), prior to P_4 initiation and 5/11 (45.5%) had *long follicular phases* (>21 days of unopposed E administration). The shortest and longest follicular phases resulting in sustained implantation were of 5 and 35 days duration, respectively. Embryo transfers were normalized to day of P_4 initiation (day 15). Embryo transfers were performed between day 15–20 with 2–3 day old (2–12 cell) embryos. Pregnancies occurred with embryo transfers on every day between day 15–20 extending the window implantation to at least 6 consecutive days.

The human endometrium is highly compliant to a wide range of E_2 and P_4 stimulation. Various doses of estrogen, with either oral, transdermal or vaginal routes of administration, are capable of producing morphologically and ultrastructurally normal endometrium. Recently we were able to show that morphological adequacy is accompanied by normal function – namely, the ability to sustain embryo implantation.

REFERENCES

1. NOYES, R. W., A. T. HERTIG & J. ROCK. 1950. Dating the endometrial biopsy. Fertil. Steril. 1: 3–25.
2. ROGERS, P. A. W. & C. R. MURPHY. 1989. Uterine receptivity for implantation: Human studies. *In* Blastocyst Implantation. Koji Yoshinaga, Ed.: 231–238. Serono Symposium. Adams Publishing Group. Boston, MA.
3. MARTEL, D., C. MALET, J. P. GAUTRAY & A. PSYCHOYOS. 1981. Surface changes of the luminal uterine epithelium during the human menstrual cycle: A scanning electron microscopic study. *In* The Endometrium: Hormonal Impacts. J. de Brus, J. Martel & J. P. Gautray, Eds.: 15–29. Plenum Publishing Corporation, New York.
4. GURPIDE, E., S. TABANELLI, M. T. BENEDETTO & F. SCHATZ. 1989. Endometrial products with a possible role in implantation and maternal tolerance of the embryo. *In* Gift: From Basics

to Clinics. G. L. Capitano, R. H. Asch, L. DeCecco & L. Croce, Eds.: 161–174. Serono Symposia. Raven Press, New York.

5. HEFFNER, L. J., P. A. IDDENDEN & R. C. LYTTLE. 1986. Electrophoretic analyses of secreted human endometrial proteins: Identification and characterization of luteal phase prolactin. J. Clin. Endocrinol. Metab. **62**: 1288–1295.

6. GRUNFELD, L., B. SANDLER, J. FOX, C. BOYD, P. KAPLAN & D. NAVOT. 1989. Luteal phase inadequacy following completely normal follicular and periovulatory phases. Fertil. Steril. **52**: 919–923.

7. LUTJEN, P., A. TROUNSON, J. LEETON, J. FINDLAY, C. WOOD & P. RENOV. 1984. The establishment and maintenance of pregnancy using *in vitro* fertilization and embryo donation in a patient with primary ovarian failure. Nature **307**: 174–175.

8. NAVOT, D., N. LAUFER, J. KOPOLOVIC, et al. 1986. Artificially induced endometrial cycles and establishment of pregnancies in the absence of ovaries. New Engl. J. Med. **314**: 806–811.

9. NAVOT, D., T. L. ANDERSON, K. DROESCH, R. T. SCOTT, D. KREINER & Z. ROSENWAKS. 1989. Hormonal manipulation and endometrial maturation. J. Clin. Endocrinol. Metab. **68**: 801–817.

10. DROESCH, K., D. NAVOT, R. T. SCOTT, D. KREINER, H. C. LIU & Z. ROSENWAKS. 1988. Transdermal replacement in ovarian failure for ovum donation. Fertil. Steril. **50**: 931–934.

11. STEINGOLD, K., P. STUMPF, D. KREINER, H. C. LIU, D. NAVOT & Z. ROSENWAKS. 1989. Estradiol and progesterone regimens for the induction of endometrial receptivity. Fertil. Steril. **52**: 756–760.

12. JUDD, W. 1987. Efficacy of transdermal estradiol. Am. J. Obstet. Gynecol. **156**: 1326–1331.

13. SERHAL, P. F. & I. L. CRAFT. 1989. Oocyte donation in 61 patients. The Lancet **1**: 1185–1187.

14. SERHAL, P. F. & I. L. CRAFT. 1987. Ovum donation—a simplified approach. Fertil. Steril. **48**: 265–269.

15. ANDERSON, T. L. & L. H. HOFFMAN. 1984. Alterations in epithelial glycocalyx of rabbit uteri during early pseudopregnancy and pregnancy, and following ovariectomy. Am. J. Anat. **171**: 321–334.

16. MAROUDAS, N. G. 1975. Polymer exclusion, cell adhesions, and membrane fusion. Nature **254**: 695–696.

17. ANDERSON, T. C., C. CODDINGTON, M. SHEN & G. HODGEN. 1987. Defining the window of uterine receptivity: Biochemical evaluation of the endometrium. 5th World Congress on In Vitro Fertilization and Embryo Transfer, Norfolk, VA, 73 (Abstr.).

18. JANSEN, R. P. S., M. TURNER, E. JOHANNISSON, B. M. LANDGREN & E. DICZFALUSY. 1985. Cyclic changes in human endometrial surface glycoproteins: A quantitative histochemical study. Fertil. Steril. **44**: 85–91.

19. SHUR, B. D. & N. G. HALL. 1982. A role for mouse sperm surface galactosyltransferase in sperm binding to the egg zona pellucida. J. Cell Biol. **95**: 574–579.

20. CHAVEZ, D. J. 1986. Cell surface of mouse blastocysts at the trophecto-derm uterine interface during the adhesive stage of implantation. Am. J. Anat. **176**: 153–158.

21. ASCH, R., J. P. BALMACEDA, T. ORD, et al. 1988. Oocyte donation and gamete intrafallopian transfer in premature ovarian failure. Fertil. Steril. **49**: 263–267.

Endometrial Receptivities after Leuprolide Suppression and Gonadotropin Stimulation: Histology, Steroid Receptor Concentrations, and Implantation Rates

JAMES P. TONER,[a] DIMITRIOS K. HASSIAKOS,[b]
SUHEIL J. MUASHER,[a] JENG G. HSIU,[c]
AND HOWARD W. JONES, JR.[a]

[a] The Jones Institute for Reproductive Medicine
Department of Obstetrics and Gynecology
[c] Department of Pathology
Eastern Virginia Medical School
Norfolk, Virginia 23507

[b] Aretaion Hospital
Second Department of Obstetrics and Gynecology
University of Athens
76 V. Sofias Avenue
Athens, Greece 11528

INTRODUCTION

Implantation of the blastocyst is a sequence of cooperative events between the initial free conceptus in the endometrial cavity and the uterine endometrium that requires synchronous development between the two for a successful outcome.

The relative roles of pre-embryonic quality and uterine receptivity in the initiation of pregnancy remains uncertain in programs of *in vitro* fertilization and embryo transfer (IVF-ET). The fact that the survival probability of a human conceptus in normal reproduction is on the order of 20–25% and that the probability of survival in IVF is about half that[1] suggests that factors other than pre-embryo quality might be affecting IVF survival. Endometrial receptivity is certainly one factor to be considered. Unfortunately, there is but scant understanding of uterine receptivity in the human as studies have been limited by practical restrictions and ethical considerations.

Intrauterine transfer of pre-embryos in IVF programs is usually carried out 24

[a] *Address for correspondence:* James P. Toner, M.D., Ph.D., Department of Obstetrics and Gynecology, The Howard and Georgeanna Jones Institute for Reproductive Medicine, Eastern Virginia Medical School, Hofheimer Hall–6th floor, 825 Fairfax Avenue, Norfolk, VA 23507, (804) 446-8948/FAX (804)446-8998.

hours earlier than the arrival of the conceptus in the uterine cavity in natural reproduction. This discrepancy has been a cause for concern.

In a previous study[2] there was indirect evidence to suggest that pregnancy was much more likely to occur if at the time of transfer (normally day 16 of an idealized cycle) the endometrium was advanced to day 17, *i.e.*, was histologically identical to the phase of the endometrium when the conceptus reaches the uterus in normal reproduction. In that study the endometrial phase correlated well with peripheral serum P_4 on the day of transfer; however, E_2 levels were not considered. Furthermore, the type of stimulation in that study seldom resulted in follicular E_2 values >500–700pg/ml, and the luteal range was seldom >350–400pg/ml. P_4 levels seldom >40ng/ml.

With current stimulation protocols, especially with luteal leuprolide suppression, the follicular E_2 often exceeds 2500pg/ml, and the maximum luteal E_2 level is often in the 2000pg/ml range; the maximal luteal P_4 values may exceed 200ng/ml. In spite of these extremely high follicular and luteal values, transfer on day 16 seems to be efficient.

The status of the endometrium on the day of transfer using contemporary stimulation protocols has not been well characterized. It is the purpose of this study to do that and to restudy the previous material by correlating the E_2 data which was not considered in the previous study.

MATERIALS AND METHODS

Endometrial Biopsies

Endometrial biopsies were obtained from 29 women in the IVF program, and all but one (natural cycle IVF) had exogenous ovarian stimulation. In 20 cases no leuprolide was administered; in 9 it was used adjunctively (7 luteal, 2 follicular). Luteal leuprolide was begun in the preceding mid-luteal phase and continued until human chorionic gonadotropin (hCG) was administered; this regimen was applied to intermediate and high responders beginning in 1989. Follicular leuprolide, begun on cycle day 2, took advantage of the burst of gonadotropin secretion; this regimen was reserved for poor responders (day 3 serum FSH > 15mIU/ml or history of poor response). Gonadotropin stimulation (Pergonal and/or Metrodin) was begun on cycle day 3 (luteal leuprolide) or day 4 (follicular leuprolide), usually at a dose of 4 ampules per day, with subsequent step-down individualized.[3,4] Eighteen biopsies were taken before leuprolide was available (1982–1984); these were the subject of a prior report.[2] At that time all patients were treated in a step-down protocol; 6 received 3 ampules of Pergonal daily; the remainder received 2 ampules. Ovarian response consequently was not as high as is now routinely seen. In both the recent and earlier cases, P_4 supplementation was begun on idealized day 16 (day of transfer), initially at 25 mg IM daily, and 4 days later advanced to 50 mg IM daily until the pregnancy result was known.

Biopsies were taken on the morning of the planned pre-embryo transfer in 16 cases, and later in the luteal phase in 13. Some older biopsies were taken as late as the 7th post-ovulatory day. A Pipelle or Novak curette was used to sample tissue from the posterior surface of the fundus. For presentation, the day of pre-embryo transfer was standardized to day 16 (thus 2 days after follicle aspiration and 4 days after hCG). Endometrial dating was performed independently by all authors using the criteria of Noyes, Hertig, and Rock;[5] no more than 1 day of discrepancy was noted among observers for each case. Cases with discrepancy were resolved to unanimity by simultaneous review by all authors. When glandular-stromal asynchrony was observed, glandular dating was used in statistical analyses.

Estrogen and Progesterone Receptors

In 6 recent cases, a portion of the endometrial biopsy specimen was set aside for receptor analysis. Immediately after biopsy, the specimen was placed in a cryo tube and plunged into liquid nitrogen. After all specimens were collected, they were taken on dry ice to a commercial lab (Nichols), where receptor levels were determined by an assay for cytosolic concentrations.[6]

IVF Implantation Rates

To determine the potential impact of high E_2 levels on implantation, all IVF cycles (except severe male factor cases) in Norfolk in 1989 were evaluated. Cycles were divided into groups by peak E_2 and by day of biopsy E_2 or P_4. For peak E_2, a low response group ($E_2 < 500$; n = 147), an intermediate response group ($E_2 = 500-1000$; n = 298), and a high response group ($E_2 > 1000$; n = 155) were evaluated. For P_4 on cycle day 16 (standardized), a low P_4 group ($P_4 \leqslant 25$ng/ml; n = 161) and a high P_4 group ($P_4 > 25$ng/ml; n = 315) were studied. This P_4 cutoff was selected for its ability to discriminate lagging and non-lagging endometrial histology. Implantation rates were calculated for each group. A similar analysis on the same patients was performed using $E_2 > 200$pg/ml on the idealized cycle day 16 as a cutoff (>200pg/ml; n = 323; $\leqslant 200$pg/ml; n = 156).

Two subgroups of low responders whose supplemental P_4 was begun at different times in the luteal phase were also examined. All patients had received follicular leuprolide and gonadotropins. In Series 37 (Nov–Dec 1989) P_4 supplementation began on the morning of pre-embryo transfer (n = 11); in Series 38 (Jan–Mar 1990) it began 2 days earlier, on the morning of oocyte retrieval (n = 42). Implantation rates were compared for each form of P_4 supplementation.

Hormone Assays

All tests were run in duplicate on a gamma counter, using standard RIA techniques. Overall variation in the low, mid, and high ranges of the assays were 10.3% (at 49pg/ml), 7.95% (at 96pg/ml) and 5.3% (at 670pg/ml) for E_2 (Pantex, direct method), 12.4% (at 1.2ng/ml), 7.9% (at 10.9ng/ml), and 10.8% (at 25ng/ml) for P_4 (Pantex, direct method), and 13.5% (at 13.7mIU/ml), 7.2% (at 24.1mIU/ml) and 4.5% (at 69mIU/ml) for FSH (Leeco).

Statistics

The relation between endometrial histology and hormone parameters was evaluated by simple regression analysis. In every case a logarithmic transformation of the hormone values was applied, since this made the relationship more linear. Nonparametric correlation coefficients were calculated for these same relationships using Spearman's rank correlation approach. Frequency data (implantation rates and histology type) were compared using the chi-square or Fisher's exact test. All statistics were performed using Statgraphics® software on a personal computer.

RESULTS

Endometrial Histology

Endometrial histology showed a significant relationship to both E_2 and P_4 levels, and under all conditions examined: peak values, values on cycle day 16, and values on the day of biopsy (13 of 29 biopsies were taken later than day 16). TABLE 1 provides correlation coefficients between histologic day and the hormone values in each of 6 conditions. The relationships were stronger for P_4 than E_2; of the 3 days examined, hormone values on the day of biopsy were most strongly related to histology (TABLE 2).

TABLE 1. Correlation Matrix among Response Variables and Histology in IVF Cycles[a]

	Histology	Peak Values		Cycle Day 16 Values		Day of Biopsy Values	
		E_2	P_4	E_2	P_4	E_2	P_4
Histology	—	.53[c]	.49	.59[c]	.52[b]	.62[c]	.62[c]
Peak E_2	.53[c]	—	.61[b]	.81[c]	.75[c]	.84[c]	.79[c]
Peak P_4	.49	.61[b]	—	.69[b]	.92[c]	.63[b]	.77[c]
Day 16 E_2	.59[c]	.81[c]	.69[b]	—	.79[c]	.93[c]	.84[c]
Day 16 P_4	.52[b]	.75[c]	.92[c]	.79[c]	—	.80[c]	.90[c]
Biopsy day E_2	.62[c]	.84[c]	.63[b]	.93[c]	.81[c]	—	.79[c]
Biopsy day P_4	.62[c]	.79[c]	.77[c]	.84[c]	.90[c]	.79[c]	—

[a] Spearman rank correlation coefficients.
[b] $p < 0.05$.
[c] $p < 0.01$.

TABLE 2. Regression Analyses of Histology and Hormone Parameters[a]

Condition	r	R^2	df	F	*p*
Peak value					
$-E_2$	.528	27.9%	28	10.4	.003
$-P_4$	.625	39.0%	15	8.9	.009
Cycle day 16					
$-E_2$	.538	28.9%	21	8.1	.009
$-P_4$	.509	25.9%	16	5.2	.037
Day of biopsy					
$-E_2$	.548	30.0%	25	10.3	.004
$-P_4$	.634	40.3%	19	12.1	.003

[a] Regression analysis based on least squares model; hormone values log transformed. r = correlation coefficient; R^2 = amount of total variance in histology accounted for by hormone parameter; df = degrees of freedom; F = regression test statistic; *p* = significance level.

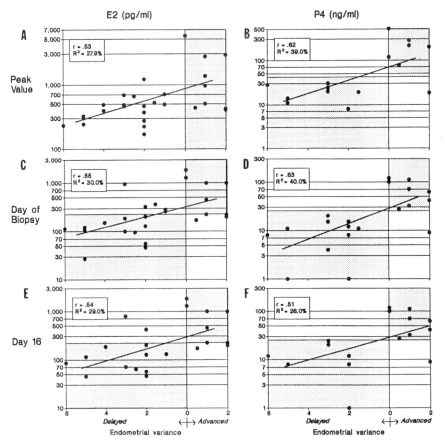

FIGURE 1. Regression plots of various hormonal features of IVF cycles versus the discrepancy between the histologic day and the actual cycle day. The actual cycle day is based on standardizing the day of embryo transfer to day 16. All hormonal values are plotted on a logarithmic scale and were entered into the regression analyses with this transformation. In each panel the sloped line represents the best fit by a least squares approach; the correlation coefficients and the R^2 values were derived from the regression analysis. When possible, a cutoff value for each hormonal parameter was selected which attempted to discriminate lagging from non-lagging endometrium. The upper right box represents cases of non-lagging endometrium above the hormonal threshold; the lower left box represents lagging endometrium below the hormonal threshold. A: Peak E_2. No threshold could be established. B: Peak P_4. C: E_2 on day of endometrial biopsy. D: P_4 on day of endometrial biopsy. E: E_2 on cycle day 16. F: P_4 on cycle day 16.

Though the relationship between peak E_2 and histology was statistically strong, there was no convenient threshold which discriminated lagging and advanced endometria (FIG. 1A). However, a peak $P_4 \geq 40$ng/ml helped differentiate 6 of 7 non-lagging endometria from all 9 lagging endometria (Fisher's exact test: $p < 0.001$; FIG. 1B).

Threshold values of E_2 and P_4 associated with non-lagging endometria were clearly discerned for both day 16 and day of biopsy values. On cycle day 16, $E_2 > 200$pg/ml discriminated 7 of 9 non-lagging endometria from 12 of 17 lagging endometria ($p = 0.025$; FIG. 1C). Similarly, $P_4 \geqslant 25ng/ml$ divided 8 of 9 non-lagging endometria from all 11 lagging endometria ($p < 0.001$; FIG. 1D).

On the day of biopsy, $E_2 \geqslant 200pg/ml$ separated 7 of 9 non-lagging endometria from 11 of 13 lagging endometria ($p = 0.006$; FIG. 1E) while $P_4 \geqslant 25ng/ml$ discriminated 8 of 9 non-lagging endometria from all 8 lagging endometria ($p < 0.001$; FIG. 1F).

The fact that the same threshold values were observed for E_2 ($>200pg/ml$) and P_4 ($>25ng/ml$) for both day 16 and day of biopsy hormone values is partly due to the fact that 15 of 28 biopsies were performed on day 16.

Without the use of luteal leuprolide, endometrial histology lagged ($\geqslant 1$ day) in all but one case. Conversely, in women treated with luteal leuprolide, none showed lagging endometrial histology.

There was a limit to the degree of histologic advancement that could be achieved. In no case was endometrial glandular development seen beyond day 18, no matter how high the hormone levels were. The endometrial stromal compartment often showed edema when high hormone levels occurred (4 of 8 cases). That is, glandular-stromal asynchrony was commonly seen in cases of high response. Glands appeared more resistant to the effects of high steroid response.

In one case of a low responder, P_4 supplementation was instituted on the day of retrieval. Histology was in phase; this was the only case in which a low responding patient had a biopsy without lag. (This case has been excluded from the preceding analyses.)

Endometrial Receptor Concentrations

Six patients were biopsied with a portion of the endometrial sample reserved for receptor levels; clinical characteristics are shown in TABLE 3. There was a range of responsiveness from typical low response (patients DM, LB, and TD) through average response (SW) to high response (PR, MP). All patients received P_4 supplementation beginning on the morning of transfer except DM, who received it from the day of retrieval (2 days earlier). Endometrial histology ranged from day 16 to 18.

E_2R was lower in low responders and higher in high responders. Patient MP appeared to be an exception in that her E_2R levels were extremely low despite high E_2 tone. It is curious that the histology in this case was not advanced, despite the extraordinarily high hormone levels.

We could not discern any relation between P_4R and the responsiveness of the ovarian stimulation, except that patient MP with markedly supraphysiologic E_2 had low P_4R levels.

Implantation Rates

TABLE 4 provides the implantation rate at three levels of E_2 response. The lowest rates were observed at intermediate levels of response (500–1000 peak E_2). This reduction was significant for leuprolide and non-leuprolide cycles compared to the high responders. The levels of E_2 and P_4 on the day 16 in these cycles also varied according to the E_2 response.

When cases were divided by the P_4 of 25ng/ml on the day of retrieval, the im-

TABLE 3. Stimulation Characteristics and Receptor Concentrations in IVF Cycles

Patient	Stimulation (# oocytes retrieved)	Peak E_2 (pg/ml)	E_2 Day of Biopsy (pg/ml)	P_4 Day of Biopsy (ng/ml)	Endo-metrial Histology (cycle day)	E_2R (fmol/mg protein)	P_4R (fmol/mg protein)
DM	6 FSH P_4 from d retrieval (3 preovs)	291	146	53	17	131	294
PR	follicular leuprolide (7 preovs)	1657	883	61	16	232	387
TD	natural cycle IVF (2 preovs)	503	QNS[a]	QNS	17	220	456
LB	luteal leuprolide (5 preovs)	420	217	41	18	133	347
SW	luteal leuprolide (6 preovs)	948	220	32	17	194	368
MP	luteal leuprolide (45 preovs)	5536	1792	100	16	<3	35

[a] QNS = quantity not sufficient.

TABLE 4. Implantation Rate Depending on Estradiol Response in IVF[a]

	$E_2 < 500$ pg/ml		$E_2 = 500$–1000 pg/ml		$E_2 > 1000$ pg/ml	
Stimulation	Peak E_2 d16 E_2 d16 P_4 (n)	Implantation % -sacs/embryo	Peak E_2 d16 E_2 d16 P_4 (n)	Implantation % -sacs/embryo	Peak E_2 d16 E_2 d16 P_4 (n)	Implantation % -sacs/embryo
Luteal leuprolide	470 173 19 (37)	14.4	936 304 40 (141)	10.2[b]	2111 692 65 (121)	14.0[b]
Follicular leuprolide	405 134 29 (17)	9.5	845 251 43 (23)	7.8	1968 644 46 (4)	11.1
No leuprolide	346 133 18 (93)	9.0	802 289 31 (134)	6.0[c]	1736 691 46 (29)	12.0[c]

[a] d16 = idealized day 16; (n) = number of patients in each group.
[b] $p < 0.01$ (chi square).
[c] $p < 0.05$ (chi square).

plantation rate was slightly higher in the higher P_4 group (10.6% *vs.* 9.7%). Using E_2 >200pg/ml on the day of retrieval to divide cases, again there was a small but non-significant trend toward higher implantation when higher E_2 was observed (11.1% *vs.* 8.3%).

Low responders who received follicular leuprolide were given P_4 beginning on the day of oocyte retrieval or the day of pre-embryo transfer. P_4 supplementation beginning on the day of oocyte retrieval was associated with an implantation rate of 10.6% (13 sacs/123 pre-embryos transferred), whereas when P_4 supplementation was not begun until the day of pre-embryo transfer, no pregnancies resulted from the transfer of 18 pre-embryos ($p > 0.05$).

DISCUSSION

The impact of controlled ovarian hyperstimulation in IVF-ET on the process of embryo implantation is a crucial issue in assisted reproduction but a difficult one to study. We examined this relationship by correlating the degree of ovarian response with implantation rate, endometrial histology, and E_2 and P_4 receptor concentrations.

We were concerned that the markedly supraphysiologic levels of E_2 and P_4 commonly seen in leuprolide pretreated patients would adversely affect implantation potential. However, under these conditions the implantation rate was not diminished, and in fact was increased in our study population. Moreover, endometrial histology was commonly advanced, a condition observed only once in low response cycles. We therefore could find no direct evidence of impaired implantation following high ovarian response, and we suspect that the histologic advancement may be beneficial.

A review of studies on endometrial biopsies performed on days 16–18 in non-transferred IVF cycles shows that 88/149 (59%) had secretory and 61/149 (41%) had proliferative endometria.[2,7-13] Thus it is not uncommon to find proliferative endometria in stimulated cycles at retrieval and transfer. Of the 64 secretory endometria, 39 (61%) were in phase for the day of biopsy while 25 (39%) were advanced. A disparity was noted between glandular epithelium and stromal maturity in some cases.[7] Sterzik *et al.*[12] noted insufficient secretory endometrium in all 17 women >35 years of age, though most showed poor ovarian response.

We observed a strong relation between various hormonal manifestations of ovarian response and endometrial histology. Others have also reported relationships between histologic maturity and various measures of ovarian response: peak preovulatory E_2 levels,[7-9] E_2 at biopsy,[11] and P_4 levels at biopsy.[2,7,11] However, some patients with proliferative endometria showed apparently adequate P_4 levels.[10,11]

We defined threshold levels of E_2 and P_4 on the day of transfer which discriminate lagging from non-lagging endometria. More than 25ng/ml of P_4 and >200pg/ml E_2 at transfer were associated with non-lagging endometria. Using this cutoff to examine implantation rates showed a small increase above these cutoffs for both E_2 and P_4.

While there is an overall correlation between hormone levels and histologic appearance, the endometrium demonstrated some limits. Glandular histology could not be advanced beyond day 18, no matter how high the E_2 and P_4 levels went. Thus there appears to be an inherent limit in the system preventing more advanced glandular changes. This might be important in ensuring better synchronization between the histologic day and normal day of embryo entry into the uterus, bringing it closer to what normally occurs in natural reproduction. We do not speculate about what might mediate this limit to glandular differentiation.

Stromal histology was also sensitive to peripheral E_2 and P_4 levels but did not demonstrate the same limit as glandular histology. Stroma showing a pattern as late as day 20 was seen in cases of high steroid response. This suggests that different controls exist which regulate the rate of glandular and stromal changes.

Endometrial E_2 and P_4 receptor concentrations were examined in a limited number of patients. E_2R was somewhat higher when ovarian response was high. P_4R showed no discernable pattern. However, in the single case of extremely high response (peak $E_2 = 5536$ pg/ml), both E_2R and P_4R were very low. In conjunction with non-advanced histology observed in this case, this suggests that there may be a threshold level of E_2 (or P_4) which down-regulates receptor concentrations and prevents advanced histological changes. Thus there may be level of high response which prevents appropriate histologic differentiation and impairs implantation.

Prior studies on the window of uterine receptivity have suggested that days 17–19 are optimal for embryo transfer. This is primarily based on donor egg data: in patients with ovarian failure receiving donor eggs while on E_2 and P_4 replacement, endometria histologically developed to days 17–19 are more likely to result in implantation.[14,15] Based on the present data, we infer that implantation is improved when ovarian response is high; this ensures that the endometrial histology is not lagging (i.e., day 16 or beyond).

To accelerate endometrial maturation and reproduce the desired physiological state, P_4 support has been given by others before oocyte retrieval and even before hCG administration.[7,13,16] Howles et al.[16] noted an improvement in the pregnancy rate per embryo transfer in cycles supplemented with P_4 compared to non-supplemented cycles (i.e., 39% vs. 23%, respectively). Ben-Nun et al.[7] reported no alteration in oocyte maturation, fertilization, or cleavage rates when P_4 was given 12 hours before hCG compared to controls; nonetheless, the pregnancy rate per embryo transfer in P_4 treated cycles was 41.2% vs. 23.5%, respectively. In our one case of a low response cycle in which P_4 supplementation was given earlier (day of retrieval), the histology was in phase. This was our only case of a low response cycle demonstrating non-lagging endometrium.

SUMMARY

The effect of markedly supraphysiologic levels of E_2 and P_4 on the endometrium was assessed by examining endometrial histology, E_2 and P_4 receptor concentrations, and embryo implantation rates in IVF cycles with and without leuprolide use. Results suggest that 1) the high ovarian response common in leuprolide pretreated cycles can advance endometrial histology, but only up to a certain limit, 2) $P_4 > 25$ ng/ml or $E_2 > 200$ pg/ml on the day of transfer was associated with non-lagging endometria, 3) implantation rate in high response cycles is not impaired and may be increased, 4) earlier P_4 supplementation in low response cycles may be beneficial, 5) extraordinarily high response ($E_2 > 5000$ pg/ml) may be detrimental to implantation, and 6) the optimal histology for implantation appears to be at least day 16.

ACKNOWLEDGMENTS

We thank Debi Jones for supplying summary data on implantation and Charlotte Schrader, Ph.D. for editorial review.

REFERENCES

1. BOKLAGE, C. E. 1990. Survival probability of human conceptions from fertilization to term. Int. J. Fertil. **35:** 75–94.
2. GARCIA, J. E., A. A. ACOSTA, J. G. HSIU & H. W. JONES, JR. 1984. Advanced endometrial maturation after ovulation induction with human menopausal gonadotropin/human chorionic gonadotropin for *in vitro* fertilization. Fertil. Steril. **41:** 31–35.
3. MUASHER, S. J., J. E. GARCIA & Z. ROSENWAKS. 1985. The combination of follicle-stimulating hormone and human menopausal gonadotropin for the induction of multiple follicular maturation for *in vitro* fertilization. Fertil. Steril. **44:** 66ff.
4. VEECK, L. L., J. W. E. WORTHAM, J. WITMEYER, B. A. SANDOW, A. A. ACOSTA, J. E. GARCIA, G. S. JONES & H. W. JONES, JR. 1983. Maturation and fertilization of morphologically immature human oocytes in a program of *in vitro* fertilization. Fertil. Steril. **39:** 594ff.
5. NOYES, R. W., A. T. HERTIG & J. ROCK. 1950. Dating the endometrial biopsy. Fertil. Steril. **1:** 3–25.
6. EHRLICH, C. E., P. M. YOUNG & R. E. CLEARY. 1981. Cytoplasmic progesterone and estradiol receptors in normal, hyperplastic, and carcinomatous endometria: Therapeutic implications. Am. J. Obstet. Gynecol. **141:** 539ff.
7. BEN-NUN, I., Y. GHETLER, R. JAFFE, A. SIEGAL, H. KANETI & M. FEJGIN. 1990. Effect of preovulatory progesterone administration on the endometrial maturation and implantation rate after *in vitro* fertilization and embryo transfer. Fertil. Steril. **53:** 276–281.
8. COHEN, J. J., C. DEBACHE, F. PIGEAU, J. MANDELBAUM, M. PLACHOT & J. DE BRUX. 1984. Sequential use of clomiphene citrate, human menopausal gonadotropin in human *in vitro* fertilization. II. Study of luteal phase adequacy following aspiration of the preovulatory follicle. Fertil. Steril. **42:** 360–365.
9. FORMAN, R. G., B. EYCHENNE, C. NESSMANN, R. FRYDMAN & P. ROBEL. 1989. Assessing the early luteal phase in *in vitro* fertilization cycles: relationship between plasma steroids, endometrial receptors, and endometrial histology. Fertil. Steril. **51:** 310–316.
10. FRYDMAN, R., J. TESTART, P. GIACOMINI, M. C. IMBERT, E. MARTIN & K. NAHOUL. 1982. Hormonal and histological study of the luteal phase in women following aspiration of the preovulatory follicle. Fertil. Steril. **38:** 312–317.
11. PORTUONDO, J. A., J. L. CARONERO, M. D. ROMAN, A. A. ACOSTA & J. G. HSIU. 1986. Luteal phase after follicle aspiration for oocyte retrieval in clomiphene citrate stimulated cycles. Infertility **9:** 199–215.
12. STERZIK, K., C. DALLENBACH, V. SCHNEIDER, V. SASSE & G. DALLENBACH-HELLWEG. 1988. *In vitro* fertilization: the degree of endometrial insufficiency varies with the type of ovarian stimulation. Fertil. Steril. **50:** 457–462.
13. TROUNSON, A., D. HOWLETT, P. ROGERS & H. O. HOPPEN. 1986. The effect of progesterone supplementation around the time of oocyte recovery in patients superovulated for *in vitro* fertilization. Fertil. Steril. **45:** 532–535.
14. NAVOT, D., N. LAUFER, J. KOPOLOVIC, R. RABINOWITZ, A. BIRKENFELD, A. LEWIN, M. GRANAT, E. J. MARGALIOTH & J. G. SCHENKER. 1986. Artificially induced endometrial cycles and establishment of pregnancies in the absence of ovaries. N. Engl. J. Med. **31:** 806–811.
15. ROSENWAKS, Z. 1987. Donor eggs: Their application in modern reproductive technologies. Fertil. Steril. **47:** 895–909.
16. HOWLES, C. M., M. C. MACNAMEE & R. G. EDWARDS. 1988. Progesterone supplementation in the late follicular phase of an in-vitro fertilization cycle: A 'natural' way to time oocyte recovery? Hum. Reprod. **3:** 409–412.

The Endometrium in Human Assisted Reproduction

ETTORE CITTADINI[a] AND ROBERTO PALERMO

Istituto Materno Infantile
Università degli Studi di Palermo
Palermo, Italy

The assessment of endometrial function in physiological conditions is one of the most controversial areas in reproduction, and the situation is further complicated in human assisted reproduction by the multitude of variables associated with any form of treatment.

So-called medically assisted reproduction implies different degrees of intervention, which are intended to overcome an identified or even a non-identified factor of reproductive failure, but these interventions may potentially alter endometrial receptivity for adequate implantation. Thus, when we select an infertile female patient with evident ovarian function, either normal or abnormal, for a specific assisted reproductive treatment, the first "manipulation" we do, to improve the chance of establishing pregnancy, is controlled ovarian hyperstimulation: a key and critical step between the selection of patients and the adoption of one of the treatment techniques (FIG. 1).

Different strategies are adopted for inducing multiple follicular growth. The protocols mainly used are the combination of clomiphene citrate (CC) with human menopausal gonadotropins (hMG), the combination of hMG with gonadotropin releasing hormone agonists (GnRH-a) or hMG alone. Whichever protocol is used, the expected multiple follicular growth will produce supraphysiological levels of estradiol during the follicular phase and the resulting multiple corpora lutea will produce supraphysiological levels of estradiol and progesterone during the luteal phase.

Another important aspect regarding the endometrial environment, which differentiates *in vitro* fertilization with intrauterine embryo transfer from other techniques and natural conception, is the different timing of arrival of embryos into the uterine cavity and the different developmental stage of the embryo at that time. In fact, in spontaneous conception, and we have to suppose the same situation exists after the replacement of embryos or gametes into the tubes, a morula or an early blastocyst will arrive into the uterine cavity 5–6 days after the ovulation. In *in vitro* fertilization (IVF) embryos at 4–8 blastomeric stage are usually replaced into the uterine cavity 48 hours after the oocyte retrieval.

Most studies designed to investigate endometrial function have been conducted in IVF and embryo transfer (ET) studies, so we have to keep in mind these points in reviewing this topic.

---

[a] *Address for correspondence:* Ettore Cittadini, M.D., Direttore Clinica Ostetrica e Ginecologica (R), Istituto Materno Infantile, via Cardinale M. Rampolla, 1, 90100 Palermo, Italy.

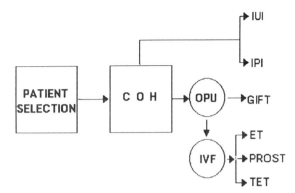

FIGURE 1. Critical steps of assisted reproductive technologies. *Abbreviations:* COH = controlled ovarian hyperstimulation; OPU = oocyte pick-up; IUI = intrauterine insemination; IPI = intraperitoneal insemination; GIFT = gamete intra-fallopian transfer; IVF = *in vitro* fertilization; ET = embryo transfer; PROST = pronuclear state transfer; TET = tubal embryo transfer.

HORMONAL STUDIES

Ovarian steroid secretion is of crucial importance for the development of an adequate endometrial environment for implantation. With any strategy used for inducing multiple follicular growth, different patterns of estradiol responses may be observed during the follicular phase.[1,2] Regular and constant rise of plasma estradiol (E_2) until the day after human chorionic gonadotropin (hCG) injection is associated with the highest pregnancy rate, while the success rate declines with follicular phase E_2 patterns consistent with an inadequate or insufficient follicular stimulation and growth.

Conflicting results have been reported in regard to the correlation between the absolute values of plasma E_2 concentrations in the preovulatory period of stimulated cycles and the chance of pregnancy after ET. Significantly better results have been observed in patients defined as high responders ($E_2 > 900$pg/ml at hCG day), compared with intermediate ($E_2 = 400–900$pg/ml) or low ($E_2 < 400$pg/ml) responders.[3] By contrast, Forman and coworkers[4] recently reported in a large series a marked decrease of pregnancy rate when the concentrations of plasma E_2 were above the 90th percentile of the population studied, corresponding to an E_2 level higher than 2,300pg/ml. But was relevant in that study that the cycles in which 3 to 4 embryos were transferred no difference in pregnancy rate could be observed among all estradiol intervals compared to the transfer of 2 embryos. This suggests that a reduced endometrial receptivity may be offset by the increase in the number of embryos available for implantation. Looking at the E_2 levels during the follicular phase in pregnant and non-pregnant patients undergoing IVF and ET, we did not observe statistically significant difference in a retrospective study of 1000 IVF cycles using concomitant GnRH-a and hMG for ovarian stimulation (FIG. 2). However, E_2 values were always considerably higher than in spontaneous cycles.

Plasma steroid concentrations are evidently conditioned by the implantation, and we did not observe significant differences in E_2 and progesterone (P) plasma levels before day 8 after the day of hCG administration (FIG. 3). By day 8 of the luteal phase,

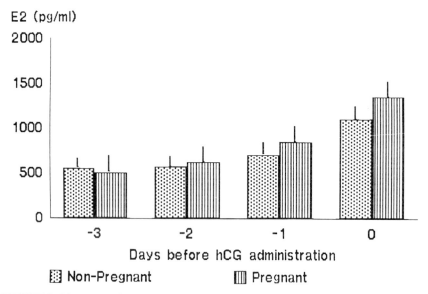

FIGURE 2. Plasma estradiol values (mean $\pm$ SE) in pregnant and non-pregnant IVF cycles during follicular phase.

E_2 concentrations were significantly higher in pregnant patients as compared with non-pregnant. There was no significant difference in P concentrations throughout the early and mid-luteal phase, while in the late luteal phase P levels were consistently higher in pregnant patients by day 8 of the luteal phase.

On the other hand, the indispensability of P secretion by the corpus luteum (CL) has been demonstrated in human spontaneous conception.[5] Lutectomy on about day 19 of pregnancy is associated with a drop in E_2 and P levels and generally results in abortion. The administration of E_2 alone to lutectomized humans maintains normal serum levels of the hormone but abortion occurs in the presence of low P levels. The administration of P maintains normal serum P levels and pregnancy can be sustained in spite of precipitous decline in serum E_2 levels.

The quality of the conceptus and the response of the corpus luteum in the peri-implantation period certainly plays an important role for establishing the receptivity of endometrium for implantation. Earlier rescue of the CL reflects a good quality embryo and may be crucial for achieving pregnancy in assisted reproduction. Liu and coworkers[6] have recently demonstrated that in IVF cycles a significantly higher proportion of term pregnancies had the CL rescue on or before day 12 of the luteal phase as opposed to a later rescue in miscarriages. In that study it was also reported that in all pregnancies implantation was evident before CL rescue as assessed by plasma hCG. This seems to indicate that implantation is essential for CL rescue and implies an embryo signal. Liu's data are consistent with the data relating embryo quality, as assessed by morphological criteria, to the rate of pregnancy after ET. Hill and co-workers[6] have recently reported that patients who conceived after ET had a significantly higher number of "good quality" embryos replaced than those patients who did not conceive.

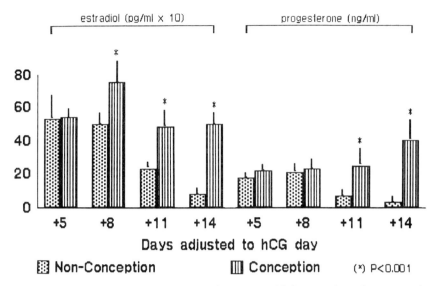

FIGURE 3. Plasma estradiol and progesterone values (mean ± SE) in conception and non-conception IVF cycles during luteal phase.

HISTOLOGICAL STUDIES

Several studies have addressed histological patterns of endometrium in stimulated cycles for IVF and ET.[7-13] Endometrial biopsies are usually done in the luteal phase of stimulated cycles without ET. The rate of abnormalities reported is very high, ranging from 28% to 76% (TABLE 1). However, it is remarkable how widely different are the criteria used for the definition of abnormalities: some studies[8,11,13] utilized exact histological dating as the measure of normalcy, whereas other studies[9,12] described different degrees of histological alterations without any temporal correlation. However, even when similar criteria were used, the results were still discrepant and these discrepancies can be at least partially explained by the differences in the stimulation

TABLE 1. Luteal Phase Endometrial Histology in Stimulated Cycles

Author	Year	No. of Patients	Day of EB[a]	Abnormal Dating (%)
Frydman et al.[7]	1982	25	17	28
Garcia et al.[8]	1984	22	14–16	73
Cohen et al.[9]	1984	19	16–18	63
Salat-Baroux et al.[10]	1984	32	21	35
Graf et al.[11]	1986	25	23–25	76
Sterzik et al.[12]	1988	58	11–18	70
Forman et al.[13]	1989	14	16	71

[a] EB = endometrial biopsy.

protocols used and different patient population. In addition, most studies do not describe detailed hormonal characteristics of the studied cycles.

Garcia's study[8] described 21 patients who had endometrial biopsy on the luteal phase in the stimulated cycle for IVF without ET. Significant differences were found in P levels and patterns between cycles in which the endometrial biopsies were in phase compared to an advanced endometrium. Pregnancies occurred in cycles with similar hormonal patterns as found in advanced biopsies. Garcia's conclusion was that an advanced endometrium may enhance implantation. The main difficulty in this study is the fact that cycles that did not result in pregnancy also had a similar hormonal pattern.

The study by Cohen and coworkers[9] illustrated the wide range of E_2 and P that will still create what they call a "suitable" endometrium for implantation. The "unsuitable" endometrium was associated to a trend for both lower E_2 and P. However, the values of these steroids overlap with the values resulting in normal endometrium.

What is the potential effect of the ovarian stimulants used for inducing multiple follicular growth?

Few studies have addressed this point. Sterzik's study[12] described a wide range of endometrial insufficiency highly related to the use of CC either alone or in combination with hMG, as opposed to the use of hMG alone. More recently different results have been reported by Forman and coworkers.[13] They observed that ovarian stimulation determines an advanced endometrium in most of the cases regardless of the stimulation protocol, but the endometrial histology could be related to the absolute values of preovulatory E_2 and P levels on day 16 of the stimulated cycle: more than 500pg/ml of preovulatory E_2 and more than 11ng/ml of day 16 P were associated with an advanced endometrium. In addition, in this study, low concentration of both endometrial receptors for estrogens and P were associated with most advanced endometrium regardless the type of stimulation.

A potential direct effect of CC on endometrium has to be considered. Birkenfield and coworkers[14] demonstrated inappropriate secretory changes of endometrial gland on biopsies made on the mid- to late-follicular phase of cycles stimulated with CC, even the presence of very low (preovulatory) plasma levels of P. Considering the absence of follicular luteinization, these changes have to be determined by the anti-estrogenic effect of CC at the level of endometrial estrogen receptors. A different mechanism may be advocated for abnormalities of the endometrium using the association of CC and hMG: in these cycles a subtle luteinization may be observed in the preovulatory period as opposed to hMG only stimulation, and this may be related to the well-known increase of plasma gonadotropins associated with CC administration determining that subtle luteinization in the presence of high estrogen produced by hMG-stimulated follicles.[15] Extremely interesting are the data recently published by Ben-Nun and coworkers[16] who studied the effect of a daily dose of P with administration starting 10 hours before hCG injection in stimulated cycles for IVF. As expected, significantly higher P levels were induced in the treatment cycles group in comparison with control group. Endometrial biopsies done 48 hours after follicular aspiration (in patients without ET) showed an evident discrepancy between glandular and stromal maturation in the treatment group, and this finding was quite constant being observed in 6 out of 9 biopsies. What is really interesting in this study is the fact that clinical pregnancy rate per ET was significantly higher for the treatment group (FIG. 4) and is possible to hypothesize that the glandulo-stromal discrepancy of endometrial maturation could be present in the conception cycles after ET.

The importance of these histological findings remains questionable, and all these

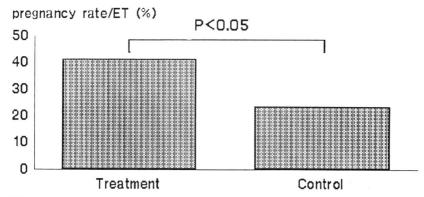

FIGURE 4. Pregnancy rate per embryo transfer in patients undergoing preovulatory progesterone supplementation (from Ben-Nun *et al.*, 1990[16]).

data together strongly suggest that morphological criteria may be insufficient to define the adequacy of endometrial maturation for implantation.

REFERENCES

1. DLUGI, A. M., N. LAUFER, A. H. DE CHERNEY N. J. MacLUSKY, F. P. HASELTINE, M. L. POLAN, H. C. B. TARLATZIS & F. NAFTOLIN. 1984. Fertil. Steril. **41**: 530–537.
2. JONES, H. W., JR., G. S. JONES, M. C. ANDREWS, A. ACOSTA, C. BUNDREN, J. E. GARCIA, B. SANDOW, L. L. VEECK, C. WILKES, J. WITMYER, J. E. WORTHAM & G. WRIGHT. 1982. Fertil. Steril. **38**: 14–19.
3. JONES, H. W., JR., A. ACOSTA, M. C. ANDREWS, J. E. GARCIA, G. S. JONES, T. MANTZAVINOS, J. McDOWELL, B. SANDOW, L. L. VEECK, T. WHIBLEY, C. WILKES & G. WRIGHT. 1983. Fertil. Steril. **40**: 317–323.
4. FORMAN, R., N. FRIES, J. TESTAR, J. BELAISH-ALLART, A. HAZOUT, R. FRYDMAN. 1988. Fertil. Steril. **49**: 118–122.
5. CSAPO, A. I. & M. PULKINEN. 1978. Obstet. Gynecol. Surv. **33**: 69–77.
6. HILL, G. A., M. FREEMAN, M. C. BASTIAS, B. J. ROGERS, C. M. HERBERT, III, K. G. OSTEEN & A. C. WENTZ. 1989. Fertil. Steril. **52**: 801–806.
7. FRYDMAN, R., J. TESTAR, P. GIACOMINI, M. C. IMBERT, E. MARTIN & K. NAHOUL. 1982. Fertil. Steril. **38**: 312–317.
8. GARCIA, J. E., A. A. ACOSTA, J. HSIU & H. W. JONES, JR. 1984. Fertil. Steril. **41**: 31–35.
9. COHEN, J. J., C. DEBACHE, F. PIGEAU, J. MANDELBAUM, M. PLACHOT & J. DE BRUX. 1984. Fertil. Steril. **42**: 360–365.
10. SALAT-BAROUX, J. P. GIACOMINI & D. CORNET. 1984. Fertil. Steril. **41** (abstr.): 16s.
11. GRAF, M. J., J. V. REYNIAK, P. BATTLE-MUTTER & N. LAUFER. 1988. Fertil. Steril. **49**: 616–619.
12. STERZIK, K., C. DALLENBACH, V. SCHNEIDER, V. SASSA & G. DALLENBACH-HELLWEG. 1988. Fertil. Steril. **50**: 457–463.
13. FORMAN, R. G., B. EYECHENNE, C. NESSMANN, R. FRYDMAN & P. ROBEL. 1989. Fertil. Steril. **51**: 310–316.
14. BIRKENFELD, A., D. NAVOT, I. S. LEVIJ, N. LAUFER, K. BEIER-HELLWIG, C. GOECKE, J. G. SCHENKER & H. M. BEIER. 1986. Fertil. Steril. **45**: 462–468.
15. BIRKENFELD, A., S. MOR-JOSEPH, J. EZRA, A. SIMON & D. NAVOT. 1990. Hum. Reprod. In press.
16. BEN-NUN, I., Y. GHETLER, R. JAFFE, A. SIEGAL, H. KANETI & M. FEJGIN. 1990. Fertil. Steril. **53**: 276–281.

Etiology and Histogenesis of Endometriosis

W. PAUL DMOWSKI[a]

*Institute for the Study and Treatment of Endometriosis
and Rush Medical College
Chicago, Illinois 60614*

INTRODUCTION

Endometriosis, ever since Sampson first coined its name in the 1920s,[1] has remained a perplexing, poorly understood disease of the female reproductive system. It is usually defined as a misplaced, *i.e.*, outside of the uterine cavity, growth of the endometrial tissue. The disease affects women in the reproductive years, limits their fertility, and seriously impairs their health, although it is not life threatening. It is not known why only some women develop endometriosis, but it is well established that its persistence and spread are stimulated by the cyclic secretion of ovarian hormones.

The true incidence of endometriosis is unknown. The prevalence in various groups of women ranges between 0 and 50%. It is estimated that in the general female population, the prevalence of endometriosis is at least 1%. Interestingly, in women with affected first degree relatives, the prevalence of endometriosis is about 7 times higher, suggesting that the disease may be transmitted in a polygenetic/multifactorial mode.[2] It has been suggested that the frequency of endometriosis has dramatically increased during recent years. This may merely be the result of more frequent use of diagnostic laparoscopy, or the increase in the prevalence may be real.[3]

HISTOGENESIS OF ENDOMETRIOSIS

During the first half of this century, several theories were proposed to explain the process through which endometriosis develops, and clinical as well as experimental evidence has since accumulated in support of each of these concepts. The most popular, and currently the most acceptable, is that proposed by Sampson.[4] He postulated that fragments of the uterine endometrium, transported through the fallopian tubes in a retrograde manner at the time of the menstrual flow, implant in the peritoneal cavity, giving origin to endometriosis. Clinical and experimental studies confirm that shed endometrial fragments are viable and that retrograde tubal transport takes place, lending credence to Sampson's theory.

[a] *Address for correspondence:* W. Paul Dmowski, M.D., Ph.D., Institute for the Study and Treatment of Endometriosis, Grant Hospital, 550 W. Webster Ave., Chicago, IL 60614, (312)883-3881.

The theory that endometriosis develops through the process of metaplasia was postulated by Meyer[5] at the beginning of this century. According to this theory, repeated irritation of the celomic epithelium by a variety of factors (*e.g.*, infectious stimuli) can induce metaplastic changes in the totipotential celomic cells, resulting in their transformation into endometrial tissue. The concept of metaplasia is supported by individual case reports of endometriosis in women with primary amenorrhea and without functional uterine endometrium and endometriosis of the urinary bladder in men after prostatectomy and orchiectomy and prolonged treatment with estrogens (for review see ref. 6).

The "induction concept" suggests that chemical substances liberated from the uterine endometrium but not the endometrium itself may stimulate undifferentiated mesenchyme to undergo metaplastic transformation into endometrial glands and stroma.[7] In support of this concept, Merrill[8] demonstrated in rabbits and monkeys that cell-free endometrial extracts stimulated development of lesions resembling endometriosis in the adjacent connective tissue.

ETIOLOGY OF ENDOMETRIOSIS

The etiology of endometriosis is unknown. If Sampson's theory is accepted, retrograde tubal flow and factors causing ectopic dissemination of the endometrial fragments (*e.g.*, iatrogenic) may be considered as primary determinants in the development of endometriosis. Yet, retrograde transport of the endometrial fragments has been demonstrated in women not affected by endometriosis, and uterine endometrium when experimentally transferred into ectopic locations did not implant in all cases.

If laparoscopy is performed during menses, retrograde blood flow can be demonstrated in about 90% of women.[9] Blood in the peritoneal cavity during menses has also been observed in more than 80% of women on peritoneal dialysis.[10] Endometrial cells have been isolated from the peritoneal fluid of as many as 50% of women with and without endometriosis,[11] and endometrial fragments have been demonstrated histologically in the lumen of the fallopian tubes.[12] These data indicate that the retrograde tubal transport of endometrial cells and fragments during the menstrual flow is a phenomenon common to all menstruating females.

If the retrograde transport of endometrial fragments into the peritoneal cavity is a common phenomenon, why is the prevalence of endometriosis in the general female population only 1%?

CHANGES IN THE IMMUNE SYSTEM ASSOCIATED WITH ENDOMETRIOSIS

During the past decade, evidence has accumulated linking endometriosis with alterations in the immune system. Changes in both cell mediated and humoral immunity in rhesus monkeys and in women with endometriosis have been observed by several investigators. Furthermore, it has been reported that rhesus monkeys given total body exposure to proton irradiation[13] or treated chronically with polychlorinated biphenyls (PCBs)[14] developed endometriosis more frequently than normal controls. It is possible that suppression of the immune system by systemic irradiation or by PCBs, both of which have immunosuppressive properties, facilitates implantation of endometrial fragments in ectopic locations and results in the development of endometriosis.

Changes in Humoral Immunity in Endometriosis

Several studies by different investigators indicate high frequency of circulating auto-antibodies in women with endometriosis. Startseva in 1980[15] reported increased B cell activity; Weed and Arguembourg[16] in the same year provided evidence for the presence of anti-endometrial antibodies reacting with the uterine endometrium; and Mathur and coworkers[17] two years later identified IgG and IgA autoantibodies against ovarian and endometrial tissues in the sera and various body fluids of women with endometriosis. In subsequent studies, other investigators using hemagglutination, immunodiffusion, and immunofluorescence techniques confirmed the high frequency of antiendometrial antibodies in the serum, peritoneal fluid and endometrial tissue from women with endometriosis.[18-21]

In addition to antiendometrial antibodies, autoantibodies against phospholipids and other chemical substances integral to the cell structure, have also been identified in women with endometriosis. Gleicher and associates[22] studied 31 women with endometriosis; 65% had IgG and 45% had IgM autoantibodies to at least 1 of 16 antigens investigated. Most frequently detected were autoantibodies to phospholipids, particularly phosphatidyl serine, histones, and nucleotides. Such multiple autoantibodies suggest polyclonal B-cell activation. We confirmed these observations; in a group of 20 women with laparoscopically diagnosed and staged endometriosis, 50% had autoantibodies against five or more of the 45 cell antigens tested.[23]

Danazol, a synthetic steroid derivative used commonly in the management of endometriosis, is capable of suppressing abnormal autoantibodies in several autoimmune diseases including idiopathic thrombocytopenic purpura (ITP) and systemic lupus erythematosus (SLE). In endometriosis, 6 months treatment with danazol decreased IgG, IgM, and IgA levels, and suppressed elevated autoantibodies. Interestingly, treatment with GnRH agonists, although clinically as effective as with danazol, did not have significant effects on the immunoglobulin or autoantibody levels.

Changes in Cell-mediated Immunity

It is possible that both humoral and cell-mediated immunity is altered in endometriosis. In rhesus monkeys with spontaneous endometriosis, we observed decreased *in vivo* reactivity to intradermal injection of autologous endometrial antigens (measured as intensity of perivascular lymphocytic infiltration) compared with normal controls.[24] *In vitro* lymphocyte proliferation in response to the same autologous endometrial antigens was also less pronounced in monkeys with endometriosis. In women with endometriosis, cytotoxicity assays using peripheral lymphocytes and autologous ^{51}Cr-labeled endometrial cells as the target cells demonstrated decreased target cell lysis with differences between subjects and controls most significant among patients with moderate and severe endometriosis.[25] Tests for nonspecific immune function were comparable between subjects and controls, suggesting that both monkeys and women with endometriosis were otherwise identical immunologically.

In the peritoneal cavity, macrophages which originate from peripheral blood monocytes play a major role in maintaining homeostasis. They remove red blood cells, damaged tissue fragments and most likely endometrial cells that gain access to the peritoneal cavity through fallopian tubes. Several studies indicate that in endometriosis the concentration and total number of peritoneal macrophages and their activational status are increased.[26,27] Peritoneal macrophages also produce higher levels of IL-1[28] and fibronectin,[29] the later of which may contribute to the development of peritoneal adhesions.

In addition to phagocytic activities, peritoneal macrophages may also regulate other events in the peritoneal cavity by release of products such as cytokines, prostaglandins, growth factors, complement components, and hydrolytic enzymes. Furthermore, macrophages release low levels of reactive oxygen metabolites, such as superoxide anion, hydrogen peroxide and singlet oxygen.

The generation of reactive oxygen products can be estimated by measuring light emission or chemiluminescence. We have reported that in endometriosis, resting chemiluminescence of peritoneal macrophages is significantly increased, indicating the increase in their activational status.[30] Furthermore, peripheral blood monocytes from women with endometriosis, when stimulated, demonstrated significantly higher chemiluminescence. Similarly, peripheral monocytes from women with endometriosis also displayed higher production of IL-1 *in vitro*.[31] These studies indicate that endometriosis may be a systemic disorder of the immune system rather than a local, gynecologic disease.

Our ongoing research indicates that the cytotoxicity of peritoneal macrophages is impaired in endometriosis. This defect, which is most pronounced in severe endometriosis, seems to be prostaglandin dependent. With addition of indomethacin to the *in vitro* culture, we could significantly increase the suppressed cytotoxic activity of peritoneal macrophages from women with severe endometriosis.

ENDOMETRIOSIS AS A DISEASE OF THE IMMUNE SYSTEM: A HYPOTHESIS

The data reviewed above seem to indicate that the immune system plays a role in the pathophysiology of endometriosis, although the exact mechanism of this involvement is not clear. In rhesus monkeys, treatment with immunosuppressive agents seems to be followed by increased frequency of endometriosis, although specific changes in the immune system have not been identified. In women with endometriosis, the most consistent changes in the immune function are observed in the monocyte/macrophage system. Peritoneal macrophages are increased in number and activational status, but their cytotoxic activities are suppressed, especially in severe endometriosis. These functional, although not numerical changes may also be observed in peripheral monocytes before they become sequestered in the peritoneal cavity. The observation that indomethacin is capable of reversing the cytotoxic exhaustion of the peritoneal macrophages, suggests that this change may be prostaglandin dependent. The autoantibodies are present in the peripheral circulation and in various body fluids in about 50 to 60% of affected patients. Some of these autoantibodies are directed against endometrial antigens, others against chemical substances which are the integral part of the cell structure. Interestingly, a drug that is therapeutically effective in endometriosis seems to also have immunoregulatory effects, and is capable of autoantibody suppression.

The recognition and tolerance of self-antigens are two hallmarks of the immune system. A critical feature of an immune response is that effector mechanisms are directed against foreign but not self, antigens. An immune response to self antigens typically results in the development of autoimmune diseases. However, the concept that the immune response is directed exclusively against foreign antigens is changing slowly. The aberrant or abnormal cells, such as senescent or cancer cells, that in the strictest sense are self-antigens, are eliminated by the immune system. There is also evidence suggesting that the growth of normal autologous cells in ectopic locations is limited by the immune system. The auto-transplants, such as skin will more likely engraft near donor sites[32] and testes of dogs when surgically transferred into the peritoneal cavity, undergo lymphocytic infiltration resulting in tissue destruction.[33]

It is possible that endometriosis is an autoimmune disease, not unlike SLE, with which it seems to be frequently associated. Increased immunoglobulin levels and high frequency of autoantibodies indicate polyclonal activation of B cells. Other characteristics of autoimmune diseases, such as female preponderance, familial occurrence, tissue damage, multi-organ involvement, and evidence for antigen-antibody reaction are also present in endometriosis. Furthermore, treatment with danazol inhibits autoantibody production and brings about clinical improvement in several autoimmune disorders as well as in endometriosis.

Alternatively, it is possible that endometriosis is a disorder of immune surveillance and destruction of ectopic endometrial cells. It is possible that the healthy immune system prevents ectopic implantation of the endometrial cells transported outside of the uterine cavity through fallopian tubes, blood or lymphatic vessels. Endometriosis therefore would indicate an alteration in the immune function which could be transmitted genetically. According to this concept, endometrial cells or fragments displaced into the peritoneal cavity of healthy women are "disposed of" by the local immune system, consisting primarily of the peritoneal macrophages. Endometriosis may develop when the peritoneal "disposal system" is defective and permits implantation of the endometrial cells or fragments. It is also possible that endometriosis may develop if the peritoneal "disposal system" is overwhelmed by the increased retrograde transport due to the obstructed menstrual flow, as in cervical stenosis. The changes in the humoral immunity would then be secondary to deficient cellular mechanisms. A possible scenario is that in the peritoneal cavity endometrial cells are processed by activated macrophages and presented to the T cells. Under the influence of macrophage-released cytokines such as IL-1 and IL-2, T cells proliferate and differentiate into functional subsets of cells with helper, suppressor, suppressor-inducer, and cytotoxic properties. A host of T cell–derived factors then play a critical role in the activation of B cells from the resting state into a proliferative state and into further differentiation and antibody secretion. The activated B cells then produce autoantibodies against endometrial cells or against endometrial cell-derived phospholipids, histones, or nucleotides. Autoantibodies may in turn reduce fertility by interfering with ovum capture or implantation as well as by increasing the frequency of abortions.

REFERENCES

1. SAMPSON, J. A. 1925. Am. J. Obstet. Gynecol. **10:** 649.
2. SIMPSON, J. L., S. ELIAS, L. R. MALINAK & V. C. BUTTRAM. 1980. Am. J. Obstet. Gynecol. **137:** 327.
3. HOUSTON, D. E. 1984. Epidemiol. Rev. **6:** 167.
4. SAMPSON, J. A. 1921. Arch. Surg. **3:** 245.
5. MEYER, R. 1919. Zentralbl. Gynaekol. **36:** 745.

6. DMOWSKI, W. P. & E. RADWANSKA. 1984. Acta Obstet. Gynecol. Scand. (Suppl.) **123**: 29.
7. LEVANDER, G. 1941. Arch. Klin. Chir. **202**: 497.
8. MERRILL, J. A. 1966. Am. J. Obstet. Gynecol. **94**: 780.
9. HALME, J., M. G. HAMMOND, J. F. HULKA, S. G. RAJ & L. M. TALBERT. 1984. Obstet. Gynecol. **64**: 151.
10. BLUMENKRANTZ, M. J., R. N. GALLAGHER, R. A. BASHORE & H. TENCKHOFF. 1981. Obstet. Gynecol. **57**: 667.
11. KONINCKX, P. R., P. IDE, W. VANDENBROUCKE & I. A. BROSENS. 1980. J. Reprod. Med. **24**: 257.
12. RIDLEY, J. H. 1968. Obstet. Gynecol. Surv. **23**: 1.
13. WOOD, D. H., M. G. YOCHMOWITZ, Y. L. SALMON, R. L. EASON & R. A. BOSTER. 1983. Aviat. Space Environ. Med. **54**: 718.
14. CAMPBELL, J. S., J. WONG, L. TRYPHONAS, *et al.* 1985. Proc. Ont. Assoc. Pathol.
15. STARTSEVA, N. V. 1980. Akush. Ginekol. (Mosk.) **3**: 23.
16. WEED, J. C. & P. C. ARGUEMBOURG. 1980. Clin. Obstet. Gynecol. **23**: 885.
17. MATHUR, S., M. R. PERESS, H. O. WILLIAMSON, C. D. YOUMANS, S. A. MANEY, A. J. GARVIN, P. F. RUST & H. H. FUDENBERG. 1982. Clin. Exp. Immunol. **50**: 259.
18. SAIFUDDIN, A., C. H. BUCKLEY & H. FOX. 1983. Int. J. Gynecol. Pathol. **2**: 255.
19. BADAWY, S. Z., V. CUENCA & A. STITZEL. 1984. Obstet. Gynecol. **63**: 271.
20. WILD, R. A. & C. A. SHIVERS. 1985. Am. J. Reprod. Immunol. Microbiol. **8**: 84.
21. KREINER, D., F. B. FROMOWITZ, D. A. RICHARDSON & D. KENIGSBERG. 1986. Fertil. Steril. **46**: 243.
22. GLEICHER, N., A. EL-ROEIY & E. CONFINO. 1987. Obstet. Gynecol. **7**: 115.
23. EL-ROEIY, A., W. P. DMOWSKI, N. GLEICHER, E. RADWANSKA, L. HARLOW, Z. BINOR, I. TUMMON & R. RAWLINS. 1988. Fertil. Steril. **50**: 864.
24. DMOWSKI, W. P., R. W. STEELE & G. F. BAKER. 1981. Am. J. Obstet. Gynecol. **141**: 377.
25. STEELE, R. W., W. P. DMOWSKI & D. J. MARMER. 1984. Am. J. Reprod. Immunol. **6**: 33.
26. HANEY, A. F., J. J. MUSCATO & J. B. WEINBERG. 1981. Fertil. Steril. **35**: 696.
27. HALME, J., S. BECKER & R. WING. 1984. Am. J. Obstet. Gynecol. **148**: 85.
28. FAKIH, H., B. BAGGETT & G. HOLTZ, K. Y. TSANG, J. C. LEE & H. O. WILLIAMSON. 1987. Fertil. Steril. **47**: 213.
29. KAUMA, S., M. R. CLARK, C. WHITE & J. HALME. 1988. Obstet. Gynecol. **72**: 13.
30. ZELLER, J. M., I. HENIG, E. RADWANSKA & W. P. DMOWSKI. 1987. Am. J. Reprod. Immunol. Microbiol. **13**: 78.
31. PARVIZI, S. T., P. JENSEN, A. DECHERNEY. March, 1988. Proc. 35th Annual Meeting, Society for Gynecologic Investigation, Baltimore, MD. Abstract 450, p. 284.
32. STEELE, R. W., J. W. EICHBERG & R. L. HERBERLING. 1976. J. Med. Primatol. **6**: 119.
33. SHIRAI, M., S. MATSUSHITA & M. KAGAYAMA, S. ICHIJO & M. TAKEUCHI. 1966. Tohoku. J. Exp. Med. **90**: 363.

Experimental Endometriosis in Monkeys

ROBERT S. SCHENKEN

Division of Reproductive Endocrinology and Infertility
Department of Obstetrics and Gynecology
The University of Texas Health Science Center at San Antonio
7703 Floyd Curl Drive
San Antonio, Texas 78284-7836

ROBERT F. WILLIAMS AND GARY D. HODGEN

The Jones Institute for Reproductive Medicine
Department of Obstetrics and Gynecology
Eastern Virginia Medical School
855 W. Brambleton Ave., Suite B
Norfolk, Virginia 23510

INTRODUCTION

Endometriosis is a common gynecologic disorder that is associated with several distressing, debilitating symptoms. The classic symptoms reported by women having endometriosis include pelvic pain, dyspareunia, dysmenorrhea, and infertility. Although the incidence and severity of these symptoms have been well described, our understanding of the pathophysiologic mechanism(s) is incomplete. In fact, it has yet to be established that endometriosis actually causes any of the symptoms that are so common ascribed to it in women.[1]

Despite the absence of evidence for a specific cause-and-effect relationship, it is widely believed that the symptoms of endometriosis are a result of ectopic endometrial tissue. To investigate this in women would require longitudinal, controlled, and invasive experiments that would obviously be ethically unacceptable. Accordingly, numerous animal models have been developed to simulate endometriosis in women. These models have been primarily used to study the effects of drugs and hormones on endometriotic implants and to clarify the mechanism(s) of infertility due to endometriosis. To establish an animal model for the human disease, the model must evoke the symptoms of the disease. In regards to endometriosis and infertility, surgical transplantation of endometrium to the peritoneal cavity in rats, rabbits, and monkeys has consistently resulted in reduced fecundity.[2-4] Of all these models, the monkey represents the most suitable because of its endocrinologic and menstrual cycle similarity to women and because spontaneous endometriosis is known to occur in monkeys. Here, we will review our initial studies on the surgical induction of endometriosis in monkeys as a model to study the effects of ectopic endometrial implants on fertility.

MATERIAL AND METHODS

Twenty-one adult female cynomolgus monkeys (*Macaca fascicularis*) demonstrating menstrual regularity were selected for the study. Housing, feeding, and general husbandry practices have been described previously.[5]

Surgical Induction of Endometriosis

Using ketamine (Vetalar®, Parke-Davis, Morris Plains, NJ) anesthesia (15 mg/kg), blood was collected daily on days 8 to 14 of the menstrual cycle via venipuncture and serum assayed for 17β-estradiol (E_2) by radioimmunoassay (RIA). Laparotomy, using the same anesthetic, was then performed 3 to 5 days after the preovulatory serum E_2 peak. All animals with obvious pelvic adhesions or without an ovulatory stigma were excluded from the study. At laparotomy, care was taken to avoid contaminating the abdominal cavity with blood. Prior to any surgical manipulation, the pelvic organs were irrigated with 3.0 ml of normal saline and the fluid was collected in a heparinized syringe. The peritoneal washings were then centrifuged at $1200 \times g$ for 15 minutes and stored at $-15°C$. A 1-cm vertical fundal hysterotomy was performed and ~ 100 mg of endometrium was dissected from the myometrium and placed in sterile 0.9% saline. The uterine incision was closed in one layer with 4-0 Vicryl (Ethicon, Somerville, NJ) suture. In 11 animals, the endometrial tissue was minced and injected subperitoneally into the vesicouterine fold, uterine incision, right and left broad ligaments, and cul-de-sac. In ten animals, the endometrial tissue was discarded, and ~ 1 g of omental adipose tissue was resected, minced in sterile 0.9% saline, and injected into the same five sites. The abdominal incision was then closed in layers.

During the subsequent menstrual cycle, laparotomy was performed 3 to 5 days after the midcycle E_2 peak. Peritoneal washings were collected as described above. The presence of viable endometrial and adipose tissue and the extent of adhesion formation were noted. The endometrial and adipose tissue implants were biopsied, and a portion of tissue was fixed in 10% formalin for histologic examination after hematoxylin and eosin staining. The remaining specimen was washed with cold Tyrode's solution and stored at $-15°C$. The American Fertility Society classification for pelvic endometriosis, modified to correct for the smaller size of the pelvic organs in the monkey, was used to stage the disease.[6]

Fertility Studies

During three subsequent menstrual cycles, blood was collected every other day during the early follicular and luteal phases of the cycle and daily on cycle days 8 to 14. Blood sampling was discontinued at the time of the next menses or, in the absence of menses, on cycle day 42. Serum was frozen at $-15°C$ until assayed for luteinizing hormone (LH), follicle-stimulating hormone (FSH), E_2, and progesterone (P) by RIA.[7] An aliquot of serum was obtained from all periovulatory samples for daily E_2 determination. RIA for macaque chorionic gonadotropin (mCG) was performed on all blood samples after cycle day 24.[8]

All females were time-mated for 2 to 3 days with males of proven fertility. Matings were conducted near midcycle, beginning on the first day after the serum E_2 peak.

Laparotomy was performed 3 to 5 days after the preovulatory peak in serum E_2 in each study cycle. Pelvic findings were recorded in detail, the presence or absence of a stigma of ovulation was noted, and peritoneal washings were collected.

In the absence of menses and with a positive mCG, rectal palpation was performed (after 40 to 45 days of gestation) to confirm continuation of an intrauterine pregnancy. Pregnancies were allowed to progress to term without subsequent intervention.

Cycles were defined as ovulatory when an ovulatory stigma was present and serum P levels were >3 ng/ml at 5 to 10 days after the LH surge.[7] Absence of a stigma of ovulation in association with luteal phase serum P levels >3 ng/ml was the criterion used to document a luteinized unruptured follicle (LUF). Cycles were defined as anovulatory when luteal phase serum P levels remained <3 ng/ml and no ovulatory stigma was present. Luteal phase defect (LPD) was defined in cases where the luteal phase length was <10 days and the P secretion (integrated area under the curve) <50% of the mean for all study cycles. Luteal phase mCG values >50 µg/ml were considered chemical pregnancies.[8]

To determine the effect of pelvic adhesions on fertility, we correlated the location of moderate or severe peritubal or periovarian adhesions with the location of the corpus luteum during each ovulatory cycle. A specific cycle was recorded as having adhesions only when peritubal or periovarian adhesions were present ipsilateral to the corpus luteum.

Prostaglandin Assays

Tissue samples were thawed and homogenized in cold Tyrode's solution containing 10 µg/ml of indomethacin. All tissue samples and peritoneal washings were extracted, chromatographed, and assayed for prostaglandin $F_{2\alpha}$ ($PGF_{2\alpha}$) and prostaglandin E (PGE) by RIA as previously described.[9] Inter-assay and intra-assay coefficients of variation, respectively, were 9.8% and 9.9% for $PGF_{2\alpha}$ and 5.7% and 11.6% for PGE. The sensitivity was 60 pg per tube for both $PGF_{2\alpha}$ and PGE. Protein content of the tissue samples was determined by the method of Lowry et al.[10]

Statistical Analysis

The Fisher exact probability test was used to compare menstrual cycle characteristics and pregnancy rates. Student's t-test was used to determine differences in duration of the follicular and luteal phase endocrine profiles and gonadotropin and steroid secretion (area under the curve). Student's paired t-test was also used to compare prostaglandin levels in peritoneal washings before and after tissue autografts. Analysis of variance and Dunnett's test were used to compare differences in tissue sample prostaglandin content and prostaglandin levels in peritoneal washings during study cycles. A difference was considered statistically significant when its p value was <0.05.

RESULTS

Macroscopic and Microscopic Examination

Macroscopic examination confirmed the presence of viable tissue in all 11 monkeys with endometrial autografts. The implants ranged in size from 1 to 4 mm in diameter

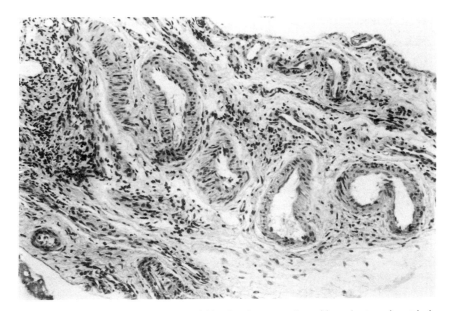

FIGURE 1. Photomicrograph of endometrial implant in one monkey with moderate endometriosis. Notice the presence of both endometrial glands and stroma (hematoxylin and eosin, original magnification, ×100). (From Schenken, R. S., R. H. Asch, R. F. Williams & G. D. Hodgen. 1984. Etiology of infertility in monkeys with endometriosis: Luteinized unruptured follicles, luteal phase defects, pelvic adhesions, and spontaneous abortions. Fertil. Steril. 41: 122. Reproduced with permission of the publisher, The American Fertility Society.)

and appeared as well-vascularized, reddish nodules or hemosiderin-like deposits. Two animals developed cystic adnexal masses that contained hemorrhagic, thick fluid ("chocolate cysts"). Pelvic adhesions were present in varying degrees. Most animals developed "puckering" of the peritoneum surrounding the implants, fine peritubal or periovarian adhesions, or dense fibrotic adnexal adhesions. Using a modification of The American Fertility Society classification, the endometriosis was staged as mild in five animals, moderate in four, and severe in two.

Microscopic examination of implants in all 11 animals revealed endometrial glands and stroma (FIG. 1). Hemosiderin-laden macrophages and areas of fibrosis were often observed. Endometrial cyst walls were lined with low cuboidal epithelium and sparse endometrial glands.

Macroscopic examination of adipose tissue autografts revealed the presence of normal-appearing vascularized tissue that was indistinguishable from surrounding subperitoneal fat. Adhesions were noted to involve the uterine incision and omentum in several animals. Adnexal adhesions developed in only one animal.

Microscopic examination of fat implants showed normal adipose tissue in five monkeys and evidence of endometrial glands or hemosiderin-laden macrophages, usually near the fundal scar, in five animals. These animals were classified as controls with adipose tissue only (n = 5) and animals with microscopic endometriosis (n = 5).

TABLE 1. Prostaglandin Concentrations[a] in Peritoneal Washings before and after Tissue Autografts[b]

Group	n	$PGF_{2\alpha}$ Before	$PGF_{2\alpha}$ After	PGE Before	PGE After
Adipose tissue	5	0.201 ± 0.091	0.282 ± 0.085	1.065 ± 0.332	0.067 ± 0.363
Endometriosis					
Microscopic	5	0.205 ± 0.085	0.215 ± 0.115	0.728 ± 0.239	0.884 ± 0.224
Mild	5	0.307 ± 0.080	0.580 ± 0.114	1.511 ± 0.472	1.733 ± 0.424
Moderate	4	0.186 ± 0.016	0.539 ± 0.114^c	1.189 ± 0.617	1.072 ± 0.095
Severe	2	0.180 ± 0.010	0.619 ± 0.050^c	0.566 ± 0.010	0.553 ± 0.111

[a] Values expressed as nanograms of prostaglandins per milliliter of peritoneal washing (mean ± SEM).

[b] Adapted from Schenken, R. S., R. H. Asch, R. F. Williams & G. D. Hodgen. 1984. Etiology of infertility in monkeys with measurement of peritoneal fluid prostaglandins. Am. J. Obstet. Gynecol. **150:** 349.

[c] $p < 0.05$ versus before.

Tissue Prostaglandin Levels

The concentration of $PGF_{2\alpha}$ and PGE in peritoneal washings before and after tissue autografts is presented in TABLE 1. The peritoneal-washing $PGF_{2\alpha}$ and PGE concentrations were not significantly altered after adipose tissue implantation, despite the presence of microscopic endometriosis in 5 of 10 monkeys. All monkeys with ectopic endometrial autografts demonstrated increased $PGF_{2\alpha}$ concentrations in peritoneal washings, but this increase was significant only in monkeys with moderate and severe disease. In contrast to $PGF_{2\alpha}$, PGE concentrations in peritoneal washings were not significantly changed after endometrial implantation.

The $PGF_{2\alpha}$ and PGE content in autograft biopsy specimens is shown in TABLE 2. Adipose tissue autografts contained 0.020 ± 0.005 ng of $PGF_{2\alpha}$ per milligram of protein ($\pm$ SEM), whereas endometrial tissue autografts contained 0.049 ± 0.009, 0.035 ± 0.008, and 0.037 ± 0.005 ($\pm$ SEM) ng of $PGF_{2\alpha}$ per milligram of protein in monkeys with mild, moderate, and severe endometriosis, respectively. The increased

TABLE 2. Prostaglandin Content[a] in Tissue Autografts[b]

Group	n	$PGF_{2\alpha}$	PGE
Adipose tissue	5	0.020 ± 0.005	0.066 ± 0.027
Endometriosis			
Microscopic	5	0.020 ± 0.005	0.085 ± 0.032
Mild	5	0.049 ± 0.009^c	0.088 ± 0.021
Moderate	4	0.035 ± 0.008^c	0.099 ± 0.032
Severe	2	0.037 ± 0.005^c	0.097 ± 0.052

[a] Values expressed as nanograms of prostaglandin per milligram of protein (mean ± SEM).

[b] Adapted from Schenken, R. S., R. H. Asch, R. F. Williams & G. D. Hodgen. 1984. Etiology of infertility in monkeys with measurement of peritoneal fluid prostaglandins. Am. J. Obstet. Gynecol. **150:** 349.

[c] $p < 0.05$ versus adipose tissue.

$PGF_{2\alpha}$ content in ectopic endometrium was significantly greater than in adipose autografts ($p < 0.05$). Although a trend toward greater PGE content in endometrial autografts, compared to adipose autografts, was apparent, the difference was not significant ($p > 0.05$).

Menstrual Cycle Characteristics, Endocrine Profiles, and Peritoneal-Washing Prostaglandin Levels

The total number of cycles studied and cycle characteristics for each group are presented in TABLE 3. The number of cycles studied was similar in all groups when corrected for the number of animals in each group. The percentage of ovulatory cycles was similar in control monkeys (79%), monkeys with microscopic endometriosis (80%), and those with mild endometriosis (82%). However, monkeys with moderate and severe endometriosis demonstrated a lower incidence of ovulatory cycles, 46% and 50%, respectively; the difference was due solely to the greater incidence of LUF in these monkeys.

The endocrine profiles and duration of the follicular and luteal phases during ovulatory cycles in control monkeys and animal with mild, moderate, or severe endometriosis demonstrated no significant differences in the following: 1) follicular or luteal phase lengths; 2) serum gonadotropins, as determined by follicular phase LH/FSH ratio or follicular phase LH and FSH secretion; 3) midcycle LH and FSH surge; and 4) serum steroids, as determined by midcycle E_2 peak or luteal phase E_2 and P secretion.

The $PGF_{2\alpha}$ and PGE concentrations in peritoneal washings during the study cycle and presented in TABLE 4. Analysis of variance did not show any significant differences ($p > 0.10$) between study cycle groups in monkeys with endometrial autografts.

TABLE 3. Total Number of Study Cycles in which Monkeys were Time-mated and Incidence of Ovulation, Anovulation, LUF, and LPD[a]

Group	Total Cycles	Ovulatory Cycles[b]	Anovulatory Cycles[c]	LUF[d]	LPD[e]
Adipose tissue	14	11 (79%)	1 (7%)	0 (0%)	2 (14%)
Endometriosis					
Microscopic	15	12 (80%)	1 (6%)	0 (0%)	2 (13%)
Mild	11	9 (82%)	2 (18%)	0 (0%)	0 (0%)
Moderate	11	5 (46%)	1 (9%)	5 (46%)[f]	5 (46%)[g]
Severe	6	3 (50%)	0 (0%)	3 (50%)[f]	0

[a] Adapted from Schenken, R. S., R. S. Asch, R. F. Williams & G. D. Hodgen. 1984. Etiology of infertility in monkeys with endometriosis: Luteinized unruptured follicles, luteal phase defects, pelvic adhesions, and spontaneous abortions. Fertil. Steril. **41:** 122.

[b] Luteal phase serum P > 3 ng/ml, ovulatory stigma present.

[c] Luteal phase serum P < 3 ng/ml, ovulatory stigma absent.

[d] Luteal phase serum P > 3 ng/ml, ovulatory stigma absent.

[e] Luteal phase length <10 days and P secretion <50% of mean for all cycles.

[f] $p < 0.01$ versus animals with adipose tissue implants.

[g] All five cycles with an LUF demonstrated an LPD.

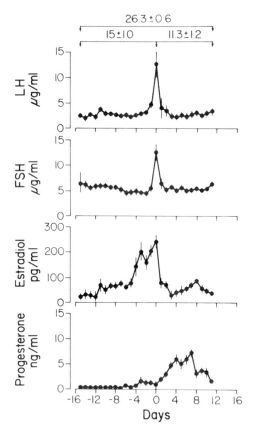

FIGURE 2. Endocrine profile and duration of follicular and luteal phases during cycles with an LUF without LPD in monkeys having moderate and severe endometriosis (total cycles, 3). (From Schenken, R. S., R. H. Asch, R. F. Williams & G. D. Hodgen. 1984. Etiology of infertility in monkeys with endometriosis: Luteinized unruptured follicles, luteal phase defects, pelvic adhesions, and spontaneous abortions. Fertil. Steril. **41**: 122. Reproduced with permission of the publisher, The American Fertility Society.)

Luteinized Unruptured Follicle and Inadequate Luteal Phase

An LUF was noted in 5 of 10 cycles in monkeys with moderate endometriosis and three of six cycles in animals with severe disease. An LUF was never present in control animals or animals with microscopic and mild endometriosis. The incidence of an LUF was significantly greater ($p < 0.01$) in animals with moderate and severe endometriosis, as compared with control animals (TABLE 3). Cycles with an LUF were never associated with a serum mCG >50 µg/ml or clinical evidence of pregnancy.

Although each individual monkey with moderate and severe endometriosis demonstrated an LUF during at least one study cycle, the occurrence of LUF was random. That is, in an individual animal, a cycle with an LUF might be followed by a cycle with an obvious ovulatory stigma, or vice versa. The size or location of endometrial implants or pelvic adhesions did not correlate with the occurrence of an LUF, except in one animal. In this monkey, an ovarian endometrioma was noted adjacent to an LUF during two study cycles. An LPD was present in 5 of the 8 cycles with an LUF.

The endocrine profiles of cycles with an LUF, but without an LPD, are presented in FIGURE 2. There was no significant difference in these cycles, as compared with

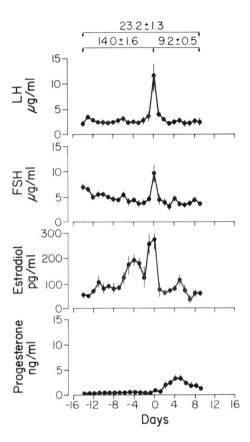

FIGURE 3. Endocrine profile and duration of follicular and luteal phases during cycles with both an LUF and LPD in monkeys exhibiting moderate endometriosis (total cycles, 5). (From Schenken, R. S., R. H. Asch, R. F. Williams & G. D. Hodgen. 1984. Etiology of infertility in monkeys with endometriosis: Luteinized unruptured follicles, luteal phase defects, pelvic adhesions, and spontaneous abortions. Fertil. Steril. **41:** 122. Reproduced with permission of the publisher, The American Fertility Society.)

normal ovulatory cycles, with regard to follicular phase length, FSH/LH ratios, LH or FSH secretion, midcycle E_2 surge, the "preovulatory" peak of LH and FSH, luteal phase length, or P and estrogen secretion in the luteal phase. Similarly, the endocrine profile in monkeys with an LUF and LPD demonstrated no significant endocrine abnormalities, except for shortened luteal phase and diminished P secretion (FIG. 3).

An LPD was noted during two cycles in the group with adipose tissue implants and two cycles in the group with microscopic endometriosis. However, none of these cycles were associated with an LUF.

There was a trend ($p = 0.07$) toward a greater $PGF_{2\alpha}$ concentration in peritoneal washings obtained during cycles characterized by a luteinized unruptured follicle as compared to normal ovulatory cycles (TABLE 4).

Pelvic Adhesions

Significant pelvic adhesions were present in 3 of 11 cycles in the adipose tissue group, 3 of 5 cycles in monkeys with moderate endometriosis, and 2 of 3 cycles in monkeys with severe endometriosis. None of the cycles resulted in a term intrauterine

TABLE 4. Prostaglandin Concentrations[a] in Peritoneal Washings during Study Cycles in Monkeys with Endometrial Autografts[b]

	Ovulatory	Anovulatory	Luteinized Unruptured Follicle	Luteal Phase Defect	Adhesions
$PGF_{2\alpha}$	0.448 ± 0.065	0.597 ± 0.133	0.569 ± 0.050^c	0.535 ± 0.074	0.589 ± 0.165
PGE	0.669 ± 0.173	0.844 ± 0.228	0.617 ± 0.209	0.993 ± 0.572	0.762 ± 0.302
n	17	3	8	5	5

[a] Values expressed as nanograms of prostaglandins per milliliter of peritoneal washing (mean ± SEM).

[b] Adapted from Schenken, R. S., R. H. Asch, R. F. Williams & G. D. Hodgen. 1984. Etiology of infertility in monkeys with measurement of peritoneal fluid prostaglandins. Am. J. Obstet. Gynecol. 150: 349.

[c] $p = 0.07$ versus ovulatory cycles.

pregnancy (TABLE 5). When adnexal adhesions were not present ipsilateral to the corpus luteum, there was no significant difference in pregnancy rates between the control group with adipose tissue (38%) and the endometriosis group (33%).

Chemical and Term Pregnancy

In each of the groups of monkeys with adipose tissue, microscopic endometriosis, and mild endometriosis, 3 of 5 monkeys carried a pregnancy to term. In contrast, only 1 of 6 animals with moderate or severe endometriosis delivered at term.

A luteal phase serum mCG >50 µg/ml was detected in 18 of the 57 study cycles

TABLE 5. Effect of Pelvic Adhesions on Term Pregnancy Rates during Ovulatory Cycles[a]

Group	Ovulatory Cycles[b]	Ovulatory Cycles with Adhesions[c]	Term Intrauterine Pregnancies[d]	Ovulatory Cycles without Adhesions[e]	Term Intrauterine Pregnancies[f]
Adipose tissue	11	3	0 (0%)	8	3 (38%)
Endometriosis					
Microscopic	12	0	0 (0%)	12	3 (27%) ⎫
Mild	9	0	0 (0%)	9	3 (33%) ⎬ 33%
Moderate	5	3	0 (0%)	2	1 (50%) ⎭ 33%
Severe	3	2	0 (0%)	1	0 (0%)

[a] Adapted from Schenken, R. S., R. S. Asch, R. F. Williams & G. D. Hogden. 1984. Etiology of infertility in monkeys with endometriosis: Luteinized unruptured follicles, luteal phase defects, pelvic adhesions, and spontaneous abortions. Fertil. Steril. 41: 122.

[b] Luteal phase serum P > 3 ng/ml, ovulatory stigma present.

[c] Adhesions present ipsilateral to the corpus luteum.

[d] Percentage of ovulatory cycles with adhesions.

[e] No adhesion or adhesion contralateral to the corpus luteum.

[f] Percentage of ovulatory cycles without adhesions.

TABLE 6. Chemical (Luteal Phase Serum mCG > 50 µg/ml) and Term Pregnancy Rates during Ovulatory Cycles[a]

Group	Total Cycles	Luteal Phase mCG > 50 µg/ml (% of total cycles)	Term Intrauterine Pregnancies (% of mCG > 50 µg/ml)
Adipose tissue	14	6 (42)	3 (50)
Endometriosis			
Microscopic	15	6 (40)	3 (50)
Mild	11	4 (36) } 21%	3 (75) } 67%
Moderate	11	1 (9) }	1 (100) }
Severe	6	1 (17) } 12%[b]	0 (0) } 50%
Total	57	18 (32)	10 (56)

[a] Adapted from Schenken, R. S., R. S. Asch, R. F. Williams & G. D. Hogden. 1984. Etiology of infertility in monkeys with endometriosis: Luteinized unruptured follicles, luteal phase defects, pelvic adhesions, and spontaneous abortions. Fertil. Steril. **41**: 122.

[b] $p < 0.05$ versus animals with adipose tissue implants.

(TABLE 6). The incidence of a chemical pregnancy was similar in monkeys with adipose tissue implants, microscopic endometriosis, and mild endometriosis. The lower chemical pregnancy rate in animals with moderate and severe endometriosis was statistically significant, as compared with control animals with adipose tissue ($p < 0.05$).

Ten of the 18 cycles with a diagnosed chemical pregnancy resulted in a term intrauterine pregnancy, suggesting that embryonic death occurred in 8 fertile menstrual cycles. The incidence of pregnancy loss was not significantly different among the groups, and none of the animals demonstrated clinical evidence of spontaneous abortion or preterm delivery.

TABLE 7 summarizes the concentrations of $PGF_{2\alpha}$ and PGE in peritoneal washings obtained during normal ovulatory cycles in relation to subsequent chemical and term pregnancies. Luteal phase serum mCG concentrations were >50 µg/ml in six cycles. Of these six chemical pregnancies, two monkeys spontaneously aborted and four delivered normal, viable offspring at term. The $PGF_{2\alpha}$ and PGE concentrations in peritoneal washings from monkeys that subsequently aborted were not significantly different from those of monkeys that delivered at term.

DISCUSSION

The rat, rabbit, and monkey have been used to study the effect of endometriosis on fertility.[2-4] Although each model has specific advantages with respect to availability, cost, and other factors, the monkey offers distinct advantages, in that 1) endometriosis can be surgically induced with a high success rate and 2) the reproductive functions of monkeys are very similar to those of human beings, allowing more realistic extrapolation of findings to the clinical setting.

In this study, surgical induction of endometriosis was successful in all animals autografted with endometrial tissue. Histologic examination of the implants demonstrated endometrial glands and stroma in all cases. Animals with adipose tissue autografts did not develop macroscopic endometriosis; however, implants in 5 of 10 ani-

TABLE 7. Prostaglandin Concentrations[a] in Peritoneal Washings during Ovulatory Cycles in Relation to Chemical and Term Pregnancies

		mCG > 50 µg/ml	
	mCG < 50 µg/ml	Spontaneous Abortion	Term Delivery
PGF$_{2\alpha}$	0.458 ± 0.096	0.422 ± 0.299[c]	0.455 ± 0.028
PGE	0.478 ± 0.123	0.997 ± 0.366[c]	0.566 ± 0.112
n	11	2	4

[a] Values expressed as nanograms of prostaglandins per milliliter of peritoneal washing (mean ± SEM).

[b] Adapted from Schenken, R. S., R. H. Asch, R. F. Williams & G. D. Hodgden. 1984. Etiology of infertility in monkeys with measurement of peritoneal fluid prostaglandins. Am. J. Obstet. Gynecol. 150: 349.

[c] $p > 0.05$ versus monkeys with mCG > 50 µg/ml and term delivery.

mals were noted to have microscopic foci of endometrial glands and stroma. This may represent either coelomic metaplasia or inadvertent spill of endometrial tissue at the time of hysterotomy and resection of endometrial tissue.

The incidence of anovulatory cycles in control monkeys and monkeys with endometriosis was similar when anovulation was determined by absence of an ovulatory stigma and luteal phase serum P levels <3 ng/ml. Previous studies in human beings have suggested an increased incidence of anovulatory cycles with all stages of endometriosis. Soules et al. [11] described a 17% incidence of ovulatory disturbance in women with endometriosis, and Acosta et al. [12] reported a 27% incidence of anovulation in 107 women with endometriosis. The lower incidence of assigned anovulation in our study may have resulted from the separate classification of animals with an LUF and LPD.

The "LUF syndrome" describes an infertile woman with regular menses and presumptive evidence of ovulation, but without release of an ovum. Brosens et al. [13] observed this phenomenon at laparoscopy in 21% of patients with endometriosis, but in only 6% of control patients. However, this relationship of LUF to infertility with endometriosis remains speculative, as other investigators have demonstrated a similar incidence of LUF in patients with and without endometriosis. [1,16] This discrepancy may be due to the timing of laparoscopy; that is, the laparoscopy may have been performed after the stigma had undergone epithelial regeneration. It is clear from our findings that an LUF frequently occurred in monkeys with moderate endometriosis (46%) and severe endometriosis (50%). Because an LUF was not observed in animals with adipose tissue autografts, microscopic or mild endometriosis, or in cycles prior to the induction of moderate or severe endometriosis, it appears that an LUF is a major cause of infertility in monkeys with endometriosis. In animals with severe endometriosis, an LUF was noted in two cycles involving the same ovary bearing an endometrioma. Apart from this animal, however, the location of the endometriosis or pelvic adhesions could not be correlated with the occurrence of an LUF. Furthermore, the occurrence of an LUF was sporadic in monkeys with endometriosis and not consistently present in consecutive cycles.

The role of LPD in infertility with endometriosis is unclear. Grant, in his study of luteal function in women with endometriosis, [14] reported that 45% of patients had evidence of LPD. Hargrove and Abraham[15] also demonstrated that mean P levels were lower and E_2 levels were higher during the luteal phase of women with endometriosis. However, others[14,16,17] have argued that the corpus luteum in women with endometriosis is not defective. In our study, an LPD was noted during two cycles in control animals, two cycles in animals with microscopic endometriosis, and five cycles in animals with moderate endometriosis. In monkeys with moderate endometriosis, an LUF was present in all cycles with LPD. Interestingly, the aberrant follicular phase endocrine profile normally found in monkeys with LPD was not present in monkeys with endometriosis and LPD.[7]

Pelvic adhesions in patients with endometriosis may affect fertility by preventing ovum pickup or gamete transport. This cause-and-effect relationship is difficult to refute in patients with moderate or severe endometriosis and extensive pelvic adhesions. In our study, no term pregnancies resulted when adnexal adhesions were noted on the same side as the ovary having the ovulatory stigma. In contrast, when adnexal adhesions were not present, the incidence of a term pregnancy was similar in monkeys with endometriosis and in control monkeys with adipose tissue implants. These preliminary findings are consistent with studies in rabbits and suggest that when normal follicular rupture occurs in monkeys with endometriosis, it is the location of pelvic adhesions and not endometriosis per se that impairs fertility.[18]

Studies in women with mild endometriosis have demonstrated that pregnancy rates after expectant management are similar to pregnancy rates after medical or surgical therapy.[19–21] Our data support this interpretation, in that chemical pregnancy rates per cycle in animals with microscopic endometriosis (40%) and mild endometriosis (36%) were not significantly different from the term pregnancy rate in control animals (42%). In contrast, chemical pregnancy rates were lower in animals with moderate and severe endometriosis and in association with the highest incidence of LUF and pelvic adhesions. In addition to the lower incidence of chemical pregnancies in animals with moderate and severe endometriosis, monkeys in these groups demonstrated a lower incidence of term pregnancies per cycle, compared with control animals. Although the mechanism of this reduced apparent early pregnancy rate is unknown, it may be related to an increase in peritoneal fluid macrophages. These cells have a higher capacity to phagocytize human spermatozoa than do macrophages from women without endometriosis, and may reduce fertility by preventing fertilization.[1,22]

In some studies, the incidence of spontaneous abortion in patients with endometriosis is reported to be increased. However, in a carefully controlled study, the incidence of spontaneous abortion was not significantly different between patients with treated and untreated endometriosis.[23] In our study, monkeys with mild, moderate, and severe endometriosis were noted to have luteal phase serum mCG values consistent with conception during six cycles. Because only four term intrauterine pregnancies occurred, we estimated that the spontaneous abortion rate was 33%. In animals with adipose tissue implants and microscopic endometriosis, 6 of 12 cycles having mCG values >50 µg/ml resulted in term pregnancies, or a spontaneous abortion rate of 50%. The high incidence of spontaneous abortion in both the endometriosis and control groups may be due to the small sample size. Based on this limited observation, the presence of endometriosis in monkeys did not appear to increase the incidence of spontaneous abortion.

The present data in monkeys clearly suggest a relationship between endometriosis and elevated concentrations of peritoneal fluid $PGF_{2\alpha}$, but not PGE. The $PGF_{2\alpha}$ concentrations in peritoneal washings were increased significantly ($p < 0.05$) in animals with moderate and severe endometriosis. That this increase was not secondary to the surgical manipulation is indicated by the absence of a similar increase in $PGF_{2\alpha}$ after adipose tissue autografts in control monkeys. Furthermore, $PGF_{2\alpha}$ concentrations in peritoneal washings of monkeys with ectopic endometrial autografts were significantly greater than in monkeys with adipose tissue autografts. Analysis of the prostaglandin content in biopsy specimens from both types of tissue autografts demonstrated a greater $PGF_{2\alpha}$ content in endometrial implants as compared to adipose tissue implants, suggesting that the observed increase in peritoneal fluid $PGF_{2\alpha}$ was due to the presence of viable ectopic endometrial tissue.

Demonstration of a causal relationship between endometriosis and peritoneal fluid prostaglandins is not sufficient to establish a cause-and-effect relationship between prostaglandins and infertility associated with endometriosis. Although $PGF_{2\alpha}$ concentrations in peritoneal washings of cycles with luteinized unruptured follicles, luteal phase defects, and adhesions were increased in comparison with those of ovulatory cycles, the difference was not statistically significant. Furthermore, a relationship between spontaneous abortion and prostaglandin concentrations in peritoneal washings was not established in these primates. We acknowledge that certain differences between this laboratory model and clinical endometriosis may also exist. Accordingly, appropriate caution should be used in interpreting these findings.

In summary, we have described the surgical induction of endometriosis in monkeys. This primate model for endometriosis seems well suited for studying the mechanisms of infertility associated with endometriosis. Here, impaired fertilization and term pregnancy rates in monkeys with endometriosis were apparent only in association with moderate or severe disease. Our findings indicate that impaired fertility is mediated by failure of follicular rupture (LUF) and pelvic adhesions; however, unidentified factors that inhibit fertilization may also be important. LPDs in the absence of an LUF, anovulation, and spontaneous abortion were not principal factors contributing to infertility specifically in monkeys with endometriosis. Although peritoneal-washing PG levels are increased in monkeys with endometrial autografts compared to those with adipose autografts, PG levels did not correlate with the etiology of infertility in monkeys with surgically induced endometriosis.

REFERENCES

1. BURNS, W. N. & R. S. SCHENKEN. 1989. Pathophysiology. *In* Endometriosis: Contemporary Concepts in Clinical Management. R. S. Schenken, Ed., Chapter 3: 83–126. J. B. Lippincott Company, Philadelphia, PA.
2. VERNON, M. W., K. GRAVES, M. J. JAWAD & E. A. WILSON. 1983. The surgical induction of endometriosis in the rat. Presented at the Thirtieth Annual Meeting of the Society for Gynecologic Investigation, March 17–20, Washington, D.C., Abstract 171.
3. SCHENKEN, R. S. & R. H. ASCH. 1980. Surgical induction of endometriosis in the rabbit: Effects on fertility and concentrations of peritoneal fluid prostaglandins. Fertil. Steril. **34:** 581–587.
4. SCHENKEN, R. S., R. H. ASCH, R. F. WILLIAMS & G. D. HODGEN. 1984. Etiology of infertility in monkeys with endometriosis: Luteinized unruptured follicles, luteal phase defects, pelvic adhesions, and spontaneous abortions. Fertil. Steril. **41:** 122–130.
5. GOODMAN, A. L., C. C. DESCALZI, D. K. JOHNSON & G. D. HODGEN. 1977. Composite pattern of circulating LH, FSH, estradiol and progesterone during the menstrual cycle in cynomolgus monkeys. Proc. Soc. Exp. Biol. Med. **155:** 479–481.
6. AMERICAN FERTILITY SOCIETY. 1979. Classification of endometriosis. Fertil. Steril. **32:** 633–634.
7. WILKS, J. W., G. D. HODGEN & G. T. ROSS. 1979. Endocrine characteristics of ovulatory and anovulatory menstrual cycles in the rhesus monkey. *In* Human Ovulation. E. S. E. Hafez, Ed.: 205–218. Elsevier-North Holland Biomedical Press, Amsterdam.

8. HODGEN, G. D., W. W. TULLNER, J. L. VAITUKAITIS, D. N. WARD & G. T. ROSS. 1974. Specific radioimmunoassay of chorionic gonadotropin during implantation in rhesus monkeys. J. Clin. Endocrinol. Metab. **39**: 457–464.

9. HARPER, M. J. K., G. VALENZUELA, B. J. HODGSON & T. M. SILER-KHODR. 1979. Contraceptive properties of endotoxin in rabbits. Fertil. Steril. **31**: 441–447.

10. LOWRY, D. H., N. J. ROSEBROUGH, A. L. & R. J. RANDALL. 1951. Protein measurement with the Folin phenol reagent. J. Biol. Chem. **193**: 265–275.

11. SOULES, M. R., L. R. MALINAK, R. BURY & A. POINDEXTER. 1976. Endometriosis and anovulation: a coexisting problem in the infertile female. Am J. Obstet. Gynecol. **125**: 412–417.

12. ACOSTA, A. A., V. C. BUTTRAM, P. K. BESCH, L. R. MALINAK, R. R. FRANKLIN & J. D. VANDERHEYDEN. 1973. A proposed classification of pelvic endometriosis. Obstet. Gynecol. **42**: 19–25.

13. BROSENS, I. A., P. R. KONINCKX & P. A. CORVELYN. 1978. A study of plasma progesterone, oestradiol 17β, prolactin and LH levels, and of the luteal phase appearance of the ovaries in patients with endometriosis and infertility. Br. J. Obstet. Gynaecol. **85**: 246–250.

14. GRANT, A. 1966. Additional sterility factors in endometriosis. Fertil. Steril. **17**: 514–519.

15. HARGROVE, J. T. & G. E. ABRAHAM. 1980. Abnormal luteal function in endometriosis. Fertil. Steril. (Abstr) **34**: 302.

16. DMOWSKI, W. P., R. RAO & A. SCOMMEGNA. 1980. The luteinized unruptured follicle syndrome and endometriosis. Fertil. Steril. **33**: 30–34.

17. WENTZ, A. C. 1980. Premenstrual spotting: Its association with endometriosis but not luteal phase inadequacy. Fertil. Steril. **33**: 605–607.

18. SCHENKEN, R. S. & M. D. WALTERS. 1986. Ovulation and tubal ovum transport in rabbits with endometriosis. Presented at the 33rd Annual Meeting of the Society for Gynecologic Investigation, Toronto, Ontario, Canada, March 19–22, Abstract #361P.

19. HULL, M. E., K. S. MOGHISSI, D. F. MAGYAR & M. F. HAYES. 1987. Comparison of different treatment modalities of endometriosis in infertile women. Fertil. Steril. **47**: 40–44.

20. SCHENKEN, R. S. & L. R. MALINAK. 1982. Conservative surgery versus expectant management for the infertile patient with mild endometriosis. Fertil. Steril. **37**: 183–186.

21. SEIBEL, M. M., M. J. BERGER, F. G. WEINSTEIN & M. L. TAYMOR. 1982. The effectiveness of danazol on subsequent fertility in minimal endometriosis. Fertil. Steril. **38**: 534–537.

22. HANEY, A. F., M. A. MISUKONIS & J. B. WEINBERG. 1983. Macrophages and infertility: Oviductal macrophages as potential mediators of infertility. Fertil. Steril. **39**: 310–315.

23. METZGER, D. A., D. L. OLIVE, G. F. STOHS & R. R. FRANKLIN. 1986. Association of endometriosis and spontaneous abortion: Effect of control group selection. Fertil. Steril. **45**: 18–22.

Tissue Factors Influencing Growth and Maintenance of Endometriosis[a]

CORRADO MELEGA,[b] MARCO BALDUCCI,[b]
CARLO BULLETTI,[b] ANDREA GALASSI,[c]
VALERIO M. JASONNI,[b] AND CARLO FLAMIGNI[b]

[b]Reproductive Medicine Unit
Department of Obstetrics and Gynecology
University of Bologna
Via Massarenti 13
40138 Bologna, Italy

[c]Department of Pathology
Bassano del Grappa General Hospital
Via delle Fosse
36061 Bassano del Grappa (VI), Italy

INTRODUCTION

Endometriosis is a common pathology during reproductive years consisting in ectopia of the endometrium, normally localized only in the uterine cavity. Endometriosis shares, with the eutopic endometrium, many morphological aspects but differs in its biological behavior. We must underline that this "dislocation" of the endometrial tissue is a disease because of its consequences on fertility and woman's well-being. In this century many studies have been carried out in an attempt to gain an understanding of histogenesis of this disease, but it still remains unclarified. It is accepted that estrogen is the most important factor involved in the appearance, growth, and maintenance of this tissue. Estrogen's mechanism of action on target tissues has not been fully explained,[1-4] but its presence is the necessary condition for endometriotic support;[5] for this reason, most common therapies are aimed at decreasing plasma estrogen levels to mimic a condition of hypoganadotropic hypogonadism.[6,7] Ectopic and eutopic endometrium are not synchronized in their histologic changes; ectopic tissue implants present a maturation disorder and it is possible to find glands with different degrees of differentiation and organization in the same implant.[8] Complete secretory modifications are rarely found in endometriosis. Electron microscopic appearance and nuclear estrogen-binding studies distinguish ectopic endometrium implant from uterine endometrium. Furthermore, the unusual sensitivity to sex steroids is documented by the variable presence of estrogen and progesterone receptors, (ER and PR) that are lower

[a] This work was supported by the University of Bologna (grant n. 89020729), the Regione Emilia Romagna (grant n. 89.02089), the Italian National Research Council (grants n. 88.00662.44 and n. 88.00451.04) and the Associazione per la Ricerca sul Cancro nella Donna.

[b] Author to whom correspondence should be addressed; (Tel. (51) 343934; FAX (51) 342820).

than in the endometrium.[9] Cyclic variations of ER and PR have not been observed in endometriosis during the menstrual cycle. Some enzymatic activities seem to distinguish ectopic tissue from eutopic.[10-12]

In this study we investigated the presence of EGFr and of receptors for estrogen and progesterone in eutopic and ectopic endometrium before and after treatment with Danazol or the gonadotropin releasing hormone analogue (GnRHa), Buserelin. In all eutopic endometria epidermal growth factor receptors (EGFr), ER, and PR were present, but not in all cases of endometriosis. In eutopic and ectopic endometrium both therapies caused a decrease in staining for all antigens tested, but some cases remained EGFr positive and ER negative.

MATERIALS AND METHODS

Endometrial and endometriosis tissue samples were obtained at S. Orsola General Hospital, University of Bologna, from 41 patients undergoing laparoscopy for pelvic endometriosis. The staging of Endometriosis was obtained using the American Fertility Society [AFS] classification:[13] Stage I n. 4, Stage II n. 17, Stage III n. 20. Patients underwent laparoscopy twice, before and at the end of the hormonal treatment, in order to remove all remaining endometriotic implants and to collect samples of endometriotic tissue. Specimens of eutopic and ectopic endometrium were collected simultaneously at the time of laparoscopy. Endometrial biopsies were obtained by using a Novak curette. At the time of the first diagnostic laparoscopy all patients were in the late proliferative phase (days 10–14). All patients gave their informed consent to participate in this study. The mean age was similar in both study groups 30.1 ± 4 (group I) and 28.9 ± 4.4 (group II). No patient had taken hormonal treatment for at least four months before this study. All patients (n. 41) were nulligravid and were referred to us for infertility or pelvic pain. Twenty-eight of 41 patients received drug therapy: patients of group I (n. 16) received subcutaneous (300 to 500 µg twice a day for 15 days) and subsequently intranasal (1200 µg/day up to 6 months) Buserelin, while patients of group II (n.12) received Danazol (600 mg/day for 6 months). Plasma levels of E_2, P, FSH, LH were evaluated by RIA using routine methods before and during hormone treatment to verify ovarian suppression. All patients began therapy on the first day of the menstrual cycle. Specimens of ectopic endometrium were obtained from the ovary, the corpus uteri, the broad ligament and the cul-de-sac and from the uterosacral area. Tissue samples were processed for routine diagnostic procedure and for immunohistochemical detection of EGFr, ER, and PR. Tissue samples for histological diagnosis were fixed in 10% buffered formalin, embedded in paraffin, cut in serial sections about 6 µm thick and stained with hematoxylin and eosin. The timing of eutopic and ectopic endometrial tissues were performed using the method of Noyes, *et al.*[14] Tissue samples for the immunohistochemical study were frozen in liquid nitrogen, lightly fixed at $-20°C$ in acetone for EGFr, in paraformaldehyde 4% in 0.1 mol/l PBS for ER, and in pycric acid paraformaldehyde for PR. Sections 10 µm thick were then obtained. Endogenous peroxidase was inhibited in 3% H_2O_2 in methanol for 5 minutes at room temperature. Sections were dehydrated in graded alcohol and in three washes in PBS for 5 minutes each. Preincubation at room temperature was performed using normal rabbit serum (Sigma Clinical Co., St. Louis, MO) diluted 1/10 for 30 minutes. Primary antisera were: monoclonal mouse anti-human epidermal growth factor receptor (Cambridge Research Laboratories, Cambridge, UK); monoclonal anti-human estrogen receptor (Abbott, North-Chicago, Ill.); monoclonal anti-human progesterone receptor (Trans-Bio, Paris, France). The antisera dilution was 1/60 for EGFr, 1/10 for ER and 1/30 for PR. The antisera were incubated for 30 minutes at room temperature, and "overnight" at +4°C for PR and ER. The secondary antiserum, biotinylated rabbit anti-mouse was purchased from Sclavo, Siena, Italy and used diluted 1/50 for 30 minutes. Streptavidin-biotinylated peroxidase complexes (Sclavo) were diluted 1/100 and incubated for 30 minutes at room temperature. Stained with a solution of DAB-H_2O_2 (50 mg of diamino-benzidine in 50 ml of PBS added to 50 ml of H_2O and 50 µl of H_2O_2 at 36% nuclear staining). Then slides were rinsed in tap water before dehydration in ethanol and xylene and mounting with Permount (Fisher Scientific Fair Lawn, NJ). The analysis of results was carried out using the McNemar χ^2 test.

RESULTS

After therapy, in patients of group I plasma levels of FSH, LH, E2 and P were similar (p N.S.) to those detected in the clinical condition of hypogonadotropic hypogonadism (E_2 = 16.4 pg/ml $\pm$ 0.7 pg/ml, P = 0.4 ng/ml $\pm$ 0.1 ng/ml, FSH = 3.6 mUI $\pm$ 0.9 mUI, LH = 4.1 mUI/ml $\pm$ 1.5 mUI/ml) and similar findings were found in patients of group II (E_2 = 28 pg/ml $\pm$ 14 pg/ml, P = 0.4 ng/ml $\pm$ 0.07 ng/ml, FSH = 4.1 mUI/ml $\pm$ 3 mUI/ml, LH = 7.1 mUI/ml $\pm$ 4.4 mUI/ml). A clear dissociation in the immunohistochemical response to the antisera for EGFr, PR, and ER was observed between the eutopic and ectopic endometrium (TABLE 1). All endometrial specimens (100%) collected before treatment, were EGFr, ER, and PR positive. EGFr staining was present in glandular and endothelial cells. Er and PR were present in nucleus of both glandular and stromal cells. The parallel evaluation of endometriotic tissues revealed immunostaining for EGFr in 49% of cases, a moderate

TABLE 1. Epidermal Growth Factor Receptor (EGFr), Estrogens Receptor (ER), Progesterone Receptor (PR) in Eutopic and Ectopic Endometrium: Histological and Immunohistochemical Response to Danazol or GnRH Analogue

	Number of Cases		Number of Histochemical Positive Cases (%)		
	Cases Tested	Histological Diagnosis[a]	EGFr	ER	PR
Endometrium					
Before treatment	41	P 41	41 (100)	41 (100)	41 (100)
After treatment[b]					
Group 1	16	A 16	0 (0)	0 (0)	4 (25)
Group 2	12	A 12	0 (0)	0 (0)	0 (0)
Endometriosis					
Before treatment	41	P 34, S 7	29 (71)	22 (59)	20 (49)
After treatment[b]					
Group 1	16	P 3, A 13	4 (25)	4 (25)	1 (6)
Group 2	12	S 3, A 9	2 (17)	2 (17)	1 (8)

[a] P = proliferative; S = secretory; A = atrophic.
[b] Group 1 = GnRHa; Group 2 = Danazol.

positivity in 22% of cases, and a total absence of immunohistochemical response in 29% of cases (TABLE 1). At the end of treatment, the macro and microscopic appearance of the explants were similar in all treated women. However, the number of cases that exhibited immunohistochemical staining for EGFr, ER, and PR antisera, decreased dramatically both in the eutopic and ectopic endometrium after therapy with Danazol as well as with GnRHa (TABLE 2). In 75% of cases in group I and in 83% of cases of group II we observed the contemporary disappearance of EGFr and ER, associated with an endocrinological condition of hypogonadotropic hypogonadism. Finally after therapy we observed a positive immunostaining for EGFr and a negative reaction for ER in 17% (group I) and in 25% (group II) of cases. TABLE 2 shows the response of eutopic and ectopic endometrium to Danazol and GnRH in terms of variation of the immunohistochemical staining for EGFr, PR, and ER antisera. In endometrium we observed reduction of positive cases in both study groups. The complete disappearance of positivity was observed only for EGFr and ER in group I and for EGFr, Er, and PR in group II. The immunohistochemical response of endometriosis was lower than that of endometrium. The statistical analysis of positive cases before therapy versus the positive cases after therapy showed a significant reduction of all receptors studied except for ER in endometriosis in both study groups (TABLE 2).

DISCUSSION

Although initiation of endometriosis does not seem to depend on ovarian steroids, its growth and maintenance do. That is why several medical treatments were proposed to mimic ovarian quiescence.[6] GnRH analogues cause FSH and LH suppression and indirectly an ovarian quiescence,[7] while Danazol induces only[15] a relative hypogonadotropic state because it diminishes the mid-cycle FSH and LH surge without having

TABLE 2. Epidermal Growth Factor Receptor (EGFr), Estrogens Receptor (ER), Progesterone Receptor (PR) and their Relation with Therapy[a] in Eutopic and Ectopic Endometrium

	Number of Immunohistochemical Positive Cases (%)					
	EGFr		ER		PR	
	Before Treatment	After Treatment	Before Treatment	After Treatment	Before Treatment	After Treatment
Endometrium						
Group 1	$p < 0.001$		$p < 0.01$		$p < 0.05$	
	16	0 (0)	16	0 (0)	16	4 (25)
Group 2	$p < 0.005$		$p < 0.005$		$p < 0.005$	
	12	0 (0)	12	0 (0)	12	0 (0)
Endometriosis						
Group 1	$p < 0.05$		$p < 0.05$		$p < 0.05$	
	16	4 (25)	3	4 (66)	9	1 (11)
Group 2	$p < 0.05$		$p < 0.05$		$p < 0.05$	
	12	2 (17)	9	2 (40)	9	1 (11)

[a] Group 1 = GnRH; Group 2 = Danazol.

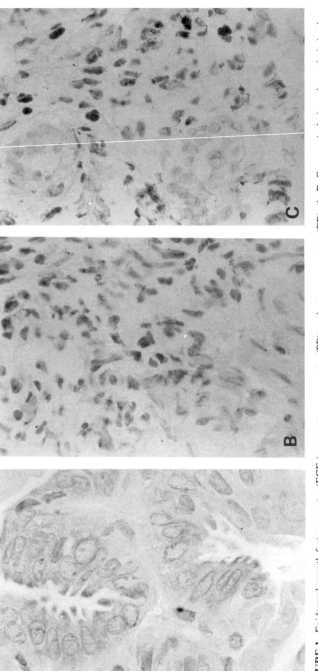

FIGURE 1. Epidermal growth factor receptor (EGFr), progesterone receptor (PR), and estrogen receptor (ER): A, B, C respectively in endometriotic implants and D, E, F in eutopic endometrium.

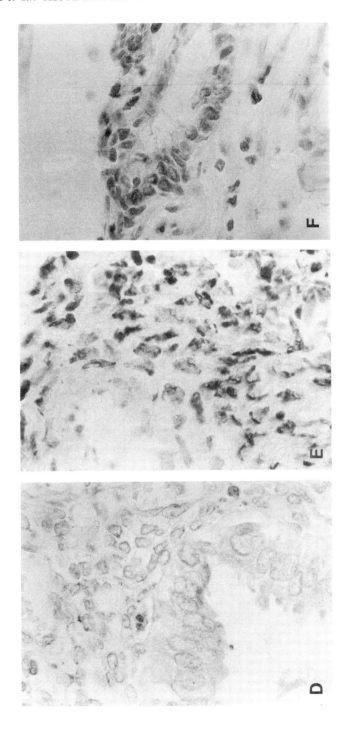

any effects on basal levels.[16] However, the relative hypogonadotropic state induced by Danazol is sufficient to reduce serum estradiol levels[17] that, in turn, could inhibit growth of ectopic endometrium. Furthermore, Danazol has a direct effect on endometriotic implants[1,18] possibly through interaction with steroid receptors;[19,20] Danazol suppresses growth of endometrial cells cultured *in vitro.*[21] Although progestins like medical oophorectomy were shown to be ideal methods for relieving symptoms related to endometriosis, they do lead to an incomplete suppression of endometriotic foci and there is a 5-year recurrence in up to 40% of patients.[22] The normal response of endometriotic tissue is unpredictable, and the specific mechanism whereby estrogens modulate cell proliferation is not fully understood.[2] Recent studies have hypothesized that estrogens may act indirectly and directly:

1. indirectly, by inducing synthesis and/or release of growth factors that cause cell proliferation;[3,4] and
2. directly, by inducing synthesis and secretion of growth factors on the part of the estrogen target cells themselves.

In the present study we did not find a uniform positivity in the immunohistochemical reaction for EGFr, ER and PR antisera for eutopic and ectopic endometrium. The endometriotic implants did not show immunostaining in several tissue samples, while a complete (100%) positivity was found when EGFr, ER, and PR antisera were used in the endometrium. The immunohistochemical staining for EGFr, ER, and PR in eutopic and ectopic endometrium with both GnRH and Danazol was significantly decreased. A reduction of staining for ER antiserum was found in both eutopic and ectopic endometria after treatment with both drugs. The reduction of ER and PR after treatment with GnRHa may be due to the indirect ovarian steroid suppression, while Danazol could act directly or indirectly with similar results. EGF is a potent mitogen of various cells *in vitro* and *in vivo*; in fact it binds to its receptor on the cell surface, is internalized and degraded by lysosomal enzyme,[23,24] resulting in the activation of tyrosine kinase system. EGF can regulate the expression of specific genes and thus cause cellular differentiation[25,26] through a positive or negative control. Eutopic endometrium is a target and/or source tissue for multiple hormones, including estrogens, progesterone and protein hormones, like growth factors. The response to hormones is often maintained in eutopic and ectopic endometrium,[1,27] and the suppression of ovarian steroid secretion causes beneficial effects for patients with endometriosis. However, the high percentage of recurrence rates observed and the failure of both medical castration and progestin therapy (with direct efficacy on human endometrium) to completely suppress the foci of endometriosis,[28] suggests the hypothesis of autocrine and/or paracrine release of factors which may lead to the growth and maintenance of endometriosis.[3,4] In the present study, about 80% of cases EGFr positive become negative in close association with the disappearance of ER. EGFr, ER, and PR immunoreactivity in the proliferative and secretory phases of menstrual cycle is not related in eutopic and ectopic endometrium. However, after 6 months of therapy, approximately 20% of cases showed EGFr positive and ER negative endometriotic specimens. The clinical regression of endometriosis after both therapies is associated with a reduction in the EGFr and PR immunoreactivity. Since PR is a marker on E_2 action, its reduction confirms the reduction of E_2 secretion and the parallel decrease in EGFr suggests some relationship between estrogens and possible peptide control of endometrial growth. The persistence of about 20% of EGFr positive and ER negative cases after both therapies suggests that growth and maintenance of these endo-

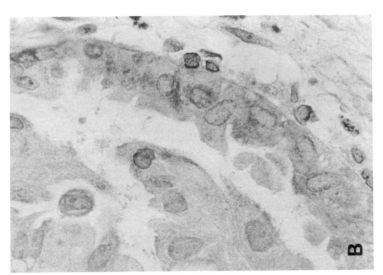

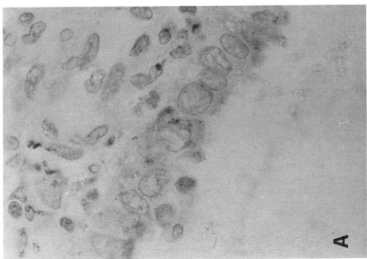

FIGURE 2. Immunohistochemical revelation of EGFr and ER after treatment with Danazol (600 mg/day for 6 months) in human endometriotic implants. Absence of immunostaining for ER (A) is shown in one case of positivity of reaction for EGFr (B).

metriotic implants may be regulated mainly by peptide hormones (EGF) rather than steroid hormones (estrogens) (FIGS. 1 and 2).

SUMMARY

The unpredictable response of endometriosis to steroids and its recurrence after therapy, led us to hypothesize a possible further control of this pathology by factors other than steroids. The presence of estrogen, progesterone and epidermal growth factor receptors (ER, PR, EGFr) was evaluated using immunohistochemistry before and after therapy with Danazol or a gonadotropin-releasing hormone analogue (GnRHa), Buserelin. EGFr, ER and PR were present in 100% of endometrial specimens, and in 71%, 29% and 49% of endometriotic implants, respectively. Danazol and GnRHa reduced immunohistochemical staining for EGFr antisera in the endometrial and endometriotic specimens. About 21% of endometriosis were EGFr positive and ER negative, suggesting a potential role of epidermal growth factor in growth and maintenance of endometrial ectopia.

REFERENCES

1. BULLETTI, C., A. GALASSI, M. BALDUCCI, M. C. GELLI, V. M. JASONNI, C. MELEGA & C. FLAMIGNI. 1988. Direct effects of danazol on endometriosis tissue. *In* The Management of Endometriosis. J. A. Rock & K. W. Schweppe, Eds.: 61–72. The Parthenon Publishing Group. Casterton Hall, Carnforth, Lancs. LA 6 2LA, UK.
2. SOTO, A. M. & C. SONNENSCHEIN. 1987. Cell proliferation of estrogen sensitive cells: The case for negative control. Endocrinol. Rev. 8: 44–52.
3. SIRBASKO, D. A. 1978. Estrogen induction of growth factors specific for hormone-responsive mammary, pituitary and kidney tumour cells. Proc. Natl. Acad. Sci. USA 75: 3786–3790.
4. FITZPATRICK, S. L., J. BRIGHTWELL, J. WITTLIFF, H. BARROWGS & G. S. SCHULTZ. 1984. Epidermal growth factor binding by breast tumour biopsies and relationship to estrogen receptor and progestin receptor levels. Cancer Res. 44: 3448–3453.
5. BERQVIST, A., K. CARLSTROM, S. JEPPSSON, S. KULLANDER & O. LJUNGBERG. 1981. Histochemical localization of specific estrogen and progesterone binding in human endometrium and endometriotic tissue. A preliminary report. Acta Obstet. Gynecol. (Suppl.) 123: 15–21.
6. GREENBLATT, R. B., W. P. DMOWSKY, V. B. MAHESH & H. F. L. SCHOLER. 1971. Clinical study with an antigonadotropin, Danazol. Fertil. Steril. 22: 102–112.
7. LEMAY, A., R. MAHEUX, N. FAUREN, C. JEAN & A. T. A. FAZEKAS. 1984. Reversible hypogonadism induced by a luteinizing hormone-releasing hormone (LH-RH) agonist (Buserelin) as a new therapeutic approach for endometriosis. Fertil. Steril. 41: 863–871.
8. LESSEY, B. A., D. A. METZEGER, A. F. HANEY & K. S. MCCARTY. 1989. Immunohistochemical analysis of estrogen and progesterone receptors in endometriosis: Comparison with normal endometrium during the menstrual cycle and the effect of medical therapy. Fertil. Steril. 51: 409–415.
9. PRAKASH, S., H. ULFELDER & B. R. COHEN. 1965. Enzyme-histochemical observation on endometriosis. Am. J. Obstet. Gynecol. 91: 990–997.
10. KAUPPILA, A., P. VIERIKKO, H. ISOTALO & L. RONNEMBERG. 1984. Cytosol estrogen and progestin receptor concentration and 17β-hydroxysteroid dehydrogenase activities in the endometrium and endometriotic tissue: Effects of hormonal treatment. Acta Obstet. Gynecol. Scand. (Suppl) 123: 45–52.
11. VIERIKKO, P., A. KAUPPILA, L. RONNBERG & R. VIHKO. 1985. Steroidal regulation of endometriosis tissue: Lack of induction of 17β-hydroxysteroid dehydrogenase activity by progesterone, medroxyprogesterone acetate, or danazol. Fertil. Steril. 43: 218–226.

12. MAGUN, B. E., L. M. MATRISIAN & G. T. BOWDEN. 1980. Epidermal growth factor. J. Biol. Chem. **225**: 6373–6381.
13. AMERICAN FERTILITY SOCIETY. 1985. Revised American Fertility Society classification of endometriosis. Fertil. Steril. **43**: 351–352.
14. NOYES, R. W., A. T. HERTIG & J. ROCK. 1950. Dating the endometrial biopsy. Fertil. Steril. **1**: 3–25.
15. DI ZEREGA, G. S., D. L. BARBER & G. D. HODGEN. 1980. Endometriosis role of ovarian steroids in initiation, maintenance and suppression. Fertil. Steril. **33**: 649–653.
16. FLOYD, W. S. 1980. Danazol: Endocrine and endometrial effect. Int. J. Fertil. **25**: 75–80.
17. WOOD, G. P., L. H. WU, G. L. FLICKINGER & G. MIKKAIL. 1975. Hormonal changes associated with danazol therapy. Obstet. Gynecol. **45**: 302–304.
18. DICKEY, R. P., S. N. TAYLOR & D. N. CUROLE. 1984. Serum estradiol and danazol. I. Endometriosis response, side effects, administration interval, concurrent spironolactone and desamethasone. Fertil. Steril. **42**: 709–716.
19. HENIG, I., R. G. RAWLINS, H. P. WEINRIB & W. P. DMOWSKY. 1988. Effects of Danazol, gonadotropin-releasing hormone agonist, and estrogen/progestogen combination on experimental endometriosis in the ovariectomized rat. Fertil. Steril. **49**: 349–355.
20. CHAMNESS, G. C., R. H. ASCH & C. J. PAUERSTEIN. 1980. Danazol binding and translocation of steroid receptors. Am. J. Obstet. Gynecol. **136**: 426–429.
21. TAMAYA, T., K. WADA, J. FUJIMOTO, T. YAMADA & H. OKADA. 1984. Danazol binding to steroid receptors in human uterine endometrium. Fertil. Steril. **41**: 732–735.
22. NOVAK, E. & O. A. DE LIMA. 1948. A correlative study of adenomyosis and pelvic endometriosis with special reference to the hormonal reaction of ectopic endometrium. Am. J. Obstet. Gynecol. **56**: 634–644.
23. CARPENTER, G. 1979. Epidermal growth factor. Ann. Rev. Biochem. **48**: 193–216.
24. RHEINWALD, J. C. & H. GREEN. 1977. Epidermal growth factor and the multiplication of cultured human epidermal keratinocytes. Nature. **265**: 421–424.
25. HAPGOOD, J., T. A. LIBERMANN, Y. L. YARDEN, A. B. SCHREIBER, Z. NAOR & J. SCHLESSINGER. 1983. Monoclonal antibodies against epidermal growth factor receptor induce prolactin synthesis in cultured rat pituitary cells (GH3). Proc. Natl. Acad. Sci. USA. **80**: 6451–6455.
26. NISOLLE-POCHET, M., F. CASANAS-ROUX & J. DONNEZ. 1988. Histologic study of ovarian endometriosis after hormonal therapy. Fertil. Steril. **49**: 423–426.
27. SUN, T. T. & H. GREEN. 1977. Cultured epithelial cells of cornea, conjunctive and skin: Absence of marked intrinsic divergence of their differentiated states. Nature **269**: 489–492.
28. ROSE, G. I., M. DOWSETT, J. E. MUDGE, J. O. WHITE & S. L. JEFFCOATE. 1988. The inhibitor effects of danazol, danazol metabolites, gestrinone and testosterone on the growth of human endometrial cells in vitro. Fertil. Steril. **49**: 224–228.

Role of Peritoneal Inflammation in Endometriosis-associated Infertility

JOUKO HALME

Department of Obstetrics and Gynecology
Division of Reproductive Endocrinology and Fertility
University of North Carolina at Chapel Hill
Chapel Hill, North Carolina 27599-7570

IS ENDOMETRIOSIS ASSOCIATED WITH INFERTILITY?

An association between endometriosis and infertility is generally assumed, but most of the studies or surveys suggesting this have been based on retrospective or cross-sectional analysis. There are several reasonable arguments against such association, however. Firstly, since prevalence estimates of endometriosis in healthy, potentially fertile women range from 2–18 percent,[1,2] there is no certainty that the approximately 4.5–33.3 percent reported prevalence in infertile women is significantly higher.[3] Secondly, it has been suggested that infertility may precede the development of endometriosis. If true, it may cast a doubt on our thinking on the pathogenetic mechanisms, but would not dispute the existence of an association. Finally, since several good studies have indicated that treatment of minimal to mild endometriosis leads to no better chances of pregnancy than expectant management this has raised doubts whether such an association really exists.[4-6] An excellent randomized study by Hull *et al.*[6] clearly demonstrated that placebo was as efficacious as two accepted therapeutic regimens, danazol and medroxyprogesterone acetate, in leading to pregnancy. However, this is not a strong argument since poor treatment results may only reflect our inability to treat the disease sufficiently with the existing modalities.

The evidence for a close association between infertility and endometriosis includes the recognized relative high prevalence of this disease in patients laparoscoped for long-term unexplained infertility and the fact that even after acceptable treatment with surgical or medical modalities (or placebo) the fecundability of these patients remains ⅓ to ½ of healthy fertile women.[7] The strongest data indicating a significant association comes from a study by Jansen,[8] who prospectively laparoscoped women requesting artificial insemination with donor sperm as treatment for male factor infertility. In women who were found to have minimal endometriosis it was left untreated and all women were started on monthly inseminations. A life-table analysis clearly demonstrated a significantly reduced monthly fecundability in women with endometriosis as compared to other women in this series. Summarizing the foregoing arguments one tends to believe that there really is a close association between relative subfertility and even minimal stages of endometriosis.

POSSIBLE MECHANISMS OF INFERTILITY

In reviewing the existing information regarding the myriad of mechanisms proposed to explain the infertility in patients with endometriosis it's hard to be very specific since there are in excess of 200 studies addressing the issue.[9] Abnormalities in virtually every step in the female reproductive process have been suggested as the cause of infertility (TABLE 1). Although anatomic factors at least in higher stages of endometriosis on one hand and ovulatory and/or hormonal dysfunction and possibly abnormal fertilization on the other may be important in some women with endometriosis they do not serve as adequate explanations for subfertility in most patients with minimal to mild disease. This review will focus on studies about mechanisms that involve the peritoneal microenvironment and its possible alterations and having the potential to lead to reproductive failure very early in the preconceptional or preimplantation period.

INFLAMMATION IN THE PERITONEAL FLUID

There are several physiologic sources for an inflammatory response in the peritoneal environment. Retrograde menstruation occurs in essentially all menstruating women who have open fallopian tubes and certainly provides such an inflammatory stimulus.[10] Rupture of the preovulatory follicle leads to the release of follicular contents and often bleeding that have the potential for initiating a local inflammatory reaction. So do spermatozoa, which represent foreign material in themselves but may in addition carry associated microbial pathogens.[11] Nonphysiologic sources of inflammation include an altered biologic response by ectopic endometrial implants in the pelvis and their possible secretion of compounds such as prostaglandins[12] or cytokines[13] that can influence the inflammatory response by the host. *In situ* menstruation and possible local "breakthrough bleeding" may also be important sources for inflammation. In our studies we documented a highly significant increase in the presence of blood in the peritoneal fluid in women with endometriosis as compared to other women when they were laparoscoped during the nonperimenstrual part of their cycle[10] (FIG. 1).

Since the macrophage is the predominant nucleated cell in the peritoneal fluid it probably represents the first-line host response to an inflammatory stimulus.[14] Attracted by chemotaxis, these cells extravasate through small pores in the vessel wall and enter the peritoneal cavity to perform their phagocytic and secretory functions (FIG. 2). Both autocrine and paracrine mechanisms are involved in the cell-cell communication and modification of the cellular interactions. Inflammation mediators or cytokines that mediate such interactions include Interleukin 1 (IL-1), Transforming Growth Factor-β (TGF-β), and Tumor Necrosis Factor-α (TNF). In addition, Fibro-

TABLE 1. Proposed Mechanisms for Infertility in Endometriosis

Anatomic factors
Ovulatory/Hormonal dysfunction
Abnormal fertilization
Early pregnancy loss
Altered peritoneal fluid inflammatory response

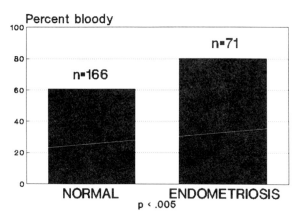

FIGURE 1. Evidence for increased bleeding into the peritoneal fluid in women with endometriosis on days 7–26 of cycle.

blast Growth Factor and Platelet derived Growth Factor provide mitogenic stimuli to fibroblastic cells and have been shown to be produced by macrophages as well.[15] The recognized results of this inflammatory cascade of events are increased vascularity by angiogenesis and synthesis of new connective tissue that may lead to the formation of adhesions.

Evidence for the existence of local inflammation in the peritoneal environment in infertile women and particularly in those with endometriosis is rather abundant. Numerous studies have indicated high levels of prostanoids in the peritoneal fluid (see ref. 12). Bioactivity of IL-1,[16] Interleukin 2 (IL-2) and TNF have been reported in the peritoneal fluid.[13,17,18] Increased vascularity in and around endometriotic lesions in the pelvis is a well-known phenomenon that can be demonstrated even histologically and indicates the presence of angiogenesis. The volume of peritoneal fluid is significantly increased both in women with endometriosis and with unexplained infertility.[19–21]

Finally and most importantly, the total number of peritoneal macrophages is significantly increased in patients with endometriosis indicating the presence of an enhanced inflammatory environment.[21,24]

As a reflection of the increased inflammatory environment increased peritoneal volume appears to have a detrimental impact on fecundability. Syrop *et al.*[25] found that in patients with endometriosis it took a significantly longer time to achieve pregnancy for those patients with peritoneal fluid volumes exceeding 12 ml as compared to those with less fluid. Hormonal suppression of endometriosis by progestin treatment has recently been shown to result in significant decreases of these inflammatory parameters. Haney and Weinberg[26] found that the volume of peritoneal fluid decreased in every patient being treated with medroxyprogesterone acetate. Similarly, the total peritoneal macrophage count fell significantly in most patients with this treatment.

In view of these data it appears quite likely that endometriosis is associated with an inflammatory exudate in the peritoneal compartment. What are then the possible mechanisms how these inflammatory changes negatively impact on the reproductive process?

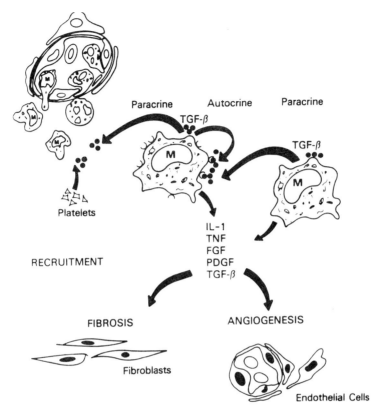

FIGURE 2. Role of macrophages and cytokines in the inflammatory response. TGF-β is released by platelets and acts as a chemo-attractant to recruit monocytes. Autocrine and paracrine mechanisms are involved in the cellular interactions and secretion of monokines and growth factors that lead to angiogenesis and fibroblast proliferation.

DIRECT TESTING OF TOXICITY

Several lines of evidence have accumulated in recent years to document with direct experimentation in various test systems that peritoneal fluid from patients can possess such toxicity. Generally, these studies require gametes or tissues from other species for testing except in the case of human sperm function, human semen being readily available.

One of the more interesting studies is by Suginami *et al.*,[27,28] who developed an *in vitro* test of fimbrial function by utilizing the fimbriae of golden hamsters and standardized conditions where the fimbriae capture oocyte-cumulus complexes from superovulated mice. By adding peritoneal fluid from various patients he was able to demonstrate inhibitory activity in these samples. This OCI (Ovum Capture Inhibitor) activity was found to be significantly more associated with endometriosis. The source of this activity is not known, but it appears to be a large molecular weight protein labile at high temperature. His studies have also suggested that this compound attaches to the fimbrial surface and forms a physical barrier that interferes with the fimbrial function. Danazol appears to decrease the level of OCI in the peritoneal fluid in patients with endometriosis.[29]

Peritoneal macrophages and peritoneal lymphocytes constituting the vast majority of nucleated cells in the peritoneal fluid have been implicated through various mechanisms in mediating adverse effects on the reproductive process. Either direct phagocytosis, cellular cytotoxicity or release of harmful secretory products by these cells have been suggested to be operative.

It is clear that macrophages are primarily responsible for physiologic phagocytosis of cellular debris, including sperm, in the pelvis. In view of this several studies have attempted to find evidence for abnormal or increased sperm phagocytosis in peritoneal fluid of patients with infertility and endometriosis (TABLE 2). So far, out of four studies addressing this issue directly three have found significant increase over patients without endometriosis.[30-33] However, one study examining macrophage phagocytosis of zymosan particles did not find an increase by peritoneal macrophages in these patients.[34]

The ready availability of murine embryos and their wide-spread use in quality-control of media in laboratories involved in in vitro–fertilization have made it possible to test effects of peritoneal fluid or macrophage-conditioned media on the in vitro development of mouse embryos (TABLE 3). Several studies have examined this recently and two studies with peritoneal fluid find a toxic effect associated with endometriosis,[35,36] two find no such effect.[32,37] One in vivo study in a rabbit model stands alone and finds reduced implantation sites in normal rabbits when they are injected with peritoneal fluid from donor rabbits that have experimentally induced endometriosis.[38] When macrophages from women with endometriosis were incubated in vitro and the conditioned medium was tested for embryotoxicity, one study did[39] and two other

TABLE 2. Evidence for Macrophage Phagocytosis in Endometriosis

	Increased Phagocytosis	Target
Muscato et al., 1982	yes	sperm
London et al., 1985	yes	sperm
Awadalla et al., 1987	no	sperm
Halme et al., 1984	no	zymosan

TABLE 3. Evidence for Embryo Toxicity in Endometriosis

	Increased Toxicity	Model	Source
Morcos et al., 1985	yes	2-cell mouse embryo	PF[a]
Hahn et al., 1986	yes	in vivo rabbit	PF
Hill et al., 1987	yes	2-cell mouse embryo	MCM
Schneider et al., 1987	no	4-cell mouse embryo	MCM
Sims et al., 1988	no	1-cell mouse embryo	PF
Prough et al., 1988	yes	2-cell mouse embryo	PF
Awadalla et al., 1987	no	2-cell mouse embryo	PF
Awadalla et al., 1987	no	2-cell mouse embryo	MCM

[a] PF = peritoneal fluid; MCM = macrophage conditioned medium.

studies did not find such toxicity.[32,40] One more recent study by Schneider et al.[41] detected no adverse effects on murine embryos when they were incubated with in vitro–activated monocytes. The reasons for these discrepant findings are unclear and well-founded doubts have been raised about the lack of sensitivity of the murine embryo model in prediction of toxicity towards human embryos. For obvious reasons human embryos are not and will not be easily available for appropriate testing.

Since peritoneal fluid or the fallopian tube being in direct contact with the peritoneal fluid are the sites where fertilization of the egg by the spermatozoan takes place,[42] several investigators have addressed the issue of sperm toxicity in patients with endometriosis (TABLE 4). Sperm motility, sperm velocity, sperm survival and zona-free hamster egg penetration and effects by either peritoneal fluid or macrophage conditioned media have been studied. Altogether five studies demonstrate a significant degree of sperm toxicity[43–47] while three studies show no increased toxicity[48–50] in endometriosis as compared to patients with unexplained infertility or with adhesions or fertile donors. It thus appears that indeed sperm toxicity may well be an important mechanism by which the local inflammatory reaction in endometriosis will negatively impact on reproduction.

POSSIBLE MEDIATORS OF INFERTILITY

In order to narrow down the specific substance responsible for anti-fertility effects, attempts have been made to test several cytokines, secretory products of either macrophages or lymphocytes, directly for adverse effects in vitro. Hill et al.[39] tested various concentrations of IL-1, Interferon-γ (I-γ), IL-2 and TNF and found significant embryotoxicity only by TNF and I-γ. IL-1 and IL-2 were recently found to exhibit no such effect by Schneider et al.[41] These two compounds appear therefore unlikely to be responsible for deleterious effects, although a preliminary study by Fakih et al.[16] had so suggested.

TNF-α and I-γ remain the two potential cytokines exhibiting gamete toxicity present in the peritoneal fluid of patients with endometriosis. No information so far is available about interferon levels in peritoneal fluid, but recently two studies have examined the presence of TNF-α related cytotoxicity in patients with and without endometriosis. Eisermann et al.[51] demonstrated increased TNF activity in peritoneal fluid of patients with severe but not with milder forms of endometriosis. More recently, the author's own studies[13] revealed a significantly increased level of cytotoxicity in the peritoneal

TABLE 4. Evidence for Sperm Toxicity in Endometriosis

	Increased Toxicity	Model	Source
Oak et al., 1985	yes	sperm motility	PF[a]
Chacho et al., 1986, 1987	yes	sperm/hamster ova	MCM
Sueldo et al., 1987	yes	mouse sperm ova	PF
Muse et al., 1986	no	sperm motility	PF
Roh et al., 1989	no	sperm motility	PF
Eisermann et al., 1988	yes	sperm motility	PF
Halme & Hall, 1982	no	sperm/hamster ova	PF

[a] MCM = macrophage conditioned medium; PF = peritoneal fluid.

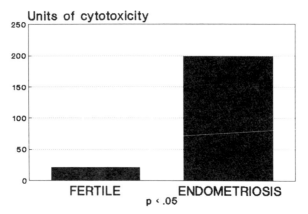

FIGURE 3. Tumor necrosis factor activity in peritoneal fluid of patients with and without endometriosis (Fertile, n = 16, Endo, n = 34). Statistical analysis based on log transformed values.

fluid of patients with mild endometriosis as compared to fertile women (FIG. 3). In addition, the macrophage-conditioned medium of endometriosis patients significantly more often exhibited this activity than either fertile women or women with unexplained infertility without endometriosis (FIG. 4).

Additional evidence to support the role of TNF in endometriosis-associated subfertility comes from a recent study by Eisermann *et al.*[57] who demonstrated that peritoneal fluid from endometriosis patients exhibited spermotoxicity that was directly proportional to the level of TNF-α measured in the fluid samples. Total motility, sperm velocity, and zona-free hamster egg penetration were all affected in a dose-dependent fashion.

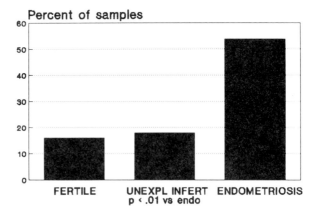

FIGURE 4. Proportion of samples releasing significant tumor necrosis factor activity *in vitro* by peritoneal macrophages of patients with and without endometriosis (Fertile, n = 13, Unexplained Infertility, n = 11, Endo, n = 33). Statistical evaluation with Chi-square analysis.

SUMMARY

This paper has discussed the evidence for the presence of infertility in patients with endometriosis and more critically reviewed some of the studies that have addressed the impact of various potential local peritoneal mechanisms that may lead to subfertility. Substantial evidence supports the notion that patients with endometriosis have reduced fecundability. Although several mechanisms, including, *e.g.*, anatomic factors and ovulatory dysfunction, are possible, recent studies have pointed towards local inflammatory cells and their secretory products as being important mediators of subfertility. Ample evidence exists for the presence of an altered peritoneal inflammatory environment in patients with endometriosis. In addition, *in vitro* studies have identified peritoneal macrophages and their secretory products, specifically TNF-α as the most likely contributors to the reduced fecundability through effects on sperm function.

REFERENCES

1. STRATHY, J. H., C. A. MOLGAARD, C. B. COULAM, *et al.* 1982. Fertil. Steril. **38**: 667–670.
2. DODGE, S. T., R. S. PUMPHREY & K. MIYAZAWA. 1986. Fertil. Steril. **45**: 774–777.
3. GOLDMAN, M. B. & D. W. CRAMER. 1990. *In* Current concepts in Endometriosis. D. R. Chadha & V. C. Buttram, Jr., Eds.: 15–31. Alan R. Liss, Inc., New York.
4. SEIBEL, M. M., M. J. BERGER, F. G. WEINSTEIN & M. L. TAYLOR. 1982. Fertil. Steril. **38**: 534–538.
5. BAYER, S. R., M. M. SEIBEL, D. S. SAFFAN, M. J. BERGER, *et al.* 1988. J. Reprod. Med. **33**: 179–183.
6. HULL, M. E., K. S. MOGHISSI, D. F. MAGYAR & M. F. HAYES. 1987. Fertil. Steril. **47**: 40–44.
7. COOKE, I. D., R. A. SULAIMAN & E. A. LENTON. 1981. Clin. Obstet. Gynecol. **8**: 531–540.
8. JANSEN, R. P. S. 1986. Fertil. Steril. **46**: 141–143.
9. BURNS, W. N. & R. S. SCHENKEN. 1989. *In* Endometriosis: Contemporary Concepts in Clinical Management. R. S. Schenken, Ed.: 83–126. J. B. Lippincott Co., Philadelphia, PA.
10. HALME, J., M. G. HAMMOND, J. F. HULKA, S. G. RAJ & L. M. TALBERT. 1984. Obstet. Gynecol. **64**: 151–154.
11. BAGASRA, O., M. FREUND, J. WEIDMAN & G. HARLEY. 1988. J. AIDS **1**: 431–458.
12. SYROP, C. H. & J. HALME. 1987. Fertil. Steril. **48**: 1–9.
13. HALME, J. 1989. Am. J. Obstet. Gynecol. **161**: 1718–1725.
14. HALME, J., S. BECKER & S. HASKILL. 1987. Am. J. Obstet. Gynecol. **156**: 783–788.
15. HALME, J., S. WHITE, S. KAUMA, J. ESTES & S. HASKILL. 1988. J. Clin. Endocrinol. Metab. **66**: 1044–1049.
16. FAKIH, H., B. BAGGETT, G. HOLTZ, K-Y TSANG, *et al.* 1987. Fertil. Steril. **47**: 213–217.
17. HILL, J. A. & D. J. ANDERSON. 1989. Am. J. Obstet. Gynecol. **161**: 861–864.
18. EISERMANN, J., M. J. GAST, J. PINEDA, R. R. ODEM & J. L. COLLINS. 1988. Fertil. Steril. **50**: 573–579.
19. DRAKE, T. S., S. A. METZ, G. M. GRUNERT & W. F. O'BRIEN. 1980. Fertil. Steril. **34**: 280–282.
20. OAK, M. K., E. N. CHANTLER, C. A. V. WILLIAMS & M. ELSTEIN. 1985. Clin. Reprod. Fertil. **3**: 297–302.
21. SYROP, C. H. & J. HALME. 1987. Obstet. Gynecol. **69**: 416–418.
22. HANEY, A. F., J. J. MUSCATO & J. B. WEINBERG. 1981. Fertil. Steril. **35**: 696–701.
23. OLIVE, D. L., J. B. WEINBERG & A. F. HANEY. 1985. Fertil. Steril. **44**: 772–777.
24. HALME, J., S. BECKER, M. G. HAMMOND, M. H. G. RAJ & S. RAJ. 1983. Am. J. Obstet. Gynecol. **145**: 333–337.
25. SYROP, C. H. & J. HALME. 1986. Fertil. Steril. **46**: 631–635.
26. HANEY, A. F. & J. B. WEINBERG. 1988. Am. J. Obstet. Gynecol. **159**: 450–454.
27. SUGINAMI, H., K. YANO, K. WATANABE & S. MATSUURA. 1986. Fertil. Steril. **46**: 1140–1146.
28. SUGINAMI, H. & K. YANO. 1988. Fertil. Steril. **50**: 648–653.

29. SUGINAMI, H., K. YANO, N. NAKAHASHI & Y. TAKEDA. 1990. *In* Current Concepts in Endometriosis. D. R. Chadha & V. C. Buttram, Jr., Eds.: 81–97. Alan R. Liss, Inc., New York.
30. MUSCATO, J. J., A. F. HANEY & J. B. WEINBERG. 1982. Am. J. Obstet. Gynecol. **144:** 503–510.
31. LONDON, S. N., A. F. HANEY & J. B. WEINBERG. 1985. Fertil. Steril. **43:** 274–278.
32. AWADALLA, S. G., C. I. FRIEDMAN, A. U. HAQ, S. I. ROH, *et al.* 1987. Am. J. Obstet. Gynecol. **157:** 1207–1214.
33. SAMEJIMA, T., H. MASUZAKI, T. TSHIMARU & T. YAMABE. 1989. Asia-Oceanic J. Obstet. Gynecol. **15:** 175–181.
34. HALME, J., S. BECKER & R. WING. 1984. Am. J. Obstet. Gynecol. **148:** 85–90.
35. MORCOS, R. N., W. E. GIBBONS & W. E. FINDLEY. 1985. Fertil. Steril. **44:** 678–683.
36. PROUGH, S. G., R. R. YEOMAN & S. AKSEL. 1988. Annual Meeting of the American Fertility Society, Atlanta, GA, October 10–13, P-097.
37. SIMS, J. A., J. W. E. WORTHAM, JR., D. A. KALLENBERGER, *et al.* 1988. Annual Meeting of the American Fertility Society, Atlanta, GA, October 10–13, P-021.
38. HAHN, D. W., R. P. CARRAHER, R. G. FOLDESY, *et al.* 1986. Am. J. Obstet. Gynecol. **155:** 1109–1113.
39. HILL, J. A., F. HAIMOVICI & D. J. ANDERSON. 1987. J. Immunol. **139:** 2250–2254.
40. SCHNEIDER, E. G., A. E. DANIELE & M. L. POLAN. 1987. Annual Meeting of the American Fertility Society, Reno, NV, September 28–30, A047.
41. SCHNEIDER, E. G., D. R. ARMANT, T. S. KUPPER & M. L. POLAN. 1989. Biol. Reprod. **40:** 825–833.
42. HANEY, A. F., M. A. MISUKONIS & J. B. WEINBERG. 1983. Fertil. Steril. **39:** 310–315.
43. OAK, M. K., E. N. CHANTLER, C. A. WILLIAMS, *et al.* 1985. Clin. Reprod. Fertil. **3:** 297–302.
44. CHACHO, K. J., M. S. CHACHO, P. J. ANDRESEN & A. SCOMMEGNA. 1986. Am. J. Obstet. Gynecol. **154:** 1290–1295.
45. CHACHO, K. J., P. J. ANDRESEN & A. SCOMMEGNA. 1987. Fertil. Steril. **48:** 694–696.
46. SUELDO, C. E., H. LAMBERT, A. STEINLEITNER, *et al.* 1987. Fertil. Steril. **48:** 697–699.
47. EISERMANN, J., K. B. REGISTER, R. C. STRICKLER & J. L. COLLINS. 1989. J. Androl. **10:** 270–274.
48. HALME, J. & J. L. HALL. 1982 Fertil. Steril. **37:** 573–576.
49. MUSE, K., S. ESTES, M. VERNON, P. ZAVOS, *et al.* 1986. Annual Meeting of the American Fertility Society, Toronto, Ont., September 27–October 2, P-286.
50. ROH, S. I., D. L. FULGHAM, G. E. HOFMANN, *et al.* 1989. Annual Meeting of the Society for Gynecologic Investigation, San Diego, CA, March 15–18, A-124.
51. EISERMANN, J., B. CANTOR, H. LAMBERT & J. L. COLLINS. 1989. Annual Meeting of the American Fertility Society, San Francisco, CA, November 13–16, P-024.

Efficacy and Endocrine Effects of Medical Treatment of Endometriosis

GIAN BENEDETTO MELIS,[a] VALERIO MAIS,
ANNA MARIA PAOLETTI, SILVIA AJOSSA, AND
STEFANO GUERRIERO

Department of Obstetrics and Gynecology
University of Cagliari, School of Medicine
09126 Cagliari, Italy

PIERO FIORETTI

Department of Obstetrics and Gynecology
University of Pisa, School of Medicine
Via Roma 67
56100 Pisa, Italy

INTRODUCTION

Over the last 30 years a variety of non-surgical methods have been proposed for curing and controlling endometriosis. First, the combination of an estrogen and a progestogen, or "pseudopregnancy," has been used for many years;[1,2] then "pseudomenopause" therapy has been proposed, after Greenblatt *et al.*[3] published the first clinical studies with the "antigonadotropin," danazol.

Danazol has been reported to reduce LH and FSH concentrations in castrated rats and monkeys, as well as in postmenopausal women.[4,5] However, this drug does not modify basal gonadotropin concentration or gonadotropin response to exogenous gonadotropin-releasing hormone (GnRH), although it blunts the midcycle gonadotropin surge.[4,5] Moreover, danazol is metabolized to approximately 60 different molecules after its administration by the oral route, and some of these metabolites are known to be hormonally active.[5] Therefore, it seems inappropriate to refer to danazol as "antigonadotropin," because of its complex pharmacology.[5]

Recently, other compounds having "antigonadotropin" properties have been tested for the medical management of endometriosis. Gestrinone, one of these drugs, has been reported to be clinically effective at relatively low dosages,[6,7] and to blunt the preovulatory gonadotropin surge.[8] However, basal gonadotropin levels are not modified by chronic gestrinone administration in premenopausal women,[8] and the drug has been also reported to have anti-estrogen, anti-progesterone, androgenic, and progestogenic effects on peripheral or central steroid receptors.[6-8]

Finally, "medical oophorectomy" therapy using GnRH-agonists has been shown

[a] *Address for correspondence:* Gian Benedetto Melis, MD, Professor, Clinica Ostetrica e Ginecologica, Università di Cagliari, Ospedale S. Giovanni di Dio, Via Ospedale 46, 09126 Cagliari, Italy.

to be a promising approach to medical treatment of endometriosis.[9] With chronic administration of GnRH-agonists, after an initial stimulation phase, gonadotropin secretion is progressively suppressed because of pituitary desensitization, leading to blockage of follicular maturation and estrogen secretion.[9,10]

The present controlled trial was conducted to compare the efficacy and the endocrine effects of chronic treatment with danazol, gestrinone, or the GnRH-agonist, Buserelin, in women with pelvic endometriosis diagnosed and scored by laparoscopy. To compare the effects of the three drugs on hypothalamic-pituitary function, gonadotropin response to exogenous GnRH was evaluated before, during, and one month after the end of the treatment.

MATERIALS AND METHODS

Thirty patients, 18 to 45 years of age, were included in the study. All subjects had regular menstrual cycles and pelvic endometriosis diagnosed and scored, according to the Revised American Fertility Society Classification:1985,[11] by a laparoscopy or laparotomy performed 2 to 6 months before the beginning of the study. The patients were randomly divided into three groups and each group was treated for six months with one of the following drugs. In all subjects, treatment was started during the early follicular phase (day 1–4 of the cycle). Ten subjects received gestrinone orally at a dose of 2.5 mg twice weekly. Ten subjects received danazol orally at a dose of 600 mg/day (200 mg three times a day). Ten subjects received buserelin at a dose of 300 µg twice a day subcutaneously for the first month, and 400 µg three times a day intranasally for the following five months.

During the early follicular phase (day 3–7) of the menstrual cycle preceding the beginning of treatment, all patients underwent a preliminary endocrine evaluation. The subjects were hospitalized at 8:00 A.M. at 8:30 A.M. a polyethylene catheter was inserted in a antcubital vein and kept patent by a slow saline infusion. At 9:00 A.M. a blood sample was obtained to evaluate basal gonadotropin (LH,FSH), 17β-estradiol (E_2) and progesterone (P) levels. Thereafter, 100 µg of GnRH were intravenously injected. Blood samples were then collected 15, 30, 60, and 90 min after GnRH injection to measure plasma LH and FSH concentration.

The same endocrine evaluation was performed after 1, 2, 3, and 6 months of treatment. At the same time intervals the patients also underwent a clinical evaluation. At each visit, the subjects were asked about timing and occurrence of vaginal bleeding, dysmenorrhea, dyspareunia, pelvic pain, and side-effects attributable to therapy. During the study the patients were not taking other drugs that could interfere with endocrine function and used barrier contraceptives.

Plasma LH, FSH, E_2, and P were measured by previously described radioimmunological methods.[12]

The statistical analysis was performed by analysis of variance and multiple range testing. To evaluate GnRH-stimulated gonadotropin release, the integrated gonadotropin secretion was calculated by the method of triangulation on data normalized as the net change over the value immediately before GnRH injection (zero time). Net change values were connected by straight line segments, and the area under these segments was calculated using the trapezoidal technique.

RESULTS

The three drugs used for medical management of endometriosis showed a similar clinical efficacy. In all groups of subjects dysmenorrhea and pelvic pain were similarly relieved during treatment. A second-look laparoscopy performed one month after the end of treatment in 6 patients treated with gestrinone, 5 patients treated with buserelin, and 5 patients treated with danazol demonstrated a significant reduction of endometriosis score. Only three patients, one in each group, showed a significant weight gain. All patients showed a reduction of breast tissue without significant differences among the three groups. All patients treated with gestrinone or danazol, showed acne and seborrhea. On the contrary, hot flushes were reported by all patients, but their frequency and intensity were significantly greater in the group treated with buserelin. As for menstrual cyclicity, all subjects treated with buserelin reported one episode of menstrual bleeding 10 to 15 days after the beginning of treatment and thereafter became amenorrheic. Nine of the ten patients treated with danazol became amenorrheic after the first month of treatment and only one had irregular scanty bleeding throughout treatment duration. Two women treated with gestrinone became amenorrheic after the first month of treatment, three women after two months and one after three months. The other four subjects had irregular scanty bleeding throughout treatment duration.

The endocrine effects of the three drugs are reported in FIGURES 1 to 6 as mean

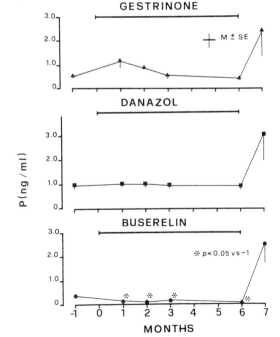

FIGURE 1. Mean ± SE basal plasma concentrations of progesterone observed before, during, and after treatment with gestrinone, danazol, or buserelin.

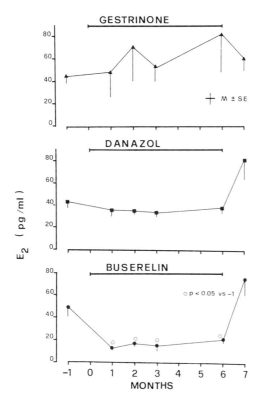

FIGURE 2. Mean ± SE basal plasma concentrations of 17β-estradiol observed before, during, and after treatment with gestrinone, danazol, or buserelin.

± SE. In all groups, plasma P concentrations remained in the follicular phase range throughout treatment, but only buserelin was able to further and significantly reduce P levels (FIG. 1).

As for E_2 secretion, gestrinone did not modify the hormone plasma levels that during treatment ranged from 49.4 ± 21.7 pg/ml to 73.3 ± 34.3 pg/ml. Also during treatment with danazol plasma E_2 concentrations were similar to those measured in the early follicular phase, ranging from 34.5 ± 3.5 pg/ml to 38.2 ± 4.3 pg/ml. Only buserelin significantly reduced plasma E_2 concentrations to postmenopausal levels (FIG. 2).

Gestrinone significantly reduced basal FSH levels, but not basal LH levels. Danazol did not modify basal concentration of both FSH and LH. Buserelin reduced both FSH and LH (FIGS. 3 and 4).

The most evident differences among the central endocrine effects of the three drugs were observed in the response of both LH (FIG. 5) and FSH (FIG. 6) to exogenous GnRH. In fact, gestrinone induced a significant increase of the response of both gonadotropins, danazol did not modify this response, and buserelin completely suppressed it. One month after the end of treatment, the response of both gonadotropins to exogenous GnRH was similar to the pretreatment one in all groups.

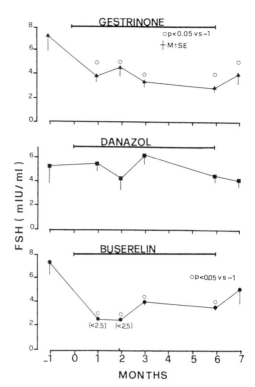

FIGURE 3. Mean ± SE basal plasma concentrations of FSH observed before, during, and after treatment with gestrinone, danazol, or buserelin.

DISCUSSION

This trial demonstrated that the three drugs used for medical treatment of endometriosis have similar clinical efficacy, but quite different endocrine effects.

In fact, buserelin reduced E_2 concentrations to postmenopausal levels by suppressing pituitary gonadotropin secretion. Therefore, the clinical efficacy of this drug probably depends on the complete blockage of ovarian function.[9,10]

By contrast, danazol inhibited ovulation, but did not modify basal plasma gonadotropins or their response to exogenous GnRH. Moreover, E_2 levels remained in the early follicular phase range throughout treatment. Thus, the clinical efficacy of this drug seems to depend not only on its antigonadotropic properties, but also on the androgenic, progestogenic effects of either danazol or its metabolites at central or peripheral level.[5] This complex mechanism of action could also explain the reduction of breast tissue and the appearance of hot flushes with plasma E_2 levels similar to those observed in the early follicular phase of the normal menstrual cycle.

As for gestrinone, the drug seems to have a progestomimetic effect at central level, since it reduces basal plasma FSH levels, but enhances the response of both gonadotropins to exogenous GnRH administration.[13] Therefore, suppression of midcycle

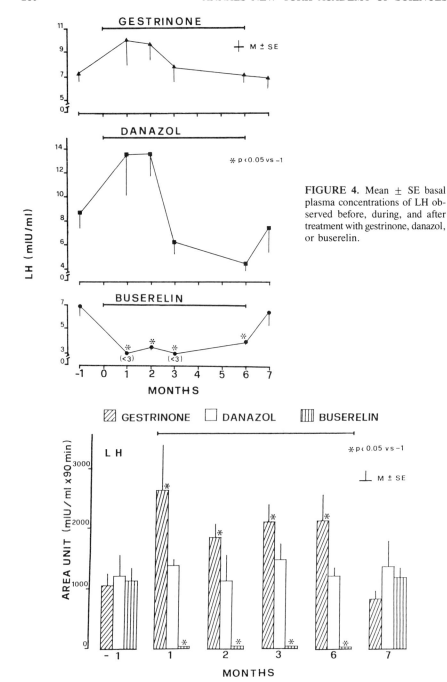

FIGURE 4. Mean ± SE basal plasma concentrations of LH observed before, during, and after treatment with gestrinone, danazol, or buserelin.

FIGURE 5. Mean ± SE integrated LH secretion (mIU/ml × 90 min) after injection of exogenous GnRH (100 μg, i.v. bolus) observed before, during, and after treatment with gestrinone, danazol, or buserelin.

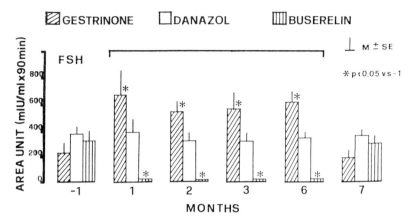

FIGURE 6. Mean $\pm$ SE integrated FSH secretion (mIU/ml $\times$ 90 min) after injection of exogenous GnRH (100 µg, i.v. bolus) observed before, during, and after treatment with gestrinone, danazol, or buserelin.

LH and FSH surge could depend on a blockage of pituitary sensitivity more than on a reduction of pituitary reserve.[13] The efficacy of gestrinone treatment in the management of endometriosis could then rely on its peripheral actions.[6-8] The reduction of mammary gland tissue and the appearance of hot flushes with plasma E_2 levels greater than 50 pg/ml also suggest that gestrinone might have a quite complex pharmacology.

REFERENCES

1. KISTNER, R. W. 1958. The use of newer progestins in the treatment of endometriosis. Am. J. Obstet. Gynecol. **75:** 264–278.
2. KISTNER, R. W. 1975. Management of endometriosis in the infertile patient. Fertil. Steril. **26:** 1151–1161.
3. GREENBLATT, R. B., L. P. DMOWSKI, U. MAHESH & H. F. C. SCHOLER. 1971. Clinical studies with an antigonadotrophin-danazol. Fertil. Steril. **22:** 102–113.
4. DMOWSKI, W. P. 1979. Endocrine properties and clinical application of danazol. Fertil. Steril. **31:** 237–251.
5. BARBIERI, R. L. & K. J. RYAN. 1981. Danazol: Endocrine pharmacology and therapeutic applications. Am. J. Obstet. Gynecol. **141:** 453–463.
6. COUTINHO, E. M. 1982. Treatment of endometriosis with gestrinone (R-2323), a synthetic antiestrogen, antiprogesterone. Am. J. Obstet. Gynecol. **144:** 895–898.
7. VENTURINI, P. L., S. BERTOLINI, M. C. MARRÉ BRUNENGHI, A. DAGA, V. FASCE, A. MARCENARO, M. CIMATO & L. DE CECCO. 1989. Endocrine, metabolic, and clinical effects of gestrinone in women with endometriosis. Fertil. Steril. **52:** 589–595.
8. ROBYN, C., J. DELOGNE-DESNOECK, P. BOURDOUX & G. COPINSCHI. 1984. Endocrine effects of gestrinone. *In* Medical Management of Endometriosis. J. P. Raynaud, T. Ojasoo & L. Martini, Eds.: 207–221. Raven Press. New York, NY.
9. LEMAY, A., R. MAHEUX, R. FAURE, N. JEAN & C. FAZEKAS. 1984. Reversible hypogonadism induced by a luteinizing hormone-releasing hormone (LH-RH) agonist (Buserelin) as a new therapeutic approach for endometriosis. Fertil. Steril. **41:** 863–871.

10. LEMAY, A., J. SANDOW, M. BUREAU, R. MAHEUX, J. Y. FONTAINE & P. MERAT. 1988. Prevention of follicular maturation in endometriosis by subcutaneous infusion of luteinizing hormone-releasing hormone agonist started in the luteal phase. Fertil. Steril. **49:** 410–417.
11. THE AMERICAN FERTILITY SOCIETY. 1985. Revised American Fertility Society classification of endometriosis: 1985. Fertil. Steril. **43:** 351–352.
12. MAIS, V., G. B. MELIS, A. M. PAOLETTI, F. STRIGINI, D. ANTINORI & P. FIORETTI. 1986. Prolactin-releasing action of a low dose of exogenous gonadotropin-releasing hormone throughout the human menstrual cycle. Neuroendocrinology **44:** 326–330.
13. WANG, C. F., B. L. LASLEY, A. LEIN & S. S. C. YEN. 1976. The functional change of the pituitary gonadotrophs during the menstrual cycle. J. Clin. Endocrinol. Metab. **42:** 718–728.

Endometrial Effects of Danazol in Perimenopausal Abnormal Bleeding

U. MONTEMAGNO, G. DE PLACIDO, N. COLACURCI,
AND F. ZULLO

Department of Obstetrics and Gynecology
II School of Medicine of Naples
Naples, Italy

INTRODUCTION

Danazol (D), a 2-3 isoxazol derivative of 17-ethinyltestosterone, is routinely used for the treatment of endometriosis[1] and is known to suppress menstrual bleeding.[2] Endometrial effects of D are not only related to the well-known inhibition of the hypothalamic pituitary function and ovarian steroid synthesis, but they seem to be primarily determined by a direct action on the endometrium.[3] In fact, D binds to progesterone receptors (PR) and inhibits 17-β-hydroxy-steroid-dehydrogenase[4] and steroid sulfatase activity[5] in human endometrium. The effectiveness of D in treatment of perimenopausal abnormal bleeding has been confirmed in many trials.[6-7] The demonstration of antiproliferative activity on human endometrial cancer cells *in vivo*[8] and on adenomatous hyperplasia *in vivo*,[9] together with the histologic observation that D induces rapid atrophic changes whereas a marked decidual reaction is found through progestin treatment, suggest a difference in the effect of D and typical progestins on endometrial tissue. In this regard we have considered useful to evaluate clinically, hysteroscopically and histopathologically the efficacy of D 200 mg daily for 3 months in the treatment of perimenopausal abnormal bleeding sustained by endometrial hyperplasia without cytologic atypia[10] in patients at their first therapeutic approach (group A) and in women already treated by progestin with persistance of the disease or recurrence within two months (group B). In addition a further endometrial antiproliferative mechanism of action of D, probably in relation with its immunosuppressive activity is indirectly shown by means of a primary endometrial cell culture conditioned by medium from peritoneal macrophages cultured *in vitro*.

MATERIALS AND METHODS

Subjects and Clinical Protocols

We have treated by 200 mg daily of D 42 patients with perimenopausal abnormal bleeding underlying an endometrial hyperplasia without cytologic atypia and not previously treated (group A) and 23 women with uterine bleeding already treated by Norethisterone and/or Medroxyprogesterone but with a persistance or recurrence of symptoms within two months (group B). Each patient underwent a hysteroscopic examination with guided endometrial biopsy before starting treatment. The treatment was monitored by: 1) a subjective semiquantitative evaluation of bleeding during treatment and in a follow up to 12 months; 2) hysteroscopically before, at the end of treatment, and in a follow up to 12 months; 3) histopathologically before and after treatment. Side effects and adverse reactions were carefully evaluated.

Experimental Section

On the basis of a previous experience[11] in which we showed that D, at a concentration of 10^{-6}M, significantly reduced the phagocytic ability of peritoneal macrophages *in vitro*, we wanted to see if the steroid is able to decrease the secretion of growth factors[12,13] by these immune cells and how such an immunosuppressive effect can be related to endometrial proliferation *in vitro*. Macrophages derived from peritoneal fluid collected laparoscopically with an average yield of 5×10^5 cells/ml. Cells were put in RPMI medium with 5% FBS steroid free, washed, centrifuged, and resuspended to a final concentration of 1×10^6 per dish using 24-well tissue culture plates in 1.5 ml of medium. Cultures were washed 2 hours after plating to separate nonadherent cells, and then incubated for 48 hours. Then supernatants were recovered and frozen at $-80°C$ or immediately used. In some of these cultures, after separating nonadherent cells, D was added at different concentrations washing and changing medium 24 hours later. Then macrophages were cultured for 48 hours when supernatants were recovered. Endometrial cells derived from biopsy specimens sampled in the luteal phase and immediately put in ice-cold 1:1 mixture of DMEM and Ham's-F-12. Samples were dissected and a separation between stromal and epithelial cells was performed following the Osteen technique[14] with some slight modifications.[15] Essentially the method was based on three consecutive incubations in medium containing 0.5% collagenase and 0.05% DNAase followed by differential sedimentation of epithelial cells at unit gravity and by selective attachment of stromal cells to plastic cultureware. At the end of separation both epithelial and stromal cells were plated at a final density of 5×10^5 cells/ml in 24-well plates in DMEM-F-12 with 10% charcoal extracted FBS for 48 hours (T_0). Cultures were washed and incubated in medium with 2% steroid free FBS for 48 hours (T_f). Cell counts were performed on day 2 and day 4 of culture. At T_0 different amounts (10–60% vol/vol) of supernatant from macrophage culture previously treated or not with different concentrations of D were added to the endometrial cell cultures. Viability of cell cultures were assessed by Trypan blue exclusion.

RESULTS AND DISCUSSION

In group A (TABLE 1) there was a subjective significant decrease of bleeding in 38 out of 41 patients (88.2%), and this result remained unchanged (84.3%) 2 months after discontinuation of treatment, while 4 months after (24.9% of recurrence) and up to 12 months the abnormal bleeding reappeared in 56.2% of women. In TABLE 2 is shown how in group B (patients not responding to progestins) the persistence of heavy blood loss at the end of treatment was 22.7%; this can be considered a very good result considering patients as a control for themselves. This result was practically unchanged 2 months later (27%), with a significant increase in recurrence at 4 (49.9%)

TABLE 1. Blood Loss and Days of Bleeding in Group A

| | Pretreatment n (%) | End of Treatment n (%) | Months Posttreatment | | |
			2 n (%)	4 n (%)	Up to 12 n (%)
Blood Loss					
Flooding	19 (45)	–	1 (3)	2 (7)	4 (25)
Heavy	23 (55)	3 (7)	3 (9)	6 (18)	6 (31)
Normal	–	33 (81)	25 (79)	18 (69)	6 (38)
Spotting	–	2 (5)	1 (3)	1 (3)	1 (8)
Amenorrhea	–	3 (7)	2 (8)	1 (3)	–
Number of Patients	42	41	32	28	16
Days of Bleeding (mean ± SD)	8.9 ± 3.7	5.2 ± 3.4	5.4 ± 3.8	6.3 ± 4.8	6.9 ± 3.7

and up to 12 months (55.3%). Hysteroscopically in only two patients in group A (4.8%) and two patients in group B (9%) did the hyperplastic picture not revert at the end of treatment, and one of these four patients was a false positive on the basis of the biopsy result (TABLE 3). The hysteroscopic follow-up showed a rapid appearance of hypoatrophic pictures with a progressive increase in the normal findings both proliferative and secretive, but also with a meaningful reappearance of hyperplasia up to 60% at 4 and 12 months (TABLE 4).

The comparison of hysteroscopic findings with histopathologic pictures shows clearly a good correlation with just 1 hysteroscopic false positive, 2 false negative, and 2 not diagnostic exams (TABLE 5). The most interesting aspect of this comparison is the invaluable importance of the hysteroscopy in the diagnosis of hypoatrophia, which is very often undiagnosed bioptically for inadequate sampling.

The most frequent side effects during this treatment were weight gain, muscle cramps, headache and acne, but in only two cases was it necessary to stop treatment (TABLE 6).

Our data clearly show the efficacy of the regimen of D 200mg daily in the treatment of perimenopausal abnormal bleeding, as indicated in previous reports too,[6,7,9] but

TABLE 2. Blood Loss and Days of Bleeding in Group B

| | Pretreatment n (%) | End of Treatment n (%) | Months Posttreatment | | |
			2 n (%)	4 n (%)	Up to 12 n (%)
Blood Loss					
Flooding	8 (38)	1 (5)	2 (9)	3 (17)	3 (26)
Heavy	14 (81)	4 (18)	4 (18)	6 (33)	8 (53)
Normal	–	14 (63)	14 (83)	8 (44)	3 (28)
Spotting	–	1 (5)	1 (5)	–	–
Amenorrhea	–	2 (9)	1 (5)	1 (6)	1 (7)
Number of Patients	23	22	22	18	15
Days of Bleeding (mean ± SD)	8.5 ± 4.1	5.9 ± 2.2	6.4 ± 3.6	6.8 ± 4.3	7.6 ± 3.8

TABLE 3. Hysteroscopic Findings before (T_0) and at the End of Treatment (T_1) with Danazol 200 mg Daily for 3 Months

Hysteroscopic Finding	T_0		T_1	
	Group A n (%)	Group B n (%)	Group A n (%)	Group B n (%)
Hyperplasia	39 (92.8)	22 (95.6)	2 (4.8)	2 (9.0)
Hypo-atrophy	—	—	32 (78.0)	16 (72.7)
Normotrophy	2 (4.7)	—	6 (14.6)	4 (18.1)
Not diagnostic	1 (2.3)	1 (4.3)	1 (2.4)	—
TOTAL	42	23	41	22

TABLE 4. Hysteroscopic Follow-up at 2 Months (T_2), 4 Months (T_3) and up to 12 Months (T_4) after Treatment with Danazol 200 mg Daily for 3 Months

Hysteroscopic Finding	T_2		T_3		T_4	
	Group A n (%)	Group B n (%)	Group A n (%)	Group B n (%)	Group A n (%)	Group B n (%)
Hyperplasia	2 (11.1)	3 (20.0)	4 (28.5)	3 (27.2)	9 (60.0)	5 (62.5)
Hypo-atrophy	10 (55.5)	8 (53.3)	4 (28.5)	2 (18.1)	2 (13.3)	1 (12.5)
Normotrophy						
Proliferative	4 (22.2)	3 (50.0)	4 (28.5)	4 (36.3)	3 (20.0)	2 (25.0)
Secretory	2 (11.1)	1 (6.6)	2 (14.2)	2 (18.1)	5 (33.3)	—
Not diagnostic	—	—	—	—	—	—
TOTAL	18	15	14	11	15	8

TABLE 5. Comparison between Hysteroscopic Findings and Histopathologic Pictures before (T_0) and after Treatment (T_1)

Histopathologic Appearance	Hysteroscopic Finding									
	Hyperplasia		Hermotrophy		Hypo-atrophy		Not diagnostic		TOTAL	
	T_0	T_1	T_0	T_1	T_0	T_1	T_0	T_1	T_0	T_1
Adenomatous hyperplasia	9	2	—	—	—	—	—	—	9	2
Glandular hyperplasia	21	1	2	—	—	—	2	—	25	1
Gland. cystic hyperplasia	31	—	—	—	—	—	—	—	31	—
Proliferative (a) with fibrotio stroma (b)	—	1a	—	7b	—	—	—	—	—	8
Irregular maturation	—	—	—	2	—	—	—	1	—	3
Atrophic	—	—	—	—	—	18	—	—	—	18
Atrophic with stroma pseudodecidualization	—	—	—	1	—	11	—	—	—	12
Inadequate sampling	—	—	—	—	—	19	—	—	—	19
TOTAL	61	4	2	10	—	48	2	1	65	63

TABLE 6. Side Effects during Treatment

	Month 1 n (%)	Month 3 n (%)
Weight gain	7 (10.7)	5 (7.9)
Headache	3 (4.6)	3 (4.7)
Nausea or vomiting	3 (4.6)	–
Acne	3 (4.6)	4 (6.3)
Hirsutism	1 (1.5)	1 (1.5)
Muscle cramps	4 (6.1)	2 (3.1)
Hot flushes	3 (4.6)	3 (4.7)
Skin rash	1 (1.5)	–
Voice change	1 (1.5)	1 (1.5)
Edema	2 (3.0)	–
Decreased breast size	3 (4.6)	4 (6.3)
TOTAL	65	63

they also point out the effectiveness of this steroid in those forms not responding to progestins, confirming indirectly the existence of additional mechanisms of antiproliferative action on the endometrium if compared to progestogens. In order to verify the hypothesis of an antiproliferative effect mediated by the immunosuppressive activity of this steroid, we have used an experimental model of primary endometrial cell cultures conditioned by supernatants from peritoneal macrophages cultured *in vitro* with or without D. The rationale underlying this hypothesis was to test the ability of D to inhibit the secretion of growth factors stimulating the endometrial proliferation by uterine immune cells.

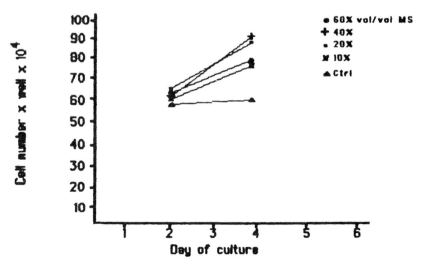

FIGURE 1. Epithelial cells growth with the addiction of different concentration of supernatant from a peritoneal macrophage culture (MS).

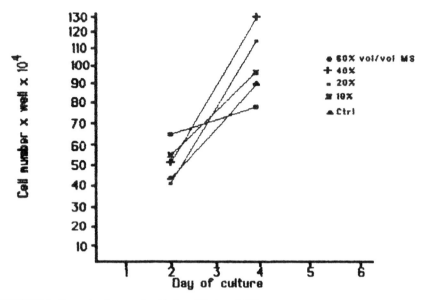

FIGURE 2. Stromal cells growth with the addiction of different concentration of supernatant from a peritoneal macrophage culture (MS).

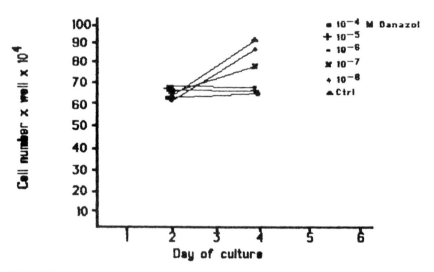

FIGURE 3. Epithelial cells with the addiction of 40% vol/vol of supernatant from a peritoneal macrophage culture previously treated with different concentration of Danazol.

Our results with this model have shown a marked increase in proliferation when adding to endometrial epithelial cells an aliquot of 40% in volume of supernant from the peritoneal macrophage culture (FIG. 1). We have used peritoneal samples as a source of macrophages because they can be easily collected and because they seem to be strictly related to the resident immune cells in human endometrium.[15] Using endometrial stromal cells the increase induced by macrophage supernatant was not so evident, probably in relation to the more active early proliferation to confluence of these cells *in vitro* (FIG. 2). When we have used supernatants of macrophages previously exposed to different concentrations of D, we have demonstrated a significant decrease in the proliferation with the peak at $10^{-6}M$ concentration of D (FIG. 3).

In conclusion, our clinical data strongly suggest the presence of other mechanisms of endometrial antiproliferative effect of D in addition to the progestin-like ones. Among these further mechanisms, our preliminary results using a conditioned endometrial primary cell culture seem to show the importance of the inhibition in the production of growth factors by local immune cells exerted by D.

REFERENCES

1. DMOWSKI, W. P. 1971. Endocrine properties and clinical application of D. Fertil. Steril. **31**(3): 237–251.
2. LUCIANO, A. A. 1982. A guide to managing endometriosis. Contemp. Obstet. Gynecol. **19**(5): 211–234.
3. BARBIERI, R. L. & K. J. RYAN. 1981. D endocrine pharmacology and therapeutic applications. Am. J. Obstet. Gynecol. **149**(4): 453–463.
4. KOKKO, E., O. JANNE, A. KAUPPILA, L. RONNBERG & R. VIHKO. 1982. D has progestin like actions on the human endometrium. Acta Endocrinol. **99**: 588–593.
5. CARLSTRÖM, K., A. DOBERL, A. POUSETTE, G. RANNEVIK & N. WILKING. 1984. Inhibition of steroid sulfatase activity by D. Acta Obstet. Gynecol. Scand. **123**: 107.
6. LAMB, M. P. 1987. D in menorrhagia: A double-blind placebo-controlled study. J. Obstet. Gynecol. **7**: 212–216.
7. FLAMIGNI, C., V. IASONNI, C. BULLETTI & G. FUSCHINI. 1986. Efficacia e tollerabilita' del D nel trattamento della sindrome menorragica: studio multicentrico. Minerva Ginecol. **38**: 1–8.
8. IKEGAMI, H., N. TARAKAWA, I. SHINIZU, T. AONO, O. TANIZAWA & K. MATSUMOTO. 1986. D binds to progesterone receptors and inhibits the growth of human endometrial cancer cells in vitro. Am. J. Obstet. Gynecol. **155**(4): 857–861.
9. TERAKAWA, N., M. INOUE, I. SHIMIZU, H. IKEGAMI, T. MIZUTANI, M. SAKATA, D. TANIZAWA & K. MATSUMOTO. 1988. Preliminary report on the use of D in the treatment of endometrial adenomatous hyperplasia. Cancer **62**: 2618–2621.
10. FERENCZY, A. & M. GELFAND. 1989. The biologic significance of cytologic atypia in progestogen-treated endometrial hyperplasia. Am. J. Obstet. Gynecol. **1**: 126.
11. ZULLO, F., D. L. FULGHAM, S. I. ROH, G. DE PLACIDO & N. J. ALEXANDER. 1989. Decreased sperm phagocytic ability of peritoneal macrophages from women with endometriosis, using danazol and 6-methyl-prednisolone. Gamete Physiology, Serono Symposia, Newport Beach, CA, USA, November 6–10, 1988. Abstract Book, Abst. 56.
12. HALME, J., M. G. HAMMOND & C. S. SYROP. 1985. Macrophages modulate human granulosa luteal progesterone production. J. Clin. Endocrinol. Metab. **61**: 912.
13. HALME, J., S. BECKER & S. HASKILL. 1987. Altered maturation and function of peritoneal macrophages: Possible role in pathogenesis of endometriosis. Am. J. Obstet. Gynecol. **156**: 783.
14. OSTEEN, K. G., G. A. HILL, J. T. HARGREVE & F. GASTEIN. 1989. Development of a method to isolate and culture highly purified populations of stromal and epithelial cells from human endometrial biopsy specimens. Fertil. Steril. **52**(6): 965.
15. ZULLO, F., K. G. OSTEEN, G. D. HODGEN & T. L. ANDERSON. 1989. Development of a model

for isolation and culture of endometrial epithelial and stromal cells from the non-human primate. Society for Gynecological Investigation, San Diego, CA, USA, March 15–18, 1989. Abstract book, Abst. 77.

16. KREIGE, H., H. J. RADZUN, K. HEIDORN, M. R. PARWORESCH & L. METTLER. 1989. Expression of the M-CSF-gene and C-FMS-proto-oncogene in human tissue macrophages. J. Reprod. Immunol. July 1989 (Suppl.): 184.

Immunological Treatment of Implantation Failure

G. DE PLACIDO, F. ZULLO, N. COLACURCI,
D. PERRONE, A. NAZZARO, F. PAOLILLO, AND
U. MONTEMAGNO

Department of Obstetrics and Gynecology
II School of Medicine
Naples, Italy

INTRODUCTION

The non-rejection of the implanting blastocyst is one of the most fascinating topics in reproductive immunology. The interest in it has enormously increased in the last years since, with the development of the *in vitro* fertilization–embryo transfer (IVF-ET) technique, the great number of very early abortions (biochemical pregnancies) has become apparent;[1,2] thus, the implantation rate must be considered as the real limiting factor in all the assisted reproductive techniques. It seems likely that several immunological mechanisms such as the modification of the mother immune response by hormones and by non-hormonal substances, fetal and maternal suppressor cells, and maternal blocking antibodies are involved in the maintenance of pregnancy.[3-5] An immunological recognition of the blastocyst has been claimed to be a necessary prerequisite for a successful pregnancy. It has been further postulated that failure in this immunological recognition could lead to repeated unexplained abortions.[6] So far immunization treatment of women with recurrent abortion has been introduced, using different protocols: third party leukocytes,[7] husband's leukocytes,[6] or trophoblast membrane preparation.[8] Recently, a passive immunization treatment by using Ig from a donor pool (IVIG) has been proposed as well, which should provide immunological protection of pregnancy in the same way as the previous techniques.[9]

Considering the very high reliability of this technique, which has no side effects, a pilot study was undertaken to examine the possibility to extend this treatment to two other groups: 1) women with two or more previous very early pregnancy failures (including biochemical pregnancies) following assisted reproductive techniques; 2) women with repeated (n ≥ 3) unsuccessful embryo transfers either uterine or tubal. So far we have treated 19 women (12 group A and 7 group B) obtaining 5 ongoing pregnancies out of a total of nine positive β-HCG.

MATERIALS AND METHODS

Inclusion criteria for the passive immunization protocol were: 1) women with two or more previous very early pregnancy failures (including biochemical pregnancies)

TABLE 1. Results Obtained Using the Intravenous Immunoglobulin Protocol

Patients	Cause of Infertility	Previous Attempts	Current Attempts	Results
1	Tubal	3 UET[a] 2 BP	IVF	No pregnancy
2	Male Factor	4 IUI 3 DIPI 2 UET 1 TET 1 BP	ZIFT	No pregnancy
3	Unexplained	4 IUI 3 UET	ZIFT	Ongoing pregnancy (14 week)
4	Unexplained	4 DIPI 1 UET 2 TET	ZIFT	No pregnancy
5	Tubal	3 UET 1 EA	IVF	Ongoing pregnancy (16 week)
6	Unexplained	5 IUI 3 DIPI 2 GIFT 1 BP 1 UET 1 EA	ZIFT	Ongoing pregnancy (8 week)
7	Tubal + male factor	3 UET	IVF	No pregnancy
8	Unexplained	3 DIPI 3 GIFT 1 BP 1 UET 1 EA	ZIFT	Early abortion (7 week)
9	Unexplained	4 IUI 3 DIPI 2 UET 1 TET 2 BP	ZIFT	No pregnancy
10	Unexplained	4 DIPI 1 UET 2 TET	ZIFT	Ongoing pregnancy (20 week)
11	Tubal	4 UET 1 EA 1 BP	IVF	No pregnancy
12	Unexplained	4 DIPI 3 UET	ZIFT	No pregnancy
13	Unexplained	3 IUI 2 DIPI 1 GIFT 1 UET 2 EA	ZIFT	No pregnancy
14	Unexplained	4 IUI 3 DIPI 2 UET 1 TET 1 BP	ZIFT	Ongoing pregnancy (15 week)
15	Tubal + male factor	3 UET 1 BP	IVF	No pregnancy
16	Unexplained	3 IUI 3 DIPI 1 GIFT 1 EA 1 UET 1 BP	ZIFT	Biochemical pregnancy
17	Unexplained	2 IUI 4 DIPI 1 GIFT 1 EA 1 UET 1 BP	ZIFT	Biochemical pregnancy
18	Unexplained	4 IUI 3 DIPI 2 UET 1 TET 1 BP	ZIFT	No pregnancy
19	Tubal	3 UET 1 BP	IVF	Early abortion (7 week)

[a] *Abbreviations:* IUI = IntraUterine Insemination; DIPI = Direct IntraPeritoneal Insemination; UET = Uterine Embryo Transfer; TET = Tubal Embryo Transfer; EA = Early Abortion; BP = Biochemical Pregnancy.

TABLE 2. Differences in One Way MLC in Women with Habitual Abortion/Failure of Implantation

Responder Lymphocytes[a]	Stimulator Lymphocytes[b]	cpm in AB Serum[c]	Autologous Serum[c] (% of Stimulation in AB Serum)	Responder Lymphocytes[a]	Stimulator Lymphocytes[b]	cpm in AB Serum[c]	Autologous Serum[c] (% of Stimulation in AB Serum)
Women				Women			
1	—	400	115	11	—	314	91
	Own husband	25623	42		Own husband	41107	55
	Pool	41428	65		Pool	42818	18
2	—	1635	132	12	—	667	105
	Own husband	73777	38		Own husband	73777	65
	Pool	41653	71		Pool	41654	41
3	—	4200	96	13	—	1647	87
	Own husband	82200	111		Own husband	60553	161
	Pool	92428	103		Pool	52709	95
4	—	425	128	14	—	1564	94
	Own husband	17959	76		Own husband	44775	123
	Pool	34427	43		Pool	250774	117
5	—	1259	155	15	—	1791	116
	Own husband	62505	74		Own husband	83155	36
	Pool	42169	59		Pool	76459	21
6	—	679	108	16	—	3659	133
	Own husband	34258	144		Own husband	78924	39
	Pool	48519	112		Pool	91932	46
7	—	1259	89	17	—	473	152
	Own husband	72917	122		Own husband	29942	18
	Pool	84215	139		Pool	84421	80
8	—	318	141	18	—	987	85
	Own husband	54156	24		Own husband	141180	143
	Pool	92818	57		Pool	105492	109
9	—	1250	88	19	—	893	126
	Own husband	116790	46		Own husband	59004	23
	Pool	201123	32		Pool	201135	19
10	—	1647	157				
	Own husband	95150	129				
	Pool	68617	86				

[a] 2×10^5 cell/well. [b] Cells treated with mitomycin C, 2×10^5/well. [c] Mean of sextuplet.

following assisted reproductive techniques; 2) women with repeated (n ≥ 3) unsuccessful embryo transfers either uterine or tubal. Informed consent was obtained from 19 women: 12 in group A and 7 in group B. The Intra-Venous Immunoglobulin (IVIG) protocol we have adopted has been: 20g of human Ig from a pool of 100 donors (Endobulin, Immuno) in slow infusion at the beginning of ovarian hyperstimulation by exogenous gonadotropins for IVF, followed by a second dose of 15g at the moment of positive β-HCG and then every 3 weeks up to week 20. The blocking capacity of sera was investigated in one way mixed lymphocytes culture (MLC): lymphocytes were separated by Ficoll gradient centrifugation and then transferred in RPMI supplemented with 10% serum; all sera from patients were heat inactivated; the inhibition exerted by each single serum was determined as a percentage of the response in AB serum (100 × cpm in own serum/cpm in AB serum).

RESULTS AND DISCUSSION

By using the IVIG technique, as reported in TABLE 1, we have obtained 9 pregnancies out of a total of 19 treated women. Five of these have an ongoing pregnancy (between 8 and 20 weeks), 2 have had a biochemically detectable pregnancy and 2 a very early abortion (within 8 weeks). Four out of the 5 pregnant women had an abnormal one way MLC suggesting a deficient blocking activity in the serum. These very preliminary results seem to show a positive effect of IVIG treatment in these indications of 55.5% (5 out of 9) in a population with a well documented inability to obtain a successful implantation. Considering the MLC results (TABLE 2) we can observe a significantly higher success rate of IVIG treatment in those patients with a presumptive lower serum blocking activity. Furthermore, the IVIG technique has some important advantages over the other immunization techniques, such as simplicity of use and the absence of major side effects,[10] particularly long-term ones, both on the mother and on the fetus.

REFERENCES

1. MILLER, J. F., E. WILLIAMSON, Y. G. GORDON, J. G. GRUDZINSKAS & A. SYKES. 1980. Fetal loss after implantation: A prospective study. Lancet **1:** 554.
2. EDMONDS, D. K., K. S. LINDSAY, J. F. MILLER, E. WILLIAMSON & P. J. WOOD. 1982. Early embryonic mortality in women. Fertil. Steril. **38:** 447.
3. BEER, A. E. 1983. Immunopathologic factors contributing to recurrent spontaneous abortions in humans. Am. J. Reprod. Immunol. **4:** 182.
4. THOMAS, M. L., J. M. HARGER, D. K. WAGENER, B. S. RABIN & T. J. GILL. 1985. HLA sharing and spontaneous abortions in humans. Am. J. Obstet. Gynecol. **151:** 1053.
5. FAULK, W. P. & J. A. MCINTYRE. 1987. Role of anti-TLX antibody in human pregnancy. *In* Reproductive Immunology. D. A. Clark & B. A. Croy, Eds.: 106. Amsterdam, Elsevier Science Publications.
6. BEER, A. E. 1988. Sem. Reprod. Endocrinol. **6:** 162. Thieme Medical Publishers.
7. UNANDER, A. M. & A. LINDHOLM. 1986. Transfusions of leukocyte-rich erythrocyte concentrates: A successful treatment in selected cases of habitual abortions. Am. J. Obstet. Gynecol. **154:** 516.
8. JOHNSON, P. M., K. V. CHIA, C. A. HART, M. B. GRIFFITH & W. J. A. FRANCIS. 1988. Trophoblast membrane infusion for unexplained recurrent miscarriage. Br. J. Obstet. Gynecol. **95:** 342.
9. MUELLER-ECKHARDT, G., O. HEINE, J. NEPPERT, W. KUNZEL & C. MUELLER-ECKHARDT. 1989. Treatment of recurrent spontaneous abortion (RSA) by intravenous immunoglobulin (IVIG):

A pilot study. J. Reprod. Immunol. (Suppl. July) 4th International Congress of Reproductive Immunology; Abstract book, p. 113.

10. VARGA, P. J., Z. SZEREDAY, A. ARTNER & J. SZEKERES-BARTHO. 1989. Early pregnancy loss, premature and low birth weight delivery, and increased maternal lymphocyte cytotoxicity. Am. J. Reprod. Immunol. **19**: 136.

Steroid Therapy and the Endometrium: Biological and Clinical Implications

L. DE CECCO,[a,b] M. LEONE, D. GERBALDO,
P. L. VENTURINI, R. RISSONE, AND
M. MESSENI LEONE[c]

[b] Department of Obstetrics and Gynecology
[c] Department of Histology and Embryology
University of Genoa
Genoa, Italy

INTRODUCTION

Estrogen replacement therapy in postmenopausal women remains one of the most controversial issues in medicine, despite its widespread use for more than 40 years.[1,2] Exogenous estrogens are universally considered an established and effective treatment, not only for the acute symptoms of estrogen deficiency but also for prevention of longer-term problems such as osteoporosis, genitourinary atrophy, and cardiovascular diseases.[3-6] At the same time however, the appearance of cancer of the endometrium in estrogenically conditioned patients has been reported since 1960.[7] This prompted the addition of the natural antagonist of estrogen, progesterone, to the estrogen replacement therapy, but controversies still exist on the best progestogen to be chosen and its dosage to reduce the incidence of endometrial hyperstimulation and irregular vaginal bleeding.[8,9] Moreover we observed, like other authors, a marked interpatient variation in histological response to steroid replacement therapy.[2,10]

In this report we examined the relationship between histological findings and immunocytochemical evaluation of estradiol receptor (Er), progesterone receptor (Pr) and epidermal growth factor receptor (EGFr) during steroid replacement therapy (SRT), in order to evaluate the effect of steroids on the autocrine and paracrine regulation of menopausal endometrium.

MATERIALS AND METHODS

Nineteen women were recruited from the Menopause Center of the Department of Obstetrics and Gynecology of the University of Genoa. The average age of the subjects was 53 years; all had undergone a natural menopause and were within 20% of their ideal body weight. They were all between 2 and 3 years of their last menstrual period. Complete history and physical examination were unremarkable. All patients had a pretreatment endometrial biopsy for histological evaluation and then were di-

[a] Address for reprint requests and correspondence: Prof. Luigi De Cecco, Clinica Ostetrica e Ginecologica, Padiglione 1 Ospedale San Martino, Viale Benedetto XV, 1, 16132 Genova, Italia.

vided randomly into two groups. In group A (11 patients) Estraderm 50 µg patches (Ciba Geigy SA, Basel, Switzerland) were applied from days 1–21 of a 28-day cycle and 10 mg oral medroxyprogesterone acetate were added to the last 12 days. Group B received 0.625 mg oral conjugated equine estrogens from days 1–21 of a 28 day cycle and 10 mg oral medroxyprogesterone acetate for the last 12 days. During cycle days 22–28 the patients received no medication, and the cycle was restarted on day 1. The patients were instructed to record the onset of any vaginal bleeding. Endometrial samples were obtained with a curette from the anterior fundal region of the uterine cavity between days 17–18 of the sixth cycle of therapy. Two biopsies were obtained to assure adequate tissue for both histological review and immunocytochemical evaluation of Er, Pr and EGFr.

Immunocytochemistry

The tissue was quick-frozen on dry ice and stored at $-70\,°C$ until analyzed. Cryostate sections 8µ thick were cut and then thawed, mounted into gelatin coated glass slides, and fixed in 3.7% formaldeheide in 0.1 M/L phosphate-buffered saline (PBS) for 10 minutes. Slides were then transferred to PBS and treated with blocking reagent in the moist incubation chamber to reduce the non-specific binding of subsequent reagent. Immunostaining was performed by the peroxidase anti-peroxidase method (PAP) using a kit from Abbott Laboratories (Rome, Italy) in which the solution containing Er antibody and that containing Pr antibody were alternatively used. Duplicate sections were lightly counterstained with hematoxyline to facilitate the identification of the cells. The sites of the immunoreactive EGFr were localized using the alkaline phosphatase anti-alkaline phosphatase (APAAP) immunostaining technique (kit 67c, Dako Corp. Santa Barbara, CA, USA) with a monoclonal antibody anti-EGFr (Biomakor, Rehovot, Israel).

The resultant staining was evaluated by the distribution of staining within each tissue component and the intensity of the staining. The intensity of staining was assigned the following scores: 0 = none; 1 = weak; 2 = distinct; and 3 = strong. The histochemical score (HSCORE) was calculated as in the previous report of Lessey *et al.*,[11] using the following equation: HSCORE = Pi (i + 1) where Pi was the percentage of stained cells and i the intensity of staining. The same immunocytochemical evaluation was also performed on 5 endometrial samples obtained from premenopausal women, during proliferative phase of the menstrual cycle, undergoing hysterectomy for leyomiomata, as control. Estradiol serum levels were evaluated for each patient on the day of endometrial sampling.

RESULTS

Histological Findings

The histological patterns of pretreatment biopsies revealed atrophic endometrium (17 cases) or proliferative endometrium (2 cases). At the sixth cycle of treatment, group A endometria were atrophic (3 cases), atrophic with edematous stroma (3 cases), proliferative (2 cases), hyperplastic (2 cases) and secretive (1 case). In group B, 2 atrophic

TABLE 1. Histological Findings and Number of Cases Immunoreactive for Er, Pr and EGFr before Treatment and after Six Cycles of SRT Therapy both Percutaneous (TTS) and Oral (ECE)

Time	Histological Findings	N+ Immunoreactive Cases		
		EGFr	Er	Pr
TTS				
Pre-treatment	9 (A)[a]	0	0	0
	2 (P)	0	2	0
Post-treatment	3 (A)	0	0	0
	3 (ES)	0	3	3
	2 (P)	2	2	2
	2 (H)	2	2	2
	1 (S)	1	1	1
ECE				
Pre-treatment	8 (A)	0	0	0
Post-treatment	2 (A)	0	0	0
	2 (ES)	0	2	1
	2 (P)	2	2	2
	1 (H)	1	1	1
	1 (S)	1	1	1

[a] *Abbreviations:* A = atrophic; P = proliferative; ES = edematous stroma; H = hyperplastic; S = secretive.

endometria, 2 atrophic endometria with edematous stroma, 2 proliferative endometria, 1 hyperplastic endometrium and 1 secretive were observed (TABLE 1). In all cases we found some areas with these histological characteristics in the context of inactive endometrium.

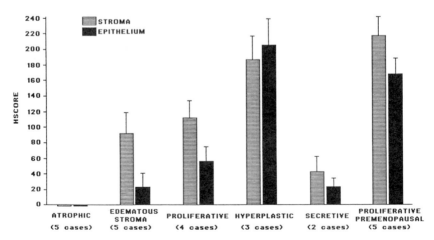

FIGURE 1. Er content of glandular epithelium and stroma in endometrium after the sixth cycle of SRT (both percutaneous and oral) using immunocytochemical analysis and mean HSCORE ($\pm$SE).

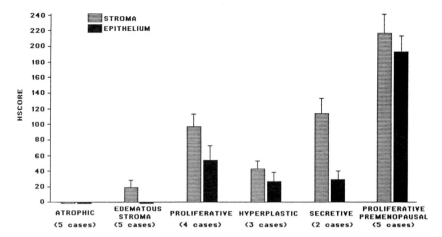

FIGURE 2. Pr content of glandular epithelium and stroma in endometrium after the sixth cycle of SRT (both percutaneous and oral) using immunocytochemical analysis and mean HSCORE (±SE).

Immunocytochemical Evaluation

Immunocytochemical staining detected well-defined patterns of receptor localization and the counterstaining with hematoxilin permitted us to clearly identify glandular cells and stromal cells.

Er and Pr were always localized within the nuclei. After six months of SRT, only atrophic endometria (5 cases) were negative for Er by immunocytochemistry (FIG. 1). H-score was always lower, however, except hyperplasia, than in normal proliferative endometrium (days 10–14 of menstrual cycle) from premenopausal women.

Pr were increased after SRT in proliferative, hyperplastic and secretive endometria, but were always lower than in normal proliferative endometrium (FIG. 2).

EGFr were always localized on the cell membranes of the endometrium, principally on the luminal surface of the glands. H-score of this growth factor receptor was increased only in proliferative, hyperplastic and secretive endometria with lower levels than in normal proliferative tissue and with the highest levels in hyperplastic endometrium (FIG. 3).

Bleeding Patterns

SRT induced both in group A patients and in group B patients withdrawal bleeding, but 15 patients had breakthrough bleeding independently of the histological findings. There was no relation between histological findings and circulating estradiol levels.

DISCUSSION

The immunocytochemical techniques used in this study permitted us to evaluate receptor distribution, both within cells and between coexistent cell types in the same target tissue.

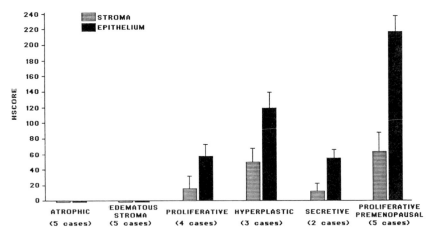

FIGURE 3. EGFr content of glandular epithelium and stroma in endometrium after the sixth cycle of SRT (both percutaneous and oral) using immunocytochemical analysis and mean HSCORE ($\pm$SE).

We observed the nuclear localization of Er and Pr as previously reported by King and Greene[12] and the localization of EGFr on cell membranes as biochemically demonstrated in the rat by Mukku and Stancel.[13]

Er and EGFr seemed to be related to the estrogen-induced modifications of the endometrium. The highest H-score for Er and EGFr was in fact found in hyperplastic endometria and the endometria which remained inactive after six months of SRT were not immunoreactive.

Interestingly hyperplastic endometrium also, showed lower H-score for Er and EGFr than normal proliferative endometrium from premenopausal women. These could be due to a dishomogeneous estrogenic priming of the endometrium. This hypothesis may be sustained by the observation of hyperplastic areas in the context of inactive endometrium.

However the presence of Er, EGFr and also Pr in these hyperplastic endometria induce us to consider these histological findings as hormone dependent; further studies should be performed to evaluate whether this SRT-induced hyperplasia has the same risks of malignant transformation as the hormone independent.

The highest levels of Pr were detected in secretive endometria. The levels were lower than in normal proliferative endometrium and we ascribe this result to the dishomogeneous response of the endometrium.

Our results suggest that the functional response of endometrium to SRT may be determined in part by fluctuations of Er and Pr levels, and in part by the action of epidermal growth factor through its receptors in the epithelial compartment.

SUMMARY

The benefits of estrogen replacement therapy in postmenopausal women include increased quality of life, relief from specific symptoms, and the prevention of osteoporosis, genitourinary atrophy, and cardiovascular diseases. Despite these advantages, this therapy has been reported to be associated with an increased frequency of endometrial hyperplasia and adenocarcinoma. In order to evaluate a possible relationship between the histological findings and stroma-derived growth regulators, 19 endometrial samples obtained from women undergoing both percutaneous ($n = 11$) and oral ($n = 8$) steroid replacement therapy were processed for histological and immunocytochemical evaluation of estrogen receptor (Er), progesterone receptor (Pr), and epidermal growth factor receptor (EGFr). Transdermal estradiol was given for 21 days and 10mg medroxyprogesterone acetate (MAP) were added to the last 12 days; conjugated equine estrogens were given for 21 days and 10mg MAP added to the last 12 days. Endometrial samples were obtained between days 17–18 of the sixth month of therapy.

Proliferative and hyperplastic endometria showed immunoreactivity against Er, Pr, and EGFr. Atrophic endometria were always negative by immunocytochemistry.

Our results suggest: 1) a relationship between histological findings and the receptor examined; 2) a crucial role for EGF in the regulation of endometrial proliferation.

REFERENCES

1. GUSBERG, S. B. 1947. Precursors of corpus carcinoma estrogens and adenomatous hyperplasia. Am. J. Obstet. Gynecol. **54:** 905–910.
2. FRASER, D. I., A. PARSONS, M. I. WHITEHEAD, J. WORDSWORTH, G. STUART & J. PRYSE-DAVIES. 1990. The optimal dose of oral norethindrone acetate for addition to transdermal estradiol: A multicenter study. Fertil. Steril. **53 (3):** 460–468.
3. STEINGOLD, K. A., L. LAUFER, R. J. CHETKOWSKI, J. D. DE FAZIO, D. W. MATT, D. R. MELDRUM & H. L. JUDD. 1985. Treatment of hot flashes with transdermal estradiol administration. J. Clin. Endocrinol. Metab. **61 (4):** 627–632.
4. HORSMAN, A., J. C. GALLAGHER, M. SIMPSON & B. E. C. NORDIN. 1977. Prospective trial of oestrogen and calcium in postmenopausal women. Br. Med. J. **2:** 789–792.
5. JUDD, H. L., R. E. CLEARY & W. T. CREASMAN. 1981. Estrogen replacement therapy. Obstet. Gynecol. **58:** 267–272.
6. ROSS, R. K., A. PAGANINI-HILL & T. M. MACK. 1981. Menopausal oestrogen therapy and protection from death from ischaemic heart disease. Lancet **1:** 858–863.
7. GUSBERG, S. B. & R. E. HALL. 1961. Precursors of corpus cancer: III. The appearance of cancer of the endometrium in estrogenically conditioned patients. Obstet. Gynecol. **17:** 397–412.
8. GELFAND, M. M. & A. FERENCZY. 1989. A prospective 1-year study of estrogen and progestin in postmenopausal women: Effects on the endometrium. Obstet. Gynecol. **74 (3):** 398–402.
9. GERBALDO, D., A. FERRAIOLO, R. CUROTTO, L. BERNARDINI, A. TRUINI & G. PESCETTO. 1989. Problematiche nella valutazione dell'endometrio post menopausale. Proceedings of *Isteroscopia e microisteroscopia oggi e domani.* Vicenza. Italy.
10. GEOFFREY, L., N. C. SIDDLE, T. A. RYDER, J. PRYSE-DAVIES & M. I. WHITEHEAD. 1986. Is provera the ideal progestogen for addition to postmenopausal estrogen therapy? Fertil. Steril. **45 (3):** 345–352.
11. LESSEY, B. A., A. P. KILLAM, D. A. METZEGER, A. F. HANEY, G. L. GREENE & K. S. McCARTY, JR. 1988. Immunohistochemical analysis of human uterine estrogen and progesterone receptors throughout the menstrual cycle. J. Clin. Endocrinol. Metab. **67 (2):** 334–340.
12. KING, W. J. & G. L. GREENE. 1984. Monoclonal antibodies localize oestrogen receptor in the nuclei of target cells. Nature **307:** 745–751.
13. MUKKU, V. R. & G. M. STANCEL. 1985. Receptors for epidermal growth factor in the rat uterus. Endocrinology **117:** 149–154.

Prevention of Postmenopausal Bone Loss and Endometrial Responses during a Two Year Prospective Study with Transdermal 17β-Estradiol and Oral Medroxyprogesterone Acetate

PIERO FIORETTI,[a] MARCO GAMBACCIANI,
ADRIANA SPINETTI, ANGELO CAGNACCI,
ANNA MARIA PAOLETTI, RENATO FELIPETTO,
AND GIAN BENEDETTO MELIS

Department of Obstetrics and Gynecology
University of Pisa, School of Medicine
Via Roma 67
56100 Pisa, Italy

INTRODUCTION

The effectiveness of oral estrogen in the prevention of postmenopausal osteoporosis is now well established.[1-3] However, the possibility of adverse metabolic effects can limit the prescription of hormone replacement therapy over the postmenopausal years.[4-7] Oral administration can induce undesirable effects on liver metabolism, and can result in subjective side effects due to estrogen overdoses.[4] In fact, most side effects and risks of estrogen replacement therapy seem to be dose- and duration dependent. Particularly, unopposed estrogen administration stimulates endometrial cells, potentially leading to endometrial hyperstimulation and hyperplasia.[4] A proliferative endometrium can progress to a cystic and adenomatous hyperplasia, that has been reported as a premalignant state. The likelihood of developing endometrial hyperplasia is directly related to the dose of estrogen.[4-7] Progestogen co-therapy can avoid the estrogen-induced endometrial hyperplasia and thus sequential progestins are prescribed in patients undergoing estrogen replacement therapy.[4-7] The recent possibility of administering 17β-estradiol via transdermal patches offers the main advantage of avoiding the first pass in the liver using low doses of the main physiological estrogen.[8,9]

The aim of this study was to evaluate the endometrial effects of transdermal estradiol plus medroxyprogesterone acetate administration and their effectiveness in the prevention of bone loss in postmenopausal women (PMW).

---

[a] Author to whom correspondence should be addressed.

MATERIALS AND METHODS

In the present study we included 37 PMW who were referred to the Menopause Clinic of our Department for the evaluation of bone mass and preventive proposals. Their mean age was 53.2 years (ranging from 47 to 60 years). All patients were post-menopausal as defined by amenorrhea for at least 6 months, a negative progesterone challenge test and plasma estradiol levels less than 25 pg/ml. The interval since the menopause was less than 6 years in all cases. Subjective symptoms were evaluated with a visuoanalogic scale (0 = no symptom, 20 = as bad as it could be). Clinical examination, mammography, blood and urine sampling, endometrial biopsy (Vabra curettage) and bone mass measurement were performed before treatment and, except mammography, every six months for the two years of therapy.

The transdermal estradiol patches were prescribed for three weeks, followed by one treatment-free week (n = 25). Each patch was designed to deliver 0.05 mg of estradiol per day, and each patch was applied for 3 days. Patients were advised to stick the patches on the lower abdomen, buttocks or thighs. Oral medroxyprogesterone acetate (MPA) 10 mg/day was prescribed daily for the first ten days of each calendar month. The control group consisted in 12 PMW receiving an oral calcium supplementation (500 mg/day). Bone density was determined by dual proton absorptiometry (I 125, Am 241, Osteoden/P NIM, Verona, Italy) obtaining quadruplicate readings at distal radius of non-dominant arm. The intra- and intermeasurement coefficients of variation were less than 2% and 3%, respectively.

Statistical analysis of the results was performed by ANOVA followed by Duncan's test, as appropriate.

RESULTS

All patients completed the study. TABLE 1 shows the endometrial findings in the hormone-treated subjects. At the pretreatment assessment no endometrium, insufficient tissue or atrophic endometrium was obtained from 13 patients. During therapy pro-liferative endometrium was the most common finding. There was no evidence of hyper-plasia in any sample (TABLE 1).

The number of days of bleeding is shown in TABLE 2. Every patient experienced withdrawal bleeding during the study. Three patients reported breakthrough bleeding

TABLE 1. Endometrial Histologic Findings before and during Cyclic Sequential Transdermal Estradiol/MPA Therapy in 25 Postmenopausal Women

	Months		
Endometrium	0	12	24
Proliferative	10	5	10
Secretory	0	5	5
Hyperplasia	2	0	0
Atrophic	6	8	5
Insufficient tissue	4	5	4
No tissue	3	2	1
TOTAL	25	25	25

TABLE 2. Characteristics of Withdrawal Bleeding in 25 PMW Patients during Transdermal Estradiol/MPA Therapy

	Months		
	6	12	24
Number of patients with bleeding	25	25	25
Number days of bleeding	5.4 ± 1.4	4.0 ± 1.8	4.0 ± 1.2
Amount of bleeding (score)	7.5 ± 2.5	6.0 ± 2.0	5.6 ± 2.0

in the first 6 months of treatment. No patient reported heavy bleeding. The majority of bleedings were moderate in intensity and predictable in duration.

Treatment with transdermal estradiol/MPA caused a slight but significant fall ($p < 0.05$) in urinary hydroxyproline excretion (TABLE 3), in comparison to the untreated controls. In the control group a significant ($p < 0.05$) decrease in forearm bone density was evident after 12 months of observation. Conversely, no significant changes in bone density was observed in the 2 year follow-up during transdermal estradiol/MPA administration (TABLE 3).

As for the side effects, five out of 25 women treated with estradiol patches developed mild skin reaction, compatible with the continuation of treatment. No other relevant side effects were reported from transdermal estradiol/MPA-treated subjects.

DISCUSSION

The results of this 2-year prospective study show that transdermal estradiol plus MPA administration is effective in preventing postmenopausal bone loss. In addition, present results confirm that the calcium supplementation alone, at least at the doses used in this study, does not prevent postmenopausal bone loss.[10]

Previous studies reported that percutaneous 17β-estradiol administration can prevent postmenopausal bone loss when it is associated with high plasma levels of 17β-estradiol (150–200 pg/mL).[11] Conversely, other authors recently reported that even

TABLE 3. Hydroxyproline (OH-P) Urinary Excretion (mg/24 h) and Distal Forearm Bone Density (BD, mg/cm^2) before and during Treatment with Calcium (controls, n=12) or Transdermal Estradiol/MPA (TTS + MPA, n=25)

	Months		
	0	12	24
OH-P			
Controls	26 ± 3	29 ± 4	30 ± 5
TTS + MPA	25 ± 3	17 ± 2^a	15 ± 3^a
B.D.			
Controls	415 ± 30	390 ± 25^a	385 ± 38^a
TTS + MPA	405 ± 28	414 ± 32	420 ± 29

^{a} $p < 0.05$ vs. corresponding pretreatment value.

the administration of lower doses of transdermal estradiol can effectively prevent the bone remodeling observed in the postmenopausal state.[12]. Our findings confirm and extend these last results, supporting the contention that the low dose (0.05 mg/day) estradiol administration can be considered effective in the prevention of postmenopausal bone loss.

The daily estradiol dose by the transdermal patch is lower than the doses usually prescribed by means of oral preparations, but is highly effective in the cure and prevention of the postmenopausal signs and symptoms.[8,9] Most clinical regimens relieve subjective symptoms, but they do differ with respect to estrogenic potency and metabolic response in various organs.[4-7]

In the mid-1980s different authors compared the clinical and endocrinological effects of transdermal estradiol with those of oral estrogen preparations, namely conjugated estrogens.[8,9] These studies demonstrated that transdermal estradiol patches provide plasma level of estradiol similar to those of early follicular phase, a physiological estradiol/estrone ratio, and does not induce estradiol accumulation.[8,9] In addition, transdermal estradiol prevents the metabolic consequences of first pass hepatic metabolism. Since an increased risk of hypertension, cholelithiasis and intravascular clotting may be considered the results of estrogen hepatic effects, transdermal estradiol administration can be seen as a step forward for a more widespread use of hormone replacement therapy in the PMW.

Protection against endometrial hyperstimulation is one of the most important goals in the study of an "ideal" hormone replacement schedule for postmenopausal women.[4] Continuous and combined estrogen-progestin therapy is effective in relieving menopausal symptoms, and prevents bone loss.[13] In addition, combined estroprogestin preparations induce endometrial atrophy in most patients, and thus prevent unwanted endometrial proliferations.[13] However, it is well known that all progestins may cause physical, metabolic, and psychological side effects. The long-term metabolic effects of continous progestogen administration need further evaluation since no data are available on the effects of continuous estroprogestin preparations on lipids and lipoproteins.[13]

In this view, the cyclical low-dose MPA administration in combination with low-dose transdermal estradiol can offer some advantages. The cyclical transdermal estradiol induces a mild endometrial proliferation in most patients, and the addition of a low dose progestogen produces an acceptable bleeding pattern, and is not associated with any degree of endometrial hyperplasia.

In conclusion present study shows that transdermal estradiol associated with MPA results in a maintenance of bone mass in postmenopausal women, inducing a safe and balanced endometrial stimulation.

REFERENCES

1. NACHTINGALL, L. E., R. H. NACHTINGALL & R. D. NACHTINGALL. 1979. Obstet. Gynecol. **53:** 277–281.
2. LINDSAY, R., D. M. HART & J. M. AITKEN. 1976. Lancet **1:** 1038–1042.
3. LINDSAY, R., D. M. HART & C. FARREST. 1980. Lancet **2:** 1151–1154.
4. HAMMOND, C. B. & W. S. MAXSON. 1986. Clin. Obstet. Gynecol. **29:** 407–430.
5. WHITEHEAD, M. I. & D. FRASER. 1987. Am. J. Obstet. Gynecol. **156:** 1313–1322.
6. DON GAMBRELL, R. 1987. Am. J. Obstet. Gynecol. **156:** 1304–1313.
7. ETTINGER, B. 1988. Obstet. Gynecol. **72:** 31S–36S.

8. PADWICK, M. I., J. ENDACOTT & M. I. WHITEHEAD. 1985. Am. J. Obstet. Gynecol. **152:** 1085–1091.
9. POWERS, M. S., L. SCHEWKEL, P. E. DARLEY, W. R. GOOD, J. C. BALESTRA & V. A. PLACE. 1985. Am. J. Obstet. Gynecol. **152:** 1099–1106.
10. NILAS, L., C. CHRISTIANSEN & P. RØDBRO. 1984. Br. Med. J. **289:** 1103–1106.
11. RIIS, B. J., D. THOMNSEN, V. STROM & C. CHRISTIANSEN. 1987. Am. J. Obstet. Gynecol. **156:** 61–65.
12. RIBOT, C., F. TREMOLLIERS, J. M. POUILLES, J. P. LOUVET & R. PEYRON. 1990. Obstet. Gynecol. **75(4):** 42S–46S.
13. WHITEHEAD, M. I., T. C. HILLARD & D. CROOK. 1990. Obstet. Gynecol. **75(4):** 59S–76S.

Estrogen, Calcium Metabolism and the Skeleton[a]

ROBERT LINDSAY AND FELICIA COSMAN

Department of Medicine
Columbia University
College of Physicians and Surgeons
New York, New York 10032

and

Department of Internal Medicine
Helen Hayes Hospital
West Haverstraw, New York 10993

INTRODUCTION

Osteoporosis is an intrinsic disorder of the skeleton, in which skeletal tissue is lost, resulting in low bone mass with an accompanying increase in the risk of fracture. The most common form of the disorder is seen in postmenopausal women. Albright[1] originally drew our attention to this some 50 years ago, yet even today there is speculation about the precise role of the menopause and estrogen in particular in the pathogenesis of the disorder. Since prevention of osteoporotic fracture is important in terms of public health,[2] it is most appropriate to consider this issue in a conference principally devoted to a discussion of the endometrium, since sex steroids appear to be powerful mediators of skeletal function and potent preventive agents for osteoporotic fracture.[3] Thus, osteoporosis prevention and treatment is an important indication for long-term therapy of the postmenopausal female with sex steroids. Their effects on the skeleton must, therefore, be considered in any discussion of the endometrial stimulation that may result from their use over several years.[4] This article reviews the evidence that sex steroid deficiency is important in the pathogenesis of osteoporosis and evaluates the beneficial effects that might be achieved with long-term therapy, considering only the skeleton as the clinical outcome.

PATHOGENESIS

Although descriptions of osteoporosis can be found in the medical literature dating back to the writings of Hippocrates, it was not until the elegant clinical studies of Albright that the relationship between ovarian failure and osteoporosis was clearly enunciated. Albright noted the increased frequency of oophorectomy among patients with osteoporotic fracture and postulated that estrogen deficiency was a principal causative factor in the skeletal changes that resulted in these fractures. Furthermore, he used estrogen as treatment for the disorder,[5] and postulated that its effects were

[a] Supported in part by NIH Grant AR39191.

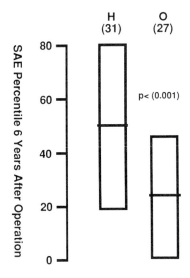

FIGURE 1. The effect of oophorectomy on bone mass in young women. H represents bone mass (mean ± SD) in premenopausal women 6 years after hysterectomy (n = 31) with ovarian conservation. O represents results from 27 women 6 years after oophorectomy.

mediated through osteoblasts, the bone-synthesizing cells. It was not until the development of techniques that allowed non-invasive estimation of bone mass in the 1960s that further investigation of the relationship between ovarian failure and skeletal metabolism could be examined in more detail.

In our early studies we demonstrated that bone mass was lower among women who had been oophorectomized prior to normal age of menopause, when compared to women of similar age who had had hysterectomy with ovarian conservation[6] (FIG. 1). Prospective data confirmed that these women were losing bone at a rate faster than either premenopausal or hysterectomized women who still had endogenous ovarian function. The rate of loss of skeletal tissue was correlated with the production of estrogen,[7] presumably from peripheral conversion of adrenal androgens. As a consequence obesity tended to be associated with a somewhat slower rate of bone loss, confirming the clinical impression that obesity is protective against osteoporotic fracture.[8]

In a somewhat similar study, Richelson and her colleagues[9] demonstrated that 50-year-old women oophorectomized on average twenty years previously had bone mass similar to women 70 years of age who had gone through a natural menopause at the average age of 50. Thus, the number of years spent in the postmenopausal state is more important in determining skeletal status than absolute age.

Prospective data from other studies have confirmed our observation that rate of loss is dependent on endogenous estrogen supply.[10] There appear to be differences in the sensitivity of different parts of the skeleton to estrogen withdrawal, with bone loss being seen earlier in the primarily trabecular bone of the spine (prior to overt menopause) and later in cortical bone. Circulating levels of 17β-estradiol below 40 pg/ml appear to be critical, resulting in bone loss at almost all sites in the skeleton.[10,11]

Animal data also support the concept that ovarian removal results in loss of bone tissue, even though no entirely satisfactory model for osteoporosis has been described.

Data from rodents and dogs indicate increased loss of bone in oophorectomized animals when compared with sham operated groups.[12,13]

The elegant studies of Heaney[14-16] have demonstrated that there occur across the menopause significant changes in calcium movement into and out of the skeleton. However, the increment in efflux of calcium from bone was found to be greater than the increase in influx and thus net bone loss occurs. These alterations in skeletal metabolism are accompanied by reduction in the efficiency of calcium absorption across the intestine and increased excretion of calcium in urine. Thus the postmenopausal state creates inefficiency in the utilization of dietary calcium. The primary mechanism is thought to be occurring within the skeleton since primary alterations in calcium homeostasis in the gut or kidney would produce different secondary responses in the organism (FIG. 2) than those occurring in the postmenopausal state.

Bone loss has been found in all postmenopausal populations studied. Recent data suggest that bone mass measurements can be used clinically to determine individual susceptibility to fracture.[17,18] Fracture prevalence and incidence are clearly related to bone mass. In prospective studies, a single determination of bone mass predicts the risk of future fracture. These data are important since they support assessment of individual patients for fracture risk during the asymptomatic phase of bone loss, or around the time of menopause. The high risk population can therefore be targeted for intervention.

PREVENTION

Given the ubiquitous nature of the studies demonstrating loss of bone mass among postmenopausal women, it is perhaps not surprising that estrogen therapy reduces the rate of bone loss in this population.[19-22] In our original controlled studies, we demonstrated that estrogen intervention completely inhibited bone loss measured by

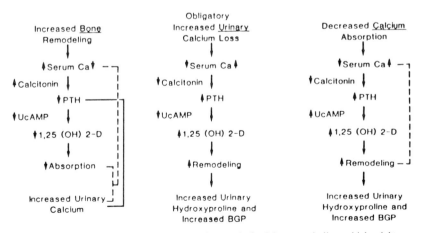

FIGURE 2. Postulated impairments in hormonal control of calcium metabolism which might occur after menopause and account for the observed changes in mineral and skeletal homeostasis.

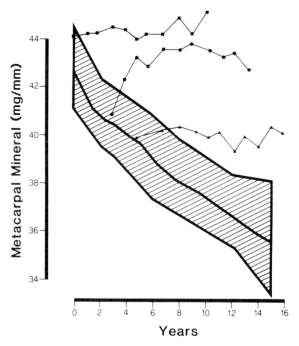

FIGURE 3. Long-term prevention of bone loss by estrogen. The hatched area represents the placebo (mean ± SD) using a prospective controlled study in oophorectomized women. The 3 lines show the mean values only for 3 estrogen-treated groups; treatment initiated at the time of oophorectomy (*squares*), 3 years after (*circles*), or 6 years after oophorectomy (*triangles*). Bone loss is prevented in all 3 situations, however, the earlier treatment is begun, the better the outcome, in terms of bone mass after 10 years of therapy. (From LINDSAY, R. 1988. *In* Osteoporosis II: 508–512. Used with permission.)

single photon absorptiometry. Estrogen effects were not dependent on the elapsed time between ovarian failure and the introduction of treatment.[23] In the early data, we examined the effects in women up to six years after ovarian failure (FIG. 3), and more recently have shown estrogen effects in women up to 75 years of age with an average duration of 12 years after menopause. The effects persist for as long as therapy is given, at least up to 15 years. When treatment is discontinued, bone loss begins again at a rate that is parallel to that seen immediately after oophorectomy.[24] Numerous other studies have confirmed our findings.

The biochemical sequelae in calcium homeostasis seen following ovarian failure are reversed by estrogen therapy. There is improvement in calcium transport across the intestine and reduction in calcium loss through the kidney.[14–16] Biochemical indicators of skeletal remodeling are reduced by estrogens, demonstrating their important effects on bone. Again, these biochemical sequelae are evident for as long as treatment is provided.[20]

The skeleton appears to be extremely sensitive to exogenous estrogen. The minimum effective dose for conjugated equine estrogen, the most commonly used estrogen

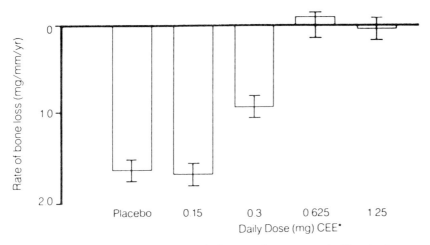

FIGURE 4. Rates of bone loss during 2 years in 5 groups of women treated with a placebo or one of several doses of conjugated equine estrogens. (From LINDSAY, R., *et al.* 1984. Obstet. Gynecol. **63**: 759. Used with permission.)

for replacement therapy (FIG. 4) in the USA, is 0.625 mg/day.[25] Data also show that other estrogens that increase circulating 17β-estradiol levels above 40 pg/ml may provide sufficient estrogen to reduce the rate of bone loss. The route of administration is not important, and all routes are effective if sufficient estrogen is provided.[26]

A number of epidemiological studies have demonstrated that provision of estrogen to postmenopausal women is associated with a reduction in the risk of osteoporotic fracture.[27-29] The best documented is the reduction in the risk of hip fractures, which are the most important of the osteoporotic fractures in terms of their public health impact. The data available suggest that estrogen exposure is associated with a reduction in risk of about 50%. Perhaps not surprisingly the most beneficial effects are seen when estrogens are introduced close to menopause. The required duration of treatment to demonstrate effects on hip fracture risk appears to be 5–10 years. Reduction in risk for Colles' fracture has also been shown in epidemiological data. It has been more difficult, however, to demonstrate prevention of vertebral crush fractures, principally since many of these are asymptomatic and even when associated with sudden back pain, rarely require hospital admission. One cross-sectional evaluation of chest radiographs obtained in postmenopausal women enrolled in a Health Maintenance Program found a reduction in vertebral fracture prevalence of about 60%.[30] Our prospective data suggested that long-term estrogen therapy is associated with almost a 90% reduction in radiographic vertebral abnormalities.[20]

TREATMENT

Comparatively few studies have addressed treatment of established osteoporosis, although estrogens have been approved for use in this disorder for some time. Two groups have shown that estrogens can retard bone loss in patients at least up to 70 years of age.[31,32] Recently we completed a controlled study of estrogen intervention in patients with the established syndrome.[33] We compared estrogen (given with a progestogen to patients with an intact uterus) and calcium supplementation to bring total intake to 1500 mg/day with calcium supplementation alone. The results were dramatic. Estrogen (conjugated equine estrogen 0.625 mg/day) prevented loss of bone in both lumbar spine and femoral neck while those patients given calcium alone continued to lose bone mass at both sites (FIG. 5). Two other studies[31,32] have now demonstrated somewhat similar findings in patients with osteoporosis. It is yet to be shown, however, that the reduced loss of skeletal tissue results in reduction of fracture recurrence.

MODE OF ACTION

It is still not entirely clear how estrogens act upon the skeleton. The recent finding of estrogen receptors in bone cells increases the possibility that estrogens act directly on bone.[34,35] However, the cells which appear to have receptors, although in low number, are osteoblasts or osteoblast-like cells, while estrogens reduce activation frequency and rate of resorption[20] when given *in vivo*. It is possible that osteoblasts are responsible for control of activation, but for reduction in resorption one must speculate a second messenger that is secreted by osteoblasts to control osteoclast activity. Such activity has not been demonstrated *in vitro*. Potential local modulators of estrogen action include insulin-like growth factor (IGF-1), interleukins (either IL-1 or IL-6), transforming growth factor-beta (TGF-β), or prostaglandins (especially PGE-2). This is an area of marked scientific interest at present. *In vitro* experiments have demon-

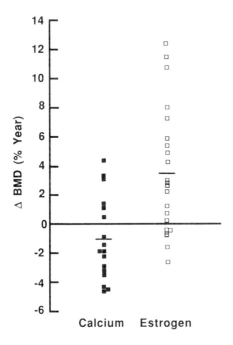

FIGURE 5. Individual changes in bone mass in women given estrogen (*open squares*) plus calcium (total intake 1500 mg/day) and in women given only calcium supplements (1500 mg/day total intake).

strated physiological responses of osteoblast-like cells to appropriate concentrations of estrogen, including alterations in growth rate, and increased synthesis of procollagen and alkaline phosphatase, and it is indeed tempting to postulate that these cells may also mediate the effects on osteoclasts.

Indirect action of estrogen on bone has fallen out of favor at present because of the interest in the action on osteoblasts. However, indirect effects are not excluded by evidence of direct action of the hormones on bone cells. Some evidence supports the concept that estrogens will stimulate the production of endogenous calcitonin, and it has been postulated that the inhibition of bone resorption following estrogen administration is consequent upon increased circulating levels of calcitonin,[36] whose only apparently important physiological action is inhibition of osteoclastic bone resorption. Because of difficulties in measurement of calcitonin, further data are required to support this concept.

REFERENCES

1. ALBRIGHT, F., F. BLOOMBERG & P. H. SMITH. 1940. Postmenopausal osteoporosis. Trans. Assoc. Am. Phys. **55:** 298–305.
2. CUMMINGS, S. R., S. M. RUBIN & D. BLACK. 1990. The future of hip fractures in the United States. Clin. Orthop. Rel. Res. **252:** 163–166.
3. LINDSAY, R. 1988. Sex steroids and osteoporosis. *In* Osteoporosis: Etiology, Diagnosis and Management. B. L. Riggs & L. J. Melton, III, Eds.: 333–358, Raven Press. New York.
4. WEISS, N. S., D. R. SZEKELY, R. DALLAS, M. S. ENGLISH, I. ABRAHAM & A. I. SCHWEID. 1979. Endometrial cancer in relation to patterns of menopausal estrogen use. J. Am. Med. Assoc. **242:** 261–264.
5. ALBRIGHT, F. 1947. The effect of hormones on osteogenesis in man. Recent Prog. Horm. Res. **1:** 293–353.
6. AITKEN, J. M., D. M. HART, J. B. ANDERSON, R. LINDSAY & D. A. SMITH. 1973. Osteoporosis after oophorectomy for non-malignant disease. Br. Med. J. i: 325–328.
7. LINDSAY, R., J. R. T. COUTTS, A. SWEENEY & D. M. HART. 1977. Endogenous oestrogen and bone loss following oophorectomy. Calcif. Tissue Res. **22:** 213–216.
8. SAVILLE, P. D. 1979. Observations on 80 women with osteoporotic spine fractures. *In* Osteoporosis. U. Barzel, Ed.: 38–46. Grune and Stratton. New York.
9. RICHELSON, L. S., H. W. WAHNER, L. J. MELTON & B. L. RIGGS. 1984. Relative contributions of aging and estrogen deficiency to postmenopausal bone loss. New Engl. J. Med. **311:** 1273–1275.
10. SLEMENDA, C., S. L. HUI, C. LONGCOPE & C. C. JOHNSTON. 1987. Sex steroids and bone mass; A study of changes about the time of the menopause. J. Clin. Invest. **80:** 1261–1269.
11. JOHNSTON, C. C., S. L. HUI, R. M. WITT, R. APPLEDORN, R. S. BAKER & C. LONGCOPE. 1985. Early menopausal changes in bone mass and sex steroids. J. Clin. Endocrinol. Metab. **61:** 905–911.
12. LINDSAY, R., D. M. HART, J. M. AITKEN & D. PURDIE. 1978. The effect of ovarian sex steroids on bone mineral status in the oophorectomized rat and in the human. Postgrad. Med. **54S:** 50–58.
13. SNOW, G. R. & C. ANDERSON. 1986. The effect of 17 beta estradiol and progestogen on trabecular bone remodeling in the dog. Calcif. Tiss. Int. **39:** 198–205.
14. HEANEY, R. P., R. R. RECKER & P. D. SAVILLE. Calcium balance and calcium requirements in middle-aged women. Am. J. Clin. Nutr. **30:** 1603–1611.
15. HEANEY, R. P., R. R. RECKER & P. D. SAVILLE. 1978. Menopausal changes in calcium balance performance. J. Lab. Clin. Med. **92:** 953–963.
16. HEANEY, R. P., R. R. RECKER & P. D. SAVILLE. Menopausal changes in bone remodeling. J. Lab. Clin. Med. **92:** 964–970.
17. HUI, S. L., C. W. SLEMENDA & C. C. JOHNSTON, JR. 1989. Baseline measurement of bone mass predicts fracture in white women. Ann. Intern. Med. **111:** 355–361.
18. WASNICH, R. D., P. D. ROSS, L. K. HEILBRUN & J. M. VOGEL. 1985. Prediction of post menopausal fracture risk with use of bone mineral measurements. Am. J. Obstet. Gynecol. **153:** 745–751.

19. LINDSAY, R., J. M. AITKEN, J. B. ANDERSON, D. M. HART, E. B. MACDONALD & A. C. CLARK. 1976. Long-term prevention of postmenopausal osteoporosis by oestrogen. Lancet i: 1038-1041.
20. LINDSAY, R., D. M. HART, C. FORREST & C. BAIRD. 1980. Prevention of spinal osteoporosis in oophorectomized women. Lancet ii: 1151-1154.
21. RECKER, R. R., P. D. SAVILLE & R. P. HEANEY. 1977. The effect of estrogens and calcium carbonate on bone loss in postmenopausal women. Ann. Intern. Med. 87: 649-655.
22. HORSMAN, A., J. C. GALLAGHER, M. SIMPSON, & B. E. C. NORDIN. 1977. Prospective trial of estrogen and calcium in postmenopausal women. Br. Med. J. 2: 789-792.
23. LINDSAY, R., D. M. HART, H. ABDALLA & F. AL-AZZAWI. 1987. Inter-relationship of bone loss and its prevention and fracture expression. In Osteoporosis. C. Christiansen, J. S. Johansen & B. J. Riis, Eds.: 508-512. Osteopres, Denmark.
24. LINDSAY, R., D. M. HART, A. MACLEAN, A. C. CLARK, A. KRASZEWSKI & J. GARWOOD. 1978. Bone response to termination of oestrogen treatment. Lancet i: 1325-1327.
25. LINDSAY, R., D. M. HART & D. M. CLARK. 1984. The minimum effective dose of estrogen for prevention of postmenopausal bone loss. Obstet. Gynecol. 63: 759-763.
26. STEVENSON, J. C., M. P. CUST, K. F. GANCAR, et. al. 1990. A comparison of the effects of transdermal and oral estrogen replacement therapy on bone density in the spine and proximal femur in postmenopausal women. In press.
27. WEISS, N. S., C. L. URE & J. H. BALLARD. Decreased risk of fractures of the hip and lower forearm with postmenopausal use of oestrogen. New Engl. J. Med. 303: 1195-1198.
28. KREIGER, N., J. L. KELSEY & T. R. HOLFORD. 1982. An epidemiological study of hip fracture in postmenopausal women. Am. J. Epidemiol. 116: 141-148.
29. HUTCHINSON, T. A., J. M. POLANSKY & A. R. FEINSTEIN. 1979. Postmenopausal oestrogens protect against fracture of hip and distal radius. Lancet ii: 705-709.
30. ETTINGER, B., H. K. GENANT & C. E. CANN. 1985. Long-term estrogen therapy prevents bone loss and fracture. Ann. Intern. Med. 102: 319-324.
31. JENSEN, G. F., C. CHRISTIANSEN & I. TRANSBOL. 1982. Treatment of postmenopausal osteoporosis. A controlled therapeutic trial comparing oestrogen/gestagen, 1,25-dihydroxyvitamin D and calcium. Clin. Endocrinol. 16: 515-524.
32. QUIGLEY, M. E. T., B. L. MARTIN, A. M. BURNIER & P. BROOKS. 1987. Estrogen therapy arrests bone loss in elderly women. Am. J. Obstet. Gynecol. 156: 1516-1523.
33. LINDSAY, R. & J. F. TOHME. 1990. Estrogen treatment of patients with established postmenopausal osteoporosis. Obstet. Gynecol. 76: 1-6.
34. KOMM, B. S., C. M. TERPENING, D. J. BENZ, et al. 1988. Estrogen binding, receptor mRNA, and biologic response in osteoblast-like osteosarcoma cells. Science 241: 81-84.
35. ERIKSSEN, E. F., D. S. COLVARD, N. J. BERG, et al. 1988. Evidence of estrogen receptors in normal human osteoblast-like cells. Science 241: 84-86.
36. LINDSAY, R. 1988. Sex steroids in the pathogenesis and prevention of osteoporosis. In Osteoporosis: Etiology, Diagnosis, and Management. L. J. Melton, III, Ed.: 333-358.

Decidual Activation in Parturition: Examination of Amniotic Fluid for Mediators of the Inflammatory Response[a]

PAUL C. MACDONALD, S. KOGA,[b] AND

M. LINETTE CASEY

The Cecil H. and Ida Green Center for Reproductive Biology Sciences and
The Departments of Obstetrics-Gynecology and Biochemistry
The University of Texas Southwestern Medical Center
5323 Harry Hines Boulevard
Dallas, Texas 75235

INTRODUCTION

During the past three decades, many investigators have sought to define the mechanism(s) by which parturition is initiated through the identification of an increase in production of a particular uterotonin (uterine contractant) before the onset of labor. Searches for increases in such an agent have included evaluations of maternal blood and urine, amniotic fluid, fetal blood, and even maternal tissues, *e.g.*, myometrium, cervix, and decidua. The increased production of a uterotonin has been an attractive hypothesis because of the well-established pharmacological utility of the administration of oxytocin or prostaglandins in inducing labor. Indeed, spontaneous parturition at term does not differ appreciably from that induced late in human pregnancy by way of the intravenous infusion of either oxytocin or prostaglandins. But regrettably, a clear-cut increase in the level of a potent uterotonin in any biological compartment before the onset of labor has not been demonstrated. Nonetheless, there have been several provocative findings that serve to keep alive the belief, if not singularly the hope, that such an agent will be identified.

In the case of oxytocin, there is a large increase in the number of oxytocin receptors in myometrial tissue of women (and in other species as well) late in pregnancy.[1,2] And, there is an appreciable increase in the concentration of oxytocin in plasma of pregnant women during the second stage of labor and in the early postpartum period.[3,4] These findings have prompted renewed interest in the role of oxytocin in the initiation of parturition. For example, it has been suggested that a significant rise in the concentration of oxytocin in blood is not necessarily obligatory if the increase in uterine responsiveness to oxytocin is sufficiently great, *i.e.*, by way of increased oxytocin receptors.

[a] This study was supported, in part, by USPHS Grant NIH 5-P50-HD11149 and March of Dimes National Foundation Grant No. 5-622.

[b] Mr. Koga was a predoctoral fellow supported, in part, by The Chilton Foundation, Dallas, Texas.

Seemingly, the case for prostaglandins, in particular PGE_2 and $PGF_{2\alpha}$, in serving some obligatory role in parturition is even stronger. For example, several sets of findings have been cited in favor of a role for the prostaglandins in the biomolecular processes of parturition: (1) the levels of prostaglandins (or metabolites thereof) are increased in amniotic fluid and maternal plasma and urine during labor, (2) prostaglandins, administered by several routes (intravenous, intramuscular, intraovular, extraovular, or vaginally) will induce labor at any stage of gestation, and, (3) the administration of inhibitors of prostaglandin synthesis will delay the onset of parturition, arrest preterm labor, and delay the abortion induction time (for review see ref. 5). If the data for all of these lines of evidence are correct (and correctly interpreted), the case for some obligatory role for prostaglandins in the initiation of parturition seems assured. Based on this supposition, it would be important to define the tissue source of prostaglandin(s) that is produced in increased amounts during (or before) the onset of parturition in the hopes of defining the mechanism(s) by which the increase in prostaglandin formation is induced. Generally, the prostaglandins that have been identified as increased during parturition, heretofore, were restricted to PGE_2 and $PGF_{2\alpha}$ and metabolites thereof (for reviews see refs. 5 and 6). More recently, increases in the concentration of selected leukotrienes also have been identified.[7] In the case of the prostaglandins, the levels of PGE_2 and $PGF_{2\alpha}$ are increased in amniotic fluid during labor; and, these increases appear to parallel the duration or progress of labor.[8-10] In addition, increases in the levels of the metabolite, PGFM (15-keto, 13,14-dihydro-$PGF_{2\alpha}$), also are found in the amniotic fluid and in maternal plasma during labor.[11] Interestingly, no increases in the concentration of PGE_2 metabolites have been identified in maternal plasma during parturition.[12,13]

The precise nature of the prostaglandins and metabolites identified in amniotic fluid during labor are of signal interest. Namely, there is an increase in both PGE_2 and $PGF_{2\alpha}$ (as well as PGFM). This finding may serve to identify the tissue origin of the prostaglandins that accumulate in amniotic fluid during parturition. This obtains because of the specific nature of the prostaglandin synthesizing capacity of the tissues contiguous with the amniotic fluid, *i.e.*, the amnion, chorion laeve, and uterine decidua parietalis. Whereas the prostaglandin synthesis capability of the amnion is great[14,15] — provided arachidonic acid is supplied in the medium of amnion tissue or cells (or in amniotic fluid)[16-17] — this tissue produces almost exclusively PGE_2.[14,15] Therefore, the amnion cannot be the site of origin of $PGF_{2\alpha}$ or PGFM that enters the amniotic fluid during parturition. The same is true of the chorion laeve.[15] Namely, chorion laeve also produces PGE_2 but not $PGF_{2\alpha}$. Therefore, of the tissues contiguous with amniotic fluid, namely, amnion, chorion laeve, and decidua, only decidua produces $PGF_{2\alpha}$.[15]

The possibility was entertained that the decidua may convert PGE_2 of fetal membrane origin to $PGF_{2\alpha}$ by way of the action of the enzyme 9-ketoreductase. We found that 9-ketoreductase enzyme activity was demonstrable in microsomal preparations of uterine decidua;[18] but, the specific activity of this enzyme was far less than was that of 15-hydroxy prostaglandin dehydrogenase[15] and therefore was not likely to account for significant conversion of PGE_2 to $PGF_{2\alpha}$ in this tissue. But more than this, there was no conversion of PGE_2 to $PGF_{2\alpha}$ by intact decidual cells or endometrial stromal cells (the progenitors of decidual cells) in culture.[18] We also explored the possibility that $PGF_{2\alpha}$ may arise in fetal urine. And whereas we found that $PGF_{2\alpha}$ was present in human fetal urine, the amounts contained therein may account for the $PGF_{2\alpha}$ in amniotic fluid before the onset of labor but not the amounts present during labor.[19]

These several findings taken together are suggestive that during parturition there is activation of the decidua parietalis in such a manner as to produce $PGF_{2\alpha}$, part of which is metabolized to PGFM or else enters amniotic fluid as $PGF_{2\alpha}$. The central question, however, is the precise role of $PGF_{2\alpha}$ (or decidual activation for that matter) in the initiation or maintenance of human parturition. In particular, does the activation of decidua parietalis occur before or after the onset of labor? And, is decidual activation a necessary, *i.e.*, obligatory phenomenon in the initiation or maintenance of parturition? Or, contrarily, is the activation of a selected portion of the decidua parietalis a natural accompaniment of the labor process, *e.g.*, after exposure of the fetal membranes with attached decidua parietalis (with dilatation of the cervix) to bioactive agents present in cervical or vaginal secretions.

Decidual Parietalis

It is important to recognize that the fetal membranes, which are avascular structures in the human, are contiguous with amniotic fluid on the one side and with the decidua parietalis on the other. In particular, this anatomical arrangement does not include the decidua basalis, which is contiguous with the intervillous blood and the villous trophoblasts of the placenta. Because of this anatomic arrangement, together with the avascular nature of the human fetal membranes, the amniotic fluid, fetal membranes, and uterine decidua parietalis constitute a unique paracrine system between fetal and maternal tissues.[20] After blastocyst implantation, the developing blastocyst (embryo) becomes covered with endometrium (decidua); and this portion of the decidua becomes the decidua capsularis as the embryo expands to occupy the endometrial cavity. The decidua capsularis, because of the expanding embryo/fetus, ultimately is deprived of its blood supply and by the time that the fetus/amniotic sac has expanded to fill the endometrial cavity, it has largely disintegrated. The decidua parietalis develops from that portion of the endometrium distal (lateral) to the invading trophoblasts, which become the villous placenta. Ultimately, the expanding fetal mass/amniotic sac come to embrace and fuse with the decidua parietalis. At the very lowermost pole of the fetal membranes-decidua parietalis, *i.e.*, that portion that will reside over the internal os of the cervix, the blood supply to the decidua parietalis is severely limited.

Decidual Parietalis and Cervical Dilatation

As the cervix dilates, exposing the fetal membranes-decidua parietalis, the portion of decidua that has stripped away and remained attached to the membranes (*i.e.*, that from the lower uterine segment) also is severely denuded of blood supply. Before cervical dilatation, the cervix is functionally closed by way of a tortuous, narrow canal that is filled with cervical secretions (cervical mucous). But as the cervix dilates, the fetal membranes-decidua parietalis complex becomes exposed to the secretions of the cervix and vagina and to the bioactive agents that exist therein. At this time, the membranes with contiguous decidua are actually swept over these secretions during body movement and thus are in continuous and intimate contact with whatever agents may be present therein. The microbial flora of the vagina and cervix is extensive and varied in all women; and in some, gram negative microorganisms of many types are present in abundance. It is quite clear, therefore, that with exposure of the membranes-decidua parietalis **after** dilatation of the cervix, there may be an acute inflammatory response initiated not only by the microorganisms but by mediators of the inflammatory response including endotoxins [lipopolysaccharides (LPS)], cytokines [*e.g.*, interleukin-1 (IL-1), tumor necrosis factor-α (TNF-α), and interleukin-6 (IL-6)], which likely are present normally in the vaginal secretions in response to the microorganisms present in this space.

Exposed Fetal Membranes-Decidua Parietalis and the Inflammatory Response

The inflammatory response is characterized by rapid onset. For example, increases in the mRNA for IL-1, TNF-α, and IL-6 are evident within 15 minutes of exposure of cells to selected stimuli, e.g., LPS. And maximum rates of formation of these cytokines may be evident within 4 h. The inflammatory response also is characterized by increased hydrolysis of glycerophospholipids giving rise to free arachidonic acid and, in selected tissues, products of arachidonic acid including prostaglandins and leukotrienes.

It seems reasonable to presume, therefore, that increases in the levels of cytokines and products of arachidonic acid could follow the exposure of the fetal membranes-decidua parietalis to bioactive agents present in the vagina, agents known to evoke an inflammatory response. If this were the case and if this were shown to be the cause of the increase in prostaglandins in the amniotic fluid during labor, it follows that the increase in PGE_2, $PGF_{2\alpha}$, and PGFM may be a normal accompaniment of the labor process, namely cervical dilatation with exposure of the fetal membranes to bioactive agents in the vagina, and not an event that precedes or indeed is obligatory for labor.

Accumulation of Bioactive Mediators of the Inflammatory Response in Amniotic Fluid during Labor

In another chapter in this volume of the *Annals*, evidence is presented that the decidua as well as progenitor cells of the decidua (endometrial stromal cells in culture) respond to LPS and other mediators of the inflammatory process by forming prostaglandins, in particular, PGE_2, $PGF_{2\alpha}$, and the cytokines, IL-1β and IL-6.[21] And, we have shown previously that the same is true in the case of TNF-α.[22] In addition, the fetal membranes will respond to selected mediators of the inflammatory response by producing prostaglandins and IL-6 as well as endothelin, a potent contractant for smooth muscle.[23] Therefore, it is within the capacity of the exposed fetal membranes-decidua parietalis to respond to stimuli present in the vagina by the production of cytokines and prostaglandins once this tissue unit is exposed after cervical dilatation to bioactive agents in the vaginal secretions.

MATERIALS AND METHODS

Tissues

Decidua parietalis tissue and villous placental tissue were obtained at term at the time of vaginal delivery or at the time of cesarean section conducted prior to the onset of labor. In addition, decidua vera and villous placental tissues were obtained at mid-trimester of pregnancy at the time of elective termination of pregnancy. Consent to use these tissues was obtained from the pregnant woman prior to the conduct of the procedure. Decidua parietalis was removed from the fetal membranes by use of forceps. The tissues were placed on ice and dissected within minutes of delivery.

In some experiments, explants of decidua parietalis were placed in organ culture. Tissue pieces (approximately 50 mg wet weight) were placed in culture medium (1 ml) that consisted of Waymouth enriched medium and fetal bovine serum (10%, v/v). The tissue explants were maintained at 37°C in an atmosphere of CO_2 (5%) in air for 1–24 h in the presence of various test agents. Thereafter, the tissues and the media were collected and processed according to the experimental paradigm.

Quantification of IL-1β by ELISA

Decidual tissue or villous trophoblast tissues were homogenized by use of a teflon-glass homogenizer in Dulbeccos phosphate buffered saline that contained CHAPS (9 mM) and phenylmethylsulfonyl fluoride (PMSF, 1 mM). The homogenates were incubated at 4°C in an ice bath for 90 min and then centrifuged for 2 min in a microfuge; the supernatant fraction was frozen at −20°C prior to conduct of the ELISA.

IL-1β was quantified by use of an ELISA kit purchased from Cistron Biotechnology (Pine Brook, NJ). The PMSF/CHAPS extraction buffer was used as the diluent for the standard curve (5–600 pg/assay well) and for aliquots (10–100 µl) of the cell extract. In some experiments, IL-1β in the culture media was quantified; in such cases, Waymouth enriched culture medium that contained fetal bovine serum was used as the assay diluent. Intraassay and interassay coefficients of variation were 10 and 12%, respectively. Parallelism was maintained for the assay of IL-1β in homogenates or culture media in various volumes. The amount of IL-1β in the homogenates or culture media is expressed as a function of the amount of total protein quantified by the method of Lowry *et al.*[24] with bovine serum albumin as standard.

Analysis of IL-1β mRNA

Total RNA was prepared by extraction of the tissue with guanidinium thiocyanate as described by Chirgwin *et al.*[25] The RNA was purified by centrifugation through cesium chloride; in some experiments, poly(A +) RNA was prepared by chromatography on oligo-dT cellulose as described.[26] The RNA was size fractionated on agarose (1%) gels and transferred electrophoretically to nylon membranes. The membranes were baked at 80°C *in vacuo* for 2 h. A cDNA probe for IL-1β (1.7 kb) was isolated from *E. coli* that contained the pIL-1b-47 plasmid (pBR322), provided to us by Michael Tocci (Merck, Sharp, Dohme, Rahway, NJ). Prehybridizations were conducted by incubation of the membranes for 4–24 h at 42°C in prehybridization buffer comprised of 5 × SSC, 10 × Denhardt solution, formamide (50%, v/v), dextran sulfate (5%, w/v), NaH_2PO_4 (50 mM), and salmon sperm DNA (0.5 mg/ml). Hybridizations are conducted for 16 h at 42°C in buffer composed of 5 × SSC, 2 × Denhardt solution, formamide (50%, v/v), dextran sulfate (10%, w/v), NaH_2PO_4 (20 mM), salmon sperm DNA (0.1 mg/ml), and cDNA probe (5–15 µCi) radiolabeled with [α-³²P]dCTP by the random hexamer priming method. Thereafter, the blots were washed with 2 × SSC and SDS (0.1%, w/v) for 30 min at room temperature, twice with 0.1 × SSC and SDS (0.1%, w/v) for 15 min at room temperature, and 2–4 times with 0.1 × SSC and SDS (0.1%, w/v) for 30 min at 65°C. The membranes were blotted on filter paper, sealed in a plastic bag, and exposed to film for autoradiography at −70°C.

Immunoisolation of Newly Synthesized IL-1β from Decidual/Chorion Tissue Explants

Explants of decidua parietalis (with adherent chorion laeve) were placed in organ culture in serum-free Waymouth enriched culture medium that contained human serum albumin (0.4%, w/v). [35S]Methionine (1 mCi in 5 ml) was added to the culture media and the explants were incubated for 10 h at 37°C in an atmosphere of CO_2 (5%) in air. Thereafter, the tissues were homogenized in PMSF/CHAPS-containing buffer. The homogenates were processed for immunoisolation of IL-1β as described previously[17] using rabbit anti-human IL-1β polyclonal antibody (Cistron Biotechnology, Pine Brook, NJ; diluted 1:10) as the immunoprecipitating antiserum. The immunoisolated proteins were separated by sodium dodecyl sulfate-polyacrylamide gel electrophoresis (on 12.5% gels); thereafter, the gel was dried and exposed to film for autoradiography. Authentic protein standards that were used as recovery markers included rabbit muscle phosphorylase b (97.4 kDa), bovine serum albumin (66.2 kDa), ovalbumin (42.7 kDa), bovine carbonic anhydrase (31.0 kDa), soybean trypsin inhibitor (21.5 kDa), and hen egg white lysozyme (14.4 kDa).

Western Analysis of IL-1β in Decidua/Chorion Explants

Explants of decidua parietalis with adherent chorion laeve tissue were incubated in the presence of LPS (1 μg/ml; E. coli 055:B5) for 16 h. Thereafter, the tissues were collected and homogenized in PMSF/CHAPS-containing buffer. The homogenates were clarified by centrifugation in a microfuge for 10 min. Proteins in the supernatant fluid were separated by sodium dodecyl sulfate-polyacrylamide gel electrophoresis on 12.5% gels. Thereafter, the proteins were transferred electrophoretically to nitrocellulose membranes. The nitrocellulose papers were incubated in a solution that contained powdered milk (1%, w/v) as a blocker of nonspecific binding; then, the papers were incubated in the same buffer that contained rabbit anti-human IL-1β polyclonal antibody (Cistron Biotechnology, Pine Brook, NJ; diluted 1:20) antiserum. Finally, the nitrocellulose paper was incubated with [125I]protein A. The paper was exposed to film for autoradiography.

RESULTS

Expression of IL-1β mRNA in Decidua

We found that IL-1β mRNA is expressed in decidua parietalis tissue obtained from normal pregnancies at term. In decidual tissues obtained from three separate pregnancies delivered electively by cesarean section, the level of expression of IL-1β mRNA was similar to that in decidual tissue obtained from three separate pregnancies delivered vaginally (FIG. 1). In one sample of decidual tissue obtained at vaginal delivery,

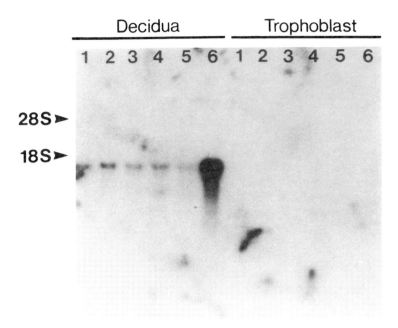

FIGURE 1. IL-1β mRNA expression in human, term decidua parietalis tissues. Total RNA (10μg per lane) from decidua parietalis and villous trophoblast tissues of normal pregnancies obtained at term at the time of elective cesarean section (*lanes 1-3*) or spontaneous vaginal delivery (*lanes 4-6*) was evaluated. A cDNA probe for IL-1β hybridized with a single species of mRNA, approximately 1.8 kb in length, in decidual tissue samples. The point of migration of 28 S and 18 S ribosomal subunits is indicated.

the level of mRNA was considerably greater than that in the other samples evaluated. It is of potential importance that in this pregnancy, labor was prolonged. In villous placental tissue obtained from these same six pregnancies, IL-1β mRNA was not detected (FIG. 1). Similar findings were obtained in analyses of additional pregnancies conducted in this manner (data not shown).

To investigate the possibility that IL-1β mRNA was expressed in placental tissue in levels that were detectable by more sensitive means, we conducted another study. Specifically, we evaluated the expression of IL-1β mRNA in villous placental tissue obtained at spontaneous vaginal delivery using poly(A+) RNA. Again, we were unable to detect IL-1β mRNA in this RNA preparation, even after long exposure times; the presence of mRNA on these northern blots was confirmed by the demonstration of mRNA for β-actin after very short exposure times with a cDNA probe of similar specific activity (FIG. 2). Thus, we conclude that little or no IL-1β mRNA is expressed in human villous placental tissue.

To evaluate the possibility that IL-1β mRNA expression in decidua parietalis was a consequence of activation of the tissue at the site of exposure after cervical dilation, we conducted another study. Decidua parietalis/chorion tissue was obtained from five normal, term pregnancies delivered vaginally after the spontaneous onset of labor. The tissue was obtained from the area of fetal membranes that made up the forebag

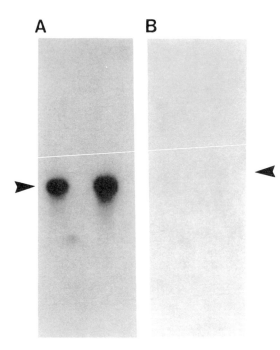

FIGURE 2. Little or no IL-1β mRNA expression in human villous placental tissue. Poly(A+) RNA was prepared from villous placental tissue obtained at term at the time of spontaneous vaginal delivery. 20μg or 40μg of poly(A+) RNA was applied to the left and right lanes, respectively, of a gel. The blot was probed first for IL-1β (*panel B*) and then for β-actin (*panel A*). The cDNA probes were estimated to be of similar specific activity. The blot shown in panel A was exposed to film for 3.5 h; that shown in panel B was exposed to film for 48 h.

or else from an area of the fetal membranes that was distal to the site of membrane rupture. We found that IL-1β mRNA expression was greater in the tissue obtained from the forebag area in 4 of 5 pregnancies (FIG. 3). Thus, it is possible that activation of decidua and thereby increased expression of IL-1β mRNA is effected in decidual tissue that is remaining at the site of the forebag exposed to vaginal bioactive agents. More specifically, the possibility exists that with dilatation of the cervix, there is induction of IL-1β mRNA as a consequence of exposure of the tissue to vaginal contents, which include bacterial products as well as IL-1β *per se*, both of which are potent stimuli of IL-1β production.

IL-1β Protein Expression in Decidua

We conducted several studies to evaluate the possibility that IL-1β protein is synthesized in decidual tissue. First, we immunoisolated a newly synthesized, [^{35}S]methionine-labeled protein of approximately 34 kDa from decidua/chorion laeve tissue homogenate using anti-IL-1β antibody (FIG. 4). In addition, by western immunoblot analysis of tissue homogenates, we demonstrated the presence of immunoreactive IL-1β in decidua/chorion laeve tissue explants. Two major immunoreactive proteins were detected; the sizes of these proteins were estimated to be approximately 34 kDa and 17 kDa (FIG. 5). In explants that were incubated in the presence of LPS (1 μg/ml) for 16 h, the level of immunoreactive protein (both species) was increased (FIG. 5).

Finally, we quantified immunoreactive IL-1β in homogenates of decidua and vil-

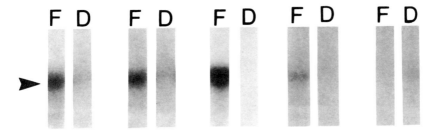

FIGURE 3. IL-1β mRNA expression in decidua parietalis/chorion tissues of five normal, term pregnancies at the time of spontaneous vaginal delivery. The tissue was obtained from the area of fetal membranes that comprised the forebag (F) or from an area of the fetal membranes that was distal (D) to the site of rupture. Total RNA (5μg per lane) was applied to each lane and probed for IL-1β. The IL-1β cDNA probe hybridized with a single species of mRNA (~ 1.8 kb, denoted by the arrow). In four of five pregnancies, the level of expression of IL-1β was greater in decidual tissue obtained from the forebag than in that obtained from the upper compartment.

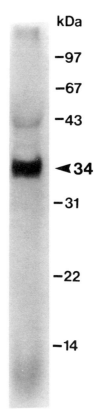

FIGURE 4. Immunoisolation of IL-1β from explants of decidua/chorion laeve tissue. A newly synthesized, [^{35}S]methionine-labeled protein of approximately 34 kDa was immunoisolated from decidua/chorion laeve tissue homogenate using anti-IL-1β antiserum.

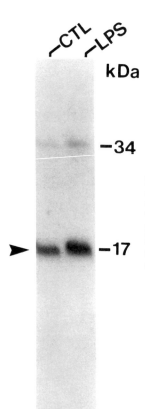

FIGURE 5. Western immunoblot analysis of IL-1β in homogenates of decidua/chorion laeve tissues. Explants of decidua/chorion laeve were incubated in the absence or presence of LPS (1μg/ml) for 16 h. Thereafter, proteins in the tissue homogenates were separated by SDS-polyacrylamide gel electrophoresis and transferred to nitrocellulose paper. By western analysis with anti-IL-1β antibody, two proteins of approximately 34 kDa and 17 kDa were detectable. The arrow denotes the point of migration of human recombinant IL-1β.

lous placental trophoblast tissues by use of an ELISA. IL-1β was present in decidua vera and villous trophoblast tissues obtained at midtrimester (n = 6) and in homogenates of decidua parietalis and trophoblast obtained at term before (n = 17) or after (n = 17) spontaneous onset of labor. The level of IL-1β was similar in decidual tissue irrespective of gestational age or the presence or absence of labor. In all cases, the level of IL-1β protein in decidua was greater than that in villous trophoblast (FIG. 6). The presence of immunoreactive IL-1β in placental tissue in the absence of demonstrable levels of mRNA is suggestive that the IL-1β originates at a site other than the syncitiotrophoblast. In other experiments, we find that immunoreactive IL-1β is not produced in isolated cytotrophoblasts; and, IL-1β mRNA is not detectable in chorion laeve tissue (data not shown). Thus, it also is unlikely that the IL-1β that is present in homogenates of placental tissue is synthesized in cytotrophoblasts.

We found that explants of decidual-chorion laeve tissue in organ culture synthesize IL-1β and secrete IL-1β into the culture media. In response to treatment with LPS, there is an increase in the level of immunoreactive IL-1β in the tissue homogenate and in the culture media (TABLE 1).

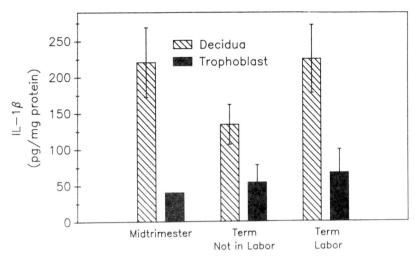

FIGURE 6. Content of immunoreactive IL-1β in decidua and villous placental trophoblast tissues. IL-1β (mean ± SEM) was quantified by ELISA in homogenates of decidua vera and villous trophoblast tissues obtained at midtrimester (n = 6) and in homogenates of decidua parietalis and trophoblast obtained at term before (n = 17) or after (n = 17) spontaneous onset of labor.

DISCUSSION

As the fetal head engages the maternal pelvis during labor with descent of the fetus, the amniotic fluid space is divided, anatomically, into two compartments. The lowermost is the forebag. This compartment of the amniotic fluid is separated from the upper compartment because of the obstruction created by entry of the fetal head into the pelvis. In primigravid women, the engagement of the fetal head commonly precedes the onset of active labor, sometimes by days or even a week or two. In multi-

TABLE 1. Production of IL-1β by Decidua-Chorion Tissue Explants

| Treatment | IL-1β Production (pg IL-1β/mg protein) | | | |
	Tissue	p value	Media	p value
Control	357 ± 63		9.95 ± 3.2	
LPS (100 ng/ml)	447 ± 56	NS	9.88 ± 25.9	$p < 0.01$
LPS (300 ng/ml)	699 ± 117	$p < 0.05$	34.87 ± 9.1	$p < 0.02$
LPS (1 µg/ml)	618 ± 59	$p < 0.05$	57.24 ± 9.7	$p < 0.005$

Explants of decidual-chorion tissue (~ 5 mg total protein) were placed in organ culture in Waymouth enriched culture media (1 ml) that contained fetal bovine serum (10%) ± LPS (*E. coli* 055:B5) in various concentrations. After incubation for 8 h at 37 °C in an atmosphere of CO_2 (5%) in air, the media and tissue explants were collected. Tissues were homogenized in PMSF/CHAPS–containing buffer and processed as described in MATERIALS AND METHODS. IL-1β in the media and tissue supernatants was quantified by ELISA. The study was conducted with replicates of 6 explant cultures for each treatment condition; data were analyzed by use of the Mann-Whitney U test.

parous women, the forebag compartment may be created after the onset of labor. In pregnancies with abnormal fetal presentations, such as incomplete or footling breech and transverse lie, there may be only one amniotic fluid compartment. The importance of this anatomic separation of the amniotic fluid is that during labor this compartmentalization also may come to involve a functional separation of the two compartments. If this were the case, sampling of the amniotic fluid from one of the compartments may not be representative of the accumulation of bioactive agents (which may be involved in the parturitional process) in both compartments. For example, if the forebag compartment is both anatomically and functionally separated from the upper compartment of amniotic fluid, the accumulation of bioactive agents of the inflammatory response may be confined to the forebag compartment, the lowermost pole of which (after cervical dilatation) is exposed to active mediators of inflammation present in the vagina.

The evidence in favor of decidual activation during parturition came originally from the finding of $PGF_{2\alpha}$ and PGFM in amniotic fluid during labor. We also have argued that increases in free arachidonic acid in amniotic fluid during labor likely arise from the decidua.[27] And, the accumulation of IL-1β, IL-6, and TNF-α (in some cases) also likely arises in decidua, albeit perhaps from monocytes or macrophages in or recruited to this tissue.[22] Yet, these findings, which clearly are supportive of the likelihood of decidual activation during parturition, may be interpreted as being a natural accompaniment of parturition and not involved in the process leading to the initiation of labor. The very great likelihood of activation of the lowermost pole of the fetal membranes-decidua parietalis unit by agents in the vaginal secretions is most consistent with this process being active after the cervix dilates and thereby exposes these tissues to such stimuli. And, if there is no functional or anatomical division of the amniotic fluid compartment by way of engagement of the fetal head in the maternal pelvis, the mediators of the inflammatory response may be found in all spaces of the amniotic cavity. Stated differently, if cervical dilatation precedes the formation of the anatomically distinct forebag, response of exposed decidua and fetal membranes to stimuli in vagina will give rise to prostaglandins and cytokines that will be distributed into the entire amniotic fluid that is then accessible by transabdominal or transuterine amniotic fluid sampling. If this were the case, the examination of amniotic fluids collected at the time of cesarean section during labor (after exposure of the fetal membranes-decidua parietalis by dilatation of the cervix) will give results similar to those obtained from the forebag by direct needle aspiration.

But in any event, spurious results with respect to bioactive agents of the inflammatory response almost certainly will be obtained in studies of amniotic fluids collected by amniotomy or by way of catheters placed into the uterine cavity.

Based on results obtained to date, we conclude that the evidence in favor of an accumulation of agents representative of an inflammatory response in the amniotic fluid is a consequence of exposure of the fetal membranes-decidua parietalis to mediators of the inflammatory response that are present in the vaginal secretions. Thus, these findings are the result of events that transpire after cervical dilatation and not before. Accordingly, there is as yet no firm evidence for the existence of an inflammatory response before labor or as an obligatory part of the parturitional process. Indeed, such an analysis casts great doubt on the obligatory role of prostaglandins in the parturitional event.

If this analysis were correct, it follows that there is no evidence presently for increased formation of a uterotonin before or during labor, except for the increase in oxytocin concentrations in maternal blood during the latter stages of labor. It then follows that there may be no increase in a uterotonin before the onset of labor; rather, it presently seems more plausible to presume that the central issue in parturition is related to the very efficient system for the maintenance of pregnancy. Specifically, parturition may be initiated by way of the retreat from pregnancy maintenance rather than by the independent production of a given uterotonin in increased amounts.

Heretofore, most investigations of the contents of amniotic fluid for assessments of agents that may be important in the parturitional process have involved fluids collected as follows: 1) midtrimester amniotic fluid collected by transabdominal amniocentesis; 2) amniotic fluids collected by amniocentesis in the third trimester for diagnostic purposes; 3) amniotic fluids collected at or near term by transabdominal or transuterine amniocentesis at the time of elective repeat cesarean section before the onset of labor; 4) amniotic fluid collected at the time of amniotomy conducted by transvaginal interruption of the fetal membranes surgically; and, 5) amniotic fluid collected through a catheter inserted into the uterine cavity to monitor uterine contractions. There are significant limitations to several of these collection methods. Fluids collected by amniotomy are not useful for two important reasons: First, the amniotic fluid may be representative only of the forebag compartment, which may be appreciably different from that of the upper compartment because of functional separation and direct stimulation of the lowermost membranes-decidua parietalis segment after dilatation of the cervix by agents in the vaginal secretions. Second, it is very difficult, if not impossible, to avoid contamination of amniotic fluid (collected by amniotomy) by vaginal contents. And, there is an inflammatory response in the vagina of most women represented by agents in the vaginal secretions that will contaminate such fluids. Therefore, the measurement of prostaglandins and cytokines or other agents commonly produced in response to an inflammatory response in amniotic fluid collected by amniotomy are useless. Other objections must be raised with respect to amniotic fluids collected by way of catheters inserted into the uterine cavity. After rupture of the membranes, the entire uterine cavity is potentially exposed to the bioactive agents as well as the microorganisms present in the vaginal secretions. Indeed, it is well-known that there is a direct and highly significant correlation between duration of rupture of the membranes and the development of clinical evidence of infection. Therefore, the monitoring of amniotic fluids as a function of time after rupture of the membranes is likely more representative of the monitoring of developing infections occurring as the consequence of rupture of the membranes and not the accompaniment of the labor process *per se*.

It is appreciably more difficult to obtain amniotic fluids during labor in a manner that will avoid vaginal contamination or the artifacts of infection that accompany rupture of the membranes. But, it is possible. Amniotic fluid can be obtained (albeit less frequently) from pregnancies during labor when the pregnancy is terminated by cesarean section. The major difficulty involved in the evaluation of fluids collected in this manner is to be assured that the woman was indeed in labor. In particular, cesarean sections are commonly conducted early in the presumed labor process in women who previously were delivered by cesarean section. And whereas it may seem that labor is in progress, we know from experiences with pregnancies that seemingly involved preterm labor (but delivery did not occur) that this is not necessarily the case. Thus, care must be taken to ensure that labor has indeed begun. The best indices of this are 1) cervical dilatation greater than 3 cm and 2) evidence of progressive cervical dilatation. In any event, it is prudent to compare results obtained in cases of cesarean section in labor by evaluating the results as a function of cervical dilatation or else as a function of those pregnancies less than or greater than 3 cm cervical dilatation.

A second option for evaluating bioactive agents in amniotic fluid is to collect samples by way of direct needle aspiration of the forebag. In this manner, contamination of the fluid with vaginal secretions can be largely avoided. It must be recognized, however, that amniotic fluids collected in this manner may be representative of an anatomically and functionally separated compartment of the amniotic fluid space. If this is taken into account, and the results of findings with these fluids are compared with those obtained at the time of cesarean section of pregnancies during labor, much valuable information may be obtained.

SUMMARY

The accumulation of bioactive agents (characteristic of an inflammatory-type response) in amniotic fluid is common during term and preterm labor, *viz.*, interleukin-1β (IL-1β), interleukin-6 (IL-6), and tumor necrosis factor-α (TNF-α). In addition, prostaglandins, including PGE_2, $PGF_{2\alpha}$, and PGFM, also accumulate in amniotic fluid in some cases of term and preterm labor. From these observations, a number of critical questions arise. Namely, 1) what is the tissue source of origin of these agents?; 2) what are the stimuli that evoke this inflammatory response?; and, 3) are these bioactive agents of inflammation involved in the commencement of labor or else a natural accompaniment of the parturition process? It is reasonable to suspect that the decidua is activated during parturition as the membranes-decidua are exposed after cervical dilation to the vaginal/cervical secretions. Amnion and chorion laeve, in the human, are avascular tissues that produce PGE_2 but not $PGF_{2\alpha}$. Therefore, the accumulation of $PGF_{2\alpha}$ and PGFM in amniotic fluid during labor cannot be attributed to a fetal membrane origin. Moreover, the fetal membranes and decidua do not convert PGE_2 to $PGF_{2\alpha}$. In addition, the fetal membranes do not produce mature, *i.e.*, secreted 17kD IL-1β. On the other hand, the decidua does produce $PGF_{2\alpha}$ and PGFM and is stimulated to do so by agents in the vaginal secretions, namely, bacterial endotoxin and IL-1β. After the fetal membranes and contiguous decidua are exposed during the time of cervical dilatation, these tissues are acted upon to cause 1) an influx of mononuclear phagocytes into the forebag compartment of the amniotic fluid; 2) to produce $PGF_{2\alpha}$ and PGFM; and 3) to produce cytokines, including IL-1β, IL-6, and TNF-α. Exposure of the fetal membranes-decidua to bioactive agents in vaginal/cervical secretions will effect an inflammatory response both *in vivo* and *in vitro*. We conclude that the accumulation of bioactive agents characteristic of the inflammatory response in amniotic fluid during term and preterm labor is usually an accompaniment of parturition and not its cause.

REFERENCES

1. FUCHS, A. R., F. FUCHS, P. HUSSLEIN, M. S. SOLOFF & M. J. FERNSTROM. 1982. Oxytocin receptors and human parturition: A dual role for oxytocin in the initiation of labor. Science 215: 1396–1398.
2. FUCHS, A. R., F. FUCHS, P. HUSSLEIN & M. S. SOLOFF. 1984. Oxytocin receptors in the human uterus during pregnancy and parturition. Am. J. Obstet. Gynecol. 150: 734–741.
3. LEAKE, R. D. 1983. Oxytocin. Initiation of parturition: Prevention of prematurity. *In* Report

of the Fourth Ross Conference on Obstetric Research. J. C. Porter & P. C. MacDonald, Eds.: 43–51. Ross Laboratories Publ. Columbus, OH.

4. LEAKE, R. D., R. E. WEITZMAN, T. H. GLATZ & D. A. FISCHER. 1981. Plasma oxytocin concentrations in men, nonpregnant women, and pregnant women before and during spontaneous labor. J. Clin. Endocrinol. Metab. **53**: 730–733.

5. CASEY, M. L. & P. C. MACDONALD. 1984. Endocrinology of preterm birth. Clin. Obstet. Gynecol. **27**: 562–571.

6. CHALLIS, J. R. G. & D. OLSON. 1988. Parturition. *In* The Physiology of Reproduction. E. Knobil & J. D. Neill, Eds. Vol. **2**: 2177–2216. Raven Press. New York.

7. WALSH, S. W. 1989. 5-Hydroxyeicosatetraenoic acid, leukotriene C4, and prostaglandin F2 alpha in amniotic fluid before and during term and preterm labor. Am. J. Obstet. Gynecol. **161**: 1352–1360.

8. KEIRSE, M. J. N. C., M. D. MITCHELL & A. C. TURNBULL. 1977. Changes in prostaglandin F and 13,14-dihydro-15-keto-prostaglandin F concentrations in amniotic fluid at the onset of and during labor. Br. J. Obstet. Gynaecol. **84**: 743–746.

9. DRAY, F. & R. FRYDMAN. 1976. Primary prostaglandins in amniotic fluid in pregnancy and spontaneous labor. Am. J. Obstet. Gynecol. **126**: 13–19.

10. KEIRSE, M. J. N. C. 1983. Prostaglandins during human parturition. *In* Report of the Fourth Ross Conference on Obstetric Research. J. C. Porter & P. C. MacDonald, Eds.: 137–144. Ross Laboratories Publ. Columbus, OH.

11. GHODGAONKAR, R. B., N. H. DUBIN, D. A. BLAKE & T. M. KING. 1979. 13,14-Dihydro-15-keto-prostaglandin $F_{2\alpha}$ concentrations in human plasma and amniotic fluid. Am. J. Obstet. Gynecol. **134**: 265–269.

12. BRENNECKE, S. P., B. M. CASTLE, L. M. DEMERS & A. C. TURNBULL. 1985. Maternal plasma prostaglandin E_2 metabolite levels during human pregnancy and parturition. Br. J. Obstet. Gynaecol. **92**: 345–349.

13. MITCHELL, M. D., K. EBENHACK, D. L. KRAEMER, K. COX, S. CUTRER & D. M. STRICKLAND. 1982. A sensitive radioimmunoassay for 11-deoxy-13,14-dihydro-15-keto-11,16-cycloprostaglandin E_2 biosynthesis during human pregnancy and parturition. Prostaglandin Leukotrienes Med. **9**: 549–557.

14. MITCHELL, M. D., J. BIBBY, B. R. HICKS & A. C. TURNBULL. 1978. Specific production of prostaglandin E by human amnion *in vitro*. Prostaglandins **15**: 377–382.

15. OKAZAKI, T., M. L. CASEY, J. R. OKITA, P. C. MACDONALD & J. M. JOHNSTON. 1981. Initiation of human parturition. XII. Biosynthesis and metabolism of prostaglandins in human fetal membranes and uterine decidua. Am. J. Obstet. Gynecol. **139**: 373–381.

16. CASEY, M. L., M. D. MITCHELL & P. C. MACDONALD. 1987. Epidermal growth factor-stimulated prostaglandin E_2 production in human amnion cells: Specificity and nonesterified arachidonic acid dependency. Mol. Cell. Endocrinol. **53**: 169–176.

17. CASEY, M. L., K. KORTE & P. C. MACDONALD. 1988. Epidermal growth factor-stimulation of prostaglandin E_2 biosynthesis in amnion cells: Induction of PGH_2 synthase. J. Biol. Chem. **263**: 7846–7854.

18. NIESERT, S., W. CHRISTOPHERSON, K. KORTE, M. D. MITCHELL, P. C. MACDONALD & M. L. CASEY. 1986. Prostaglandin E_2 9-keto-reductase activity in human decidua vera tissue. Am. J. Obstet. Gynecol. **155**: 1348–1352.

19. CASEY, M. L., S. I. CUTRER & M. D. MITCHELL. 1983. Origin of prostanoids in human amniotic fluid: The fetal kidney as a source of amniotic fluid prostanoids. Am. J. Obstet. Gynecol. **147**: 547–551.

20. CUNNINGHAM, F. G., N. F. GANT & P. C. MACDONALD. 1989. Williams Obstetrics. 18th edit. pp. 187–189. Appleton and Lange. Norwalk, CT.

21. SEMER, D. A., P. C. MACDONALD & M. L. CASEY. 1990. Responsiveness of endometrium to cytokines. Ann. N.Y. Acad. Sci. This volume. In press.

22. CASEY, M. L., S. M. COX, B. BEUTLER & L. MILEWICH. 1989. Cachectin/tumor necrosis factor-α formation in human decidua. J. Clin. Invest. **83**: 430–436.

23. SUNNERGREN, K. P., R. A. WORD, J. F. SAMBROOK, P. C. MACDONALD & M. L. CASEY. 1990. Expression and regulation of endothelin precursor mRNA in avascular human amnion. Mol. Cell. Endocrinol. **68**: R7–R14.

24. LOWRY, O. H., N. J. ROSEBROUGH, A. L. FARR & R. J. RANDALL. 1951. Protein measurement with the Folin pheno reagent. J. Biol. Chem. **193**: 265–275.

25. CHIRGWIN, J. M., A. E. PRZYBYLA, R. J. MacDONALD & W. J. RUTTER. 1979. Isolation of biologically active ribonucleic acid from sources enriched in ribonuclease. Biochemistry. **18:** 5294–5299.
26. SAMBROOK, J., E. F. FRITSCH & T. MANIATIS. 1989. Molecular Cloning. A Laboratory Manual, 2 edit. Cold Spring Harbor Laboratory Press. Cold Spring Harbor, New York.
27. CASEY, M. L. & P. C. MacDONALD. 1988. Biomolecular processes in the initiation of parturition: Decidual activation. Clin. Obstet. Gynecol. **31:** 533–552.

Involvement of Placental Neurohormones in Human Parturition[a]

FELICE PETRAGLIA,[b] GEORGE COUKOS,
ANNIBALE VOLPE, AND ANDREA R. GENAZZANI

Department of Obstetrics & Gynecology
University of Modena School of Medicine, Policlinico
Via del Pozzo 71
41100 Modena, Italy

WYLIE VALE

The Clayton Foundation Laboratories for Peptide Biology
Salk Institute
La Jolla, California 92037

INTRODUCTION

In vivo and *in vitro* evidence indicates that different fetal and/or local factors participate in the mechanisms regulating myometrial contractile activity. A challenging hypothesis is that a group of factors are secreted by the fetal-placental unit and act in concert, when the maturational processes of the fetus are completed.

Prostanoids have a central role in the mechanisms controlling uterine contractility and cervical softening. In particular, a role of prostaglandin (PG)E_2 and $PGF_{2\alpha}$ is suggested. A rise of PGE_2 and $PGF_{2\alpha}$ levels in the amniotic fluid precedes the appearance of uterine activity in the sheep,[1] and the level of PG metabolites rises in maternal plasma at parturition in the human.[2] Moreover, administration of drugs blocking PG synthesis, such as indomethacin and acetylsalicylic acid, blocks uterine activity and prolongs the onset of labor.[3] Specific receptors for prostaglandins have been shown in human myometrium, cervix, decidua and amnion.[4] Decidua, amnion, placenta and myometrium are all capable of producing prostanoids.[5] PGs synthesized in the amnion may cross the intermediate layers and act on the myometrium, as decidual PGs[6] do.

The possible factors that may influence the release of PG in fetal membranes and decidua are still under investigation. In several species, estrogens and progesterone seem to play a pivotal role in the control of PG synthesis and action. Progesterone decreases uterine contractility and reverses the effects of oxytocin on rodent uterine muscle, both through inhibition of PG synthesis and by direct action on oxytocin re-

[a] The present study was partially supported by the Consiglio Nazionale delle Ricerche (PF.FATMA; SP 7.2.3.), by NIH Grant No. DK 26741, and by the Clayton Foundation for Research, California Division. W. V. is a Clayton Foundation Investigator.
[b] Author to whom correspondence should be addressed.

ceptors in myometrium and decidua.[7] On the other hand, estrogens act as functional antagonists to progesterone, increasing the contractile activity of myometrium and stimulating the release of PGE_2 from human decidua cells.[8] It has been hypothesized that the balance between these two antagonistic factors influence in a paracrine and/or autocrine manner the rate of synthesis of stimulatory PG in fetal membranes and decidua. Initiation of labor, in human as well as in lower species, might depend on local events occurring in decidua, fetal membranes and placenta.[9]

Trophoblast, fetal membranes and decidua synthesize other factors that may influence both PG and steroid hormone release or may act directly on myometrium. Indeed, recent evidences suggest that locally produced peptide hormones as well as neuropeptides and cytokines may affect the mechanisms regulating the uterine contractility. In particular, the putative involvement of corticotropin-releasing hormone (CRF) and neuropeptide Y (NPY) will be presented.

CORTICOTROPIN-RELEASING FACTOR

Synthesis and Release

Human placenta synthesizes bioactive CRF, a 41 amino acid peptide, which displays identical immunological, biological and chemical characteristics to hypothalamic CRF.[10] Placenta-extracted CRF stimulates the release of ACTH and β-endorphin from cultured rat pituitary cells. A 1300 oligonucleotide CRF mRNA has been recently identified in human placenta.[11] Similarities between placental and hypothalamic CRF extend also to the transcriptional level. The structure of CRF mRNAs and the transcriptional mechanisms are similar in both sites.[12] The CRF mRNA is expressed in both cyto- and syncytiotrophoblast cells of human placenta, and appears as early as 7 weeks of gestation. Its concentration increases more than 20-fold during the last 5 weeks of pregnancy.[12] Placental CRF content increases in a parallel manner.[13] Immunohistochemical studies reveal a more intense staining of CRF antiserum in the inner layer of the placental villi, where the cyto- and intermediate trophoblast are located.[14] Recently, Jones et al.[15] have demonstrated that human amnion, chorion and decidua release immunoreactive CRF.

Placental CRF is released into the maternal bloodstream. Various findings support such a concept: (1) plasma CRF levels in pregnant women are significantly higher than in nonpregnant women; (2) immunoreactive and bioactive plasma maternal CRF levels increase progressively during pregnancy, with the highest levels occurring near term, in parallel with placental CRF content and CRF mRNA levels; (3) circulating CRF levels decrease within a few hours after placental delivery.[16-19] Moreover, the evidence that umbilical cord plasma CRF levels are 10- to 20-fold lower than in maternal plasma, and that CRF levels in umbilical vein are higher than those in umbilical arteries, suggests that placenta CRF is also released towards the fetal compartment.[18,20]

During spontaneous labor, maternal plasma CRF levels increase progressively until vaginal delivery, correlating positively with the progress of cervical dilatation.[21] The highest levels are observed during the active phase of labor.[17,21] No significant rise of circulating CRF is present in women undergoing elective cesarean section.[21] Moreover, women with preterm labor showed plasma CRF levels higher than healthy pregnant women matched for gestational age.[22] Therefore, the events associated with parturition may be associated to the activation of placental CRF release. This is further supported by the evidence that the release of immunoreactive CRF by *in vitro* preparations of human placenta and fetal membranes is greater from tissues obtained after spontaneous labor than from those collected at elective cesarean section.[15] These findings support an increased CRF release from placenta and fetal membranes during labor.

Factors Involved in the Regulation of Placental CRF

Results obtained from cultured placental tissue have shown that several factors affect the release of CRF from human placenta (FIG. 1). These factors are the same ones involved in the control of hypothalamic CRF and are also involved in the mechanisms regulating the stress-induced responses. They may derive from maternal and/or fetal bloodstream or may be locally released from placenta and fetal membranes.

Neuropeptides, such as angiotensin II (AII), arginine-vasopressin (AVP), and oxytocin (OT), which are known to increase during labor in maternal and/or fetal circulation, increase the release of placental CRF from cultured trophoblast.[23] Norepinephrine (NEpi), another circulating factor which significantly rises during labor,[24] also stimulates the release of CRF from cultured human placental cells. The effect of NEpi is reversed by prazosin, an α_1-adrenergic antagonist, or yohimbine an α_2-adrenergic receptor antagonist. The involvement of both adrenergic receptor subtypes is further supported by the evidence that methoxamine or clonidine, a α_1- and α_2-

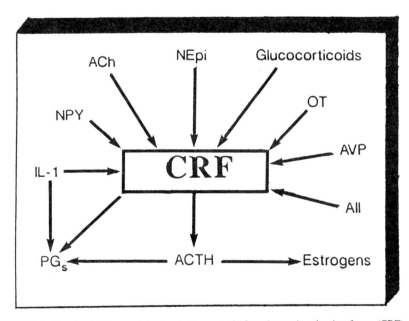

FIGURE 1. Putative factors participating to the control of corticotropin-releasing factor (CRF) release in human placenta (AII: angiotensin II; AVP: arginine-vasopressin; OT: oxytocin, NEpi: norepinephrine; Ach: acetylcholine; NPY: neuropeptide Y; IL-1: interleukin-1; PGs: prostaglandins).

adrenergic receptor agonists, respectively, stimulate CRF release from placental cells.[23]

Acetylcholine (ACh) also stimulates the output of CRF by the same cell preparations, acting via a muscarinic receptor.[23] Human placenta synthesizes ACh, contains high concentrations of ACh and of cholinergic receptors.[25] Labor is accompanied by a depletion of placental ACh, suggesting a dramatic release of the neurotransmitter.[26]

Prostanoids and cytokines, involved in the mechanisms of control of myometrial contraction, are capable to affect the release of CRF. Both PGE$_2$ and PGF$_{2\alpha}$ increase the output of CRF by human placental cells in vitro in a dose-dependent manner.[14] Furthermore, interleukin-1α (IL-1α) and IL-1β stimulate the release of CRF by placental cells.[27] The addition of IL-1β in the culture medium was followed by a two-fold increase of intracellular cyclic adenosine monophosphate (cAMP) and a fivefold increase of cyclic guanosine monophosphate (cGMP). The evidence that IL-1 stimulates the release of PG in human fetal membranes[28] and that indomethacin partially reversed the effect of IL-1β on placental cells suggests that the stimulatory action of IL-1β upon CRF release is in part mediated by prostaglandins. The presence of IL-1 has been demonstrated in human placenta, in decidua and fetal membranes and is probably due to numerous monocytes present in these tissues.[29] Recently, Romero et al.[30] proposed the participation of IL-1 in the early events triggering labor, in view of the increased amniotic fluid IL-1 levels during labor. Prostaglandins and IL-1 may represent two major local signals for CRF placental release during labor.

Finally, glucocorticoid hormones increase placental and decidual CRF release in vitro.[15,31] The addition of dexamethazone increases CRF mRNA expression in cultured human placental cells at term.[31] Glucocorticoids also stimulate CRF release from amnion, chorion and decidua.[15] Therefore, the rise of maternal and fetal circulatory cortisol at term and during labor[32,33] may represent an important factor in activating CRF release from human placenta and fetal membranes.

Biological Activity of CRF and Possible Implication in Labor

Placental CRF may act locally in regulating ACTH release or other hormonal productions but maternal and/or fetal pituitary ACTH release may also be affected. Specific CRF binding sites are present in placental tissue, and the evidence that their concentrations in specimens collected at vaginal delivery are higher than at cesarean section suggests placental cells as targets of locally released CRF.[21] Human placenta synthesizes and secretes ACTH and other proopiomelanocortin (POMC)-derived peptides.[34] The syncytiotrophoblast cells are those positively staining for these hormones.[35] The addition of synthetic CRF stimulates the release of ACTH and POMC-derived hormones from cultured human placental cells.[14,36] The effect is dose-dependent and is specifically reversed by a synthetic CRF antagonist.[14] The concentration of CRF required for 50% of maximal stimulation (EC$_{50}$) of ACTH release is higher than the EC$_{50}$ of CRF necessary to release ACTH from cultured anterior pituitary cells. The effect of CRF is mimicked by dibutyryl-cyclic AMP and forskolin, an adenylate cyclase activator, suggesting that CRF stimulates placental ACTH via the cAMP pathway.[14] Many analogies exist between placental CRF-ACTH axis and the hypothalamic-pituitary-adrenal axis, suggesting placenta as a neuroendocrine organ.[37] Epinephrine, through a β-adrenergic receptor, oxytocin, and prostaglandins are able to stimulate the release of ACTH from placental cultures.[37] The evidence that prostaglandins stimulate ACTH release via local CRF has been suggested by the results indicating that a CRF antagonist partially reverses this action.[14] These results also indicate that CRF has a paracrine or autocrine action on placental cells. Recently, Jones and Challis[38] showed that both CRF and ACTH stimulate $PGF_{2\alpha}$ and PGE_2 release from term human placenta, amnion, chorion and decidua cell preparations (FIG. 2). This effect is reversed by specific antisera. Furthermore, the effect of CRF on placenta PG release is partially inhibited by a specific ACTH antiserum, supporting that the PG stimulatory action of CRF is in part mediated by paracrine mechanisms via ACTH release. Involvement of CRF in the mechanisms regulating the increased ACTH and PG release suggests a possible role of this peptide in the mechanisms of labor. This hypothesis has been further emphasized by the recent findings of Quartero and Fry,[39] who demonstrated a priming and potentiating effect of CRF on the action of oxytocin on human isolated gestational myometrium, suggesting that CRF sensibilizes myometrium to oxytocin.

The evidence that placental CRF is released into the fetal circulation,[18,20] suggests a possible action of this peptide on the fetal pituitary-adrenal axis. CRF synergizes with AVP in increasing fetal pituitary ACTH release.[40] The hypothalamic-pituitary-adrenal axis is already mature and functioning since early second trimester in human fetus.[41] A rapid adrenal maturation is observed in lower primates before birth, in coincidence with a rise of fetal plasma and amniotic fluid cortisol levels.[42] The maturation of hypothalamic-pituitary-adrenal axis in human fetus is correlated with pulmonary maturation.[33] CRF synthesized by placenta might contribute to the activation of the fetal pituitary-adrenal axis in late pregnancy, thus participating to the mechanisms of prenatal fetal maturation. This hypothesis is true in lower species. Long-term infusion of exogenous CRF in ovine fetuses accelerates the maturation of a number

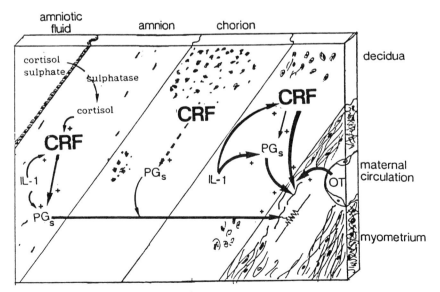

FIGURE 2. Corticotropin-releasing factor (CRF) increases prostaglandin (PGs) release from cultured human amnion, chorion and decidual cells (IL-1: interleukin-1; OT: oxytocin).

of organs and systems culminating in the premature delivery of viable lambs.[43] A possible role of CRF in the maturational processes of the human fetal lung is suggested by the evidence that in a population of pregnant women close to term, the highest CRF levels are found in those showing a lekythin:sphingomyelin ratio greater than 2 and a positive phosphatidylglycerol test.[44] Placental CRF-induced activation of fetal pituitary-adrenal axis might lead to maturation of the fetal lung and to a cortisol-induced increase of CRF output by placenta and fetal membranes. A reverberating circuit might potentiate the release of both factors, leading to activation of PG release. However, both in monkeys and in the human, the role of pituitary-adrenal axis in controlling the timing of parturition is less evident than in sheep.

An action of placental CRF on the maternal hypothalamic-pituitary-adrenal axis is suggested by the large release of CRF within maternal circulation. In spite of the presence of a binding globulin,[45-47] placental CRF may be one of the causal factors of the high ACTH and cortisol levels during pregnancy.[32] The hyperactivity of the pituitary-adrenal axis in pregnant women is supported by the lack of any inhibitory effect of glucocorticoids as well as by the failure of CRF in increasing ACTH levels.[48,49] A desensitization of pituitary CRF receptors due to the high levels of endogenous CRF may occur during pregnancy.

NEUROPEPTIDE Y

Neuropeptide Y (NPY) is a 36-amino acid peptide previously isolated in the central and peripheral nervous system.[50] NPY is widely distributed in the brain, participating in pathways influencing behavior and neuroendocrine function.[50] It is also co-localized and interacts with NEpi in the sympathetic terminations innervating the cardiovascular, respiratory, gastrointestinal, and genitourinary system.[51] Recently, immunoreactive NPY has been also evidenced in extracts of term human placenta.[52] The cyto- and intermediate trophoblast cells contain NPY. In fact, the most intense immunostaining for NPY in term placenta is found in the inner space of the villi, the periphery of the villi being only partially stained.[52] A local role of NPY in human placenta is suggested by the evidence of a single class of specific NPY binding sites largely distributed within the placental villi.[52] In preparations of cells from term human placenta, the addition of NPY stimulated the release of CRF.[52] The absence of significant change of GnRH, hCG or hPL concentrations following the addition of NPY suggests a possible specific involvement of NPY in the control of placental CRF-ACTH axis. Maternal NPY levels display a significant increase during labor. A two- to threefold rise of plasma NPY coincides with the most advanced stages of cervical dilatation and with parturition.[53] The rapid postpartum decrease supports the placental origin of the circulating NPY in pregnancy. These findings suggest an activation of NPY release from placenta during labor. Such an activation might further contribute to the dramatic increase of CRF during labor.

CONCLUSIONS

The cause-effect relationship between the dramatic increase of PG release by intra-uterine tissues and the onset of labor uterine contractile pattern is widely accepted. Prostaglandins seem to be the major autacoid drive leading to uterine contraction through a paracrine mechanism. An important role is being attributed to paracrine and/or auto-crine mechanisms occurring within placenta, fetal membranes and decidua.

The recent evidence that CRF activates the output of stimulatory PGs by human placenta, fetal membranes and decidua, as well as that it synergizes with oxytocin on myometrial contractility, suggest a possible *in vivo* role of such a peptide. CRF is synthesized by placenta, fetal membranes, and decidua. Among the factors that increase CRF release from cultured trophoblast, particular attention is devoted to NPY and IL-1.

In lower species, CRF might contribute to the synchronization between fetal mat-

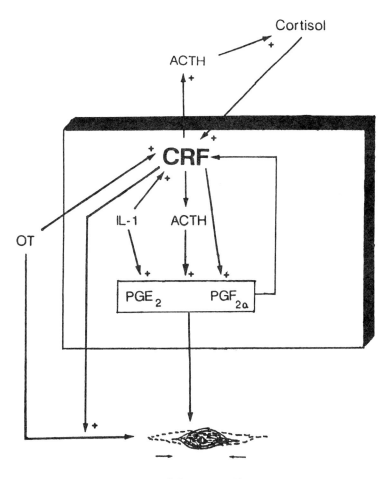

myometrial contraction

FIGURE 3. Placental corticotropin-releasing factor (CRF) may act locally in increasing ACTH, estrogen and prostaglandin release, stimulating uterine contractility and/or activating the maternal and fetal pituitary-adrenal axes (OT: oxytocin; IL-1: interleukin-1).

uration mechanisms and onset of labor, through its interaction with the fetal pituitary-adrenal axis. In primates, placental CRF participates to the mechanisms of labor, but at the present state it is difficult to predict its role in the onset of labor. Placental CRF may reinforce the endocrine responses to the stress of parturition stimulating both maternal and fetal pituitary-adrenal axes. At the same time, placental CRF may exert an important paracrine and/or autocrine action in regulating local ACTH and PG release and modulating uterine contractility (FIG. 3). It is of interest that cortisol increases placental CRF release, while CRF activates glucocorticoid secretion, as well as that PGE_2 and $PGE_{2\alpha}$ stimulate the output of CRF, while CRF stimulates the release of these eicosanoids from placenta and fetal membranes. Moreover, oxytocin stimulates the release of CRF, while CRF potentiates the effect of oxytocin on myometrium. These data suggest that CRF may participate in potentiating circuits triggered during parturition. These circuits may potentiate placental CRF release and therefore emphasize its role in the stress of parturition and in the local control of uterine contractility.

REFERENCES

1. OLSON, D. M., S. J. LYE, K. SKINNER & J. R. G. CHALLIS. 1985. Prostanoid concentrations in maternal/fetal plasma and amniotic fluid and intrauterine tissue prostanoid output in relation to myometrial contractility during the onset of adrenocorticotropin-induced preterm labor in sheep. Endocrinology 116: 389–397.

2. GREEN, K., M. BYGDEMAN, M. TOPPOZADA & N. WIQVIST. 1974. The role of prostaglandin $F_{2\alpha}$ in human parturition. Endogenous plasma levels of 15-keto-13,14-dihydro-prostaglandin $F_{2\alpha}$ during labor. Am. J. Obstet. Gynecol. 120: 25–31.

3. CHALLIS, J. R. G. & D. M. OLSON. 1988. Parturition. In The Physiology of Reproduction. E. Knobil & J. NEILL, EDS. VOL. 2: 2177–2216. Raven Press. New York.

4. GIANNOPOULOS, G., K. JACKSON, J. KREDENTSER & D. TULCHINSKY. 1985. Prostaglandin E and $F_{2\alpha}$ receptors in human myometrium during the menstrual cycle and in pregnancy and labor. Am. J. Obstet. Gynecol. 153: 904–910.

5. OKAZAKI, T., M. L. CASEY, J. R. OKITA, P. C. MacDONALD & J. M. JOHNSTON. 1981. Initiation of human parturition. XII. Biosynthesis and metabolism of prostaglandins in human fetal membranes and uterine decidua. Am. J. Obstet. Gynecol. 139: 373–381.

6. NAKLA, S., K. SKINNER, B. F. MITCHELL & J. R. G. CHALLIS. 1986. Changes in prostaglandin transfer across human fetal membranes obtained after spontaneous labour. Am. J. Obstet. Gynecol. 155: 1337–1341.

7. FUCHS, A-R., S. PERIYASAMY, M. ALEXANDROVA & M. S. SOLOFF. 1983. Correlation between oxytocin receptor concentration and responsiveness to oxytocin in pregnant rat myometrium: Effects of ovarian steroids. Endocrinology 113: 742–749.

8. OLSON, D. M., K. SKINNER & J. R. G. CHALLIS. 1983. Estradiol-17β and 1-hydroxyestradiol-17β-induced differential production of prostaglandins by cells dispersed from human intrauterine tissues at parturition. Prostaglandins 25: 639–648.

9. MITCHELL, B. F., B. CRUICKSHANK, D. McLEAN & J. R. G. CHALLIS. 1982. Local modulation of pregesterone production in human fetal membranes. J. Clin. Endocrinol. Metab. 55: 1237–1239.

10. SHIBASAKI, T., E. ODAGIRI, K. SHIZUME & N. LING. 1982. Corticotropin-releasing factor-like activity in human placental extract. J. Clin. Endocrinol. Metab. 55: 384–386.

11. GRINO, M., G. P. CHROUSOS & A. N. MARGIORIS. 1987. The corticotropin-releasing hormone gene is expressed in human placenta. Biochem. Biophys. Res. Commun. 148: 1208–1214.

12. FRIM, D. M., R. L. EMANUEL, B. G. ROBINSON, C. M. SMAS, G. K. ADLER & J. A. MAJZOUD. 1988. Characterization and gestational regulation of corticotropin-releasing hormone messenger RNA in human placenta. J. Clin. Invest. 82: 287–292.

13. SASAKI, A., P. TEMPST, A. S. LIOTTA, A. N. MARGIORIS, L. E. HOOD, S. B. H. KENT & D. T.

KRIEGER. 1988. Isolation and characterization of a corticotropin-releasing hormone-like peptide from human placenta. J. Clin. Endocrinol. Metab. **67**: 768–773.

14. PETRAGLIA, F., P. E. SAWCHENKO, J. RIVIER & W. VALE. 1987. Evidence for local stimulation of ACTH secretion by corticotropin-releasing factor in human placenta. Nature **328**: 717–719.

15. JONES, S. A., A. N. BROOKS & J. R. G. CHALLIS. 1989. Steroids modulate corticotropin-releasing hormone production in human fetal membranes and placenta. J. Clin. Endocrinol. Metab. **68**: 825–830.

16. CAMPBELL, E. A., E. A. LINTON, C. D. A. WOLFE, P. R. SCRAGGS, M. T. JONES & P. J. LOWRY. 1987. Plasma corticotropin-releasing hormone concentrations during pregnancy and parturition. J. Clin. Endocrinol. Metab. **64**: 1054–1059.

17. SASAKI, A., O. SHINKAWA, A. N. MARGIORIS, A. S. LIOTTA, S. SATO, O. MURAKAMI, M. GO, Y. SHIMIZU, K. HANEW & K. YOSHINAGA. 1987. Immunoreactive corticotropin-releasing hormone in human plasma during pregnancy, labor, and delivery. J. Clin. Endocrinol. Metab. **64**: 224–229.

18. GOLAND, R. S., S. L. WARDLAW, R. I. STARK, L. S. BROWN & A. G. FRANTZ. 1986. High levels of corticotropin-releasing hormone immunoreactivity in maternal and fetal plasma during pregnancy. J. Clin. Endocrinol. Metab. **63**: 1199–1203.

19. GOLAND, R. S., S. L. WARDLAW, M. BLUM, P. J. TROPPER & R. I. STARK. 1988. Biologically active corticotropin-releasing hormone in maternal and fetal plasma during pregnancy. Am. J. Obstet. Gynecol. **159**: 884–890.

20. NAGASHIMA, K., H. YAGI, H. YUNOKI, T. NOJI & T. KUROUME. 1987. Cord blood levels of corticotropin releasing factor. Biol. Neon. **51**: 1–4.

21. PETRAGLIA, F., L. GIARDINO, G. COUKOS, L. CALZÁ, W. VALE & A. R. GENAZZANI. 1990. Corticotropin-releasing factor and parturition: Plasma and amniotic fluid levels and placental binding sites. Obstet. Gynecol. **75**: 784–789.

22. WOLFE, C. D. A., S. PATEL, E. A. LINTON, E. A. CAMPBELL, J. ANDERSON, A. DORNHORST, P. J. LOWRY & M. T. JONES. 1988. Plasma corticotropin-releasing hormone in abnormal pregnancy. Br. J. Obstet. Gynecol. **95**: 1003–1006.

23. PETRAGLIA, F., S. SUTTON & W. VALE. 1989. Neurotransmitters and peptides modulate the release of immunoreactive corticotropin-releasing factor from human cultured placental cells. Am. J. Obstet. Gynecol. **160**: 247–251.

24. JONES, C. M. & F. C. GREISS. 1982. The effect of labor on maternal and fetal circulatory catecholamines. Am. J. Obstet. Gynecol. **144**: 149–153.

25. OLUBADEWO, J. O. & B. V. R. SASTRY. 1978. Human placental cholinergic system: stimulation secretion coupling for release of acetylcholine from isolated placental villus. J. Pharm. Exp. Ther. **204**: 433–445.

26. BRENNECKE, S. P., S. CHEN, R. G. KING & L. A. BOURA. 1988. Human placental acetylcholine content and release at parturition. Clin. Exp. Pharmacol. Physiol. **15**: 715–725.

27. PETRAGLIA, F., G. C. GARUTI, B. M. DeRAMUNDO, S. ANGIONI, A. R. GENAZZANI & M. BILEZIKJIAN. 1990. Mechanisms of action of interleukin-1β in increasing corticotropin-releasing factor and adrenocorticotropin hormone from cultured human placental cells. Am. J. Obstet. Gynecol. **163**: 1307–1312.

28. ROMERO, R., S. DURUM, C. DINARELLO, E. OYARZUN, J. C. HOBBINS & M. D. MITCHELL. 1989. Interleukin-1 stimulates prostaglandin biosynthesis by human amnion. Prostaglandins **37**: 13–22.

29. FLYNN, A., J. FINKE & M. L. HILFINKER. 1982. Placental mononuclear phagocytes as a source of interleukin-1. Science **218**: 475–476.

30. ROMERO, R., D. T. BRODY, E. OYARZUN, M. MAZOR, Y. K. WU, J. C. HOBBINS & S. K. DURUM. 1989. Infection and labor. III. Interleukin-1: a signal for the onset of parturition. Am. J. Obstet. Gynecol. **160**: 1117–1123.

31. ROBINSON, B. G., R. L. EMANUEL, D. M. FRIM & J. A. MAJZOUB. 1988. Glucocorticoids stimulate the expression of corticotropin-releasing hormone gene in human placenta. Proc. Natl. Acad. Sci. USA. **85**: 5244–5248.

32. CARR, B. R., C. R. PARKER, J. D. MADDEN, P. C. MACDONALD & J. C. PORTER. 1981. Maternal plasma adrenocorticotropin and cortisol relationship throughout human pregnancy. Am. J. Obstet. Gynecol. **139**: 416–422.

33. FENCL, M. DE M., R. J. SILLMAN, J. COHEN & D. TULCHINSKY. 1980. Direct evidence of sudden rise in fetal corticoids late in human gestation. Nature **287**: 225–226.

34. ODAGIRI, E., B. J. SHERREL, C. D. MOUNT, W. E. NICKOLSON & D. N. ORTH. 1979. Human placental immunoreactive corticotropin, lipotropin, and β-endorphin: Evidence for a common precursor. Proc. Natl. Acad. Sci. USA **76:** 2027-2031.

35. AL-TIMINI, A. & H. FOX. 1986. Immunohistochemical localization of follicle-stimulating hormone, luteinizing hormone, growth hormone, adrenocorticotrophic hormone and prolactin in the human placenta. Placenta **7:** 163-172.

36. MARGIORIS, A. N., M. GRINO, P. PROTOS, P. W. GOLD & G. P. CHROUSOS. 1988. Corticotropin-releasing hormone and oxytocin stimulate the release of placental proopiomelanocortin peptides. J. Clin. Endocrinol. Metab. **66:** 922-926.

37. PETRAGLIA, F., A. VOLPE, A. R. GENAZZANI, J. RIVIER, P. E. SAWCHENKO & W. VALE. 1990. Neuroendocrinology of human placenta. Front. Neuroendocrinol. **11:** 6-37.

38. JONES, S. A. & J. R. G. CHALLIS. 1990. Effects of corticotropin-releasing hormone and adrenocorticotropin on prostaglandin output by human placenta and fetal membranes. Gynecol. Obstet. Invest. **29:** 165-168.

39. QUARTERO, H. W. P. & C. H. FRY. 1989. Placental corticotropin releasing factor may modulate human parturition. Placenta **10:** 439-443.

40. BLUMENFELD, Z. & R. B. JAFFE. 1986. Hypophysiotropic and neuromodulatory regulation of adrenocorticotropin in the human fetal pituitary gland. J. Clin. Invest. **78:** 288-294.

41. ACKLAND, J. F., S. J. RATTER, G. L. BOURNE & L. H. REES. 1986. Corticotropin-releasing factor-like immunoreactivity and bioactivity of human fetal and adult hypothalami. J. Endocrinol. **108:** 171-180.

42. CHALLIS, J. R. G., P. HARTLEY, P. JOHNSON, J. E. PATRICK, J. S. ROBINSON & G. D. THORBURN. 1977. Steroids in the amniotic fluid of the monkey (*Macaca mulatta*). J. Endocrinol. **73:** 355-363.

43. WINTOUR, E. M., R. J. BELL, R. S. CARSON, R. J. MACISAAC, G. W. TREGEAR, W. VALE & X. M. WANG. 1986. Effect of long-term infusion of ovine corticotropin-releasing factor in the immature ovine fetus. J. Endocrinol. **111:** 469-479.

44. LAATIKAINEN, T., I. J. RAISANEN & K. SALMINEN. 1988. Corticotropin-releasing hormone in amniotic fluid during gestation and labor in relation to fetal lung maturation. Am. J. Obstet. Gynecol. **159:** 891-895.

45. ORTH, D. N. & C. D. MOUNT. 1987. Specific high-affinity binding protein for human corticotropin-releasing hormone in normal human plasma. Biochem. Biophys. Res. Commun. **143:** 411-417.

46. LINTON, E. A., C. D. A. WOLFE, D. P. BEHAN & P. J. LOWRY. 1988. A specific carrier substance for human corticotropin-releasing factor in late gestational maternal plasma which could mask the ACTH-releasing activity. Clin. Endocrinol. **28:** 315-324.

47. SUDA, T., M. IWASHITA, T. USHIYAMA, F. TOZAWA, T. SUMITOMO & Y. NAKAGAMI. 1989. Responses to corticotropin-releasing hormone and its bound and free forms in pregnant and nonpregnant women. J. Clin. Endocrinol. Metab. **69:** 38-42.

48. SMITH, R., P. C. OWENS, M. W. BRINSMEAD, B. SINGH & C. HALL. 1987. The nonsuppressibility of plasma cortisol persists after pregnancy. Horm. Metab. Res. **19:** 41-42.

49. SASAKI, A., O. SHINKAWA & K. YOSHINAGA. 1989. Placental corticotropin-releasing hormone may be a stimulator of maternal pituitary adrenocorticotropin hormone secretion in humans. J. Clin. Invest. **84:** 1997-2001.

50. O'DONOHUE, T. L., B. M. CHRONWALL, R. M. PRUSS, J. MEZEY, J. Z. KISS, L. E. EIDEN, V. J. MASSARI, R. E. TESSEL, V. M. PICKEL, D. A. DIMAGGIO, A. HOTCHKISS, W. R. CROWEL & Z. ZUKOWSKA-GROJEC. 1985. Neuropeptide Y and peptide YY neuronal and endocrine systems. Peptides **6:** 755-768.

51. STJERNQUIST, M. & C. OWEN. 1987. Interaction of noradrenalin NPY and VIP with the neurogenic cholinergic response of the rat uterine cervix in vitro. Acta Physiol. Scand. **131:** 554-562.

52. PETRAGLIA, F., L. CALZÁ, L. GIARDINO, S. SUTTON, P. MARRAMA, J. RIVIER, A. R. GENAZZANI & M. VALE. 1989. Identification of immunoreactive neuropeptide-Y in human placenta: Localization, secretion, and binding sites. Endocrinology **124:** 2016-2022.

53. PETRAGLIA, F., G. COUKOS, C. BATTAGLIA, A. BARTOLOTTI, A. VOLPE, C. NAPPI, A. SEGRE & A. R. GENAZZANI. 1989. Plasma and amniotic fluid immunoreactive neuropeptide-Y levels changes during pregnancy, labor and at parturition. J. Clin. Endocrinol. Metab. **69:** 324-328.

Evidence for 5-Hydroxyeicosatetraenoic Acid (5-HETE) and Leukotriene C₄ (LTC₄) in the Onset of Labor[a,b]

SCOTT W. WALSH

Department of Obstetrics and Gynecology
Medical College of Virginia
Virginia Commonwealth University
Box 34 MCV Station
Richmond, Virginia 23298-0034

INTRODUCTION

Prostaglandins (PGE₂, PGF$_{2\alpha}$) are produced by reproductive tissues and are important compounds in the process of labor.[1-7] They are often considered the universal mediators of parturition. The human amnion, chorion, decidua, and placenta also form the lipoxygenase compounds: hydroxyeicosatetraenoic acids (HETEs) and leukotrienes (LTs).[8-11] Preliminary evidence now suggests that they may also be involved.

In 1986, we presented the first evidence that lipoxygenase metabolites of arachidonic acid may be part of the parturitional process.[12] We demonstrated that 5-HETE is present in significantly higher concentrations than PGF$_{2\alpha}$ in the amniotic fluid of chronically catheterized rhesus monkeys, and that 5-HETE concentrations progressively increase with the onset of labor. In 1987, Romero *et al.* reported that 12-HETE, 15-HETE, and LTB₄ are present in human amniotic fluid at term, and are significantly higher in women that are in labor as compared to women not in labor.[13] In 1988, it was reported that *in vitro* synthesis of LTB₄, LTD₄ and 11-*trans*-LTD₄ by human amnion, chorion, and decidua vera is greatly increased from tissues obtained after vaginal delivery as opposed to tissues obtained during elective cesarean section before the onset of labor,[11] and in 1989 that human umbilical concentrations of LTB₄ and LTD₄ are significantly higher after spontaneous vaginal delivery than during cesarean section before labor.[14] 15-HETE and LTB₄ also increase in association with intra-amniotic infection and preterm labor,[15] and group B streptococcus stimulates the release of PGE₂ and of di- and mono-hydroxylated HETEs from term human amnion cells in culture.[16]

The following study reports sequential measurements of amniotic fluid concentrations of 5-HETE and LTC₄ in relation to PGF$_{2\alpha}$ concentrations preceding term and preterm labor in chronically catheterized rhesus monkeys.

[a] This study was previously presented in part at the 33rd Annual Meeting of the Society for Gynecologic Investigation, March 19–22, 1986, Toronto (Abstract #31); the 35th Annual Meeting of the Society for Gynecologic Investigation, Baltimore, March 17–20, 1988 (Abstract #372); and at the First European Congress on Prostaglandins in Reproduction, July 6–9, 1988, Vienna, Austria.

[b] Supported by Grant HD20973 from the National Institute of Child Health and Human Development.

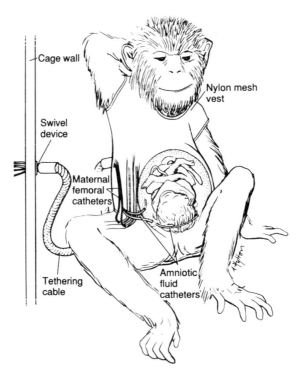

FIGURE 1. Schematic representation of the tether preparation used for chronically catheterized pregnant rhesus monkeys. (For a detailed description of the preparation see ref. 17.)

MATERIALS AND METHODS

Five healthy, pregnant rhesus monkeys (*Macaca mulatta*) of known gestational age weighing between 6.3–8.6 kg were obtained from the California Primate Research Center, Davis, California through its contract with the National Institute of Child Health and Human Development. The animals were maintained in accordance with the NIH Guide for the Care and Use of Laboratory Animals (NIH Publication No. 85-23, 1985). Surgical procedures, animal care, tether preparation (FIG. 1), sample collection and radioimmunoassays were described in the original publication of this study.[17]

Monitoring of Uterine Contractility

Uterine activity was constantly monitored by changes in intrauterine pressure. One of the amniotic fluid catheters was attached to a pressure transducer and amniotic fluid pressure changes were recorded with a 4-channel recorder (Model 7754B System, Hewlett-Packard Co.). At least four distinct patterns of amniotic fluid pressure changes were observed (FIG. 2), and were arbitrarily designated as "minimal," "moderate," "heavy," or "labor."

Uterine Contractility
(Amniotic Fluid Pressure)

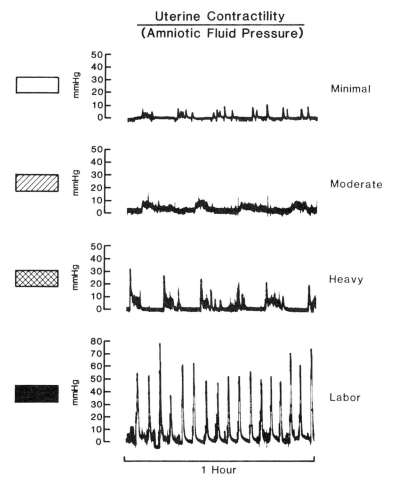

FIGURE 2. Uterine contractility patterns as determined by changes in amniotic fluid pressure. See text for descriptions of each pattern. (Reprinted from ref. 17 with permission.)

The "minimal" uterine contractile pattern appeared to be spontaneous, uncoordinated contractions. They were very low in amplitude (usually less than 5 mmHg) and of short duration (approximately 30 sec). Their frequency was variable, sometimes 4 or 5 contractions occurred one right after the other, but other times there would be a several minute gap between contractions.

"Moderate" uterine contractility was characterized by low-grade increases of amniotic fluid pressure (5–10 mmHg) with a duration of 3–6 minutes. They occurred at a frequency of 3–4 per hour.

The amniotic fluid pressure pattern of the "heavy" contractions appeared to be a progression of the "moderate" contractions. The "heavy" contractions were characterized by a very sharp initial increase in amniotic fluid pressure of approximately 20–40 mmHg in amplitude lasting less than 1 minute. Amniotic fluid pressure then decreased to approximately 10 mmHg and remained relatively constant at this amplitude for 3–6 minutes before returning to baseline. "Heavy" contractions occurred at a frequency of approximately 6 per hour. Both the "moderate" and "heavy" types of uterine contractility fit the definition of "contractures" proposed by Nathanielsz *et al.*[18]

The "heavy" type of uterine contractile pattern almost always preceded the onset of labor contractions. "Labor" contractions were high in amplitude (40–80 mmHg), short in duration (1 min), high in frequency (approximately 24 per h) and generally occurred at night (21:00 h to 06:00 h).

RESULTS AND DISCUSSION

Mean amniotic fluid concentrations at the time of intrauterine surgery are shown in TABLE 1. 5-HETE and LTC_4 were present in the amniotic fluid at this time, but $PGF_{2\alpha}$ was not. This is similar to the human in that LTC_4, but not $PGF_{2\alpha}$, is present in amniotic fluid at midgestation (unpublished observations). Δ-6-*Trans*-LTB_4, LTB_4 and LTD_4 are also present in human amniotic fluid at midgestation.[19] $PGF_{2\alpha}$ was nondetectable after intrauterine surgery despite periods of uterine contractility that were moderate to heavy (FIGS. 3–7). Therefore, $PGF_{2\alpha}$ could not have been responsible for these contractions. $PGF_{2\alpha}$ levels remained nondetectable until 1 to 2 weeks before delivery.

It was surprising that $PGF_{2\alpha}$ was absent after surgery, because in the human, amniotomy results in increased plasma concentrations of PGF metabolite[20] so one would expect an increase in prostaglandin production after intrauterine surgery. However, there is an important difference between the two observations. Amniotomy in the human was done at term, whereas intrauterine surgery in the monkey was done preterm. One can conclude from these data that the 5-lipoxygenase and glutathione S-transferase enzymes necessary for the synthesis of 5-HETE and LTC_4, respectively, are present preterm and before the onset of labor. The data also suggest that the cyclooxygenase enzyme responsible for $PGF_{2\alpha}$ in amniotic fluid may not be present or is in some way suppressed until term or the onset of labor.

Administration of indomethacin after intrauterine surgery to inhibit uterine contractility was of little value because $PGF_{2\alpha}$ was not present. 5-HETE and/or LTC_4 concentrations actually increased during or shortly after indomethacin infusion in three monkeys, #18,764, #16,586 and #17,720 (FIGS. 3, 5, and 7). This suggests that indomethacin might have caused a shunting of arachidonic acid from the cyclooxygenase pathway to the lipoxygenase pathway. The two animals that delivered prematurely (#18,764 and #17,720) also received the most indomethacin infusions, and their li-

TABLE 1. Amniotic Fluid Concentrations

	Intrauterine Surgery	Labor
5-HETE	4.4 ± 0.8 ng/ml	40 ± 8 ng/ml[a]
LTC_4	2.5 ± 0.7	20 ± 4[b]
$PGF_{2\alpha}$	ND	5.4 ± 2.1

[a] Significantly higher than LTC_4 and $PGF_{2\alpha}$.
[b] Significantly higher than $PGF_{2\alpha}$.

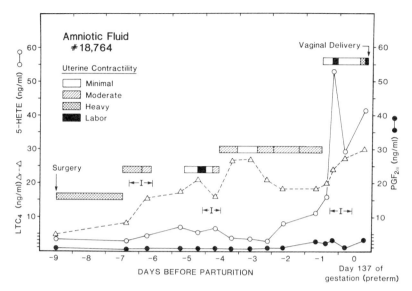

FIGURE 3. Amniotic fluid concentrations of 5-HETE, LTC₄ and PGF₂ₐ before and during preterm labor in rhesus monkey #18,764. Labor contractions were nocturnal. On Days −1 and 0, the mother demonstrated labor types of behavior characteristic of rhesus monkeys (*i.e.*, grunting, hooting, sighing, good appetite, periodically lying down on one side). A male fetus, 300g was delivered late in the evening on Day 0. I = indomethacin infusion to the mother, iv, 6mg/h. Hatch marks on X axis indicate midnight or 24:00 h. (Reprinted from ref. 17 with permission.)

poxygenase metabolites increased progressively from intrauterine surgery to vaginal delivery. Therefore, cyclooxygenase inhibition after intrauterine surgery may be counter productive. It is noteworthy that indomethacin infusion, i.v., into the mother, although effective in suppressing PGF₂ₐ, did not prevent the onset of premature labor and vaginal delivery (#18,764 and #17,720).

Approximately one week before delivery, 5-HETE and LTC₄ concentrations increased sharply in association with the appearance of a nocturnal pattern of labor contractions (FIGS. 3–6). A nocturnal pattern of uterine contractility is characteristic of rhesus monkeys during labor and is associated with a live fetus and a nocturnal rhythm in fetal adrenal activity.[21-24] We first reported that labor contractions were nocturnal in rhesus monkeys in 1980,[21] but it is now recognized that women also have a nocturnal rhythm of uterine activity when allowed to deliver on their own.[25]

The concentrations of 5-HETE and LTC₄ increased in all animals before and during labor, regardless of whether labor was term or preterm, or whether the fetus was alive or dead. This was not true of PGF₂ₐ. There was little or no change in amniotic fluid levels of PGF₂ₐ in monkey #16,586 (FIG. 5) with term labor. In monkey, #17,720 (FIG. 7), prostaglandin synthesis was suppressed with indomethacin to concentrations ≤0.08 ng/ml, but preterm labor still occurred and the animal delivered vaginally. These two animals demonstrate that labor contractions and vaginal delivery can occur without increased prostaglandin production as evidenced by amniotic fluid concentrations of PGF₂ₐ. Although it is possible uterine tissue levels of prostaglan-

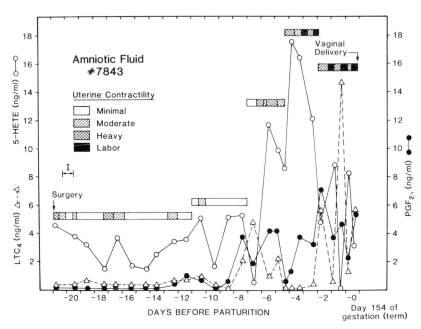

FIGURE 4. Amniotic fluid concentrations of 5-HETE, LTC$_4$, and PGF$_{2\alpha}$ before and during term labor in rhesus monkey #7843. There was a nocturnal labor contraction pattern from Day -4 to Day 0. The mother started showing labor behavioral characteristics on Day -5 that continued through delivery. The amniotic fluid samples collected on Day 0 contained blood (approximately 4% red blood cells per ml of fluid). At approximately 22:00 h of Day 0 a male fetus weighing 350g was delivered. I = indomethacin infusion to the mother, iv, 6mg/h. Hatch marks on X axis indicate midnight or 24:00 h. (Reprinted from ref. 17 with permission.)

dins were sufficient to stimulate uterine contractions, this is unlikely because intravenous infusion of indomethacin would have inhibited prostaglandin synthesis in tissues, as well as prostaglandin levels in a fluid compartment, such as the amniotic fluid.

Amniotic fluid eicosanoid concentrations sometimes fluctuated markedly from day to day and even within the same day. If similar fluctuations occur in human amniotic fluid, it would explain the large concentration variations reported for the human where only a single sample of amniotic fluid is collected from each patient.[13,15,26,27] The fluctuations in eicosanoid concentrations cannot be explained by a nonspecific factor, such as a change in amniotic fluid volume or osmolality, because 5-HETE, LTC$_4$ and PGF$_{2\alpha}$ concentrations did not always change in the same direction (FIGS. 3–7). For example, sometimes LTC$_4$ concentrations increased while 5-HETE and PGF$_{2\alpha}$ concentrations decreased, sometimes 5-HETE decreased while LTC$_4$ and PGF$_{2\alpha}$ increased, sometimes 5-HETE and LTC$_4$ changed without a change in PGF$_{2\alpha}$, and sometimes they all increased or decreased together. This suggests there are both common and separate regulatory mechanisms for the lipoxygenase and cyclooxygenase metabolites of arachidonic acid.

An increase in the osmolality of the amniotic fluid is a possible stimulus for the

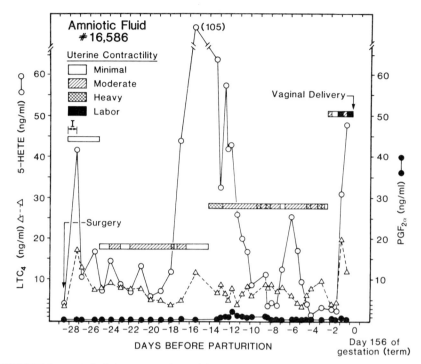

FIGURE 5. Amniotic fluid concentrations of 5-HETE, LTC$_4$ and PGF$_{2\alpha}$ before and during term labor in rhesus monkey #16,586. A nocturnal labor contraction pattern was present from Day -2 to Day 0. The mother demonstrated behavior characteristic of labor on Day -14 and again on Days -1 and 0. At approximately 10:00 h on Day 0 a female fetus weighing 400g was born. I = maternal indomethacin infusion, iv, 6mg/h. Hatch marks on X axis indicates midnight or 24:00 h. (Reprinted from ref. 17 with permission.)

synthesis of arachidonic acid metabolites from the amnion and chorion, but this cannot explain the results of this study. Changes in the amniotic fluid osmolality were not related to either the fluctuations in concentrations of the amniotic fluid eicosanoids or the marked increase in their concentrations with the onset of labor (FIGS. 8 and 9).

The source of 5-HETE and LTC$_4$ in amniotic fluid is not known. Human amnion, chorion, decidua, and placenta can synthesize HETEs and LTs,[8-11] so one or more of these tissues could be the source of the amniotic fluid lipoxygenase metabolites. Monocytes that infiltrate the decidua during pregnancy are another possible source.[28] Fetal excretion of lipoxygenase metabolites into the amniotic fluid is also possible because various fetal tissues, including kidney, liver and lung, can form lipoxygenase products.[9]

Leukotrienes synthesized by intrauterine tissues are probably not secreted into the maternal circulation. This is evidenced by the fact that systemic blood pressure did not decrease during labor (FIGS. 8 and 9) when the concentrations of LTC$_4$ were increasing greatly. If leukotrienes were secreted, then maternal blood pressure should

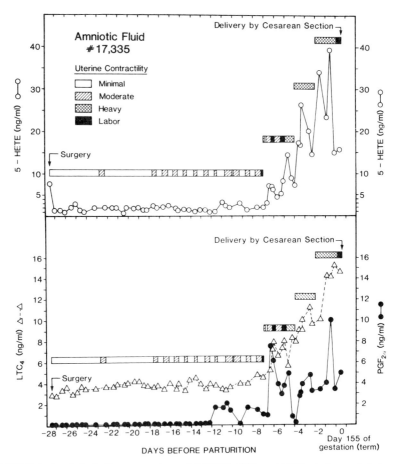

FIGURE 6. Amniotic fluid concentrations of 5-HETE, LTC_4 and $PGF_{2\alpha}$ before and during term labor in rhesus monkey #l7,335. There was a circadian rhythm in uterine activity between Days −18 to −9. The contractions were moderate during the day, usually occurring between 06:00 h and 09:00 h. On Day −8 nocturnal labor contractions began and continued until Day −5. During this time the mother's behavior was characteristic of labor. From Day −5 to Day −1 there was constant heavy uterine contractions. On Day 0, labor began at approximately 04:00 h and continued until cesarean section at 13:00 h. On Day −9 the amniotic fluid was more yellowish than previously (probably meconium stained). On Days −8 and −7 the fluid was yellowish, tinged with red. From the evening of Day −7 to Day −3 the amniotic fluid contained blood (approximately 4.2%–6.7% red blood cells per ml of fluid). By Day 0 the amniotic fluid contained thick, black blood and the mother was exhausted and experiencing labor contractions every minute. The cervix was fully effaced. Oxytocin was given several times to assist in labor, but was unsuccessful. A cesarean section was done at 13:00 h. A dead, macerated female fetus was delivered. Judging from the state of maceration, the fetus had been dead *in utero* for at least 3 to 4 days. Hatch marks on X axis indicate midnight or 24:00 h. (Reprinted from ref. 17 with permission.)

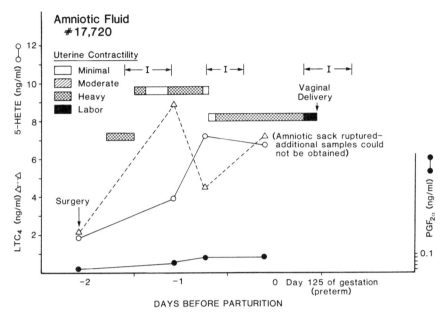

FIGURE 7. Amniotic fluid concentrations of 5-HETE, LTC$_4$ and PGF$_{2\alpha}$ before and during preterm labor in rhesus monkey #17,720. Uterine contractility was heavy at the time the amniotic fluid catheters were connected to the pressure transducer and recorder. Labor and vaginal delivery occurred two days after intrauterine surgery despite nightly indomethacin infusions that kept PGF$_{2\alpha}$ levels suppressed to $\leqslant 0.08$ ng/ml (Note change of scale for PGF$_{2\alpha}$). There was no circadian pattern for uterine contractility. On Day 0 the amniotic fluid sac ruptured in the early afternoon. The animal went into labor at approximately 19:30 h and delivered vaginally a female fetus, 300g, on Day 126 of gestation. I = indomethacin infusion, iv, 6mg/h. Hatch marks on X axis indicate midnight or 24:00 h. (Reprinted from ref. 17 with permission.)

have declined because injection of LTB$_4$, LTC$_4$ or LTD$_4$ into the lower vena cava of pregnant or postpartum rhesus monkeys causes blood pressure to fall.[29] Preliminary observations in human pregnancy also suggest that intra-uterine leukotrienes are not secreted into the mother's circulation during labor because maternal plasma concentrations of LTB$_4$ and LTD$_4$ were not increased by labor.[30]

LTC$_4$ is a potent stimulator of smooth muscle contractility.[31-35] In the guinea pig uterus, LTC$_4$ is equal in potency to PGF$_{2\alpha}$, but weaker than PGE$_2$, in stimulating contractions.[36] LTC$_4$ was not found to stimulate contractions of the human uterus *in vitro* in one report;[37] however, the investigators used doses lower than those demonstrated to stimulate uterine contractility in the guinea pig. Concentrations of LTC$_4$ in human amniotic fluid are higher for women in labor than for women not in labor at term.[27] Both the guinea pig uterus and human uterus contain receptors for LTC$_4$.[38,39]

5-HETE produces a dose-dependent increase in human myometrial contractility *in vitro*,[40] and amniotic fluid 5-HETE concentrations are higher at term for women in labor than women not in labor.[26] In the monkey, amniotic fluid concentrations of 5-HETE were several-fold higher than PGF$_{2\alpha}$ concentrations. Because both 5-HETE

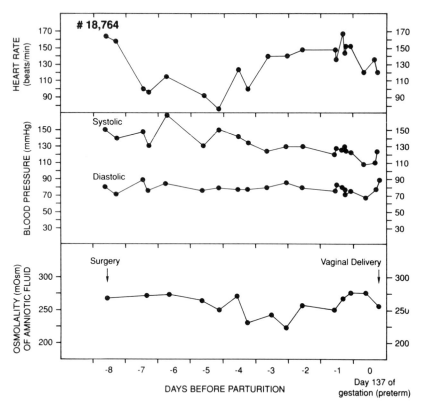

FIGURE 8. Maternal heart rate, blood pressure and amniotic fluid osmolality in rhesus monkey #18,764 who delivered preterm. Hatch marks on X axis indicate midnight or 24:00 h.

and LTC$_4$ stimulate myometrial contractility, it is likely that they act in concert with PGF and PGE to stimulate uterine contractions during parturition.

5-HETE (as well as 12- and 15-HETE) may play an important role in the parturitional process other than stimulation of uterine contractions. Most studies on parturition focus on compounds or mechanisms relating to uterine contractility, but there are other aspects to parturition that are physiologically important. For example, the HETEs are best known for their chemokinetic and chemotaxic actions on white blood cells.[41,42] Mononuclear phagocytes (especially the immature ones), as well as leukocytes, increase in human maternal peripheral blood in association with labor,[43,44] and the cytotoxic activity of human lymphocytes increases significantly at the time of labor.[45] It is possible that intrauterine production of HETEs acts as a signal to recruit white blood cells to the uterus and to activate them, there to augment prostaglandin and leukotriene production and act as a first line of defense against any infection that might enter the uterus from the vagina during or after delivery.

Teleologically this makes good sense. At the time of vaginal delivery there is an open route for bacteria to enter the uterus from the vagina. Those individuals who

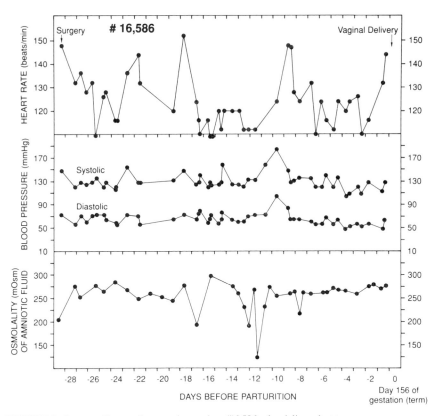

FIGURE 9. Same as FIGURE 8 except in monkey #16,586 who delivered at term.

developed the capacity to recruit additional white blood cells to line the uterine lumen before delivery would be able to immediately kill any bacteria that entered the uterus. Those individuals who did not develop this capacity and recruited white blood cells only after the uterus was infected, would have either died or the resultant scar tissue in the uterus would have made the individual infertile. In either case, the genetic information would not have been carried on to future generations.

Liggins[46] has likened cervical ripening at the time of labor as an inflammatory reaction. It may be that the entire parturitional process is an inflammatory reaction as suggested by Mitchell *et al.*[47]

The findings of the present study challenge the dogma that prostaglandins are the universal mediators of uterine contractility and parturition for several reasons: 1) Moderate to heavy uterine contractions were present after preterm intrauterine surgery despite the fact that PGF₂ₐ levels were not detectable. 2) Inhibition of prostaglandin synthesis with indomethacin did not prevent premature labor and delivery. 3) Labor and vaginal delivery occurred in two animals without an increase in PGF₂ₐ. 4) Labor contractions and vaginal delivery occurred in one animal even though prostaglandin synthesis was suppressed with indomethacin.

SUMMARY

Arachidonic acid is metabolized by cyclooxygenase leading to prostaglandins (PG), and by lipoxygenases leading to hydroxyeicosatetraenoic acids (HETE) and leukotrienes (LT). PGs are potent uterine constrictors. 5-HETE and LTC_4 also stimulate uterine contractions, but their role in labor is not known. To estimate the activities of these pathways before parturition and their relationship to uterine contractility, amniotic fluid (AF) concentrations of 5-HETE, LTC_4 and $PGF_{2\alpha}$ were determined in 5 chronically catheterized rhesus monkeys. Uterine contractility was continually assessed by changes in AF pressure. *Results*: AF concentrations at the time of intrauterine surgery were 4.4 ± 0.8 ng/ml for 5-HETE and 2.5 ± 0.7 ng/ml for LTC_4. $PGF_{2\alpha}$ levels were nondetectable. Indomethacin infusion into the mother, although effective in suppressing $PGF_{2\alpha}$ levels, did not prevent the onset of premature labor and vaginal delivery in 2 animals. $PGF_{2\alpha}$ did not increase in 1 monkey with term labor. Approximately 1 week before delivery, 5-HETE and LTC_4 concentrations increased sharply in all animals in association with a nocturnal pattern of labor contractions. Peak AF concentrations during labor were 5-HETE: 40 ± 8 ng/ml, LTC_4: 20 ± 4 ng/ml, and $PGF_{2\alpha}$: 5.4 ± 2.1 ng/ml. *Comment*: LTC_4 and 5-HETE stimulate uterine contractility *in vitro*, and probably act in concert with PGF and PGE to stimulate uterine contractions during parturition. HETEs may also act as a signal to recruit white blood cells to the uterus and to activate them, there to augment PG and LT production and act as a first line of defense against any infection that might enter the uterus from the vagina during or after delivery. *Conclusions*: 1) 5-HETE and LTC_4, but not $PGF_{2\alpha}$, are associated with uterine contractility after preterm intrauterine surgery. Surprisingly, AF $PGF_{2\alpha}$ levels were nondetectable for 1 to 2 weeks after surgery. 2) 5-HETE and LTC_4 are present in higher concentrations than $PGF_{2\alpha}$ in AF. 3) 5-HETE, LTC_4 and $PGF_{2\alpha}$ all increase with the onset of labor. AF concentrations of 5-HETE and LTC_4 are significantly higher than $PGF_{2\alpha}$ before and during term and preterm labor. 4) Labor can occur with suppressed $PGF_{2\alpha}$ levels, but with increasing 5-HETE and LTC_4 levels. 5) These data suggest that 5-HETE and LTC_4 are important components of the parturitional process, and they challenge the dogma that PGs are the universal mediators of labor.

REFERENCES

1. MITCHELL, M. D. 1987. Occurrence and measurement of eicosanoids during pregnancy and parturition. *In* Eicosanoids and Reproduction. K. Hiller, Ed.: 89–107, MTP Press, Ltd. Lancaster.
2. CHALLIS, J. R. G. 1984. Disorders of parturition. *In* Maternal-Fetal Medicine. Principles and Practices. R. K. Creasy & R. Resnik, Eds.: 401–414, W. B. Saunders Co. Philadelphia.
3. NOVY, M. J. & G. C. LIGGINS. 1980. Role of prostaglandins, prostacyclin and thromboxanes in the physiologic control of the uterus and in parturition. Semin. Perinatol. 4(1): 45–66.
4. MACDONALD, P. C. & J. PORTER, Eds. 1983. Initiation of Parturition: Prevention of Prematurity, Report on the Fourth Ross Conference on Obstetric Research: 1–184, Ross Laboratories, Columbus, OH.
5. LIGGINS, G. C., C. S. FORSTER, S. A. GRIEVES & A. L. SCHWARTZ. 1977. Control of parturition in man. Biol. Reprod., 16(1): 39–56.
6. LIGGINS, G. C., R. J. FAIRCLOUGH, S. A. GRIEVES, J. Z. KENDALL & B. S. KNOX. 1973. The mechanism of initiation of parturition in the ewe. Recent Prog. Horm. Res. 29: 111–159.
7. WALSH, S. W. 1989. Prostaglandins in Pregnancy. *In* Gynecology and Obstetrics. J. J. Sciarra,

Ed. Vol. 5. Reproductive Endocrinology, Infertility and Genetics, L. Speroff & J. L. Simpson, Eds. Ch. 5.043:1–21. J. B. Lippincott Co. Philadelphia.

8. SAEED, S. A. & M. D. MITCHELL. 1982. Formation of arachidonate lipoxygenase metabolites by human fetal membranes, uterine decidua vera and placenta. Prostaglandins Leukotrienes Med. 8(6): 635–640.

9. MITCHELL, M. D., S. P. BRENNECKE, S. A. SAEED & D. M. STRICKLAND. 1985. Arachidonic acid metabolism in the fetus and neonate. In Biological Protection with Prostaglandins. M. M. Cohen, Ed. Vol. 1: 27–44. CRC Press, Inc. Boca Raton, FL.

10. WALSH, S. W. & V. M. PARISI. 1990. Eicosanoids and hypertension in pregnancy. In Eicosanoids in Reproduction. M. D. Mitchell, Ed.: 249–272. CRC Press Inc., Boca Raton, FL.

11. PASETTO, N., E. PICCIONE, C. TICCONI, L. LENTI, A. ZICARI & G. PONTIERI. 1988. Synthesis of leukotrienes by human fetal membranes and decidua vera: Relationship with labour. XIth European Congress of Perinatal Medicine, Rome, Italy, :439–442.

12. WALSH, S. W., S. R. YOUNG & E. J. STOCKMAR. 1986. Increased 5-lipoxygenase activity precedes labor. 33rd Annual Meeting of the Society for Gynecologic Investigation, Toronto, Ontario (Abstract #31).

13. ROMERO, R., M. EMAMIAN, M. WAN, C. GRZYBOSKI, J. C. HOBBINS & M. D. MITCHELL. 1987. Increased concentrations of arachidonic acid lipoxygenase metabolites in amniotic fluid during parturition. Obstet. Gynecol. 70(6): 849–851.

14. PASETTO, N., E. PICCIONE, C. TICCONI, G. PONTIERI, L. LENTI & A. ZICARI. 1989. Leukotrienes in human umbilical plasma at birth. Br. J. Obstet. Gynaecol. 96: 88–91.

15. ROMERO, R., R. QUINTERO, M. EMAMIAN, M. WAN, C. GRZYBOSKI, J. C. HOBBINS & M. D. MITCHELL. 1987. Arachidonate lipoxygenase metabolites in amniotic fluid of women with intraamniotic infection and preterm labor. Am. J. Obstet. Gynecol. 157(6): 1454–1460.

16. BENNETT, P. R., M. P. ROSE, L. MYATT & M. G. ELDER. 1987. Preterm labor: Stimulation of arachidonic acid metabolism in human amnion cells by bacterial products. Am. J. Obstet. Gynecol. 156(3): 649–655.

17. WALSH, S. W. 1989. 5-Hydroxyeicosatetraenoic acid, leukotriene C$_4$ and prostaglandin F$_{2\alpha}$ in amniotic fluid before and during term and preterm labor. Am. J. Obstet. Gynecol. 161(5): 1352–1360.

18. NATHANIELSZ, P. W., E. R. POORE, A. BRODIE, N. F. TAYLOR, G. PIMENTEL, J. P. FIGUEROA & D. FRANK. 1984. Update on the molecular events of myometrial activity during pregnancy. In Research in Perinatal Medicine (I), P. W. Nathanielsz & J. T. Parer, Eds.: 87–111. Perinatology Press. Ithaca, NY.

19. LENTI, L., A. ZICARI, G. PONTIERI, C. TICCONI, A. PIETROPOLLI, E. PICCIONE & N. PASETTO. Leukotrienes in human amniotic fluid at midgestation. Clin. Chem. Enzymol. Commun. In press.

20. MITCHELL, M. D., A. P. F. FLINT, J. BIBBY, J. BRUNT, J. M. ARNOLD, A. B. M. ANDERSON & A. C. TURNBULL. 1977. Rapid increases in plasma prostaglandin concentrations after vaginal examination and amniotomy. Br. Med. J. 2(6096): 1183–1185.

21. NOVY, M. J., S. W. WALSH & M. J. COOK. 1980. Chronic implantation of catheters and electrodes in pregnant nonhuman primates. In Animal Models in Fetal Medicine. P. Nathanielsz, Ed.: 133–168. Elsevier/North Holland Biomedical Press. Amsterdam.

22. DUCSAY, C. A., M. J. COOK, S. W. WALSH & M. J. NOVY. 1983. Circadian patterns and dexamethasone-induced changes in uterine activity in pregnant rhesus monkeys. Am. J. Obstet. Gynecol. 145: 389–396.

23. TAYLOR, N. F., M. C. MARTIN, P. W. NATHANIELSZ & M. SERON-FERRÉ. 1983. The fetus determines circadian oscillation of myometrial electromyographic activity in the pregnant rhesus monkey. Am. J. Obstet. Gynecol. 146: 557–567.

24. WALSH, S. W., C. A. DUCSAY & M. J. NOVY. 1984. Circadian hormonal interactions among the mother, fetus, and amniotic fluid. Am. J. Obstet. Gynecol. 150: 745–753, 1984.

25. SMOLENSKY, M. H. 1983. Aspects of human chronopathology. In Biological Rhythms and Medicine: Cellular, Metabolic, Physiopathologic and Pharmacologic Aspects. A. Reinberg & M. H. Smolensky, Eds.: 131–209. Springer-Verlag. New York.

26. ROMERO, R., Y. K. WU, M. MAZOR, J. C. HOBBINS & M. D. MITCHELL. 1989. Amniotic fluid concentration of 5-hydroxyeicosatetraenoic acid is increased in human parturition at term. Prostaglandins. Leukotrienes Essent. Fatty Acids 35(2): 81–83.

27. ROMERO, R., Y. K. WU, M. MAZOR, J. C. HOBBINS & M. D. MITCHELL. 1988. Increased amniotic fluid leukotriene C_4 concentration in term human parturition. Am. J. Obstet. Gynecol. 159(3): 655–657.

28. SMARASON, A. K., A. GUNNARSSON, J. H. ALFREDSON & H. VALDIMARSSON. 1986. Monocytosis and monocytic infiltration of decidua in early pregnancy. J. Clin. Lab. Immunol. 21(1): 1–5.

29. WALSH, S. W. & V. M. PARISI. 1989. Leukotrienes, but not hydroxyeicosatetraenoic acids, lower blood pressure in pregnant and postpartum rhesus monkeys. Clin. Exp. Hypertens. [B] Hypertens. Pregnancy B8: 305–329.

30. PASETTO, N., E. PICCIONE, C. TICCONI, L. LENTI, A. ZICARI & G. PONTIERI. 1988. Leukotrienes and labour: Maternal plasma levels. New Trends Gynaecol. Obstet. 4: 41–46.

31. PIPER, P. J. 1984. Formation and actions of leukotrienes. Physiol. Rev. 64: 744–761.

32. SAMUELSSON, B. 1983. Leukotrienes: Mediators of immediate hypersensitivity reactions and inflammation. Science 220(4597): 568–575.

33. YOKOCKI, K., P. M. OLLEY, E. SIDERIS, F. HAMILTON, D. HUHTANEN & F. COCEANI. 1982. Leukotriene D_4: A potent vasoconstrictor of the pulmonary and systemic circulation in the newborn lamb. In Leukotrienes and other Lipoxygenase Products, Advances in Prostaglandin, Thromboxane, Leukotriene Research. B. Samuelsson & R. Paoletti, Eds. Vol. 9: 211–214. Raven Press. New York.

34. SOIFER, S. J., R. D. LOITZ, C. ROMAN & M. A. HEYMANN. 1985. Leukotriene and organ antagonists increase pulmonary blood flow in fetal lambs. Am. J. Physiol. 249(3): H570–H576.

35. WALSH, S. W. & V. M. PARISI. 1986. The role of arachidonic acid metabolites in preeclampsia. Semin. Perinatol. 10(4): 334–355.

36. WEICHMAN, B. M. & S. S. TUCKER. 1982. Contraction of guinea pig uterus by synthetic leukotrienes. Prostaglandins 24(2): 245–253.

37. BRYMAN, I., S. HAMMARSTRÖM, B. LINDBLOM, A. NORSTRÖM, M. WIKLAND & N. WIQVIST. 1985. Leukotrienes and myometrial activity of the term pregnant uterus. Prostaglandins 30(6): 907–911.

38. BRAY, M. A. 1985. Leukotriene receptors. In Leukotrienes in Cardiovascular and Pulmonary Function. A. M. Lefer & M. H. Gee, Eds.: 17–28. Alan R. Liss, Inc. New York.

39. CHEGINI, N. & CH V. RAO. 1988. The presence of leukotriene C_4- and prostacyclin-binding sites in nonpregnant human uterine tissues. J. Clin. Endocrinol. Metab. 66(1): 76–87.

40. BENNETT, P. R., M. G., ELDER & L. MYATT. 1987. The effects of lipoxygenase metabolites of arachidonic acid on human myometrial contractility. Prostaglandins 33(6): 837–844.

41. GOETZL, E. J., D. W. GOLDMAN, P. H. NACCACHE, R. I. SHA'AFI & W. C. PICKETT. 1982. Mediation of leukocyte components of inflammatory reactions by lipoxygenase products of arachidonic acid. In Leukotrienes and Other Lipoxygenase Products, Advances in Prostaglandin, Thromboxane, Leukotriene Research, B. Sammuelsson & R. Paoletti, Eds. Vol. 9: 273–282. Raven Press. New York.

42. STENSON, W. F. & C. W. PARKER. 1984. Leukotrienes. Adv. Internal. Med. 30: 175–199.

43. BUCHAN, G. S., B. L. GIBBINS & J. F. T. GRIFFIN. 1985. The influence of parturition on peripheral blood mononuclear phagocyte subpopulations in pregnant women. J. Leukocyte Biol. 37(2): 231–242.

44. ACKER, D. B., M. P. JOHNSON, B. P. SACHS & E. A. FRIEDMAN. 1985. The leukocyte count in labor. Am. J. Obstet. Gynecol. 153: 737–739.

45. SZEKERES-BARTHO, J., P. VARGA & A. S. PACSA. 1986. Immunologic factors contributing to the initiation of labor-lymphocyte reactivity in term labor and threatened preterm delivery. Am. J. Obstet. Gynecol. 155(1): 108–112.

46. LIGGINS, G. C. 1981. Cervical ripening as an inflammatory reaction. In The Cervix in Pregnancy and Labour. D. A. Ellwood & A. B. M. Anderson, Eds.: 1–9. Churchill Livingstone. Edinburgh.

47. MITCHELL, M. D., D. M. STRICKLAND, S. P. BRENNECKE & S. A. SAEED. 1983. New aspects of arachidonic acid metabolism and human parturition. In Initiation of Parturition: Prevention of Prematurity, Report of the Fourth Ross Conference on Obstetric Research. P. C. MacDonald & J. Porter, Eds.: 145–153, Ross Laboratories. Columbus, OH.

The Role of Systemic and Intrauterine Infection in Preterm Parturition

ROBERTO ROMERO, CECILIA AVILA,
CAROL ANN BREKUS, AND RAFFAELLA MOROTTI

Department of Obstetrics and Gynecology
Yale University School of Medicine
New Haven, Connecticut 06510

INTRODUCTION

A growing body of evidence suggests that infection is associated with preterm labor and delivery.[1-3] This chapter will review this evidence and discuss the proposed cellular and biochemical mechanisms by which infection may lead to parturition.

Three lines of evidence support a role for infection in the onset of labor: 1) the administration of bacteria or bacterial products to animals results in either abortion or labor[4-11]; 2) systemic maternal infections such as pyelonephritis, pneumonia and typhoid fever are associated with the onset of labor[12-24]; and 3) localized intrauterine infection is associated with preterm labor and delivery.

ANIMAL EXPERIMENTATION

In 1944, Zahal and Bjerknes demonstrated that the injection of Shigella and Salmonella endotoxin into mice and rabbits was capable of inducing abortion.[5] Takeda and Tsuchiya confirmed this observation using *E. Coli* endotoxin in pregnant mice and rabbits.[6,7] Subsequently, several investigators have replicated these findings using different animal species.[8-10] Furthermore, immunization of animals with an anti-endotoxin antibody ameliorates this biological effect.[25] The mechanisms of endotoxin-induced abortion appear to be mediated by prostaglandins (PG), as the concentration of PGDF increases in serum, endometrium and urine after the administration of Salmonella endotoxin to pregnant mice on day 16.[11] Furthermore, pre-treatment of the animals with indomethacin reduced the endotoxin induced abortion rate from 51.2% to 18%.[11] Recently, a model of ascending infection has been developed by placing bacteria through a hysteroscope into the uterine cavity of rabbits.[26]

SYSTEMIC MATERNAL INFECTION

Systemic maternal febrile infections such as pneumonia, pyelonephritis, malaria and typhoid fever have been associated with preterm labor and delivery. The rate of preterm delivery associated with maternal pneumonia ranges from 15% to 48%.[12-15] Although the advent of antibiotic treatment has dramatically reduced maternal mortality from this condition, it has not affected the rate of preterm delivery. While in the pre-antibiotic era pyelonephritis was associated with preterm delivery, in the post-antibiotic era this condition is associated with preterm labor but not preterm delivery.[16-19] Similarly, typhoid fever in the pre-antibiotic era carried a 60% to 80% risk of abortion and preterm labor, but this risk has decreased after the introduction of antibiotic therapy.[20-22] Malaria during pregnancy has also been associated with a 50% rate of preterm delivery.[23] However, chemoprophylaxis seems to protect patients from preterm delivery.[24] Collectively, these data provide support for the concept that severe untreated systemic maternal infection is associated with preterm labor and delivery and that treatment may decrease the rate of preterm delivery in some cases (*e.g.*, pyelonephritis, typhoid fever) but not in others (*e.g.*, pneumonia). The mechanisms involved in the initiation of labor in the setting of systemic infections have not been studied in the human. However, wide clinical experience indicates that maternal fever is associated with increased uterine activity. This effect has been demonstrated with parenteral administration of endotoxin to women at term. A two- to threefold increase in uterine activity was noted during the chill period (15 to 60 minutes), and uterine activity gradually diminished.[27] Since parenteral administration of endotoxin to animals and humans results in the production and release of cytokines and this, in turn, can stimulate PG production, we have proposed that these products mediate the increase in uterine activity in the setting of febrile maternal infection.[28]

Intrauterine Infection

Despite the important role of systemic maternal infection in the etiology of preterm labor, these diseases are rare, and therefore, their attributable risk to preterm delivery is low. Recently, the association between intrauterine infection and preterm labor and delivery has become a major focus of investigation.

The amniotic cavity is normally sterile. Microbial invasion of the amniotic cavity can occur after rupture of membranes and even with intact membranes. To accurately assess the microbiologic state of this cavity, the method of amniotic fluid collection is critical. The two methods generally used are transabdominal amniocentesis and transcervical retrieval, either by needle puncturing of the membranes or by aspiration through an intrauterine catheter. Transcervical amniotic fluid collection is associated with an unacceptable risk of contamination with vaginal flora; therefore, when analyzing the prevalence of microbial invasion of the amniotic cavity in term and preterm labor, we will only review studies in which amniotic fluid was obtained by transabdominal amniocentesis.

There is disagreement in the literature regarding the terminology used to describe microbial invasion of the uterine cavity during pregnancy. We have previously employed the term "intraamniotic infection" to indicate the presence of a positive amniotic fluid culture for microorganisms regardless of the presence or absence of clinical signs or symptoms of infection. The term "clinical chorioamnionitis" refers to the clinical syndrome associated with microbial invasion of the amniotic cavity. Manifestations include: maternal fever, uterine tenderness, foul-smelling vaginal discharge, fetal tachycardia and maternal leukocytosis.[29] This clinical syndrome appears only in a small fraction of women with microbial invasion of the amniotic cavity. In a recent study, we found that only 12.5% of women with preterm labor (intact membranes) and a positive amniotic fluid culture had clinical chorioamnionitis.[30] The presence and severity of clinical chorioamnionitis is probably related to both microbial factors and to the host response to the infection. Microbial factors include the type and virulence of the microorganism, inoculum size and pathway of infection (hematogenous vs. ascending infection). Host factors include the local and systemic cytokine response to the presence of infection and the systemic effects of these products on the host.

Microorganisms may gain access to the amniotic cavity and fetus using any of the following pathways: 1) by ascending from the vagina and the cervix; 2) by hematogenous dissemination through the placenta (transplacental infection); 3) by retrograde seeding from the peritoneal cavity through the fallopian tubes; and 4) by accidental introduction at the time of invasive procedures (*e.g.*, amniocentesis, percutaneous blood sampling, chorionic villous sampling or shunting).[30-36]

Indirect evidence indicates that the most common pathway of intrauterine infection is the ascending route. This evidence includes: 1) histologic chorioamnionitis is more common and severe at the site of membrane rupture than in other locations, such as the placental chorionic plate or umbilical cord; 2) in cases of congenital pneumonia (stillbirths or neonatal), inflammation of the chorioamniotic membranes is present in the overwhelming majority of cases; 3) the bacteria identified in cases of congenital infections are similar to those found in the genital tract; and 4) in twin gestation, histologic chorioamnionitis is more common in the first-born twin and is extremely rare in the second twin only. As the membranes of the first twin are generally apposed to the cervix, this is taken as evidence in favor of an ascending infection.[30-36] This proposition is consistent with our observations of amniotic fluid microbiology in twin gestations. Indeed, in cases of microbial invasion of the amniotic cavity in twin gestation, the presenting sac was involved. When both amniotic cavities were involved, the inoculum size was larger in the presenting sac.[37]

The mechanisms responsible for preterm premature rupture of membranes (PROM) may also be associated with ascending infection. A localized infection in the choriodecidual junction can lead to rupture of membranes. Microbial invasion of the amniotic cavity may result from the spread of microorganisms from the localized choriodecidual nidus or by direct spread from the vagina through the site of rupture. Rupture of membranes can also result when ascending infection, as described in the previous paragraph, reaches the amniotic cavity in women with intact membranes. The effect of bacterial proteases and/or host products secreted in response to bacterial infection from both sides of the membranes may lead to weakening of the membranes.[38]

The Role of Intrauterine Infection in Preterm Delivery

Several lines of evidence suggest that intrauterine infection is associated with preterm labor and delivery. This evidence is derived from: 1) microbiologic studies of the amniotic cavity; 2) histopathologic examination of the placenta; and 3) clinical and laboratory evidence of infection or inflammation in patients with preterm delivery. This section will critically review this evidence.

Studies examining the clinical circumstances surrounding preterm delivery indicate that one third of all patients presenting with preterm labor have intact membranes. A second third is associated with preterm PROM, and the remaining third results from delivery because of maternal or fetal indications.[39]

To examine the role of intrauterine infection in preterm delivery, we will review the association between microbial invasion of the amniotic cavity and spontaneous preterm labor (with or without intact membranes). However, this analysis may underestimate the real contribution of intrauterine infection to the etiology of preterm delivery, since an amniotic fluid culture only reflects the microbiologic state of the amniotic cavity. If an intrauterine infection is limited to the extra-amniotic space (*e.g.*, deciduitis), it will not be detected with an amniotic fluid culture.

Intraamniotic Infection and Preterm Labor with Intact Membranes and Preterm Premature Rupture of Membranes

TABLE 1 displays the results of studies in which amniocenteses were performed on women with preterm labor and intact membranes.[30,40–51] The mean rate of positive amniotic fluid cultures was 11.9% (90/758). Women with positive amniotic fluid cultures generally did not have clinical evidence of infection at presentation, but they were more likely to subsequently develop chorioamnionitis (42.2% [38/90] vs. 4% [13/328]), to be refractory to tocolysis (62.5% [35/56] vs. 13% [36/276]) and to rupture their membranes spontaneously (20% [9/46] vs. 5.1% [15/292]) than were the women with negative amniotic fluid cultures.[3]

TABLE 2 displays the results of amniotic fluid cultures from women with preterm PROM in seven published studies.[50,52–57] Positive amniotic fluid cultures occurred in 27.9% (113/404). This figure probably underestimates the true prevalence of intraamniotic infection. Recent evidence gathered by ultrasound indicates that women with PROM and severely reduced amniotic fluid volumes have a higher incidence of intraamniotic infection.[56,58] Since these women are less likely to have an amniocentesis, the bias

TABLE 1. Intraamniotic Infection in Women with Preterm Labor and Intact Membranes as Determined by Amniotic Fluid Studies Obtained by Transabdominal Amniocentesis[a]

Author	Year	No. of Patients	Positive Cultures No.	Positive Cultures %	Clinical Chorio-amnionitis No.	Clinical Chorio-amnionitis %	PROM No.	PROM %	Refractory to Tocolysis No.	Refractory to Tocolysis %
Miller *et al.*[41]	1980	23	11	47.8	8	72.7	2/7	28.5		
Bobitt *et al.*[42]	1981	31	8	25.8	6	75.0			7/8	87.5
Wallace & Herrich[43]	1981	25	3	12.0	1	33.3				
Hameed *et al.*[44]	1984	37	4	10.8	3	75.0			3/4	75.0
Wahbeh *et al.*[45]	1984	33	7	21.2	2	28.5			4/7	57.1
Wieble & Randall[46]	1985	35	1	2.9	1	100.0				
Leigh & Garite[40]	1986	59	7	11.8	4	57.1	4/7	57.1	7/7	100.0
Gravett *et al.*[47]	1986	54	13	24.0	5	38.5			5/13	38.5
Iams *et al.*[48]	1987	5	0	0.0						
Duff & Kopelman[49]	1987	24	1	4.2	0		0/1		0/1	
Romero *et al.*[50]	1988	41	4	9.8						
Skoll *et al.*[51]	1989	127	7	5.5	1	14.3	1/7			
Romero *et al.*[30]	1989	264	24	9.1	3	12.5	2/24		9/16	56
TOTAL		758	90	11.9	38	42.2	9/46	19.6	35/56	62

[a] Table taken with permission from R. Romero & M. Mazor. 1988. Infection and Preterm Labor. Clin. Obstet. Gynecol. **31:** 553.

TABLE 2. Intraamniotic Infection in Women with Preterm PROM as Determined by Amniotic Fluid Studies Obtained by Transabdominal Amniocentesis[a]

Author	Year	No. of Patients	Positive Culture		Success Rate (%)	Clinical Chorio-amnionitis		Neonatal Infection	
			No.	%		No.	%	No.	%
Garite et al.[52]	1979	59	9/30	30.0	51	6/9	66.6	2/9	22.2
Garite & Freeman[53]	1982	207	20/86	23.2	49	11/20	55.0	5/20	25.0
Cotton et al.[54]	1984	61	6/41	14.6	69	6/6	100	1/6	16.6
Broekhuizen et al.[55]	1985	79	15/53	28.3	66	3/15	20	8/15	53.3
Vintzileous et al.[56]	1985	54	12/54	22.2	—	2/12	16.6	4/12	33.3
Feinstein et al.[57]	1986	73	12/50	20.0	68	6/12	50	5/12	41.6
Romero et al.[50]	1988	90	39/90	43.3	95	—		—	
TOTAL		623	113/404	27.9	59	34/74	45.9	25/74	33.7

[a] Table taken with permission from R. Romero & M. Mazor. 1988. Infection and preterm labor. Clin. Obstet. Gynecol. 31: 553.

in these studies is to underestimate the prevalence of infection. Another bias in these studies is that women with preterm PROM who were admitted in labor did not undergo amniocentesis. Therefore, such studies provide information about the prevalence of intraamniotic infection in women who had preterm PROM without labor. Recently, we have documented that patients who were in preterm labor on admission had a tendency to have a higher incidence of positive amniotic fluid cultures in comparison to women admitted with PROM who were not in labor (39% vs. 25%, p = 0.049). Furthermore, of patients who were not in labor on admission, 60% had a positive amniotic fluid culture when they entered active labor.[59]

Placental Chorioamnionitis

Inflammation of the placenta is a host-response mechanism to a variety of stimuli such as infection and immune injury. Traditionally, acute inflammation of the chorio-amniotic membranes has been considered an indicator of amniotic fluid infection.[2,29,31,36,60-62] This view has been based upon indirect evidence. Previous studies have demonstrated an association between acute inflammatory lesions of the placenta and the recovery of microorganisms from the subchorionic plate[63,64] and from the chorioamniotic space.[65] Bacteria have been recovered from the subchorionic plate of 72% of placentas with histologic chorioamnionitis.[63] In another study, 39.1% of chorio-amniotic membranes that showed diffuse inflammation had bacteria detected with Gram's and Grocott's stains in the histologic sections. Immunofluorescence studies with antibodies against Group B Streptococcus (GBS) and *Bacteroides fragilis* showed that 14/15 and 5/15 placentas, respectively, were positive for these organisms despite negative microbiology in most cases.[66] Furthermore, we have recently found that there is an excellent correlation between positive amniotic fluid cultures and histologic chorioamnionitis.[67]

Several studies have examined the prevalence of inflammation in placentas from women delivering preterm infants. The results of these studies have been reviewed in detail elsewhere.[3] Russell reported that histologic chorioamnionitis was more common in women who delivered prematurely than in the entire obstetrical population (18.7% [123/659] vs. 5.2% [392/7505], $p < 0.01$).[68] Using the data from the Collaborative Perinatal Project, Naeye and Peters found a higher incidence of histologic chorioamnionitis in the placentas of women delivering between 20 to 28 weeks than in the placentas of women delivering between 33 to 37 weeks (23% vs. 11%).[2] Guzick and Winn also found that histologic chorioamnionitis was significantly more common in women with preterm delivery than in women with term deliveries (38.8% [80/244] vs. 10% [253/2530], $p < 0.01$). If PROM was present, 48.6% (51/105) of all preterm deliveries had histologic chorioamnionitis. In the absence of PROM, 20.9% (29/139) of preterm deliveries had chorioamnionitis.[69]

Clinical Evidence of Chorioamnionitis

The prevalence of endometritis is higher in women delivering preterm than in women delivering at term (PROM preterm: 18.7% [38/203] vs. PROM term: 8.4% [38/454], $p < 0.001$; preterm intact membranes 13.1% [36/274] vs. 6.4% [120/1881], $p < 0.001$). Furthermore, the prevalence of endometritis is the same after preterm delivery with intact membranes as after delivery with PROM. These data suggest that postpartum infection is associated with preterm delivery.[70]

Maternal C-Reactive Protein

Subclinical infection is difficult to diagnose without amniocentesis. Acute phase reactant proteins have been utilized as a marker of clinical infection. The most widely utilized of these proteins is C-reactive protein (CRP).[71] However, CRP is a marker of host response to injury rather than a specific indicator of infection.

TABLE 3 shows the prevalence of elevated CRP in women with preterm labor and

TABLE 3. Prevalence of Maternal C-Reactive Protein in Women with Preterm PROM and in Women with Preterm Labor and Intact Membranes

| | | | | Preterm Labor | | | |
| | | | | PROM | | Intact Membranes | |
Author	Year	Definition of Positive Results	No. of Patients	No.	%	No.	%
Evans et al.[72]	1980	>2 mg/dl	36	20	55.5		
Farb et al.[73]	1983	>2 mg/dl	33			11	33.0
Hawrylyshyn et al.[74]	1983	>1.25 mg/dl	52	23	44.2		
Romem & Artal[75]	1984	>1.78–1.8 mg/dl	51	14	27.4		
Handwerker[76]	1984	–	50			15	30.0
Potkul et al.[77]	1985	>0.7 mg/dl	40			16	40.0
Dodds & Iams[78]	1987	>0.8 mg/dl	34			21	61.7
TOTAL			296	57/139	41.0	63/157	40.1

[a] Table taken with permission from: R. Romero, M. Mazor, Y. K. Wu, M. Sirtori, E. Oyarzun, M. D. Mitchell, & J. C. Hobbins. 1988. Infection in the pathogenesis of preterm labor. Semin. Perinatol. **12:** 262–279.

PROM.[72-78] The prevalence of elevated CRP is similar in women with preterm labor who are with or without PROM. An important observation is that women with preterm labor and elevated CRP are less likely to respond to tocolysis than women with normal or non-detectable serum CRP (77.7% [28/36] vs. 10.4% [5/48], respectively).[76,78] A good correlation between maternal CRP concentrations and histologic chorioamnionitis (sensitivity 88% and specificity 96%) in a population of patients with preterm PROM has also been reported.[74]

Genitourinary Infection

Colonization of the genitourinary tract with several microorganisms has been associated with prematurity, low birth weight and PROM. We have reviewed in detail the literature concerning urinary and cervico-vaginal colonization with the most common microorganisms and their relationship to preterm delivery. The interested reader is referred to this material for specific details.[3]

The relationship between asymptomatic bacteriuria and preterm delivery/low birth weight has been a controversial issue for years.[79-88] We have recently employed meta-analysis to critically review the available data and have found that women with asymptomatic bacteriuria have a higher rate of prematurity/low birth weight than nonbacteriuric women. Furthermore, eradication of asymptomatic bacteriuria with antibiotic treatment results in a reduction of the rate of preterm birth/low birth weight.[89]

There is convincing evidence of a relationship between gonorrhea and prematurity. Of five studies reviewed, four confirm this association.[90-94] Recently, attention has been called to the relationship between bacterial vaginosis and preterm delivery.[95] After reviewing the literature, we found three case-controlled studies and one cohort study that support an association between bacterial vaginosis and preterm labor.[47,95-98] The only cohort study in which enrollment occurred in early pregnancy did not show an assocation between preterm labor and bacterial vaginosis.[96]

Cervico-vaginal colonization with GBS, *Trichomonas vaginalis* and Mycoplasma species (*Mycoplasma hominis* and *Ureaplasma urealyticum*) has been implicated in the etiology of preterm birth.[47,96-124] After a critical review of the literature, we cannot conclude that there is evidence to support an association between cervico-vaginal colonization with these microorganisms and preterm birth.[3] The relationship between *Chlamydia trachomatis* infection and preterm birth is inconclusive. In seven different studies addressing the association between cervical colonization with *Chlamydia trachomatis* and preterm birth, three supported, three negated and one yielded inconclusive results.[97,98,103-107]

Neonatal Sepsis

The prevalence of neonatal sepsis is 4.3/1000 live births in premature infants, in contrast to 0.8/1000 live births for term infants.[125] Furthermore, the lower the birth weight, the higher the prevalence of sepsis (164/1000 for 1001 to 1500g; 91/1000 for 1501 to 2000g; and 23/1000 for 2001 to 2500g).[126] The conventional interpretation of these data is that premature newborns are more susceptible to infection. The observation that at least half of the cases of sepsis are diagnosed within the first 48 hours after delivery, together with the high prevalence of intraamniotic infection in women with preterm labor and preterm PROM, calls for a reappraisal of this traditional view. We would suggest that the higher prevalence of sepsis in the preterm newborn is partially attributable to a higher incidence of intrauterine infection in women in preterm labor. Furthermore, we propose that the onset of preterm labor in this subpopulation may be part of the repertoire of a host defense against infection.

THE ROLE OF ARACHIDONIC ACID METABOLITES AND CYTOKINES IN THE INITIATION OF PRETERM LABOR

Arachidonic Acid Metabolites

A solid body of evidence supports a role for products of arachidonic acid metabolism in the onset of human parturition at term. There are fewer available data, however, to support a similar role for metabolites of arachidonic acid in preterm labor.[127-134]

Prostaglandins have been measured in peripheral blood and amniotic fluid in women in preterm labor. Mitchell et al.[128] found no significant difference in peripheral plasma levels of 13, 14-dihydro-15-keto-PGF (PGFM) in women with preterm labor and in non-laboring women in late pregnancy. Moreover, plasma concentrations of PGFM were significantly lower in preterm labor than in early labor at term.[128] Subsequently, Sellers et al. were unable to demonstrate a significant difference in plasma PGFM concentrations between women in early preterm labor and in non-laboring women of similar gestational ages. Furthermore, the plasma concentrations of this compound were not different in women with preterm labor who delivered within 24 hours compared to those in preterm labor whose pregnancy continued and delivered at term.[129] In contrast, Weitz et al. found that plasma concentrations of PGFM were significantly higher in women with preterm labor who failed tocolysis and delivered a premature infant than in women responding to this treatment.[132]

Tambyraja et al.[127] found that the concentration of PGFM in amniotic fluid of women in preterm labor increased as labor progressed. They could not demonstrate any predictive value of PGFM concentrations in the outcome of preterm labor treated with salbutamol. Similarly, Nieder and Augustin could not demonstrate a significant elevation in amniotic fluid PGE_2 and PGF_2 in women with premature labor when compared to women without labor of a similar gestational age.[133] Recently, our group has shown that amniotic fluid concentrations of PGE_2 and its stable metabolite 11-deoxy-13, 14-dihydro-15-keto-11, 16-cyclo PGE_2 (PGEM-II) were significantly higher in women with preterm labor who are unresponsive to tocolysis than in those responsive to tocolysis.[134] Furthermore, women with preterm labor and intraamniotic infections had higher amniotic fluid concentrations of PGE_2, PGE-II, PGF_2 and PGFM than did women without intraamniotic infection.[135] In addition, amniotic fluid concentrations of PGE_2 and PGF_2 are increased in women with intraamniotic infection and preterm PROM in labor.[131] Therefore, there is evidence supporting the participation of PG in the mechanisms involved in the onset of parturition in women with intraamniotic infection. On the other hand, it should be stressed that similar evidence supporting a role for PG in preterm labor in the absence of intraamniotic infection is lacking.

Metabolites of arachidonic acid through the lipoxygenase pathway are also postulated to play a role in the onset and maintenance of human parturition at term.[136,137]

Since some of the arachidonate lipoxygenase metabolites may act as inflammatory mediators and can stimulate uterine contractility, they may also be involved in the mechanisms responsible for preterm labor.[138-140] Indeed, we have recently shown that the concentrations of 5-hydroxyeicosatetraenoic acid (5-HETE) are increased in the amniotic fluid of women in preterm labor leading to delivery, regardless of the presence or absence of infection.[141] This observation is potentially important because 5-HETE can stimulate uterine contractility in a dose-dependent manner.[139] Amniotic fluid concentrations of leukotriene-B4 (LTB4) and 15-HETE are also elevated in women with preterm labor and intraamniotic infection.[142] In contrast, we have not been able to demonstrate changes in the amniotic fluid concentrations of LTC4 and 12-HETE in these patients in comparison to other women in preterm labor.[142] These findings suggest that preterm labor with intraamniotic infection is associated with selective activation of the lipoxygenase pathway of arachidonic acid.

In the setting of preterm labor, there is a paucity of information known about the signals controlling bioavailability of PG and lipoxygenase metabolites of arachidonic acid. Although the signals may be similar to those operating in term labor, recent work has focused on the role of bacterial products and host mediators in the generation of PG by intrauterine tissues.

Bacterial Products

PG biosynthesis in the setting of bacterial infections may be stimulated by either bacterial or host signals secreted in response to microbial presence. The traditional explanation for the onset of labor in the setting of infection has been that bacterial products directly stimulate PG biosynthesis. Indeed, several investigators have shown that bacterial products are a source of phospholipase A2 and C and can stimulate PG production by human amnion.[143-147] We have also reported that endotoxin (lipopolysaccharide or LPS) is present in the amniotic fluid of women with gram-negative intraamniotic infections[147] and is capable of stimulating PG production by amnion and decidua.[148] Additionally, amniotic fluid concentrations of endotoxin from women with preterm labor and PROM are higher than in women with PROM and without labor.[149] However, the quantities of endotoxin required to stimulate PG production by human amnion are not generally found in the amniotic fluid of women with intraamniotic infection and preterm labor. Moreover, the overlap in endotoxin concentrations between the two groups suggests that factors other than endotoxin are involved in signalling the onset of premature labor in the setting of intraamniotic infection. Therefore, it is possible that other bacterial products may be responsible for the stimulation of arachidonic acid metabolites by intrauterine tissues or, alternatively, that host defense mechanisms are operative.

The observation that 28% to 33% of women with preterm PROM have an intraamniotic infection without labor suggests that the mere presence of microorganisms in the amniotic cavity is not sufficient to lead to the onset of labor.[52-57,59] Furthermore, there is now evidence that effects of microbial products on PG production by intrauterine tissues are more variable than previously thought.[148,150] Recently, we have examined the effect of a bacterial-conditioned media on PG production by amnion and decidua and found that the effect is highly concentration-dependent and that some microorganisms have an inhibitory rather than a stimulatory effect.[151]

Until recently, it was widely accepted that microorganisms alone were responsible for the ill effects and metabolic derangements associated with infection. It has now been established, however, that many of these ill effects are mediated by endogenous host products. A typical example of this is the pathophysiology of endotoxic shock. Bacterial endotoxin exerts its deleterious effects through the release of endogenous mediators such as tumor necrosis factor (TNF) and interleukin-1 (IL-1).

Host Products (Cytokines)

The onset of labor in the setting of infection can be considered the pathophysiologic counterpart to endotoxin shock and, thus, a host-mediated response. In view of the pivotal role of the macrophage-monocyte system in the host response against infection and tissue injury, we have proposed that secretory products of macrophage activation may signal the onset of labor in the presence of infection.[3]

Macrophages are ubiquitous cells present in the maternal (decidua), fetal and placental compartments. These cells are activated by microbial products to secrete a wide variety of mediators including IL-1, IL-6, and TNF.

IL-1, also known as endogenous pyrogen, is produced by activated monocyte/macrophage cells in response to bacterial products such as endotoxin.[152,153] IL-1 is pleotropic cytokine, which, along with TNF and IL-6, has been shown to mediate host responses to infection and injury. The biologic properties of IL-1 include the mediation of fever, actions of T and B lymphocytes, induction of collagenase activity and PG biosynthesis.[153]

Two biochemically related but distinct forms of IL-1 have been isolated: IL-1α and IL-1β. These two cytokines are the products of the different genes. They have the same molecular weight but a different isoelectric point (pI for IL-1α = 5; pI for IL-1β = 7). Despite sharing only a 25% amino acid sequence homology, IL-1α and IL-1β bind to the same receptor. These two peptides have the same spectrum of biological activities.

In 1985, we postulated that IL-1 produced by the host (fetus or mother) could serve as a signal for the initiation of human parturition.[154,155] The evidence to support this view includes: 1) IL-1 stimulates PG production by amnion, decidua and myometrium; 2) human decidua can produce IL-1 in response to bacterial products[154]; 3) amniotic fluid IL-1 bioactivity and concentrations are elevated in women with preterm labor and intraamniotic infection, in contrast to amniotic fluid from patients with preterm labor but without intraamniotic infection, which does not contain IL-1; 4) in women with preterm PROM and intraamniotic infection, IL-1 bioactivity is higher in the presence of labor[156] (these data indicate that it is not the microbial presence in the amniotic cavity but rather the host response to bacterial presence that is associated with the onset of labor); and 5) *in vitro* perfusion of human uteri with IL-1 results in the development of regular uterine contractions (unpublished data).

Another potential role of IL-1 in parturition is participation in cervical ripening. Changes in the biophysical properties of the cervix are associated with modifications in collagen and glycosaminoglycans. Experiments conducted in rabbits have shown that the uterine cervix from term pregnancies produces more IL-1-like activity than the uterine cervix from non-pregnant animals.[157]

We have also found that another monokine, TNF, may participate in the parturition associated with infection.[158] TNF is secreted by activated macrophages and has similar properties to IL-1.[152] Evidence suggesting a role for TNF in the onset of labor associated with infection includes the following: 1) TNF stimulates PG production by human amnion and decidua[158,159]; 2) TNF is produced by human decidua in response to bacterial products[159,160]; and 3) TNF is absent from normal amniotic fluid but is present in the amniotic fluid of women who have intraamniotic infection and preterm labor.[158]

Another cytokine that has been implicated as a major mediator of the host response to infection and tissue damage is IL-6.[161] This cytokine is produced by a wide variety of cells such as macrophages, fibroblasts, endothelial cells, keratinocytes and endometrial stromal cells.[160-165] IL-6 elicits major changes in the biochemical, physiologic and immunologic status of the host, including the acute-phase plasma protein response, activation of T and natural killer cells and stimulation and proliferation of immunoglobulin production by B cells. IL-6 induces the production of CRP by liver cells.[166] This may be important in the context of intraamniotic infection, as clinical studies have indicated that elevated maternal serum CRP often proceeds the development of clinical chorioamnionitis and the onset of preterm labor in women with preterm PROM.[72] We have assayed amniotic fluid IL-6 in women in preterm labor with and without intact membranes. Low levels of IL-6 were detected in the amniotic fluid of normal women in the midtrimester and third trimester of pregnancy. Women with preterm labor with intraamniotic infection had higher amniotic fluid levels of IL-6 than women in preterm labor without intraamniotic infection.[167]

Other bioactive agents secreted during the inflammatory process may also participate in this process. Platelet activating factor is present in the amniotic fluid from women with preterm labor, and this lipid is capable of stimulating PGE_2 production by amnion and of stimulating myometrial contractions directly.[168]

We have proposed a model (FIG. 1) in which the initiation of human parturition in the presence of infection is controlled by the host. Systemic maternal infections, such as pyelonephritis, or localized infections, such as deciduitis, could trigger parturition via the monocyte/macrophage system in peripheral blood and human decidua. Preterm labor can, therefore, be viewed as an event occurring when the intrauterine or maternal environment is hostile and threatens the well-being of the fetus. From this point of view, the initiation of preterm labor may have survival value.

The evidence reviewed above indicates an association between rupture of the fetal membranes and intrauterine infection. The pathophysiology of this event may be similar to that of preterm labor. The membranes are a connective tissue structure. Bacterial infection, directly or indirectly (IL-1 and TNF), may induce the release of proteases (collagenase, elastases, *etc.*) from macrophages or other cell types, which then degrade the fetal membranes and lead to rupture. The reason why some infections result in preterm labor and others in PROM remains to be determined. We view them as two different expressions of the same basic phenomenon: activation of the host-defense macrophage system. Infection seems to be only one etiology for this chain of events.

MICROBIAL INVASION OF THE AMNIOTIC CAVITY: CAUSE OR CONSEQUENCE OF LABOR?

Since the amniotic cavity is normally sterile, we have considered microbial invasion of the amniotic cavity as an abnormal finding. The data presented on TABLES 1 and 2 support an association between microbial invasion of the amniotic cavity and

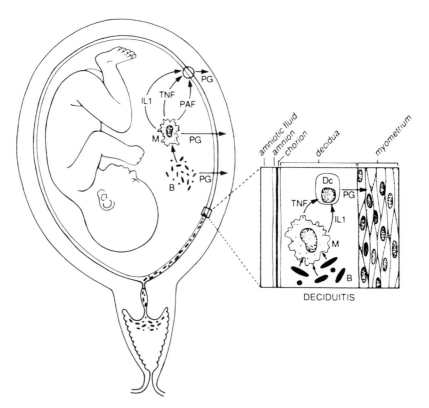

FIGURE 1. Cellular and biochemical mechanisms involved in the initiation of preterm labor in cases of intrauterine infection. Abbreviations: B = bacteria; M = monocyte/macrophage; Dc = decidua; IL-1 = interleukin-1; TNF = tumor necrosis factor/cachectin; PG = prostaglandins; PAF = platelet activating factor.

preterm labor and preterm PROM. However, these data do not provide evidence of causality. Indeed, the argument may be put forth that microbial invasion of this compartment is the consequence of labor or rupture of the membranes rather than the cause of preterm labor and preterm PROM.

Recently, we completed a study to establish the prevalence of microbial invasion of the amniotic cavity in women in spontaneous labor at term. Amniotic fluid was retrieved transabdominally in a group of women undergoing primary or repeat cesarean section in active labor or who were suspected to have preterm labor but subsequently delivered a term infant by weight and pediatric examination. We found that 18.8% (17/90) of these patients had a positive amniotic fluid culture.[169] Since the prevalence of microbial invasion of the amniotic cavity is similar in both women in term and preterm labor leading to preterm delivery, the argument could be made that microbial invasion is a phenomenon associated with labor *per se*. It is possible that microorganisms gain access to the sterile amniotic cavity when cervical dilatation exposes intact membranes to the normal vaginal flora.

Despite the similar rate of positive amniotic fluid cultures in term and preterm labor and delivery with intact membranes, there are several striking differences in these two settings. First, the innoculum size in term labor is much smaller than in preterm labor.[169] Second, the concentrations of IL-1, TNF and IL-6 are several-fold higher in the setting of preterm labor than in term labor.[170] Third, the prevalence and severity of histopathologic chorioamnionitis is much higher in preterm labor and delivery than in term gestation (23% vs. 11%).[2] Fourth, the prevalence of clinical chorioamnionitis is much higher in preterm than in term gestation.[68] Collectively, these data indicate that there are fundamental differences between microbial invasion of the amniotic cavity in the context of a term and preterm gestation. We believe that microbial invasion of the amniotic cavity can be both a cause and a consequence of labor. Ascending microbial invasion may lead to macrophage activation and parturition when present for an extended period of time. This may be a chain of events in some cases of preterm parturition and intraamniotic infection. However, if labor has already begun in the context of term or preterm gestation, secondary microbial invasion may also occur. We believe that the latter is the most likely sequence of events associated with microbial invasion during spontaneous term labor.

PRETERM LABOR AS A HETEROGENEOUS DISEASE

The traditional management of preterm labor has consisted of treatment with tocolytic agents, and often, steroid administration. This uniform approach to the problem implies that preterm labor is a unique pathologic entity for which there is a single treatment.

We view preterm labor as a pathologic event; labor may be considered as the response of the feto-maternal pair to a variety of insults (infection, ischemia, *etc.*). If these insults cannot be effectively handled in the context of a continuing pregnancy, then labor and delivery may occur. For example, several maternal infections such as pyelonephritis in the pre-antibiotic era were associated with preterm labor and delivery. Today, maternal pyelonephritis can result in preterm labor, but early antibiotic treatment prevents progression toward inevitable labor and delivery in most cases.[17-19] In the case of an intrauterine infection, the host can utilize the normal complement of host-defense mechanisms against infection (*i.e.*, specific and non-specific mechanisms) available in any other site. However, if these mechanisms fail to control the infection, labor enables the host to rid itself of the infected tissue. The presence of a second host, the fetus, adds further complexity to the solution of this problem. Nature must contend with maximizing the survival of two hosts. At term, when the fetus is mature, initiation of labor is an expedient and safe solution for both hosts. On the other hand, in the pre-viable gestation, uterine evacuation promotes maternal survival at the expense of fetal life. For these reasons, the initiation of labor in the setting of infection can be considered to have survival value.

Up to this point, this article has focused on the role of infection in preterm labor. However, infection is only one of the insults that may compromise feto-maternal survival. Placental histopathologic studies would suggest that inflammation may account for probably no more than 30% to 40% of cases of preterm delivery.[67] This estimate correlates well with our studies of amniotic fluid microbiology.[30] Therefore, other pathologic processes must be responsible for the initiation of preterm labor in the remaining cases. We have recently established that the most common non-inflammatory lesion of the placenta in the setting of preterm delivery is vascular pathology (decidual thrombosis, acute atherosis, failure of physiologic transformation of the spiral arteries, etc.).[30,171] We propose that these vascular lesions may lead to utero-placental ischemia and to the initiation of preterm labor and delivery. Clinical and experimental observations supporting this include: 1) there is an excess of intrauterine growth retardation and abruptio placenta in the setting of premature birth[66]; and 2) experimental uterine ischemia in monkeys often results in the initiation of labor.

Another distinct clinical group of patients with a potentially different mechanism for preterm labor and delivery is composed of women with congenital anomalies and polyhydramnios. Uterine overdistension may activate a uterine pressor-sensitive system capable of initiating uterine contractility and labor. This mechanism can also be invoked to explain the excess rate of preterm labor observed in multiple gestations.

Yet another potential mechanism for preterm labor and delivery is an immunologically mediated phenomenon induced by an allergic mechanism. Indeed, the uterus contains a large number of mast cells, and the trophoblast may constitute the antigen required for eliciting an allergic reaction. Garfield et al. have recently reported that products of mast cell degranulation are capable of inducing myometrial contractions.[172] We have also identified a group of patients in preterm labor with clinical and laboratory findings consistent with an allergic-mediated event.

The emerging picture is that preterm labor and delivery is a syndrome (FIG. 2). Multiple pathological processes may lead to myometrial activation and cervical ripening. This view of preterm labor has considerable implications for the diagnosis, treatment and understanding of the cellular and biochemical mechanisms responsible for the initiation of parturition.

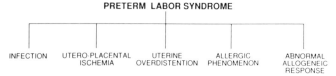

FIGURE 2. Preterm labor syndrome.

REFERENCES

1. MINKOFF, H. 1983. Prematurity: infection as an etiologic factor. Obstet. Gynecol. **62**: 137.
2. NAEYE, R. L. & E. C. PETERS. 1980. Causes and consequences of premature rupture of fetal membranes. Lancet **1**: 192.
3. ROMERO, R. & M. MAZOR. 1988. Infection and preterm labor. Clin. Obstet. Gynecol. **31**: 553.
4. BANG, B. 1897. The etiology of epizootic abortion. J. Comp. Anthol. Ther. **10**: 125–150.
5. ZAHL, P. A. & C. BJERKNES. 1943. Induction of decidua-placental hemorrhage in mice by the endotoxins of certain gram-negative bacteria. Proc. Soc. Exp. Biol. Med. **54**: 329–332.
6. TAKEDA, Y. & I. TSUCHIYA. 1953. Studies on the pathological changes caused by the injection of the Shwartzman filtrate and the endotoxin into pregnant rabbits. Jap. J. Exp. Med. **21**: 9–16.
7. TAKEDA, Y. & I. TSUCHIYA. 1953. Studies on the pathological changes caused by the injection of the Shwartzman filtrate and the endotoxin into pregnant animals. II. On the relationship of the constituents of the endotoxin and the abortion-producing factor. Jap. J. Exp. Med. **23**: 105–110.

8. RIEDER, R. F. & L. THOMAS. 1960. Studies on the mechanisms involved in the production of abortion by endotoxin. J. Immunol. **84**: 189–193.

9. MCKAY, D. G. & T.-C. WONG. 1963. The effect of bacterial endotoxin on the placenta of the rat. Am. J. Pathol. **42**: 357–377.

10. KULLANDER, S. 1977. Fever and parturition: An experimental study in rabbits. Acta Obstet. Gynecol. Scand. Suppl. **66**: 77–85.

11. SKARNES, R. C. & M. J. K. HARPER. 1972. Relationship between endotoxin-induced abortion and the synthesis of prostaglandin F. Prostaglandins **1**: 191–201.

12. FINLAND, M. & T. D. DUBLIN. 1939. Pneumococcic pneumonias complicating pregnancy and the puerperium. JAMA **112**: 1027–1032.

13. OXORN, H. 1955. The changing aspects of pneumonia complicating pregnancy. Am. J. Obstet. Gynecol. **70**: 1057–1063.

14. BENEDETTI, T. J., R. VALLE & W. J. LEDGER. 1976. Antepartum pneumonia in pregnancy. Am. J. Obstet. Gynecol. **144**: 413–417.

15. MADINGER, N. E., J. S. GREENSPOON & A. G. ELLRODT. 1989. Pneumonia during pregnancy: Has modern technology improved maternal and fetal outcome? Am. J. Obstet. Gynecol. **161**: 657–662.

16. MCLANE, C. M. & H. F. TRAUT. 1937. Relationship between infected urine and the etiology of pyelenephritis of pregnancy. Am. J. Obstet. Gynecol. **33**: 828.

17. KASS, E. 1962. Maternal urinary tract infection. New York State J. Med. **1**: 2822–2826.

18. CUNNINGHAM, F. G., G. B. MORRIS & A. MIKAL. 1973. Acute pyelonephritis of pregnancy: A clinical review. Obstet. Gynecol. **42**: 112–117.

19. FAN, Y.-D., J. G. PASTOREK, J. M. MILLER & J. MULVEY. 1987. Acute pyelonephritis in pregnancy. Am. J. Perinatol. **4**: 324–326.

20. WING, E. S. & D. V. TROPPOLI. 1930. The intrauterine transmission of typhoid. JAMA **95**: 405.

21. DIDDLE, A. W. & R. L. STEPHENS. 1938. Typhoid fever in pregnancy: Probable intrauterine transmission of the disease. Am. J. Obstet. Gynecol. **38**: 300.

22. STEVENSON, C. S., A. J. GLASKO & E. C. GILLESPIE. 1951. Treatment of typhoid in pregnancy with chloramphenicol (chloromycetin). JAMA **146**: 1190.

23. HERD, N. & T. JORDAN. 1981. An investigation of malaria during pregnancy in Zimbabwe. C. Afr. J. Med. **27**: 62–68.

24. GILLES, H. M., J. B. LAWSON, M. SIBELAS, A. VOLLER & N. ALLAN. 1969. Malaria, anaemia and pregnancy. Ann. Trop. Med. Pharmacol. **63**: 245.

25. RIOUX-DARRIEULAT, F., M. PARANT & L. CHEDID. 1978. Prevention of endotoxin-induced abortion by treatment of mice with antisera. J. Infect. Dis. **137**: 7–13.

26. DOMBROSKI, R. A., D. S. WOODWARD, M. J. K. HARPER & R. S. GIBBS. 1990. A rabbit model for bacterial-induced preterm pregnancy loss. Am. J. Obstet. Gynecol. In press.

27. SERENO, J. A., J. J. POSEIRO, Y. SICA-BLANCO & S. V. POSE. 1959. Int. Cong. Phys. Sci.

28. ROMERO, R., M. D. MITCHELL, G. W. DUFF, S. DURUM & J. C. HOBBINS. 1985. A possible mechanism for premature labor in gram-negative maternal infection: A monocyte product stimulates protaglandin release by the amnion. Presented at the 32nd Meeting of the Society for Gynecologic Investigation, Phoenix, AZ, March 20–23.

29. GIBBS, R. S., J. D. BLANCO, P. J. ST. CLAIR & Y. S. CASTANEDA. 1982. Quantitative bacteriology of amniotic fluid from women with clinical intraamniotic infection at term. J. Infect. Dis. **145**: 1–8.

30. ROMERO, R., M. SIRTORI, E. OYARZUN, *et al.* 1989. Infection and labor. V. Prevalence, microbiology, and clinical significance of intraamniotic infection in women with preterm labor and intact membranes. Am. J. Obstet. Gynecol. **161**: 817–824.

31. BLANC, W. A. 1953. Infection amniotique et neonatal. Gynaecologia **136**: 101–104.

32. BLANC, W. A. 1959. Amniotic infection syndrome: Pathogenesis, morphology and significance in circumnatal mortality. Clin Obstet. Gynecol. **2**: 705–712.

33. BLANC, W. A. 1964. Pathways of fetal and early neonatal infection: Viral placentitis, bacterial and fungal chorioamnionitis. J. Pediatr. **59**: 473–496.

34. BENIRSCHKE, K. & S. H. CLIFFORD. 1959. Intrauterine bacterial infection of the newborn infant. J. Pediatr. **54**: 11–18.

35. DRISCOLL, S. G. 1965. Pathology and the developing fetus. Pediatr. Clin. North Am. **12**: 493–514.

36. BENIRSCHKE, K. 1965. Routes and types of infection in the fetus and the newborn. Am. J. Dis. Child. **28:** 714–721.
37. ROMERO, R., S. FAYEK, C. AVILA, *et al.* 1990. The prevalence, microbiology, and clinical significance of intraamniotic infection in twin gestations with preterm labor. Am. J. Obstet. Gynecol. **163:** 757–761.
38. SCHOONMAKER, J. N., D. W. LAWELLIN, B. LUNT & J. A. McGREGOR. 1989. Bacteria and inflammatory cells reduce chorioamniotic membrane integrity and tensile strength. Obstet. Gynecol. **74:** 590–596.
39. ARIAS, F. & P. TOMICH. 1982. Etiology and outcome of low birth weight and preterm infants. Obstet. Gynecol. **60:** 277.
40. LEIGH, J. & T. J. GARITE. 1986. Amniocentesis and the management of premature labor. Obstet. Gynecol. **67:** 500–506.
41. MILLER, J. M., M. J. PUPKIN & G. B. HILL. 1980. Bacterial colonization of amniotic fluid from intact fetal membranes. Am. J. Obstet. Gynecol. **136:** 796–804.
42. BOBITT, J. R., C. C. HAYSLIP & J. D. DAMATO. 1981. Amniotic fluid infection as determined by transabdominal amniocentesis in patients with intact membranes in premature labor. Am. J. Obstet. Gynecol. **140:** 947–952.
43. WALLACE, R. L. & C. N. HERRICK. 1981. Amniocentesis in the evaluation of premature labor. Obstet. Gynecol. **57:** 483–486.
44. HAMEED, C., N. TEJANI, U. L. VERMA, *et al.* 1984. Silent chorioamnionitis as a cause of preterm labor refractory to tocolytic therapy. Obstet. Gynecol. **149:** 726–730.
45. WAHBEH, C. J., G. B. HILL, R. D. EDEN, *et al.* 1984. Intra-amniotic bacterial colonization in premature labor. Am. J. Obstet. Gynecol. **148:** 739–743.
46. WEIBLE, D. R. & H. W. RANDALL. 1985. Evaluation of amniotic fluid in preterm labor with intact membranes. J. Reprod. Med. **30:** 777–780.
47. GRAVETT, M. G., D. HUMMEL, D. A. ESCHENBACH, *et al.* 1986. Preterm labor associated with subclinical amniotic fluid infection and with bacterial vaginosis. Obstet. Gynecol. **67:** 229–237.
48. IAMS, J. D., D. H. CLAPP, D. A. CONTOS, *et al.* 1987. Does extra-amniotic infection cause preterm labor? Gas-liquid chromatography studies of amniotic fluid in amnionitis, preterm labor, and normal controls. Obstet. Gynecol. **70:** 365–368.
49. DUFF, P. & J. N. KOPELMAN. 1987. Subclinical intra-amniotic infection in asymptomatic patients with refractory preterm labor. Obstet. Gynecol. **69:** L756–L759.
50. ROMERO, R., M. EMAMIAN, R. QUINTERO, *et al.* 1988. The value and limitations of the Gram stain examination in the diagnosis of intraamniotic infection. Am. J. Obstet. Gynecol. **159:** 114–119.
51. SKOLL, M. A., M. L. MORETTI & B. M. SIBAI. 1989. The incidence of positive amniotic fluid cultures in patients in preterm labor with intact membranes. Am. J. Obstet. Gynecol. **161:** 813–816.
52. GARITE, T. J., R. K. FREEMAN, E. M. LINZEY, *et al.* 1979. The use of amniocentesis in patients with premature rupture of membranes. Obstet. Gynecol. **54:** 226–230.
53. GARITE, T. J. & R. K. FREEMAN. 1982. Chorioamnionitis in the preterm gestation. Obstet. Gynecol. **59:** 539–545.
54. COTTON, D. B., L. M. HILL, H. T. STRASSNER, *et al.* 1984. Use of amniocentesis in preterm gestation with ruptured membranes. Obstet. Gynecol. **63:** 38–43.
55. BROEKHUIZEN, F. F., M. GILMAN & P. R. HAMILTON. 1985. Amniocentesis for Gram stain and culture in preterm premature rupture of the membranes. Obstet. Gynecol. **66:** 316–321.
56. VINTZILEOS, A. M., W. A. CAMPBELL, D. J. NOCHIMSON, *et al.* 1986. Qualitative amniotic fluid volume versus amniocentesis in predicting infection in preterm rupture of the membranes. Obstet. Gynecol. **67:** 579–583.
57. FEINSTEIN, S. T., A. M. VINTZILEOS, J. G. LODEIRO, *et al.* 1986. Amniocentesis with premature rupture of membranes. Am. J. Obstet. Gynecol. **68:** 147–152.
58. GONIK, B., S. F. BOTTOMS & D. B. COTTON. 1985. Amniotic fluid volume as a risk factor in preterm premature rupture of the membranes. Obstet. Gynecol. **65:** 456–459.
59. ROMERO, R., R. QUINTERO, E. OYARZUN, *et al.* 1988. Intraamniotic infection and the onset of labor in preterm premature rupture of membranes. Am. J. Obstet. Gynecol. **159:** 661–666.
60. DRISCOLL, S. G. 1973. The placenta and membranes. *In* Obstetric and Perinatal Infections. D. Charles & M. Finland, Eds.: 529–539. Lea & Febiger, Philadelphia.

61. OVERBACH, A. M., S. J. DANIEL & G. CASSADY. 1970. The value of umbilical cord histology in the management of potential perinatal infection. J. Pediatr. **76:** 22–31.
62. MAUDSLEY, R. F., G. A. BRIX, N. A. HINTON, *et al.* 1966. Placental inflammation and infection: A prospective bacteriologic and histologic study. Am. J. Obstet. Gynecol. **95:** 648–659.
63. PANKUCH, G. A., P. C. APPELBAUM, R. P. LORENZ, *et al.* 1984. Placental microbiology and histology and the pathogenesis of chorioamnionitis. Obstet. Gynecol. **64:** 802–806.
64. AQUINO, T. I., J. ZHAN, F. T. KRAUS, R. KNEFEL & T. TAFF. 1984. Subchorionic fibrin cultures for bacteriologic study of the placenta. Am. J. Clin. Pathol. **81:** 482–486.
65. HILLIER, S. L., J. MARTIUS, M. KROHN, N. KIVIAT, K. K. HOLMES & D. A. ESCHENBACH. 1988. A case-control study of chorioamnionic infection and histologic chorioamnionitis in prematurity. N. Engl. J. Med. **319:** 972–978.
66. CHELLAM, V. G. & D. I. RUSHTON. 1985. Chorioamnionitis and funiculitis in the placentas of 200 births weighing less than 2.5 kg. Br. J. Obstet. Gynaecol. **92:** 808–814.
67. ROMERO, R., C. M. SALAFIA, A. P. ATHANASSIADIS, M. MAZOR, S. HANAOKA, J. C. HOBBINS & M. BRACKEN. 1990. The relationship between acute inflammatory lesions of the placenta and amniotic fluid microbiology. Am. J. Obstet. Gynecol. Submitted.
68. RUSSELL, P. 1979. Inflammatory lesions of the human placenta: Clinical significance of acute chorioamnionitis. Am. J. Diag. Gynecol. Obstet. **2:** 127.
69. GUZICK, D. S. & K. WINN. 1985. The association of chorioamnionitis with preterm delivery. Obstet. Gynecol. **65:** 11-16.
70. DAIKOKU, N. H., D. F. KALTREIDER, V. A. KHOUZAMI, *et al.* 1982. Premature rupture of membranes and spontaneous preterm labor: Maternal endometritis risks. Obstet. Gynecol. **59:** 13–20.
71. ABERNETHY, T. J. & O. T. AVERY. 1941. The occurrence during acute infections of a protein not normally present in blood. J. Exp. Med. **73:** 173–182.
72. EVANS, M. I., S. N. HAJJ, L. D. DEVOE, *et al.* 1980. C-reactive protein as a predictor of infectious morbidity with premature rupture of membranes. Am. J. Obstet. Gynecol. **138:** 648–652.
73. FARB, H. F., M. ARNESEN, P. GEISTLER, *et al.* 1983. C-reactive protein with premature rupture of membranes and premature labor. Obstet. Gynecol. **62:** 49–51.
74. HAWRYLYSHYN, P., P. BERNSTEIN, J. E. MILLIGAN, *et al.* 1983. Premature rupture of membranes: The role of C-reactive protein in the prediction of chorioamnionitis. Am. J. Obstet. Gynecol. **147:** 240–246.
75. ROMEM, Y. & R. ARTAL. 1984. C-reactive protein as a predictor for chorioamnionitis in cases of premature rupture of the membranes. Am. J. Obstet. Gynecol. **150:** 546–550.
76. HANDWERKER, S. M., N. A. TEJANI, U. L. VERMA, *et al.* 1984. Correlation of maternal serum C-reactive protein with outcome of tocolysis. Obstet. Gynecol. **63:** 220–224.
77. POTKUL, R. K., A. H. MOAWAD & K. L. PONTO. 1985. The association of subclinical infection with preterm labor: The role of C-reactive protein. Am. J. Obstet. Gynecol. **153:** 642–645.
78. DODDS, W. G. & J. D. IAMS. 1987. Maternal C-reactive protein and preterm labor. J. Reprod. Med. **32:** 527–530.
79. KASS, E. H. 1960. Bacteriuria and pyelonephritis of pregnancy. Arch. Intern. Med. **105:** 194–198.
80. KINCAID-SMITH, P. & M. BULLEN. 1965. Bacteriuria in pregnancy. Lancet **1:** 395–399.
81. WILSON, M. G., W. L. HEWITT & O. T. MONZON. 1966. Effect of bacteriuria on the fetus. N. Engl. J. Med. **274:** 115–118.
82. DIXON, H. G. & H. A. BRANT. 1967. The significance of bacteriuria in pregnancy. Lancet **1:** 19–20.
83. SAVAGE, W. E., S. N. HAJJ & E. H. KASS. 1967. Demographic and prognostic characteristics of bacteriuria in pregnancy. Medicine **46:** 385–407.
84. ROBERTSON, J. G., J. R. B. LIVINGSTONE & M. H. ISDALE. 1968. The management and complications of asymptomatic bacteriuria in pregnancy. Br. J. Obstet. Gynaecol. **75:** 59–65.
85. ELDER, H. A., B. A. G. SANTAMARINA, S. SMITH, *et al.* 1971. The effect of tetracycline on the clinical course and the outcome of pregnancy. Am. J. Obstet. Gynecol. **111:** 441–462.
86. BRUMFITT, W. 1975. The effects of bacteriuria in pregnancy on maternal and fetal health. Kidney Int. (suppl.) **8:** 113–119.
87. BRYANT, R. E., R. E. WINDOM, J. P. VINEYARD, *et al.* 1964. Asymptomatic bacteriuria in pregnancy and its association with prematurity. J. Lab. Clin. Med. **63:** 224–231.
88. LEBLANC, A. L. & W. J. MCGANITY. 1964. The impact of bacteriuria in pregnancy—a survey of 1300 pregnant patients. Biol. Med. **22:** 336–347.

89. ROMERO, R., E. OYARZUN, M. MAZOR, et al. 1989. Meta-analysis of the relationship between asymptomatic bacteriuria and preterm delivery/low birth weight. Obstet. Gynecol. **73:** 576–582.
90. SARREL, P. M. & K. A. PRUETT. 1968. Symptomatic gonorrhea during pregnancy. Obstet. Gynecol. **32:** 670–673.
91. HANDSFIELD, H. H., W. A. HODSON & K. K. HOLMES. 1973. Neonatal gonococcal infection: Orogastric contamination with Neisseria gonorrhea. JAMA **225:** 697–701.
92. AMSTEY, M. S. & K. T. STEADMAN. 1976. Asymptomatic gonorrhea and pregnancy. J. Am. Ven. Dis. Assoc. **33:** 14–16.
93. EDWARDS, L. E., M. I. BARRADA, A. A. HAMANN, et al. 1978. Gonorrhea in pregnancy. Am. J. Obstet. Gynecol. **132:** 637–641.
94. STOLL, B. J., W. P. KANTO, R. I. GLASS, et al. 1982. Treated maternal gonorrhea without adverse effect on outcome of pregnancy. South. Med. J. **75:** 1236–1238.
95. ESCHENBACH, D. A., M. G. GRAVETT, K. C. S. CHEN, et al. 1984. Bacterial vaginosis during pregnancy: An association with prematurity and postpartum complications. In Bacterial Vaginosis. P. A. Mardh & D. Taylor-Robinson, Eds.: 214–222. Almqvist & Wiksell, Stockholm.
96. MINKOFF, H., A. N. GRUNEBAUM, R. H. SCHWARZ, et al. 1984. Risk factors for prematurity and premature rupture of membranes: A prospective study of the vaginal flora in pregnancy. Am. J. Obstet. Gynecol. **150:** 965–972.
97. MARTIUS, J., M. A. KROHN, S. L. HILLIER, et al. 1988. Relationships of vaginal lactobacillus species, cervical Chlamydia trachomatis, and bacterial vaginosis to preterm birth. Obstet. Gynecol. **71:** 89–95.
98. GRAVETT, M. G., H. P. NELSON, T. DeROUEN, et al. 1986. Independent associations of bacterial vaginosis and Chlamydia trachomatis infection with adverse pregnancy outcome. JAMA **256:** 1899–1903.
99. BAKER, C. J., F. F. BARRETT & M. D. YOW. 1975. The influence of advancing gestation on group B streptococcal colonization in pregnant women. Am. J. Obstet. Gynecol. **122:** 820–825.
100. REGAN, J. A., S. CHAO & L. S. JAMES. 1981. Premature rupture of membranes, preterm delivery, and group B streptococcal colonization of mothers. Am. J. Obstet. Gynecol. **141:** 184–186.
101. HASTINGS, M. J. G., C. S. F. EASMON, J. NEILL, et al. 1986. Group B streptococcal colonization and the outcome of pregnancy. J. Infect. **12:** 23–39.
102. BOBITT, J. R., J. D. DAMATO & J. SAKAKINI. 1985. Perinatal complications in group B streptococcal carriers: A longitudinal study of prenatal patients. Am. J. Obstet. Gynecol. **151:** 711–717.
103. LAMONT, R. F., D. TAYLOR-ROBINSON, M. NEWMAN, et al. 1986. Spontaneous early preterm labour associated with abnormal genital bacterial colonization. Br. J. Obstet. Gynaecol. **93:** 804–810.
104. MARTIN, D. H., L. KOUTSKY, D. A. ESCHENBACH, et al. 1982. Prematurity and perinatal mortality in pregnancies complicated by maternal Chlamydia trachomatis infections. JAMA **247:** 1585–1588.
105. HARRISON, H. R., E. R. ALEXANDER, L. WEINSTEIN, et al. 1983. Cervical Chlamydia trachomatis and mycoplasmal infections in pregnancy: epidemiology and outcomes. JAMA **250:** 1721–1727.
106. ROSS, S. M., I. M. WINDSOR, R. M. ROBINS-BROWNE, et al. 1984. Microbiological studies during the perinatal period: An attempt to correlate selected bacterial and viral infections with intrauterine deaths and preterm labour. S. Afr. Med. J. **86:** 598–603.
107. SWEET, R. L., D. V. LANDERS, C. WALKER, et al. 1987. Chlamydia trachomatis infection and pregnancy outcome. Am. J. Obstet. Gynecol. **156:** 824–833.
108. KLEIN, J. O., D. BUCKLAND & M. FINLAND. 1969. Colonization of newborn infants by mycoplasmas. N. Engl. J. Med. **280:** 1025–1030.
109. BRAUN, P., L. YHU-HSIUNG, J. O. KLEIN, et al. 1971. Birth weight and genital mycoplasmas in pregnancy. N. Engl. J. Med. **284:** 167–171.
110. HARRISON, R. F., R. HURLEY & J. DeLouvois. 1979. Genital mycoplasmas and birth weight in offspring of primigravida women. Am. J. Obstet. Gynecol. **133:** 201–203.
111. ROSS, J. M., P. M. FURR, D. TAYLOR-ROBINSON, et al. 1981. The effect of genital mycoplasmas on human fetal growth. Br. J. Obstet. Gynaecol. **88:** 749–755.
112. KASS, E. H., W. M. McCORMACK, J. S. LIN, et al. 1981. Genital mycoplasmas as a cause of excess premature delivery. Trans. Assoc. Am. Physicians. **94:** 261–266.

113. UPADHYAYA, M., B. M. HIBBARD & S. M. WALKER. 1983. The role of mycoplasmas in reproduction. Fertil. Steril. **39**: 814–818.
114. McCORMACK, W. M., B. ROSNER, L. YHU-HSIUNG, *et al.* 1987. Effect on birth weight of erythromycin treatment of pregnant women. Obstet. Gynecol. **69**: 202–207.
115. SHURIN, P. A., S. ALPERT, B. ROSNER, *et al.* 1975. Chorioamnionitis and colonization of the newborn infant with genital mycoplasmas. N. Engl. J. Med. **293**: 5–8.
116. DISCHE, M. R., P. A. QUINN, E. CZEGLEDY-NAGY, *et al.* 1979. Genital mycoplasma infection: Intrauterine infection, pathologic study of the fetus and placenta. Am. Soc. Clin. Path. **72**: 167–173.
117. EMBREE, J. E., V. W. KRAUSE, J. A. EMBIL, *et al.* 1980. Placental infection with mycoplasma hominis and ureaplasma urealyticum: Clinical correlation. Obstet. Gynecol. **56**: 475–481.
118. KUNDSIN, R. B., S. G. DRISCOLL & P. A. PELLETIER. 1981. Ureaplasma urealyticum incriminated in perinatal morbidity and mortality. Science **213**: 474–476.
119. KUNDSIN, R. B., S. G. DRISCOLL, R. R. MONSON, *et al.* 1984. Association of ureaplasma urealyticum in the placenta with perinatal morbidity and mortality. N. Engl. J. Med. **310**: 941–945.
120. ZLATNIK, F. J., L. F. BURMEISTER & N. S. SWACK. 1986. Chorionic mycoplasmas and prematurity. J. Reprod. Med. **31**: 1106–1108.
121. MASON, P. R. & M. T. BROWN. 1980. Trichomonas in pregnancy. Lancet **2**: 1025.
122. ROSS, S. M. & A. V. MIDDELKOOP. 1983. Trichomonas infection in pregnancy – does it affect perinatal outcome? S. Afr. Med. J. **63**: 566–567.
123. HARDY, P. H., J. B. HARDY, E. E. NELL, *et al.* 1984. Prevalence of six sexually transmitted disease agents among pregnant inner-city adolescents and pregnancy outcome. Lancet **2**: 333–337.
124. WATTS, D. H. & D. A. ESCHENBACH. 1988. Treatment of chlamydia, mycoplasma, and group B streptococcal infections. Clin. Obstet. Gynecol. **31**: 435–452.
125. McCRACKEN, G. & H. SHINEFIELD. 1966. Changes in the pattern of neonatal septicemia and meningitis. Am. J. Dis. Child. **112**: 33–39.
126. BUETOW, K. C., S. W. KLEIN & R. B. LANE. 1965. Septicemia in premature infants. Am. J. Dis. Child. **110**: 29–41.
127. TAMBYRAJA, R. L., J. A. SALMON, S. M. M. KARIM, *et al.* 1977. F prostaglandin levels in amniotic fluid in premature labour. Prostaglandins **13**: 339–348.
128. MITCHELL, M. D., A. P. F. FLINT & J. G. BIBBY. 1978. Plasma concentrations of prostaglandins during late human pregnancy: Influence of normal and preterm labor. J. Clin. Endocrinol. Metabol. **46**: 947–951.
129. SELLERS, S. M., M. D. MITCHELL, J. G. BIBBY, *et al.* 1981. A comparison of plasma prostaglandin levels in term and preterm labour. Br. J. Obstet. Gynaecol. **88**: 362–366.
130. KARIM, S. M. & M. J. DEVLIN. 1966. Prostaglandin content of human amniotic fluid. J. Obstet. Gynaecol. Br. Commonw. **74**: 230–234.
131. ROMERO, R., M. EMAMIAN, M. WAN, *et al.* 1987. Prostaglandin concentrations in amniotic fluid of women with intra-amniotic infection and preterm labor. Am. J. Obstet. Gynecol. **157**: 1461–1467.
132. WEITZ, C. M., R. B. GHODGAONKAR, N. H. DUBIN, *et al.* 1986. Prostaglandin F metabolite concentration as a prognostic factor in preterm labor. Obstet. Gynecol. **67**: 496–499.
133. NIEDER, J. & W. AUGUSTIN. 1984. Concentrations of prostaglandins in amniotic fluid in premature labor. Z. Geburtshilfe Perinatol. **188**: 7–11.
134. ROMERO, R., Y. K. WU, M. MAZOR, J. C. HOBBINS & M. D. MITCHELL. 1988. Amniotic fluid prostaglandin E2 in preterm labor. Prostaglandins, Leukotrienes, Essen. Fatty Acids **34**: 141–145.
135. ROMERO, R., Y. K. WU, M. SIRTORI, *et al.* 1989. Amniotic fluid concentrations of prostaglandin F2 alpha, 13, 14-dihydro-15-keto-11, 16-cyclo prostaglandin E2 (PGEM-II) in preterm labor. Prostaglandins **37**: 149–161.
136. ROMERO, R., M. EMAMIAN, M. WAN, *et al.* 1987. Increased concentrations of arachidonic acid lipoxygenase metabolites in amniotic fluid during parturition. Obstet. Gynecol. **70**: 849–851.
137. ROMERO, R., Y. K. WU, M. MAZOR, *et al.* 1988. Increased amniotic fluid leukotriene C4 concentration in term human parturition. Am. J. Obstet. Gynecol. **159**: 655–657.
138. RITCHIE, D. M., D. W. HAHN & J. L. McGUIRE. 1984. Smooth muscle contraction as a model

to study the mediator role of endogenous lipoxygenase products of arachidonic acid. Life Sci. **34:** 509–513.

139. BENNETT, P. R., M. G. ELDER & L. MYATT. 1987. The effects of lipoxygenase metabolites of arachidonic acid on human myometrial contractility. Prostaglandins **33:** 837–844.

140. CARRAHER, R., D. W. HAHN, D. M. RITCHIE, *et al.* 1983. Involvement of lipoxygenase products in myometrial contractions. Prostaglandins **26:** 23–32.

141. ROMERO, R., Y. K. WU, M. MAZOR, J. C. HOBBINS & M. D. MITCHELL. 1988. Amniotic fluid 5-hydroxyeicosatetraenoic acid in preterm labor. Prostaglandins **36:** 179–187.

142. ROMERO, R., Y. K. WU, M. MAZOR, *et al.* 1989. Amniotic fluid arachidonate lipoxygenase metabolites in women with preterm labor. Prostaglandins, Leukotrienes, Essent. Fatty Acids **36:** 69–75.

143. BEJAR, R., V. CURBELO, C. DAVIS, *et al.* 1981. Premature labor: Bacterial sources of phospholipase. Obstet. Gynecol. **57:** 479–482.

144. MCGREGOR, J. A., D. LAWELLIN & A. FRANCO-BUFF. 1985. Phospholipase A2 activity of genital tract flora detected with two substrates. Society for Gynecologic Investigations, Phoenix, AZ, March 20–23.

145. LAMONT, R. F., M. ROSE & M. G. ELDER. 1985. Effects of bacterial production prostaglandin E production by amnion cells. Lancet **2:** 1131–1133.

146. BENNETT, P. R., M. P. ROSE & L. MYATT. 1987. Preterm labor: Stimulation of arachidonic acid metabolism in human amnion by bacterial products. Am. J. Obstet. Gynecol. **156:** 649–655.

147. ROMERO, R., N. KADAR, J. C. HOBBINS, *et al.* 1987. Infection and labor: The detection of endotoxin in amniotic fluid. Am. J. Obstet. Gynecol. **157:** 815–819.

148. ROMERO, R., J. C. HOBBINS & M. D. MITCHELL. 1988. Endotoxin stimulates prostaglandin E2 production by human amnion. Obstet. Gynecol. **71:** 227–228.

149. ROMERO, R., P. ROSLANSKY, E. OYARZUN, *et al.* 1988. Labor and infection ii. Bacterial endotoxin in amniotic fluid and its relationship to the onset of preterm labor. Am. J. Obstet. Gynecol. **158:** 1044–1049.

150. LAMONT, R. F., F. ANTHONY, L. MYATT, L. BOOTH, P. M. FURR & D. TAYLOR-ROBINSON. 1990. Production of prostaglandin E2 by human amnion in vitro in response to addition of media conditioned by microorganisms associated with chorioamnionitis and preterm labor. Am. J. Obstet. Gynecol. **162:** 819–825.

151. MITCHELL, M. D., S. EDWIN & R. ROMERO. 1990. Prostaglandin biosynthesis by human decidual cells: Effects of inflammatory mediators. Prostaglandins, Leukotrienes, Essen. Fatty Acids. In press.

152. DINARELLO, C. A. 1987. Clinical relevance of interleukin-1 and its multiple biological activities. Bull. Inst. Pasteur. **85:** 267–285.

153. DINARELLO, C. A. 1984. Interleukin-1. Rev. Infect. Dis. **6:** 51–95.

154. ROMERO, R., Y. K. WU, D. T. BRODY, E. OYARZUN, G. W. DUFF & S. K. DURUM. 1989. Human decidua: A source of interleukin-1. Obstet. Gynecol. **73:** 31–34.

155. ROMERO, R., S. DURUM, C. DINARELLO, *et al.* 1986. Interleukin-1: A signal for the initiation of labor in chorioamnionitis. Presented at the 33rd Annual Meeting of the Society for Gynecologic Investigation, Toronto, Ont. Canada, March 19–22.

156. ROMERO, R., D. T. BRODY, E. OYARZUN, *et al.* 1989. Infection and labor. III. Interleukin-1: a signal for the onset of parturition. Am. J. Obstet. Gynecol. **160:** 1117–1123.

157. ITO, A., D. HIRO, Y. OJIMA, *et al.* 1988. Spontaneous production of interleukin-1-like factors from pregnant rabbit uterine cervix. Am. J. Obstet. Gynecol. **159:** 261.

158. ROMERO, R., K. R. MANOGUE, M. D. MURRAY, *et al.* 1989. Infection and labor. IV. Cachectin-tumor necrosis factor in the amniotic fluid of women with intraamniotic infection and preterm labor. Am. J. Obstet. Gynecol. **161:** 336–341.

159. CASEY, M. L., S. M. COX, B. BEUTLER, L. MILEWICH & P. C. MACDONALD. 1989. Cachectin/tumor necrosis factor-formation in human decidua. J. Clin. Invest. **83:** 430–436.

160. ROMERO, R., K. MANOGUE, E. OYARZUN, Y. K. WU & A. CERAMI. 1991. Human decidua: A source of tumor necrosis factor. Eur. J. Obstet. Gynecol. Reprod. Biol.

161. GAULDIE, J., C. RICHARDS, D. HARNISH, P. LANDSCORP & H. BAUMANN. 1987. Interferon 2/B-cell hepatocyte-stimulatory factor type 2 shares identity with monocyte-derived hepatocyte stimulating factor and regulates the major acute phase protein response in liver cells. Proc. Natl. Acad. Sci. USA. **84:** 7251–7255.

162. MAY, L. T., J. GHRAYEB, U. SANTHANAM, *et al.* 1988. Synthesis and secretion of multiple forms of 2-interferon/B cell differentiation factor-2-hepatocyte stimulating factor by human fibroblasts and monocytes. J. Biol. Chem. **263:** 7760–7766.

163. MAY, L. T., G. TORCIA, F. COZZOLINO, *et al.* 1989. Interleukin-6 gene expression in human endothelial cells: RNA start sites, multiple IL-6 proteins and inhibition of proliferation. Biochem. Biophys. Res. Commun. **159:** 991–998.

164. ZHANG, Y., Y. LIN & J. VILCEK. 1988. Synthesis of interleukin-6 (interferon-2/B cell stimulatory factor 2) in human fibroblasts is triggered by an increase in intracellular cyclic AMP. J. Biol. Chem. **263:** 6177–6182.

165. KUPPER, T., K. MIN, P. B. SEHGAL, *et al.* 1989. Production of IL-6 by keratinocytes: Implications for epidermal inflammation and immunity. Ann. N.Y. Acad. Sci. **557:** 454–465.

166. TABIBZADEH, S. S., U. SANTHANAM, P. B. SEHGAL & L. T. MAY. 1989. Cytokine-induced production of interferon-2/interleukin-6 by freshly-explanted human endometrial stormal cells: Modulation by estradiol-17. J. Immunol. **142:** 3134–3139.

167. ROMERO, R., C. AVILA, U. SANTHANAM & P. B. SEHGAL. 1990. Amniotic fluid interleukin-6 in preterm labor: Association with infection. J. Clin. Invest. In press.

168. HOFFMAN, D. R., R. ROMERO & J. M. JOHNSTON. 1990. Detection of platelet-activating factor in amniotic fluid of complicated pregnancies. Am. J. Obstet. Gynecol. **162:** 525–528.

169. ROMERO, R., E. OYARZUN, J. NORES, *et al.* 1990. The prevalence, microbiology and clinical significance of intraamniotic infection in spontaneous parturition at term. Presented at the 37th Annual Meeting of the Society for Gynecologic Investigation, St. Louis, MO, March 21–24.

170. ROMERO, R., C. AVILA, R. CALLAHAN, M. MAZOR, J. C. HOBBINS & C. DINARELLO. 1990. Interleukin-1α and interleukin-1β in preterm labor and preterm premature rupture of membranes. Presented at the 10th Annual Meeting of the Society of Perinatal Obstetricians, Houston, TX, January 23–27.

171. ARIAS, F. 1990. Placental insufficiency: an important cause of preterm labor and preterm premature ruptured membranes. Presented at the 10th Annual Meeting of the Society of Perinatal Obstetricians, Houston, TX, January 23–27.

172. GARFIELD, R. E. 1989. Uterine mast cells: Immunogenic control of myometrial contractility. Presented at the 36th Annual Meeting of the Society of Gynecologic Investigation, San Diego, CA, March 15–16.

Basement Membrane in Human Endometrium: Possible Role of Proteolytic Enzymes in Developing Hyperplasia and Carcinoma

C. BULLETTI,[a,c] V. M. JASONNI,[a] V. POLLI,[a]
F. CAPPUCCINI,[a] A. GALASSI,[b]
AND C. FLAMIGNI[a]

[a] *Reproductive Medicine Unit*
Department of Obstetrics and Gynecology
University of Bologna
40138 Bologna, Italy

[b] *Department of Pathology*
Bassano del Grappa General Hospital
Via delle Fosse, 43
36061 Bassano del Grappa, (VI), Italy

INTRODUCTION

The proliferation and differentiation of human endometrium depend on the production rate of estrogens and the endometrial response to estrogens themselves.[1] Although several studies have been performed over the last two decades focusing on these topics[2,3] it is still not clear why some, but not all, women exhibit an abnormal response to estrogen. Possible mechanisms include disordered estrogen production, increased endometrium sensitivity to estrogenic stimulation and variations in estrogen influx into the endometrial gland. The effects of membrane permeability and serum protein binding on differential influx into endometrium and myometrium were previously studied[4] and disruption and/or loss of basement membrane (BM) components, in the hyperplastic and neoplastic endometrium were respectively observed[5] in close association with the increase of estrogen transport into the human endometrial hyperplasia and carcinoma.[6]

Since the BM forms a filter regulating the transport of steroid hormones between different compartments and it regulates growth and differentiation of the cells surrounding it,[7] the fragmentation and/or disruption of a barrier between estrogens and the target cells could increase the estrogen influx into the glandular epithelial cells thus affecting

[c] *Address for correspondence:* Carlo Bulletti, MD, Reproductive Medicine Unit, Dept. Ob/Gyn, University of Bologna; Via Massarenti, 13; 40138 Bologna, Italy; Tel 051-398481; FAX 051-393959.

endometrial hyperplasia and cancer. Since endometrial growth is a function of the concentration of estrogen *in situ* the factors influencing estrogen transport into this tissue may modulate endometrial growth itself.

Proteolytic enzymes such as collagenase and urokinase-type plasminogen activator may be involved in degradation of the BM.[8-11] Their activity may be under the control of a growth and inhibiting factor.[12,13] The present study was undertaken to evaluate the presence of proteolytic enzymes, EGFr and TGF-α in normal hyperplastic and neoplastic tissues.

MATERIALS AND METHODS

Endometrial samples were obtained at the S. Orsola General Hospital of the University of Bologna, Italy, by curettage or hysterectomy during routine diagnostic or therapeutic procedures, from 44 patients, aged 21 to 48 years, at different days of their menstrual cycle. All patients gave free consent to participate in this study and did not take exogenous therapy for at least 2 years before the study. Fourteen women were in the proliferative phase (days 6 to 14) and eleven were in the secretory phase. Endometrial biopsies of adenomatous hyperplasia were obtained from seven women (age 29–40) with menstrual irregularities. Twelve well-differentiated endometrial adenocarcinoma tissue samples were obtained from premenopausal women age 44 to 48. Specimens were fixed in 10% buffered formalin, embedded in paraffin and cut in serial sections about 6-μm thick and stained with Hematoxilin-Eosin for histological diagnosis. Menstrual dating was effected using the method of Noyes *et al.*[14] while endometrial hyperplasia and carcinoma were evaluated according to Di Saia and Creasman.[15]

Paraffin sections were attached to slides with polylisin for immunohistochemistry, dewaxed in xylene, and rehydrated in graded alcohol and distilled water. Endogenous peroxidase was inhibited by 10% H_2O_2 in PBS for 5 minutes. The primary antisera used were: monoclonal mouse anti-EGFr (Cambridge Res. Lab; Cambridge, UK)[16]; polyclonal rabbit anti-TGF-α (Oncogene Science Inc., USA); polyclonal rabbit anti-collagenase type IV (Garbisa, Padova, Italy)[8]; Monoclonal anti-human uPA antibody (Chemican, USA), with no cross-reaction with the tissue type plasminogen activator. Dilutions were 1/400, 1/10, 1/400 respectively for EGFr, TGF-α and collagenase; uPA was used at the concentration of 10 μg/ml. The secondary antiserum, Biotinilated rabbit anti-mouse and goat anti-rabbit, was purchased from Sclavo (Siena, Italy) and were used diluted 1/50 for 30 minutes. ABC alkaline phosphatase was purchased from Dako, Copenhagen, Denmark. Washings were made using DAB or Fast-Red GBC salt naphtol AS-BI phosphatase plus 0.01% levamisole.

RESULTS

Using the immunoperoxidase technique, collagenase does not give a positive immunoreaction in normal or abnormal endometrium, widespread moderate positivity was only detected in proliferative and hyperplastic specimens. uPA was not detectable in normal proliferative and secretory endometrium while it is clearly detectable in all specimens of adenomatous hyperplasia and adenocarcinoma (FIGS. 1 and 2) thus suggesting its role in tissue remodelling during the development of endometrial cancer.

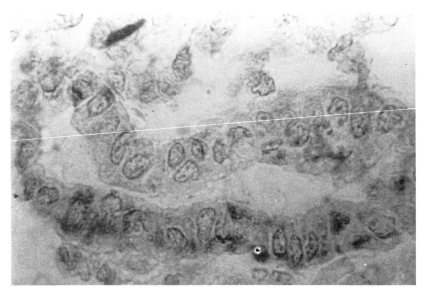

FIGURE 1. Positive immunostaining for urokinase-type plasminogen activator in typical adenomatous endometrial hyperplasia.

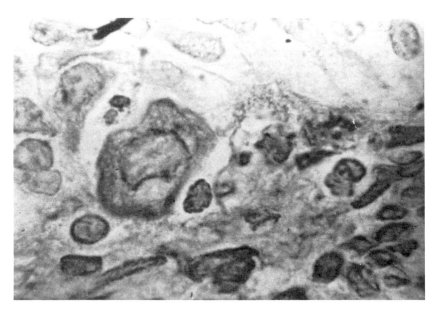

FIGURE 2. Positive immunostaining for urokinase-type plasminogen activator in well-differentiated endometrial adenocarcinoma.

Immunostaining revealed uPA presence in cytoplasmatic shape of glandular BM. Its role in BM disruption should be further considered.

DISCUSSION

Since endometrial growth is a function of the availability of estrogen in the tissue, capillary and glandular BM[4,5] plays a selective, limiting role in endometrial proliferation. To affect glandular epithelial cells, sex steroids go through different compartments. One may view these compartments as being divided by a series of BMs. One BM separates the vessels from the interstitium and a second BM separates the latter from glandular epithelial cells. Ultrafiltration is the major function of BM,[7] and alteration in the structure and function of these matrices is accompanied by an increase in permeability to proteins the size of albumin and larger. It is generally accepted that free estrogen fractions and a part of protein-bound estrogens are available in the extravascular space of the endometrium.[17-20] Alteration of BM function should increase the influx of free and protein-bound estrogens circulating in the endometrium causing abnormal endometrial growth such as hyperplasia and carcinoma.

Estrogens pass from the blood to the endometrial stroma at a higher rate in the proliferative than in the secretory phase of the menstrual cycle[4]; in endometrial hyperplasia and cancer this rate is higher than in the proliferative endometrium.[6] In the present study the urokinase-type plasminogen activator was detected in endometrial hyperplasia and adenocarcinoma but not in the normal proliferative and secretory endometrium. The uPA is over expressed in many malignancies,[21,22] but the function of uPA in human biology is not entirely clear. At present it is well documented[23,24] that the production of the widely acting serine protease, plasmin, from the inert zymogen, plasminogen, is mediated by urokinase. Plasmin has been reported to degrade the major basement membrane constituent, laminin.[25,26] The immunohistochemical detection of uPA in histological features characterized by disruption and/or absence of BM[5] and increased estrogen transportation into the tissue[6] is suggestive of a role of uPA activity in endometrial growth. Depletion of basement membrane laminin could be one of the many factors involved in steroid transport from blood to endometrial stroma and from the stroma to epithelial glandular cells.

Colonic tumors are characterized as having high levels of urokinase and this is associated with reduced amounts of laminin within basement membrane structures[27-29]; antiurokinase antibodies have been reported to reduce tumor dissemination in several systems.[30,31]

Collagenase was not completely detected by immunohistochemistry; however, its mRNA is detectable by blotting and *in situ* by hybridization (personal data). The inability of the antisera to detect this enzyme in the endometrial specimens observed may be due to the low affinity of the antisera or to proteinase inhibitors that prevent the synthesis of this protein. Amniotic membrane BM content and results obtained with proteinase inhibitors showed that inhibitors of collagenase and plasmin prevented tumor invasion of the amnion.[32] Several observations link uPA with cell growth and differentiation. A tumor cell collagenase-stimulating factor was demonstrated, and this may have an important role in inducing collagenolysis of host stroma during tumor invasion.[33] However, the available data do not include what type of functional correlation exists between growth, differentiation and plasminogen activator. uPA has recently been shown to induce human epidermal tumor cell proliferation.[34] As a

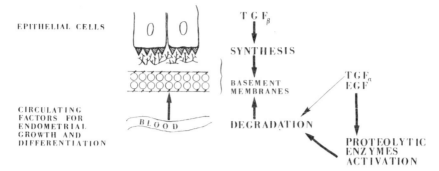

FIGURE 3. The figure shows the selective role of basement membrane encircling endometrial glands and vessels in the endometrial growth and differentiation. Basement membrane synthesis may be influenced by epithelial growth inhibiting factor (TGF-β), while its degradation may be due to proteolytic enzyme activities promoted by growth factors (EGF, TGF-α) or directly by the latter.

second role in malignancy uPA could be a factor in the autocrine growth mechanism.[11] Epidermal growth factor increases uPA[12] thus causing BM derangement by lysis of laminin and, in turn, loss of its ultrafiltration function which leads to an increase in estrogen transport into the endometrium (FIG. 3). Transforming growth factor β (TGF-β) influences the production of the extracellular matrix by increasing the production of fibronectin and procollagen.[35] TGF-β acts as a strong growth inhibitor for cells of epithelial origin but the mechanism of this growth inhibition is not understood. It is possible that the induction of extracellular matrix formation modulates the entrance of growth factors into the epithelial glandular cells which circulate in the human endometrium. A model for mechanisms controlling growth and differentiation of epithelial cells is shown in FIGURE 3.

SUMMARY

Basement membranes (BM) are elements of the extracellular matrix that are essential for growth and differentiation of tissues. Several collagenolytic enzymes of tumor cells are involved in degradation of the extracellular matrix; growth and inhibitor factors [e.g. Epidermal Growth Factor (EGF), Transforming Growth Factors α and β (TGF-α,β)] seem to be involved in the extracellular matrix formation and degradation. To establish a possible association between the presence of collagenase (C), urokinase-type plasminogen activator (uPA) and the neoplastic growth of the endometrium, 44 endometrial specimens (14 proliferative, 11 secretive, 7 adenomatous hyperplasia, 12 adenocarcinoma) were studied using immunohistochemistry with antisera for C, uPA, EGF receptors and TGF-α. Immunostaining for collagenase revealed a positive reaction in moderately differentiated adeno-carcinoma without staining the normal and hyperplastic endometrium. A progressive increase in uPA immunostaining was observed in proliferative and neoplastic endometrium. TGF-α and its receptor (EGFr) were stained in proliferative and more clearly in hyperplastic and carcinomatous endometrium. In conclusion, BM play an important role in proliferation and differentiation of human endometrium; their degradation influences estrogen transportation from blood to the stroma. Endometrial BM degradation is associated with the presence of collagenolytic enzymes and growth factors.

ACKNOWLEDGMENT

We thank Dr. Marco Balducci for his efforts in preparing histological photograms.

REFERENCES

1. LANE, G., M. C. SIDDLE, T. A. RIDER, J. PRYSE-DAVIS, R. J. B. KING & M. I. WHITEHEAD. 1983. Dose dependent effects of oral progesterone on the oestrogenized postmenopausal endometrium. Br. Med. J. 27: 1241–1246.
2. HOLINKA, C. F. & E. GURPIDE. 1980. In vivo uptake of estrone sulfate by rabbit uterus. Endocrinology 106: 1193–1197.
3. SIITERI, P. K., D. R. HEMSELL, C. L. EDWARDS & P. C. MACDONALD. 1973. Estrogens and endometrial cancer. *In* Proceedings of the Fourth International Congress of Endocrinology. R. O. Scow, Ed. Vol. 1: 1237–1239. Excerpta Medica. Amsterdam.
4. BULLETTI, C., V. M. JASONNI, P. M. CIOTTI, S. TABANELLI, S. NALDI & C. FLAMIGNI. 1988. Extraction of estrogens by human perfused uterus. Am. J. Obstet. Gynecol. : 509–515.
5. BULLETTI, C., A. GALASSI, V. M. JASONNI, G. MARTINELLI, S. TABANELLI & C. FLAMIGNI. 1988. Basement membrane components in normal hyperplastic and neoplastic endometrium. Cancer 62: 142–149.
6. BULLETTI, C., V. M. JASONNI, S. TABANELLI, P. M. CIOTTI, F. CAPPUCCINI, A. BORINI & C. FLAMIGNI. 1988. Increased extraction of estrogens in human endometrial hyperplasia and carcinoma. Cancer Detection and Prevention 13: 123–130.
7. YURCHENCO, P. D., A. C. TSILIBARY, A. S. CHARONIS & H. FURTHMAYR. 1981. Models for the self-assembly of basement membrane. J. Histochem. Cytochem. 34: 93–102.
8. GARBISA, S., C. DEGIOVANNI, G. BIAGINI, V. VASI, W. F. GRIGIONI, A. DIERRICO, A. M. MANCINI, B. DEL RE, P. L. LOLLINI, P. NANNI, G. NICOLETTI & G. PRODI. 1988. Different metastatic aggressiveness by murine TS/A clones: Ultrastructure, extracellular glycoproteins and type IV collagenolytic activity. Invasion & Metastasis 8: 177–192.
9. ELLIS, S. M., K. NABESHIMA & C. BISWAS. 1989. Monoclonal antibody preparation and purification of a tumor cell collagenase-stimulatory factor. Cancer Res. 49: 3385–3391.
10. DANO, K., P. A. ANDREASEN, J. GRONDAHL-HANSEN, P. KRISTENSEN, L. S. NIELSEN & L. SKRIVER. 1985. Plasminogen activators, tissue degradation and cancer. Adv. Cancer Res. 44: 139–239.
11. DEBRIUN, P., G. GRIFFIOEN, H. W. VARSPAGEST, J. H. VERHEIJEN, G. DOOIJWAARD, H. F. VAN DEN INGH & C. B. H. W. LAMERS. 1988. Plasminogen activators profiles in neoplastic tissue of the tumor colon. Cancer Res. 48: 4520–4524.
12. NIEDBALA, M. J. & A. SARTORELLI. 1989. Regulation by epidermal growth factor of human squamous cell carcinoma plasminogen activator-mediated meteolysis of extracellular matrix. Cancer Res. 49: 3302–3309.
13. BLASI, F. & M. P. STOPPELLI. 1989. Molecular basis for plasminogen activation surface proteolysis and their relation to cancer. *In* Growth Regulation and Carcinogenesis. W. Pentekowits, Ed. CRC Uniscience. In press.
14. NOYES, R. W., A. T. HERTIG & J. ROCK. 1950. Dating the endometrial biopsy. Fertil. Steril. 1: 3–25.
15. DI SAIA, P. J. & W. T. CREASMAN, Eds. 1984. Clinical Gynecologic Oncology. 2nd edit. C. V. Mosby. St. Louis, MO.
16. DE WEY, W. C. 1959. Vascular-extravascular exchange of I131 plasma proteins in the rat. Am. J. Physiol. 197: 423–429.
17. BULLETTI, C., V. M. JASONNI, S. LUBICZ, C. FLAMIGNI & E. GURPIDE. 1986. Extracorporeal perfusion of the human uterus. Am. J. Obstet. Gynecol. 154: 683–688.
18. STEINGOLD, K. A., W. CEFALN, W. PARDRIDGE, H. L. JUDD & G. CHANDHURI. 1986. Enhanced hepatic extraction of estrogens used for replacement therapy. J. Clin. Endocrinol. Metab. 62: 761–766.

19. VERHEUGEN, C., W. M. PARDRIDGE, H. L. JUDD & G. CHANDHURI. 1984. Differential permeability of uterine liver vascular beds to estrogens and estrogen conjugates. J. Clin. Endocrinol. Metab. **59:** 1128–1132.

20. MARKUS, G., S. CAMIOLO, S. KOHGA, J. MADEJA & A. MITTLEMAN. 1983. Plasminogen activator secretion of human tumors in short-term organ culture including a comparison of primary and metastatic tumors. Cancer Res. **43:** 5517–5525.

21. SAPPINO, A., N. BUSSO, D. BELIN & J. VASSALLI. 1987. Increase of urokinase-type plasminogen activator gene expression in human lung and breast carcinomas. Cancer Res. **47:** 4043–4046.

22. NELSON, L., J. HANSEN, L. SHRIVER, E. WILSON, K. KALTOFT, J. ZENTHEN & K. DANO. 1982. Purification of zymogen to plasminogen activator from human glioblastoma cells by affinity chromatography with monoclonal antibody. Biochemistry **21:** 6410–6415.

23. STUMP, D., M. THIENPONT & D. COLLEN. 1986. Urokinase-related proteins in human urine. J. Biol. Chem. **261:** 1267–1273.

24. LIOTTA, L., R. GOLDFARB, R. BRUNDAGE, G. SIEGAL, V. TERRANOVA & S. GARBISA. 1981. Effect of plasminogen activator (urokinase), plasmin, and thrombin on glycoprotein and collagenous components of basement membrane. Cancer Res. **41:** 4629–4636.

25. GOLDFARB, R., G. MURANO, R. BRUNDAGE, G. SIEGAL, V. TERRANOVA, S. GARBISA & L. LIOTTA. 1986. Degradation of glycoprotein and collagenous components of the basement membrane: Studies with urokinase-type plasminogen activator, thrombin and plasmin. Sem. Thrombosis Hemostasis **12:** 335–336.

26. DE BRUIN, P., G. GRIFFIOEN, H. VERSPAGET, I. VERHEIJEN & C. LAMERS. 1987. Plasminogen activators and tumor development in tumor colon: Activity levels in normal mucosa, adenomatous polyps and adenocarcinoma. Cancer Res. **47:** 4654–4657.

27. BARSKY, S., G. SIEGAL, F. JANNOTTA & L. LIOTTA. 1983. Loss of basement membrane components by invasive tumors but not by their benign counterparts. Lab. Invest. **49:** 140–147.

28. BURTIN, P., G. CHASANEL, J. FOIDART & E. MARTIN. 1987. Antigens of basement membrane and peritumoral stroma in tumor colonic adenocarcinomas: An immunofluorescence study. Int. J. Cancer **30:** 13–20.

29. OSSOWSKI, L. & E. REICH. 1983. Antibodies to plasminogen activator inhibit human tumor metastases. Cell **35:** 611–619.

30. HEARING, C., L. LAW, A. CORTI, E. ZIPELLA & F. BLASI. 1988. Modulation of metastatic potential by cell surface urokinase of murine melanoma cells. Cancer Res. **48:** 1270–1278.

31. MIGNATTI, P., E. ROBBINS & D. B. RIFKIN. 1986. Tumor invasion through the human amniotic membrane: Requirement for a proteinase cascade. Cell **47:** 487–498.

32. ELLIS, S. M., K. MABESHIMA & C. BISWAS. 1989. Monoclonal antibody preparation and purification of a tumor cell collagenase-stimulatory factor. Cancer Res. **49:** 3385–3391.

33. KIRCHEIMER, J. C., J. WOITA, G. CHRIST & B. R. BINDER. 1987. Proliferation of a human epidermal tumor cell line stimulated by urokinase. FASEB J. **1:** 125–128.

34. KESKI-OJA, J., R. RAGHOW, M. SAWDEY, D. LOSKUTOFF, A. E. POSTLETWAITE, A. A. KANG & H. L. MOSKES. 1988. Regulation of mRNAs for type-1 plasminogen activator inhibitor, fibronectin and type-1 procollagen by transforming growth factor-β. J. Biol. Chem. **263:** 3111–3115.

Growth Factors in Normal and Malignant Uterine Tissue

LIAM J. MURPHY, YUEWEN GONG,
AND LEIGH C. MURPHY

Departments of Internal Medicine, Physiology & Biochemistry
University of Manitoba
Winnipeg R3E OW3, Manitoba, Canada

BHAGU BHAVNANI

Department of Obstetrics & Gynecology
St. Micheal's Hospital
Toronto, Ontario, Canada

INTRODUCTION

Virtually all cell types in the uterus demonstrate some degree of estrogen-responsiveness and the marked atrophy of the uterus following castration would suggest that most uterine cells are in fact estrogen-dependent. Endometrial cancer arises from estrogen responsive, glandular epithelial cells. In contrast to the dramatic response of the uterus *in vivo* and the response of human endometrial cancer grown as xenografts in nude mice, human and rodent uterine cells are either unresponsive or demonstrate a poor growth response to estrogen *in vitro*.[1-4] This paradox suggests that paracrine growth factors and stromal-epithelial cell interactions are likely to be necessary components of the uterine response to estrogen. There is extensive evidence in the rodent that stromal-epithelial interaction is necessary for normal morphological development in the uterus during embryogenesis[5] and is also necessary for estrogen responsiveness of uterine epithelial cells in the neonatal mouse.[6]

While the endometrium is composed of both epithelial and stromal elements, malignant change in this tissue usually has the histological appearance of adenocarcinoma and arises from the epithelial component of the endometrium. Since stromal tissue is not a prominent morphological component of endometrial cancer histology, the requirements for stromal interaction appear to be diminished in endometrial neoplasia. Since stromal interaction appears to be an important component of the hormone responsiveness of normal uterine epithelia, malignant transformation of uterine epithelial cells may involve constitutive expression of genes which are normally part of the stromal-epithelial cell interaction. The products of these genes may represent autocrine or paracrine growth factors themselves, growth factor receptors or intracellular mediators.

A number of growth factors and growth factor receptors have been identified in human and rodent uterine tissue. These are outlined in TABLE 1. Studies in the rodent suggest that the insulin-like growth factors (IGF-I and II) and the transforming growth

TABLE 1. Growth Factor and Growth Factor Receptors in the Uterus

Growth Factors	Effect of Estrogen
EGF	Increased protein
	Increased EGF mRNA
	Proteolytic cleavage from precursor
	EGF receptors increased
	Mitogenic effects on uterine cells
IGF-I	Increased IGF-I mRNA
	Increased receptors
	Mitogenic effects in uterine tissue
IGF-II	Increased IGF-II mRNA
PDGF	Receptors present in uterine tissue
	Effects of estrogen not known
FGFs, acidic and basic	No reports to date

factor family (EGF and TGF-α) may have some role to play in the estrogen-induced uterine proliferation.

THE INSULIN-LIKE GROWTH FACTORS

Our studies in the rodent have demonstrated that the IGF-I and IGF-II are expressed in the uterus, and expression of these growth factors is estrogen-regulated. In ovariectomized rats a 10-fold increase in IGF-I mRNA abundance was seen after a single injection of 17-β estradiol. The increase in IGF-I reached a maximum at 6 h after injection and then gradually declined towards basal levels.[7] The uterine IGF-I response is direct in that it does not require continuing protein synthesis[8] and appears to be pituitary-independent.[9] Uterine IGF-II mRNA abundance also increases in response to estrogen administration to ovariectomized rats however the increase is considerably more modest than in the case of IGF-I. IGF-I is easily detectable in RNA prepared from human endometrial biopsies by Northern blot (FIG. 1). IGF-II mRNA is also present but at considerably lower levels than IGF-I. Both IGF-I and II mRNAs are abundant in human uterine leiomyomata.[11] There is no apparent difference in the abundance of IGF-I mRNA in endometrial biopsies from the secretory or proliferative phase of the menstrual cycle (FIG. 1). It should be noted that despite the obvious estrogen-dependence of IGF-I expression in the rat, there is also only a very small variation in the abundance of IGF-I throughout the estrous cycle.[10]

In the rat, *in situ* hybridization localizes the IGF-I mRNA to the stromal and myometrial cells with little expression in the luminal epithelium. In the stroma, IGF-I mRNA appears to be particularly abundant in the basal layer and in the peri-glandular stroma.[12] *In situ* localization of IGF-I expression in the human endometrium has not been reported. Although IGF-I mRNA is detectable by Northern blot analysis in human endometrial biopsies, primary cultures of either glandular epithelial or stromal cells derived from these biopsies do not have detectable levels of IGF-I or IGF-II mRNAs. This extinction of expression of these growth factors does not appear to be due to lack of stromal-epithelial cell interaction since IGF-I mRNA is not detectable in mixed

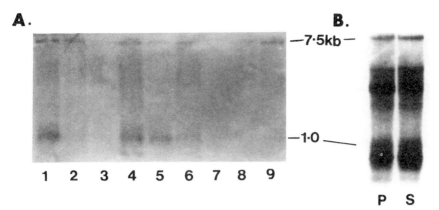

FIGURE 1. Insulin-like growth factor-I expression in human endometrium. Panel A depicts an auto-radiogram of a Northern blot where 25µg of total RNA from nine individual patient endometrial bi-opsies have been analyzed. In panel B, 50µg of poly (A⁺) RNA was prepared from pooled samples of proliferative (P) or secretory (S) endometrium and analyzed by the Northern blotting technique using a human IGF-I cDNA. Endometrial tissue was obtained by uterine currettage which was per-formed at the time of elective tubal ligation. Endometrial tissue was considered to be proliferative if obtained within 14 days of the last menses and secretory if obtained in the last 14 days of the men-strual cycle and verified by histological examination. The nitrocellulose filters were hybridized with a human IGF-I cDNA probe. The sizes of the major IGF-I transcripts were determined by comparison with the position of the 18S and 28S ribosomal RNAs.

cultures of stromal and glandular epithelial cells. It remains to be determined whether the culture of these uterine cells on more complex sub-stratums can re-activate ex-pression of the IGF-I gene as appears to be the case with various other genes.

Receptors for IGF-I have been demonstrated in uterine tissue and in the rat, these receptors are up-regulated by estrogen.[13] In organ culture, IGF-I amplifies estrogen-induced uterine DNA synthesis in rat uterine sections. This response is most marked in the presence of estrogen and in tissue derived from estrogen-pretreated rats.[12] These data suggest that IGF-I is able to function in a paracrine fashion in the uterus. This paracrine loop can be modulated by estrogen at least at two levels: enhanced expres-sion of the ligand, IGF-I and increased abundance of the receptor for this growth factor. However, the paracrine action of the IGFs in uterine tissue may be considerably more complex since at least three different IGF binding proteins are also present in uterine fluid and in uterine extracts. These binding proteins may be able to regulate the bio-availability and action of IGF-I.[14-18] The best characterized of these IGF binding pro-teins is IGFBP-1, which was originally isolated from amniotic fluid[18] and is identical to the previously described placenta protein 12.[19] It is, however, present in the non-decidualized primate and rodent uterus. In man and monkey uterine IGFBP-1 is more abundant in the luteal phase of the menstrual cycle. The physiological role of IGFBP-1 is controversial since this binding protein has been shown both to enhance and inhibit the action of IGF-I in various assay systems. A number of IGFBP-1 variants exist, including phosphorylated forms, and may account for the differences in the reported effects on IGF-I actions in different assay systems.[17] In the rat, IGFBP-1 is localized almost exclusively in the luminal and glandular epithelium whereas in man and monkey, stromal cells also express IGFBP-1. Whereas IGF-I expression is up-regulated by estrogen, in the rat expression of IGFBP-1 is suppressed. In human endometrium IGFBP-1 is more abundant in the secretory phase rather than the proliferative phase of the menstrual cycle suggesting that progesterone rather than estrogen may be the major regulator in man.[20-22]

IGFs AND IGF BINDING PROTEINS
IN ENDOMETRIAL CANCER

Two human endometrial cancer cell lines HEC 50 and the Var-1 variant of the original Ishikawa cell line have been studied in our laboratory. HEC 50 and Ishikawa cells like primary cultures of uterine epithelium do not express IGF-I or II mRNA at easily detectable levels. However, both HEC 50 and Ishikawa cells express several IGF binding proteins. In conditioned medium from HEC 50 cells IGF binding proteins with molecular weights of 30 and 24 kDa were identified by ligand blotting. The smallest of these binding proteins was the most abundant and did not react with antibodies to IGFBP-1 or 3. The 30 kDa binding protein reacted with antibody to human IGFBP-1 and IGFBP-1 mRNA was detectable in RNA prepared from HEC 50 cells. A 30 kDa binding protein was most abundant in conditioned medium from Ishikawa cells. Small amounts of 39, 40, and 42 kDa binding proteins are also present. These may represent IGFBP-3 which is known to be glycosylated and migrates in SDS gels as multiple species with apparent molecular weights of 39–42 kDa. The nature of the 30 kDa IGF binding protein present in conditioned medium from Ishikawa cells is less clear. This binding protein does not appear to be IGFBP-1 since no hybridization is seen when a human IGFBP-1 cDNA is used to probe Northern blots of Ishikawa cell RNA. Furthermore neither IGFBP-1 nor IGFBP-3 was identified in conditioned medium by Western blotting with specific antibodies to these binding proteins. It may represent IGFBP-2 which is present in fetal and neonatal rat serum but not in adult rat serum.[23] The 30 kDa binding protein present in conditioned medium from Ishikawa cells was down-regulated by incubation with insulin (FIG. 2). Insulin is also known to down-regulate IGFBP-1 in human fetal liver explants.[24] Interestingly the 30 kDa binding protein present in conditioned medium from Ishikawa cells is also down-regulated by progestins (FIG. 2). As discussed above IGFBP-1 is increased in the luteal phase of the cell cycle suggesting that progesterone may up-regulate expression of IGFBP in human endometrium.[20-23]

EGF AND THE TRANSFORMING GROWTH FACTORS

Expression of EGF and its receptor have been detected in the mouse uterus.[25,26] In this tissue, estrogen enhances both EGF and EGF-receptor mRNA abundance.[25-27] The mRNA for EGF is also detectable in RNA extracted from human endometrial biopsy tissue (FIG. 3). EGF mRNA abundance was similar in endometrium from the proliferative and secretory phase of the menstrual cycle. More detailed *in situ* hybridization studies are required to determine which cell type is responsible for EGF expression in the human endometrium and whether expression changes in certain cell populations in response to hormonal fluctuations during the menstrual cycle.

The transforming growth factors, TGF-α and TGF-β were both detectable in RNA

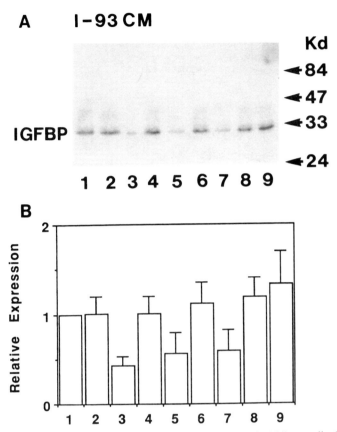

FIGURE 2. Production of insulin-like growth factor binding proteins by Ishikawa cells. 1.5 million cells were seeded in 100mm culture dishes and grown for two days in DMEM/F12 medium with 5% fetal bovine serum. After washing the monolayer twice with phosphate buffered saline, serum-free medium containing various hormones was added and conditioned for varying periods of time as indicated below. The conditioned medium was concentrated 100-fold and 15μl of the concentrated medium was analyzed by SDS-PAGE and ligand blotting using ¹²⁵I-IGF-I. The upper panel shows the autoradiogram while in the lower panel the results obtained by densitometry have been plotted as histograms. *Lane 1*, no additives conditioned for 24 hours; *lane 2*, 50μg/ml human growth hormone conditioned for 24 hours; *lane 3*, 50U/ml insulin−conditioned for 24 hours; *lane 4*, 100nM medroxyprogesterone acetate (MPA)−conditioned for 6 hours; *lane 5*, 100nM MPA−conditioned for 12 hours; *lane 6*, 100nM MPA−conditioned for 24 hours; *lane 7*, 1000nM MPA−conditioned for 24 hours; *lane 8*, 100nM MPA−conditioned for 24 hours; *lane 9*, 10nM MPA−conditioned for 24 hours.

from human endometrium (FIG. 3). The abundance of the mRNA for these growth factors was similar in proliferative and secretory endometrium. TGF-β is expressed in both stroma and glandular epithelium at approximately similar levels since it is easily detectable in RNA prepared from these cells when cultured *in vitro* (FIG. 4).

Both TGF-α and TGF-β are expressed in Ishikawa and HEC 50 human endometrial cells. TGF-α is more abundant in Ishikawa cells whereas TGF-β is more abun-

EGF

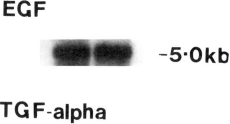

FIGURE 3. Epidermal growth factor and TGF-α expression in human endometrium. Poly (A⁺) RNA prepared from pooled human endometrial biopsy samples from the proliferative or secretory phase of the menstrual cycle were hybridized with a human EGF or TGF-α cDNA probe. The size of the transcripts were determined by comparison with the position of the 18S and 28S ribosomal RNAs.

dant in the HEC-50 cells. In complete medium containing 5% fetal calf serum, 100 nM estradiol cause a small increase in TGF-α expression in Ishikawa cells. The same concentration of tamoxifen causes a dramatic reduction in both TGF-α and TGF-β. Low concentrations (0.1–10 nM) of the synthetic progestin, medroxy progesterone acetate, was also able to inhibit TGF-β expression in both cell lines and reduced TGF-α mRNA in the Ishikawa cells (submitted for publication). These effects were seen at concentrations of medroxy progesterone acetate which significantly reduced cellular proliferation. In Ishikawa cells, the effect of medroxy progesterone acetate on TGF-α mRNA was rapid with a maximal reduction seen in 6 to 12 hours whereas the effect on TGF-β mRNA was considerably more delayed.

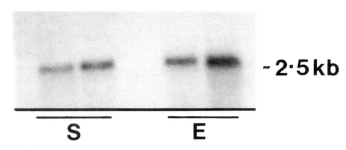

FIGURE 4. TGF-β expression in primary cultures of human endometrial stromal and glandular epithelial cells. Pure cultures of stromal (S) and glandular epithelial (E) cells were prepared by collagenase and passage through a stainless steel sieve. Total RNA was then analyzed by Northern blotting with a human TGF-β cDNA.

CONCLUSIONS

Unlike other tissues in the body where the fraction of cells which are proliferating is relatively constant, the uterus undergoes striking changes in proliferative rates in response to hormonal fluctuations which occur during the normal menstrual cycle. The most dramatic estrogen-induced changes are seen in the endometrium. However, both stromal and myometrial cells proliferate in response to estrogen, as is apparent by the hyperplasia seen in these tissues at puberty. While a dramatic uterine proliferative response to exogenous estrogen is demonstrable *in vivo*, it has been exceedingly difficult to demonstrate even minor mitogenic responses to estrogen in isolated human or rodent uterine cells in culture. An increasingly popular notion is that paracrine and/or autocrine growth factors are important in mediating the response of endocrine target tissues to trophic hormones. A considerable amount of experimental evidence has been accumulated in recent years which would support this hypothesis in the uterus. The growth factors, their receptor and the intracellular mediators responsible for the normal estrogen-induced endometrial proliferation may be constitutively expressed in endometrial cancer.

While there is good evidence that IGF-I and EGF may function as locally synthesized mediators in the rodent uterus, the evidence that these growth factors function as local estromedins in human endometrium is less clear. Our preliminary studies did not reveal any consistent difference in the abundance of the mRNAs for these growth factors in endometrium derived from the proliferative or secretory phase of the menstrual cycle. However, a more careful analysis using the *in situ* hybridization technique may identify particular cell types responding to the fluctuating levels of steroid hormones. However, even in the rodent it is unlikely that these growth factors are the only autocrine/paracrine mediators of estrogen action. It is likely that other growth factors such as platelet-derived growth factors and the fibroblast growth factors and the cytokines also have some role to play in estrogen-induced uterine proliferation.

The human endometrial cancer cells which we utilized in these studies did not express IGF-I or II. This observation is consistent with the localization of the IGFs to predominantly mesenchymal-derived tissue. The two endometrial cancer cells both express binding proteins for IGF-I however the major binding proteins present in conditioned medium from the two cell types appear to be immunologically different. In preliminary studies we were able to demonstrate that progestins, at growth inhibitor concentrations, were able to down-regulate the level of the major binding proteins in Ishikawa cell conditioned medium. The role of the IGF binding proteins remains controversial. The majority of investigators have reported inhibitory effects of the binding proteins on IGF-I action however there is at least one report which suggests that IGFBP-1 can enhance the action of IGF-I *in vitro*.[17] A more detailed study of the regulation of the binding proteins by endometrial cancer cells is currently underway to determine whether there is a correlation between the expression of the binding proteins and growth rate.

The transforming growth factors, TGF-α and TGF-β were expressed by both cell lines and in the presence of estrogen, both tamoxifen and progestins were able to reduce the levels of mRNA for each of these growth factors.

While considerable attention has been directed towards examining the effects of individual growth factors on culture cells, *in vivo* growth appears to involve a carefully orchestrated interaction of the growth factors which function both in an autocrine and paracrine fashion. Future experimentation should involve more complex experimental models involving reconstitution of the various cell types present in uterine tissue. The data generated by this type of experimentation should provide insights into the normal estrogen-induced growth response and thus be useful in designing experiments to elucidate the pathogenesis and progression of uterine cancer.

REFERENCES

1. TOMOOKA, Y., R. P. DiAUGUSTINE & J. A. McLACHLAN. 1986. Proliferation of mouse uterine epithelial cells in vitro. Endocrinology 118: 1011–1018.
2. CHEN, L., H. R. LINDNER & M. LANCET. 1973. Mitogenic action of oestradiol-17 on human myometrial and endometrial cells in long term tissue cultures. J. Endocrinol. 59: 87–97.
3. GERSCHENSON, L. E., E. CONNER & J. T. MURAI. 1977. Regulation of the cell cycle by diethylstilbestrol and progesterone in cultured endometrial cells. Endocrinology 100: 1468–1476.
4. PAVLIK, E. J. & B. S. KATZENELLENBOGEN. 1978. Human endometrial cells in primary tissue culture: Estrogen interactions and modulation of cell proliferation. J. Clin. Endocrinol. Metab. 47: 333–344.
5. CUNHA, G. R., P. YOUNG & J. R. BRODY. 1989. Role of uterine epithelium in the development of myometrial smooth muscle cells. Biol. Reprod. 40: 861–865.
6. COOKE, P. S., F. D. A. UCHIMA, D. K. FUJII, H. A. BERN & G. R. CUNHA. 1986. Restoration of normal morphology and estrogen responsiveness in cultured vaginal and uterine epithelia transplanted with stroma. Proc. Natl. Acad. Sci. USA 83: 2109–2113.
7. MURPHY, L. J., L. C. MURPHY & H. G. FRIESEN. 1988. Estrogen induces insulin-like growth factor-I expression in the rat uterus. Mol. Endocrinol. 1: 445–450.
8. MURPHY, L. J. & J. M. LUO. 1989. Effects of cycloheximide on hepatic and uterine insulin-like growth factor-I mRNA. Mol. Cell. Endocrinol. 64: 81–86.
9. MURPHY, L. J. & H. G. FRIESEN. 1988. Differential effects of estrogen and growth hormone on uterine and hepatic insulin-like growth factor-I gene expression in the ovariectomized, hypophysectomized rat. Endocrinology 122: 325–332.
10. MURPHY, L. J., L. C. MURPHY & H. G. FRIESEN. 1988. A role for the insulin-like growth factors as estromedins in the rat uterus. Trans. Assoc. Am. Physicians 99: 204–214.
11. HOPPENER, J. W. M., S. MOSSELMAN, P. J. M. ROHOLL, C. LAMBRECHTS, R. J. C. SLEBOS, P. DE PAGTER-HOLTHUIZEN, C. J. M. LIPS, H. S. JANSZ & J. S. SUSSENBACH. 1988. Expression of insulin-like growth factor-I and -II in human smooth muscle tumors. EMBO 7: 1379–1382.
12. GHAHARY, A. & L. J. MURPHY. 1990. In situ localization of the sites of synthesis and action of insulin-like growth factor-I in the rat uterus. Mol. Endocrinol. 4: 191–195.
13. GHAHARY, A. & L. J. MURPHY. 1989. Regulation of uterine insulin-like growth factor receptors by estrogen and variation throughout the estrous cycle. Endocrinology 125: 597–604.
14. MEULI, C., J. ZAPF & E. R. FROESCH. 1978. NSILA-carrier protein abolishes the action of nonsuppressible insulin-like activity (NSILA-S) on perfused rat heart. Diabetologia 14: 255–259.
15. KNAUER, D. J. & G. L. SMITH. 1980. Inhibition of biological activity of multiplication-stimulating activity by binding to its carrier protein. Proc. Natl. Acad. Sci. USA 77: 7252–7625.
16. BURCH, W. M., J. CORREA, J. E. SHIVELY & D. R. POWELL. 1990. The 25 kilodalton insulin-like growth factor (IGF)-binding protein inhibits both basal and IGF-I mediated growth of chick embryo pelvic cartilage in vitro. J. Clin. Endocrinol. Metab. 70: 173–180.
17. ELGIN, R. G., W. H. BUSBY & D. L. CLEMMONS. 1987. An insulin-like growth factor (IGF) binding protein enhances the biological response to IGF-I. Proc. Natl. Acad. Sci. USA 84: 3254–3258.
18. DROP, S. P. S., G. VALIQUETTE, H. J. GUYDA, H. J. CORVOL. M. T. CORVOL & B. I. POSNER. 1979. Partial purification and characterization of a binding protein for insulin-like activity (ILAs) in human amniotic fluid: A possible inhibitor of insulin-like activity. Acta Endocrinol. (Copenhagen) 90: 505–518.
19. KOISTINEN, R., N. KALKKINEN, M-L. HUHTALA, M. SEPPALA, H. BOHN & E-M. RUTANEN. 1986. Placental protein 12 is a decidual protein that binds somatomedin and has an identical N-terminal amino acid sequence with somatomedin-binding protein from human amniotic fluid. Endocrinology 118: 1375–1381.

20. WAITES, G. T., R. F. L. JAMES & S. C. BELL. 1988. Immunohistological localization of human endometrial secretory proteins "pregnancy-associated endometrial secretory 1-globulin" (1-PEG), an insulin-like growth factor binding protein, during the menstrual cycle. J. Clin. Endocrinol. Metab. **67**: 1100–1105.

21. BELL, S. C., S. R. PATEL, P. H. KIRWAN & J. O. DRIFE. 1986. Protein synthesis and secretion by the human endometrium during the menstrual cycle and the effects of progesterone in vitro. J. Reprod. Fertil. **77**: 221–224.

22. BELL, S. C. & H. BOHN. 1986. Immunochemical and biochemical relationship between human pregnancy-associated secreted 1- and 2-globulins (1- and 2-PEG) and soluble placental proteins (PP12 and PP14). Placenta **7**: 283–288.

23. BROWN, A. L., L. CHIARIOTTI, C. C. ORLOWSKI, T. MEHLEM, W. H. BURGESS, E. J. ACKERMAN, C. B. BRUNI & M. M. RECHLER. 1989. Nucleotide sequence and expression of a cDNA clone encoding a fetal ratbinding protein for insulin-like growth factors. J. Biol. Chem. **264**: 5148–5154.

24. LEWITT, M. S. & R. C. BAXTER. 1989. Regulation of growth hormone-independent insulin-like growth factor-binding protein (BP-28) in cultured human fetal liver explants. J. Clin. Endocrinol. Metab. **69**: 246–251.

25. DIAUGUSTINE, R. P., P. PETRUSZ, G. I. BELL, C. F. BROWN, K. S. KORACH, J. A. MCLACHLAN & C. T. TEBG. 1988. Influence of estrogens on mouse uterine epidermal growth factor precursor protein and messenger ribonucleic acid. Endocrinology **122**: 2355–2363.

26. HUET-HUDSON, Y. M., C. CHAKRABORTY, S. K. DE, Y. SUZUKI, G. K. ANDREWS & S. K. DEY. 1990. Estrogen regulates the synthesis of epidermal growth factor in mouse uterine epithelial cells. Mol. Endocrinol. **4**: 510–523.

27. LINGHAM, R. B., G. M. STANCEL & D. S. LOOSE-MITCHELL. 1988. Estrogen regulation of epidermal growth factor receptor messenger ribonucleic acid. Mol. Endocrinol. **2**: 230–235.

Human 17β-Hydroxysteroid Dehydrogenase in Normal and Malignant Endometrium[a]

R. VIHKO, O. MÄENTAUSTA, AND V. ISOMAA

Biocenter and Department of Clinical Chemistry
University of Oulu
SF-90220 Oulu, Finland

V.-P. LEHTO

Biocenter and Department of Pathology
University of Oulu
SF-90220 Oulu, Finland

K. BOMAN AND U. STENDAHL

Department of Gynecological Oncology
University Hospital
S-90185 Umeå, Sweden

PHYSIOLOGICAL FUNCTION AND POSSIBLE PATHOPHYSIOLOGICAL IMPORTANCE

17β-Hydroxysteroid dehydrogenase (17-HSD, EC 1.1.1.62) catalyzes the reversible interconversion of estrone and estradiol. There are a number of additional steroid pairs, such as androstenedione and testosterone, and dehydroepiandrosterone and 5-androstene-3β,17β-diol, the interconversion of which is dependent on this kind of enzyme activity. The terminology concerning this enzyme activity varies, and additional terms include 17-ketosteroid reductase, 17-oxidoreductase and 17β-estradiol dehydrogenase. Being obligatory for the biosynthesis of the biologically most important sex steroids, estradiol and testosterone, this enzyme activity is present in steroidogenic tissues. In addition, the enzyme activity has been detected in a number of target tissues for sex steroid action, such as the endometrium, vaginal mucosa, breast tissue, and the prostate. It has also been detected in tissues and cells, such as lung, ileum and red blood cells, which are not characteristically sex steroid–dependent. In recent measurements, using a placental cDNA probe of 17-HSD,[1] the tissue distribution of the two mRNA species detected suggested that different enzymes would be responsible for the interconversion of estrone and estradiol, and androstenedione and testosterone.

It was observed earlier that the activity of 17-HSD displays a cyclic fluctuation in the human endometrium during the menstrual cycle.[2,3] The enzyme activity is in-

[a] The research summarized in this paper was supported by the Research Council for Medicine of the Academy of Finland. The Department of Clinical Chemistry is a WHO Collaborating Centre supported by the Ministries of Education, Health and Social Affairs, and of Foreign Affairs, Finland.

duced by progesterone, and peak concentrations of the enzyme activity can be measured in the midsecretory endometrium. In superfusion experiments,[4] this increase in 17-HSD activity was shown to be associated with an increased conversion of estradiol to estrone. By this mechanism, the enzyme may have a key role in the regulation of the exposure of the endometrial cells to estrogens.[5] Estradiol, being the predominant intracellular estrogen during the proliferative phase of the cycle (see ref. 6), stimulates mitosis in endometrial cells.[7] Progesterone (and synthetic progestins) reduce mitotic activity close to zero possibly by a number of mechanisms. In addition to having an effect on the differentiation of endometrial cells to a secretory state, they reduce the concentration of estrogen receptors[8,9] and, by inducing 17-HSD activity, reduce the intracellular estradiol concentration.[4]

PURIFICATION OF PLACENTAL 17-HSD AND RAISING ANTIBODIES AGAINST THE ENZYME

17β-Hydroxysteroid dehydrogenase is an abundant protein in placental tissue, and the full term placenta contains approximately 0.7 mg of the enzyme protein/g cytosol protein. Hence, placenta is a rich source for the purification of this enzyme protein, and placental 17β-hydroxysteroid dehydrogenase has been purified to homogeneity and characterized in a number of laboratories. The enzyme consists of two identical subunits having molecular weights of 34 000–37 000 in different reports (see ref. 10).

In our work,[11] human placental 17-HSD was purified to apparent homogeneity using a three-step procedure. The placental homogenate was centrifuged and the proteins in the supernatant were fractionally precipitated by ammonium sulfate. The dissolved precipitate was dialysed and applied to a Reactive Red agarose column and the enzyme was eluted with a linear $NADP^+$-gradient. The peak enzyme fractions were pooled and applied to a DEAE-Sepharose column and eluted with a linear phosphate gradient. Peak enzyme fractions were pooled and stored at $-70°C$. Electrophoresis on polyacrylamide gels under denaturing conditions, and using silver staining, showed a single protein with an apparent molecular weight of 37 800.

Antibodies against human 17-HSD have been described by a number of groups.[11-14] These are all polyclonal antibodies and have been raised against human placental 17-HSD.

For production of polyclonal rabbit antibodies against purified placental 17-HSD in this laboratory, conventional techniques were used.[11] The antisera obtained formed a single band in immunoblotting analysis carried out using either the supernatant from the placental homogenate, or the purified enzyme preparation, indicating the high specificity of the antibody (FIG. 1). The selected antibody displayed high affinity for 17-HSD, the apparent equilibrium dissociation constant (kD) being 3.7×10^{-11}mol/L, as determined by Scatchard type analysis.[15] The addition of serial dilutions of the antiserum to the enzyme solution led to a corresponding gradual loss of enzyme activity.

IDENTITY OF PLACENTAL 17-HSD WITH ENDOMETRIAL 17-HSD

Tseng[16] reported that although the enzyme activities were very different in endometrial and placental tissues, a number of physical properties of 17-HSD from these

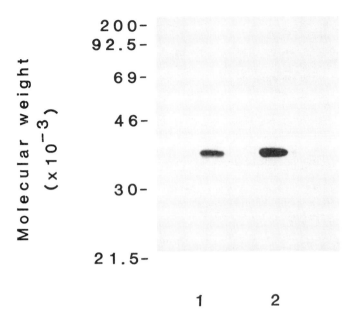

FIGURE 1. Immunoblotting analysis of a crude placental homogenate (*lane 1*) and the purified 17-HSD preparation (*lane 2*). The amount of total protein applied to lane 1 was 50μg, and that of the purified 17-HSD applied to lane 2 was 0.5μg. The dilution of the antiserum was 1:200, and the bands were visualized using protein A-peroxidase staining. From Mäentausta *et al.*,[11] with permission.

two sources were very similar. Marowitz *et al.*[12] described a possible immunological non-identity of human placental and endometrial 17-HSD, an observation that was supported by Fournet-Dulguerov *et al.*,[17] who used the same antibody.

To study further the possible identity with the endometrial enzyme of the enzyme protein purified from placental tissue, the polyclonal antibodies against placental 17-HSD raised in this laboratory, and described above, were used and immunological ligand binding and immunohistochemical assays were set up. The established sensitive radioimmunoassay used [125I]-labeled 17-HSD as a tracer, an appropriate dilution of the antibody, and solid-phase coupled double antibody for separating the antibody-bound and free fractions. The cytosol fraction (105 000 × g) of term placental tissue contained approximately 0.7mg of 17-HSD/g protein.

The sensitivity of our radioimmunoassay may explain the fact that human endometrial preparations were found to contain an immunoreactive substance. The cross-reacting substance found in our work was indistinguishable from authentic placental 17-HSD in parallelism tests based on the radioimmunoassay. There was excellent parallelism between the competition curves for [125I]-iodo-17HSD with purified 17-HSD standards and dilutions of placental and endometrial homogenates (FIG. 2).

The same antibody, following affinity purification, was used in immunohistochemical studies of the endometrium and displayed staining of the epithelial cells (FIG. 3). In addition, a several-fold increase in concentration was observed during the luteal phase as compared with the follicular phase concentrations, as evaluated by RIA,

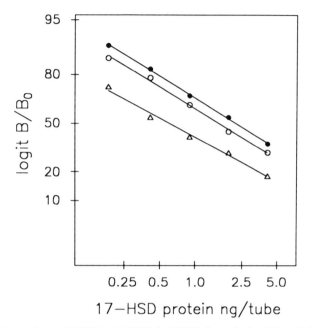

FIGURE 2. Competition of 17-HSD with [^{125}I]iodo-17-HSD for antibody binding. Labeled enzyme was incubated with the antiserum (final dilution 1:62 500) and with the indicated amounts of purified 17-HSD (*open triangles*), or of serial dilutions of the placental (*open circles*), or endometrial (*closed circles*) homogenates. The antibody-bound and -free antigens were separated by a second antibody coated onto kaolin particles. Data from Mäentausta *et al.*[11]

or from the immunohistochemical appearance of the tissue sections. These data strongly suggest that the substance measured in the endometrial specimens was 17-HSD.

CLONING AND SEQUENCING OF THE cDNA AND GENE ENCODING 17-HSD

The highly specific antiserum against placental 17-HSD was used to screen a placental cDNA library.[18] The sizes of inserts in positive clones varied from 0.8 to 1.3 kb. The largest cDNA was 1325 nucleotides long and contained an open reading frame of 987 nucleotides. The 5'- and 3'-noncoding sequences were 9 and 329 nucleotides in length, respectively. The open reading frame encoded a polypeptide of 327 amino acid residues with a predicted molecular weight of 34 853. The authenticity of the clone was verified by sequencing 23 amino acids from the N-terminal end of the purified protein and, in addition, the deduced amino acid sequence contained two peptides previously characterized from the proposed catalytic area of the placental 17-HSD enzyme protein.[19,20] Recently, two other groups have also isolated cDNA clones encoding 17-HSD using antibody and oligonucleotide screening of a placental cDNA library. The amino acid sequence of 17-HSD deduced from cDNA by Luu-The *et*

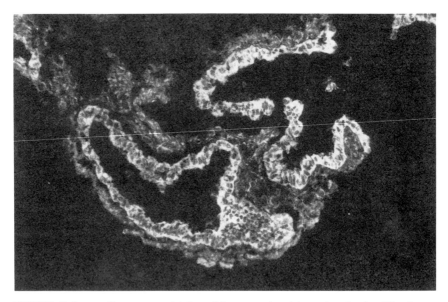

FIGURE 3. Immunofluorescence staining of human endometrium at cycle day 22 using an immunoaffinity-purified polyclonal antibody raised against purified placental 17-HSD. *Magnification:* ×250.

al.[21] agrees completely with our sequence, and the amino acid sequence determined by Gast *et al.*[13] from a cDNA clone containing almost the entire coding region had only six differences in the amino acid composition.

When cDNA encoding 17-HSD is used as a probe in Northern blot analysis of placental RNA, a major RNA species of about 1.4kb, and a minor RNA species of 2.4kb is detected (FIG. 4). Luu-The *et al.*[22] have indicated that the size difference of these two mRNA species is due to a longer 5′-nontranslated region in the 2.4kb 17-HSD mRNA. While the major mRNA starts nine nucleotides upstream of the starting codon, the minor mRNA species contains approximately 971 nucleotides upstream from the translation initiation codon. The 1.4kb and 2.4kb mRNA species are also detected in other tissues, but their relative distribution varies in different tissues. The 1.4kb mRNA is very abundant in placental and ovarian tissues. It has been suggested that the 1.4kb mRNA is present only in tissues producing estrogens,[1] but testis and prostate also contain the shorter transcript.[22] The 2.4kb mRNA species has been found in steroid-forming tissues and also in some target tissues of steroid hormone action, such as endometrium, myometrium, prostate, and breast tissue, as well as in breast and endometrial cancer cell lines. In these tissues the 2.4kb mRNA seems to be predominant.

We have assigned the gene of 17-HSD to human chromosome 17, bands q12–q21, using Southern blotting analysis of panels of different human (x) rodent somatic cell hybrids, and chromosomal *in situ* hybridization.[23] The localization of this gene on chromosome 17 has also been shown by others.[1,21]

In a recent paper, Luu-The *et al.*[22] determined the structure of two human 17-HSD genes (h17β-HSDI and H17β-HSDII). Human 17β-HSDII contained six exons and

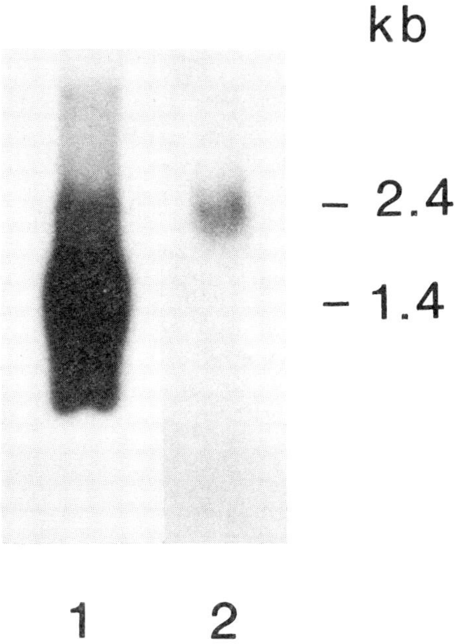

kb

FIGURE 4. Northern blot hybridization analysis of poly(A)-RNA from human placenta (*lane 1*) and the endometrial cancer cell line, RL-95-2 (*lane 2*). Total RNA was isolated as described by Davis *et al.*[31] and enriched for poly(A)-containing RNA by oligo(dT)-cellulose chromatography. *Lane 1* contains 5 μg and *lane 2* 15 μg of poly(A)-RNA. A 1.0 kb fragment of 17-HSD cDNA[18] labeled by nick translation was used as a probe.

$- 2.4$

$- 1.4$

1   2

five introns for a total length of 3250 bp, and the exon sequence was identical to the sequence of the cDNA. Comparison of the nucleotide sequence of h17β-HSDI with that of the exons and introns of the 17β-HSDII gene showed a 89% homology. It is not known whether the h17β-HSDI gene is transcribed. The sequences of cDNA clones that have been determined so far have been corresponding mRNA transcribed from h17β-HSDII gene. If the h17β-HSDI gene is also transcribed and its mRNA translated into a protein starting from corresponding AUG-codon, this mRNA would be translated into a 17-HSD having a molecular weight of about 20 000, since there is a nucleotide change in the h17β-HSDI gene that creates a stop codon at amino acid position 218.

17-HSD IN NORMAL ENDOMETRIUM

17-HSD activity increases in human endometrium during the secretory phase.[2,3,16] In these earlier studies, the activity of 17-HSD was measured in endometrial specimens at various phases of the menstrual cycle using a tracer kinetic method,[2] or a catalytic activity method[3] in these earlier studies. More than a 10-fold increase in activity occurred during the secretory phase.[16] In these studies, it was also observed that, in the normal human endometrium, epithelial glands exhibit the highest 17-HSD activity. In the stromal cells, remarkable variation in activity occurred in both proliferative and secretory endometrium, indicating that 17-HSD is present in both endometrial glands and stroma, and cyclic changes in enzyme activity occur in both types of cells. Pollow *et al.*[3] also demonstrated a cyclic change of the enzyme activity in the microsomal and mitochondrial fractions.

We measured solubilized 17-HSD concentrations by RIA in endometrium during the normal menstrual cycle. The mean concentration of the enzyme protein, measured by RIA, was 14.1 μg/g protein in specimens taken on different days over the entire cycle. These concentrations showed a significant correlation with the 17-HSD activities measured in the endometrial specimens ($r = 0.722$, $p < 0.001$, $n = 21$). Mean concentrations of the substance measured by RIA were 8.3 μg/g protein in endometrial specimens taken during the follicular phase and 22.9 μg/g protein during the luteal phase of the cycle.

Using our immunohistochemical method, we were able to demonstrate immunostaining in placental and endometrial tissues by using the same immunoaffinity purified polyclonal antibody. In the endometrium, staining intensity for 17-HSD followed the changes described for changes in the enzymatic activity during the menstrual cycle. During the proliferative phase, no staining was observed. The staining started to appear in the early secretory phase and its intensity increased strongly during the mid-secretory phase. The changes in staining intensity were closely associated with changes in the concentrations of serum progesterone and of estrogen and progestin receptors in the tissue.

Tseng and Gurpide[24] showed that blocking the protein synthesis abolished the increase in enzymatic activity, even after one day of progesterone induction, when the stimulatory effect on the enzyme was already evident. Our results[11] show that the increase in enzymatic activity is associated with an increase in enzyme protein concentration.

Pollow et al.[3] demonstrated that 17-HSD was distributed in all subcellular fractions, with the majority of the activity being present in the microsomes and mitochondria. The microsomal enzyme is bound to the membranes of endoplasmic reticulum, whereas in mitochondria the enzyme is located in the outer membranes. The cytoplasmic fractions contain less than ten percent of the total activity.

The subcellular distribution of immunologically detectable 17-HSD in the endometrium was different from the distribution of the catalytic activity. In the cytosol, microsomal and mitochondrial fractions, 47%, 36% and 17%, respectively, of the total immunologically detectable 17-HSD were observed.[11] The differences between the subcellular distributions of the enzymatic and immunoreactive activities in the endometrium cannot yet be explained. They may be due to an apparent immunological nonidentity, or they may reflect an insufficient solubilization of the mitochondrial enzyme.

17-HSD IN CANCEROUS ENDOMETRIUM

It has been amply demonstrated that the concentrations of estrogen and progestin receptors in endometrial carcinoma tissues are generally lower than those in the proliferative normal endometrium.[8,25,26] However, most of the malignant tissue specimens display these two receptors and, therefore, have the potential of being hormone dependent. In line with this, induction of 17-HSD activity has been observed in endometrial adenocarcinoma tissues. After a one-week medroxyprogesterone acetate, or danazol treatment, a significant increase in the activity of 17-HSD was observed in carcinoma specimens,[27] and the post-therapy 17-HSD activities correlated significantly with the pretreatment cytosol progestin receptor concentrations in both treatment groups. Both treatments also decreased the proliferative activity and increased the secretory activity of the malignant epithelial endometrial cells. These data[27] on female

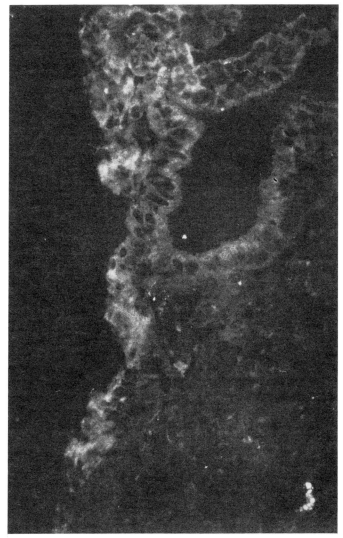

FIGURE 5. Immunofluorescence staining of human endometrial carcinoma tissue from a postmenopausal patient. The antibody against 17-HSD was as in FIGURE 3. *Magnification:* ×100.

sex steroid receptors and 17-HSD indicate that, at least in the majority of endometrial adenocarcinomas, essential features of female sex steroid action have been retained.

A critical issue in the treatment of endometrial carcinoma with progestins, however, is the duration of the therapeutic effect.[28] Data do not seem to be available on this issue using carcinoma tissue, but experiments carried out on healthy volunteers show that, despite continuous progestin administration, endometrial 17-HSD activity stays increased for only about one week to 10 days.[29,30] A period of 2 to 3 weeks of continuous progestin administration is sufficient to completely terminate the acute progestin effect reflected by the high 17-HSD activity in the endometrium.[29] Progestin action on the human endometrium has two phases: an acute stimulation of endometrial activity, followed by a reduction of endometrial metabolism, leading to atrophy of this tissue.

Immunohistochemical staining of 17-HSD in malignant endometrium does not give uniform results. Variable degrees of staining of the cells is seen, and the same specimen may display stained and unstained cells (FIG. 5). It is very likely that the heterogeneous picture that is emerging reflects the resultant of a multitude of endocrine events, in addition to a heterogeneity of the cellular population.

REFERENCES

1. TREMBLAY, Y., G. E. RINGLER, Y. MOREL, T. K. MOHANDAS, F. LABRIE, J. F. STRAUSS, III & W. L. MILLER. 1989. Regulation of the gene for estrogenic 17-ketosteroid reductase lying on chromosome 17cen→q25. J. Biol. Chem. **264:** 20458–20462.
2. TSENG, L. & E. GURPIDE. 1974. Estradiol and 20α-dihydroprogesterone activity in human endometrium during the menstrual cycle. Endocrinology **94:** 419–423.
3. POLLOW, K., H. LUBBERT, E. BOQUOI, G. KREUZER, R. JESKE & B. POLLOW. 1975. Studies on 17β-hydroxysteroid dehydrogenase in human endometrium and endometrial carcinoma. Acta Endocrinol. **79:** 134–145.
4. TSENG, L. & E. GURPIDE. 1972. Changes in the in vitro metabolism of estradiol by human endometrium during the menstrual cycle. Am. J. Obstet. Gynecol. **114:** 1002–1008.
5. SMITH, D. C., R. PRENTICE, D. J. THOMSON & W. L. HERRMAN. 1975. Association of exogenous estrogen and endometrial carcinoma. N. Engl. J. Med. **293:** 1164–1167.
6. WHITEHEAD, M. I., P. T. TOWNSEND, J. PRYSE-DAVIES, F. R. C. PATH, T. A. RYDER & R. J. B. KING. 1981. Effects of estrogens and progestins on the biochemistry and morphology of the postmenopausal endometrium. N. Engl. J. Med. **305:** 1599–1605.
7. FERENCZY, A., G. BERTRAND & M. M. GELFAND. 1979. Proliferation kinetics of human endometrium during the normal menstrual cycle. Am. J. Obstet. Gynecol. **133:** 859–867.
8. JÄNNE, O., A. KAUPPILA, K. KONTULA, P. SYRJÄLÄ & R. VIHKO. 1979. Female sex steroid receptors in normal, hyperplastic and carcinomatous endometrium. The relationship to serum steroid hormones and gonadotropins and changes during medroxy-progesterone administration. Int. J. Cancer **24:** 545–554.
9. NEUMANNOVA, M., A. KAUPPILA, S. KIVINEN & R. VIHKO. 1985. Short-term effects of tamoxifen, medroxyprogesterone acetate, and their combination on receptor kinetics and 17β-hydroxysteroid dehydrogenase in human endometrium. Obstet. Gynecol. **66:** 695–700.
10. PONS, M., S. C. NICOLAS, A. M. BOSSIOUX, B. DESCOMPS & A. CRASTES DE PAULET. 1977. Some new developments in the knowledge of human placental estradiol-17β dehydrogenase. J. Steroid Biochem. **8:** 345–358.
11. MÄENTAUSTA, O., H. PELTOKETO, V. ISOMAA, P. JOUPPILA & R. VIHKO. 1990. Immunological measurement of human 17β-hydroxysteroid dehydrogenase. J. Steroid Biochem. **36:** 673–680.
12. MAROWITZ, W., A. LOUCOPOULOS, P. G. SATYASWAROOP, E. GURPIDE, R. TODD & F. NAFTOLIN. 1980. Apparent immunologic nonidentity of human placental and endometrial 17β-estradiol dehydrogenase. Am. J. Obstet. Gynecol. **138:** 643–647.
13. GAST, M. J., H. F. SIMS, G. L. MURDOCK, P. M. GAST & A. W. STRAUSS. 1989. Isolation and

sequencing of a complementary deoxyribonucleic acid clone encoding human placental 17β-estradiol dehydrogenase: Identification of the putative cofactor binding site. Am. J. Obstet. Gynecol. **161**: 1726–1731.

14. MILEWICH, L., S. J. FORTUNATO, M. BARRIS, M. C. MABERRY, L. C. GILSTRAP & P. C. MACDONALD. 1990. 17β-Hydroxysteroid oxidoreductase activity in human maternal and umbilical cord sera. J. Steroid Biochem. **35**: 67–75.

15. SCATCHARD, G. 1949. The attraction of proteins for small molecules and ions. Ann. NY Acad. Sci. **51**: 660–672.

16. TSENG, L. 1980. Hormonal regulation of steroid metabolic enzymes in human endometrium. *In* Advances in Sex Steroid Hormone Research. J. A. Thomas & R. L. Singhalal, Eds. Vol. 4: 329–361, Urban & Schwarzenberg, Baltimore.

17. FOURNET-DULGUEROV, N., N. J. MACLUSKY, C. Z. LERANTH, R. TODD, C. R. MENDELSON, E. R. SIMPSON & F. NAFTOLIN. 1987. Immunohistochemical localization of aromatase cytochrome P-450 and estradiol dehydrogenase in the syncytiotrophoblast of the human placenta. J. Clin. Endocrinol. Metab. **65**: 757–764.

18. PELTOKETO, H., V. ISOMAA, O. MÄENTAUSTA & R. VIHKO. 1988. Complete amino acid sequence of human placental 17β-hydroxysteroid dehydrogenase deduced from cDNA. FEBS Lett. **239**: 73–77.

19. NICOLAS, J. C. & J. I. HARRIS. 1973. Human placental 17β-estradiol dehydrogenase: Sequence of the tryptic peptide containing an essential cystine. FEBS Lett. **29**: 173–176.

20. MURDOCK, G., C.-C. CHIN & J. C. WARREN. 1986. Human placental estradiol 17β-dehydrogenase: sequence of a histidine bearing peptide in the catalytic region. Biochemistry **25**: 641–646.

21. LUU-THE, V., C. LABRIE, H. F. ZHAO, J. COUET, Y. LACHANCE, J. SIMARD, G. LEBLANC, J. COTE, G. BERUBE, R. GAGNE & F. LABRIE. 1989. Characterization of cDNAs for human estradiol 17β-dehydrogenase and assignment of the gene to chromosome 17: Evidence of two mRNA species with distinct 5'-termini in human placenta. Mol. Endocrinol. **3**: 1301–1309.

22. LUU-THE, V., C. LABRIE, J. SIMARD, Y. LACHANCE, H. F. ZHAO, J. COUET, G. LEBLANC & F. LABRIE. 1990. Structure of two in tandem human 17β-hydroxysteroid dehydrogenase genes. Mol. Endocrinol. **4**: 268–275.

23. WINQVIST, R., H. PELTOKETO, V. ISOMAA, K.-H. GRZESCHIK, A. MANNERMAA & R. VIHKO. 1990. The gene for 17beta-hydroxysteroid dehydrogenase maps to human chromosome 17, bands q12-q21, and shows an RFLP with SCaI. Human Genet. **85**: 473–476.

24. TSENG L. & E. GURPIDE. 1975. Induction of human endometrial estradiol dehydrogenase by progestins. Endocrinology **97**: 825–833.

25. YOUNG, P. C., C. E. EHRLICH & R. E. CLEARY. 1976. Progesterone binding in human endometrial carcinomas. Am. J. Obstet. Gynecol. **125**: 353–358.

26. NEUMANNOVA, M., A. KAUPPILA & R. VIHKO. 1983. Cytosol and nuclear estrogen and progestin receptors and 17beta-hydroxysteroid dehydrogenase activity in normal and carcinomatous endometrium. Obstet. Gynecol. **61**: 181–188.

27. KAUPPILA, A., H. ISOTALO, S. KIVINEN, F. STENBÄCK & R. VIHKO. 1985. Short-term effects of danazol and medroxyprogesterone acetate on cytosol and nuclear estrogen and progestin receptors, 17β-hydroxysteroid dehydrogenase activity, histopathology, and ultrastructure of human endometrial adenocarcinoma. Int. J. Cancer **35**: 157–163.

28. VIHKO, R., A. ALANKO, V. ISOMAA & A. KAUPPILA. 1986. The predictive value of steroid hormone receptor analysis in breast, endometrial and ovarian cancer. Med. Oncol. Tumor Pharmacother. **3**: 197–210.

29. KOKKO, E., O. JÄNNE, A. KAUPPILA & R. VIHKO. 1982. Effects of tamoxifen, medroxyprogesterone acetate, and their combination on human endometrial estrogen and progestin receptor concentrations, 17β-hydroxysteroid dehydrogenase activity, and serum hormone concentrations. Am. J. Obstet. Gynecol. **143**: 382–388.

30. VIHKO, R., H. ISOTALO, A. KAUPPILA, L. RÖNNBERG & P. VIERIKKO. 1984. Hormonal regulation of endometrium and endometriosis tissue. *In* Medical Management of Endometriosis. J.-P. Raynaud, T. Ojasoo & L. Martini, Eds.: 79–89. Raven Press, New York.

31. DAVIS, L. G., M. D. DIBUER & J. F. BATTLEY. 1986. Basic Methods in Molecular Biology. Elsevier Science Publishing Co., New York.

Establishment and Characterization of Human Endometrial Cancer Cell Lines

HIROYUKI KURAMOTO,[a,b] MASATO NISHIDA,[c]
TAKAYUKI MORISAWA,[a,b] MIEKO HAMANO,[b]
HIROKI HATA,[a,b] YOSHIKI KATO,[a,b] EIJI OHNO,[d]
AND TOMOHIRO IIDA[e]

[a]Department of Obstetrics and Gynecology
and [b]Tissue Culture Center
School of Medicine
Kitasato University
Sagamihara 228, Japan

[c]Department of Obstetrics and Gynecology
School of Medicine
The University of Tsukuba
Tsukuba 305, Japan

[d]Department of Pathology
Kitasato University Hospital
Sagamihara 228, Japan

[e]Department of Obstetrics and Gynecology
St. Marianna University School of Medicine
Kawasaki 213, Japan

INTRODUCTION

In vitro cell culture system is one of the most convenient methods to make the detailed analysis of the normal and neoplastic cells which make up specific organs or tumors, and cell biology using culture technology is now a major research field. In the study of endometrial carcinoma this approach is no longer an exception, especially when human material is the subject for study.

The purpose of the present paper is to use our experience of culture trials of human endometrial carcinoma to clarify how human endometrial carcinoma cells are placed into *in vitro* culture systems and how their characteristic features are preserved in the *in vitro* environment. The success rates of primary cultures and transfer to successive generations leading to established cell lines are analyzed according to the histological type and grade. The growing cell types and patterns, the epithelial cells with

[a] *Address for correspondence:* Hiroyuki KURAMOTO, MD, Department of Obstetrics and Gynecology, School of Medicine, Kitasato University, 1-15-1 Kitasato Sagamihara 228, Kanagawa, Japan.

402

or without atypia, and the fibroblasts are compared morphologically and objectively with a micrometer. The analysis of the chromosome of which endometrial carcinoma is very characteristic is also worthwhile to be convinced of human origin. The cell lines of endometrial carcinoma established by our group are subject to characterization. Transplantability of the cells to heterologous animals and histological findings of the transplanted tumors are the most reliable and convincing proof of establishment of the specific cell lines. Preservation of hormone responsiveness which was inherited from its original normal endometrium is an important feature of endometrial carcinoma and must be characterized in the cell lines of the neoplasm.

MATERIALS AND METHODS PLACED IN CULTURE

A total of 210 tissue materials of endometrial carcinoma was obtained aseptically in the operating room. The culture, which was divided into 4 periods chronologically, included 54 trials during the period between 1968 and 1976, 66 during 1976 and 1985, and 45 during 1986 and 1989 in addition to 45 done by Nishida during 1980 and 1989 (TABLE 1). The monolayer culture method has been mainly adopted with the cells being digested into single cells by enzymatic agents. The plasma clot method was used for some cultures in early stages of trials.

SUCCESS RATES OF THE CULTURE

Primary Culture

Positive growth of either epithelial or fibroblastic cells was obtained in 72.1% out of 165 trials with increasing tendency from 64.8% in 1968–1976 to 88.9% in 1986–1989 (TABLE 1). Epithelial growth either with or without fibroblastic growth was realized in 56.2% out of 210 trials, whereas fibroblastic growth was observed in 61.8% of cases with an increasing tendency up to 84.4% in recent 1986–1989. Epithelial cells grown alone in a culture flask are rare, appearing in 8.6% of cases (TABLE 2), whereas a mixture of epithelial and fibroblastic growth was common (47.6% of cases), with the tendency increasing chronologically from 35.2% in 1968–1976 to 68.9% in 1986–1989. Fibroblastic cells without epithelial cells were growing in not less than 10% of the trials.

TABLE 1. Success Rates of the Primary Culture of Endometrial Carcinomas

	Cases (%) Chronologically and by Author					
	1968–1976 (Kuramoto)	1976–1985 (Morisawa, Hamano)	1986–1989 (Hamano, Iida)	SUB-TOTAL	1980–1989 (Nishida)	TOTAL
Number of Cultures	54	66	45	165	45	210
Positive Growth	35 (64.8)	44 (66.7)	40 (88.9)	119 (72.1)	–	–
Epithelial Growth	29 (53.7)	33 (50.0)	33 (73.3)	95 (57.6)	23 (51.1)	118 (56.2)
Fibroblastic Growth	25 (46.3)	39 (59.1)	38 (84.4)	102 (61.8)	–	–

TABLE 2. Success Rates and Growing-Cell Types in the Primary Culture of Endometrial Carcinomas

	Cases (%) Chronologically and by Author					
	1968–1976 (Kuramoto)	1976–1985 (Morisawa, Hamano)	1986–1989 (Hamano, Iida)	SUB-TOTAL	1980–1989 (Nishida)	TOTAL
Number of Cultures	54	66	45	165	45	210
Epithelial growth only	10 (18.5)	5 (7.6)	2 (4.4)	17 (10.3)	1 (2.2)	18 (8.6)
Both epithelial and fibroblastic	19 (35.2)	28 (42.4)	31 (68.9)	78 (47.3)	22 (48.9)	100 (47.6)
Fibroblastic only	6 (11.1)	11 (16.7)	7 (15.6)	24 (14.5)	–	

Histological Grade

The histological grades and types of original endometrial carcinoma and the success rates of the primary cultures which showed the growth of epithelial carcinoma cells with or without fibroblastic cells were analyzed chronologically. In total, well-differentiated (G1) adenocarcinoma grew successfully in 56.0% out of 75 trials, moderately differentiated (G2) adenocarcinoma in 63.6% out of 77, and poorly differentiated (G3) in 45.8% of 24 trials (TABLE 3). G3 adenocarcinoma is the most difficult in culture among the various histological grades and types, whereas adenoacanthoma and miscellaneous types reveal 54.5% and 66.7% success, respectively. There is no chronological tendency in the success rate of the cultures except for G3 carcinoma, which showed an increasing tendency to be successful.

TABLE 3. Histological Grades and Success Rates of the Primary Culture of Endometrial Carcinomas

Culture– Chronologically by Author	Histological Grades						
	G1	G2	G3	Adeno-acanthoma	Miscel-laneous	Unknown	TOTAL
1968–1976 (Kuramoto)	10/14[a] (71.4)	12/19 (63.2)	3/8 (37.5)	1/2 (50.0)	1/2 (50.0)	2/9 (22.2)	29/54 (53.7)
1976–1985 (Morisawa)	5/8 (62.5)	13/19 (68.4)	1/4 (25.0)	1/2 (50.0)	1/1 (100.0)	0	21/34 (61.8)
1976–1985 (Hamano)	4/11 (36.4)	5/13 (38.5)	2/5 (40.0)	1/3 (33.3)	0	0	12/32 (37.5)
1986–1989 (Hamano, Iida)	10/15 (66.7)	13/16 (81.3)	2/3 (66.7)	3/4 (75.0)	5/7 (71.4)	0	33/45 (73.3)
1980–1989 (Nishida)	13/27 (48.1)	6/10 (60.0)	3/4 (75.0)	0	1/2 (50.0)	0/2 (0.0)	23/45 (51.1)
TOTAL	42/75 (56.0)	49/77 (63.6)	11/24 (45.8)	6/11 (54.5)	8/12 (66.7)	2/11 (18.2)	118/210 (56.2)

[a] Successful cases/culture cases (%).

TABLE 4. Histological Grades and Success Rates of Transfer (123 Trials)

Passage Generation	Histological Grades					
	G1	G2	G3	Adeno-acanthoma	Miscel-laneous	TOTAL
Trial of culture	37	54	15	9	8	123
Primary	20 (54.1)[a]	32 (59.3)	8 (53.3)	5 (55.6)	6 (75.0)	71 (57.7)
Second	5 (13.5)	11 (20.4)	3 (20.0)	2 (22.2)	3 (37.5)	24 (19.5)
Third	3 (8.1)	6 (11.1)	2 (13.3)	1 (11.1)	1 (12.5)	13 (10.6)
Line	0 (0.0)	3 (5.6)	2 (13.3)	1 (11.1)	1 (12.5)	7 (5.7)

[a] Cases (%).

Transfer of the Culture

The success rates of transfer to successive generations more than primary culture were evaluated in the series of 123 culture trials. The success rate of primary cultures in the series was 57.7% (TABLE 4). The culture succeeded to the second generation in 19.5% out of 123 or 33.8% among successful primary cultures, whereas the third subculture was successful 10.6% of the time. Seven permanent cell lines were obtained in this series, revealing a 5.7% success rate in 123 trials. This result indicates that establishment into cell lines is a possibility in one-half of the trials if the third culture appeared successful.

Possibility of transfer depending on histological grade and type was analyzed (TABLE 4). The success rate of G1 adenocarcinoma to the second generation was 13.5% among 37 trials, whereas that of other grades and types was more than 20%. G1 carcinomas were successful to the third passage generation in 8.1% of trials, whereas others showed a rate of more than 10%. The result shows that transferring differentiated (G1) adenocarcinoma cells to successive passage generations in culture flask is quite difficult in comparison with other cell types, although the primary cultures do not much differ from each other.

Frequency of Contamination

Bacterial contamination appeared in 6 cultures (2.9%) out of 210 trials at the primary culture stage. No fungus infection was observed. Cultures of endometrial carcinoma appear quite clean as the material is obtained aseptically from an operating room.

Culture of the Normal Endometrium

The normal endometrium in various phases was cultured in the same manner for comparison with the cultures of endometrial carcinoma. All cases of 11 proliferative endometria revealed excellent growth, whereas one excellent and 4 poor growth results were obtained among 6 secretory endometria. No growth was observed in 6 endometria of the postmenopausal period. The data show that the epithelial cells of normal endometrial origin might have a great chance to grow in culture when the material was obtained from a patient who preserved the normal proliferative endometrium.

GROWING CELLS AT PRIMARY CULTURE

Cellular Morphology and Growth Patterns

Twenty-nine cultures out of the initial 54 trials were evaluated for the study. Two kinds of cells, epithelial and fibroblastic, were observed to grow *in vitro*. The morphological features of the epithelial cells grown in 29 cultures were analyzed. The common growth pattern of carcinoma cells of the endometrium is a jigsaw puzzle–like cellular arrangement due to differences of individual cell polarity (FIGS. 4, 5, and 9). The cells also disclose a wheeled pattern. A pavement cell sheet is conversely rare (FIG. 2). The statistical study revealed that all but 3 of 29 cases developed a jigsaw puzzle–like arrangement and 12 cases showed a wheeled pattern. A pavement arrangement was seen in only one case. The cultured cells gather altogether and formed a growing sheet in all but 2 cases, whereas in only 8 cases was there observed an area with a scattered arrangement without forming a sheet. The cultured epithelial cells continue to grow and pile up easily even though confluent (FIGS. 5 and 7), thus showing *in vitro* the malignant tendency of the cells in all cases. You can see not infrequently a glandular formation on the piling-up area of the better differentiated cases (FIG. 7).

Among individual cell configurations the nuclei are usually round or oval except in 2 cases; they are thick in the nuclear border and possess one or two prominent spherical nucleoli in all cases. The findings are compatible with the malignant criteria of diagnostic cytology for endometrial carcinoma,[1] in addition to the piling-up growth tendency of these cells. The presence of atypism and piling-up tendency of the adenocarcinoma cells differentiate them from the epithelial cells of the normal endometrium. Cytoplasmic vacuoles are common in endometrial carcinoma cells, being observed in all but 3 cases. In a special case with adeno-squamous mixed carcinoma, cornified square-shaped cells with abundant and non-vacuolated cytoplasms were observed in addition to typical adenocarcinoma cells. These findings suggest the detailed cellular findings correlate well with the differentiative traits of the original histology.

Differentiation between Epithelial Carcinoma and Fibroblastic Cells

Since two kinds of cells appear in the culture of endometrial carcinoma, the details of cellular configurations were measured objectively comparing epithelial carcinoma cells with fibroblasts. Three-hundred-and-sixty carcinoma cells of 12 cases in primary culture or 30 cells per case, and 100 cellular samples of fibroblasts from 2 cases were counted using a digital micrometer (OSM-D2). The mean cellular diameter of each case ranged between 28.2 and 42.4 microns, the nuclear diameter between 13.9 and 21.6 microns, the nucleolar diameter between 3.9 and 5.7 microns, and the number of nucleoli per cell between 1.0 and 2.3 (TABLE 5). The mean diameter ($M \pm SD$) of cancer cells in total was calculated as 34.3 ± 9.8 microns (TABLE 6). The nuclear diameter was 16.2 ± 2.7 microns, and the nucleolar diameter was 4.7 ± 1.0 microns. The number of the nucleoli per cell was 1.1 ± 0.5. In contrast, those of fibroblasts were 62.2 ± 24.6, 19.3 ± 4.6, 3.4 ± 0.7 and 2.2 ± 0.9 microns, respectively. These differences between 2 types of cells are significant statistically (TABLE 6). The nucleolar size of carcinoma cells is significantly larger than that of fibroblasts, whereas cellular and nuclear sizes are opposite in relationship resulting from the elongated nuclear and cellular shape of fibroblasts. It is also ascertained that a carcinoma cell

TABLE 5. *In Vitro* Cellular Features of Endometrial Carcinomas per Case

	Cellular Diameter	Nuclear Diameter	Nucleolar Diameter	No. of Nucleoli per Cell
HEC-4	38.6 ± 7.3	21.6 ± 3.3	5.7 ± 0.9	1.1 ± 0.2
HEC-7	42.4 ± 11.2	16.7 ± 2.5	5.3 ± 0.7	1.0 ± 0.2
HEC-8		13.9 ± 1.4	4.4 ± 0.6	1.0 ± 0.2
HEC-13	40.9 ± 7.5	17.6 ± 3.0	5.6 ± 0.8	1.0 ± 0
HEC-21	30.0 ± 6.9	15.8 ± 1.6	4.4 ± 0.7	1.0 ± 0.2
HEC-28	34.2 ± 7.3	15.3 ± 1.6	4.7 ± 0.5	1.0 ± 0
HEC-29		15.0 ± 1.8	4.5 ± 0.4	1.0 ± 0
HEC-30	28.2 ± 6.0	15.1 ± 1.4	4.5 ± 0.6	1.1 ± 0.2
HEC-33		15.1 ± 1.0	4.6 ± 0.6	1.0 ± 0
HEC-38	33.0 ± 9.5	14.7 ± 1.5	4.6 ± 0.6	1.0 ± 0
HEC-40	39.3 ± 12.0	17.3 ± 1.8	4.9 ± 0.7	1.1 ± 0.3
HEC-50	29.8 ± 4.5	16.0 ± 1.1	3.9 ± 0.4	2.3 ± 0.9

of the endometrium not infrequently has one single enlarged nucleolus in comparison with multiple nucleoli of a fibroblast.

Chromosome Constitution

Cytogenetic analysis of human endometrial carcinoma cells in culture was performed in 17 cases.[2] The coverslip with the cells was treated with a hypotonic solution of sodium chloride after being cultured with Colcemid. The mode of chromosome number was found to be at the diploid range in all cases, and the exact counting of the modal range revealed that the peak of the number was 46 in 75% of the analyzed cases. The distributions were even both in the hypo- and hyper-diploid areas. The karyotype analyses showed that the majority of the endometrial carcinomas presented pseudo-diploid chromosomes, revealing irregular numerical alterations of each group constitution and scattered variant chromosomes with minor structural changes. Only four cases were noted to have an unclassified chromosome with marked structural aberrations. A marker chromosome was identified in only one case, whereas no common specific chromosome was noted and the histological findings did not correlate with chromosome aberration. It is realized from our tissue culture study that carcinomas of human corpus uteri consist mainly of the cells with a pseudo-diploid chromosomal constitution.

TABLE 6. Cellular Features of Endometrial Carcinomas and Fibroblasts *in Vitro*

	Cellular Diameter	Nuclear Diameter	Nucleolar Diameter	No. of Nucleoli per Cell
Carcinoma cells	34.3 ± 9.8[a]	16.2 ± 2.7[b]	4.7 ± 1.0[b]	1.1 ± 0.5[b]
Fibroblastic cells	62.2 ± 24.6[c]	19.3 ± 4.6[c]	3.4 ± 0.7[c]	2.2 ± 0.9[c]
Significance	SIG	SIG	SIG	SIG

[a] M ± SD (n=203).
[b] M ± SD (n=360).
[c] M ± SD (n=100).
[d] SIG = significant ($p < 0.01$).

ESTABLISHMENT OF THE CELL LINES

Success Rate in the Establishment of Cell Lines

Our overall success rate for establishing the cell lines of human endometrial carcinoma has been so far 4.8% of 210 culture trials (TABLE 7). From a chronological standpoint the cultures done by Morisawa during the period between 1976 and 1985 were the most successful, revealing a 11.8% success rate.

The success rates were analyzed according to the histological grades and types of the original endometrial carcinomas. Those of the G1, G2, G3 adenocarcinoma, adenoacanthoma, and miscellaneous type appeared to be 1.3%, 5.2%, 8.3%, 18.2%, and 8.3%, respectively. The result indicates that it is quite difficult to establish the cell line of well-differentiated (G1) adenocarcinoma.

The Cell Lines Established by Our Group

Ten cell lines of human endometrial carcinoma have been established in 210 trials of the culture (TABLE 8). These include each one from G1 and serous adenocarcinomas, 4 from G2, and 2 each from G3 and adenoacanthoma of original histology. The culture materials were obtained from the primary site of the uterine corpus in all but 3 cases. The monolayer method in which the fragment of original tumor is dispersed by enzymatic agents was used for all except HEC-1, which was first placed into a plasma clot simulating to the primary culture of HeLa cells. HEC-50 was obtained from the ascitic fluid of a patient with recurrence. HEC-88nu, a cell line of adenoacanthoma, was obtained from the tumor transplanted first to nude mice. HEC-151 was from an invasive lesion of the uterine cervix. The mode of chromosomal constitution of these cell lines originated from primary site reveal mainly pseudo-or near diploid range, whereas those of metastatic or heterologous origin appear to be hyper-diploid. All of the cell lines except one which is not tried yet are transplantable to heterologous animals developing apparent tumors.

CHARACTERIZATION OF THE CELL LINES

Growth Characteristics

The cultures that grew into established cell lines have developed fairly good and constant growth from the beginning of the primary trial. No latent or degenerative phase, which is usually necessary for normal diploid cell cultures to be immortalized[3,4] has been experienced, at least in our series. It is our impression that carcinoma cells might not always need to transform their characters *in vitro* if they fit to the cultural and nutritional environment present. The growth curve is not always better in carcinoma cells than in normal cells. In our experience the growth rate of the normal endometrial cells was higher at first than that of the HEC-1 cells when both were cultured simultaneously and in the same condition.[5] The normal cells, however, went into a degenerative condition after 100 and 150 days of culture.

TABLE 7. Histological Grades and Establishment of the Cell Lines of Endometrial Carcinoma

Culture— Chronologically by Author	Histological Grades						Total No. of Cultures	Success in Establishing Line
	G1	G2	G3	Adeno-acanthoma	Miscel-laneous	Unknown		
1968–1976 (Kuramoto)	14	19 [1][a]	8 [1]	2 [1]	2	9	54 [3]	5.6%
1976–1985 (Morisawa)	8	19 [2]	4 [1]	2 [1]	1	0	34 [4]	11.8%
1976–1985 (Hamano)	11	13	5	3	0	0	32	0%
1986–1989 (Hamano, Iida)	15	16 [1]	3	4	7 [1]	0	45 [2]	4.5%
1980–1989 (Nishida)	27 [1]	10	4	0	2	2	45 [1]	2.2%
Total No. of Cultures	75 [1]	77 [4]	24 [2]	11 [2]	12 [1]	11	210 [10]	4.8%
Success in Establishing Line	1.3%	5.2%	8.3%	18.2%	8.3%	0%	4.8%	

[a] [Number of lines].

TABLE 8. Human Endometrial Carcinoma Cell Lines Established by Our Group

Name of Line	Start of Culture	Original Histology	Origin of Culture Material	Culture Method	Doubling Time (h)	Passage Generation	Chromosome Mode	Transplantability	Remarks
HEC-1	May 16, '68	G2 adenocarcinoma	Corpus	Plasma clot → Monolayer	31	409	47	+	E.P. sensitive EGFR ↑
HEC-6	June 24, '70	Adenoacanthoma	Corpus	Monolayer	52	390	46, Pseudodiploid	+	PAS
HEC-50	Aug. 7, '75	G3 adenocarcinoma	Ascites	Monolayer	30.4	472	56	+	ALP, PAS, Alcian Blue, EGFR ↑
HEC-59	Feb. 14, '78	G2 adenocarcinoma	Corpus	Monolayer	24.8	200 Frozen	47	+	ALP, PAS
Ishikawa	Oct. 21, '80	G1 adenocarcinoma	Corpus	Monolayer	28	286	46, Pseudodiploid	+	ER, PR, CA125
HEC-88nu	Dec. 2, '81	Adenoacanthoma	Tumor in nude	Monolayer	48	154	3n	+	ER, ALP, PAS, CEA
HEC-108	May 1, '84	G3 adenocarcinoma	Corpus	Monolayer	26.5	57 Frozen	48	+	PAS
HEC-116	Jan. 11, '85	G2 adenocarcinoma	Corpus	Monolayer	27.2	47	47	+	PAS
HEC-151	Nov. 29, '88	G2 adenocarcinoma	Cervix	Monolayer	38	42	3n	+	CA125, E2DH EGFR ↑
HEC-155	Jan. 24, '89	Serous adenocarcinoma	Corpus	Monolayer		11	Hyperdiploid		CA125

Morphology of Growing Cells

The carcinoma cells of the endometrium grow making a sheet with a jigsaw puzzle–like or wheel-like arrangement (FIGS. 4, 5, and 9),[6,7] and pile-up easily developing a gland-like arrangement (FIG. 7).[8] A dome- or hemicyst-like protrusion elevating from the monolayer on a culture vessel is not infrequently seen (FIG. 5).[7,9] The findings are often found in the culture of the better differentiated cases of endometrial carcinoma, and may not always be specific to endometrial carcinoma but also could be generalized findings of adenocarcinoma. In cases of the less differentiated adenocarcinoma, a pavement arrangement of the carcinoma cells is not always rare (FIG. 2).[8,10]

Elimination of Fibroblasts

An unnegligible point to establish the line is how to avoid the growth of fibroblasts. Mixed growth of epithelial and fibroblastic cells does occur not infrequently in the culture of endometrial carcinoma. Various trials using rubber policemen, time differences of digestivity between two cell types, cloning to isolate the target cells, etc. are mandatory to eliminate fibroblasts.

Chromosome Analysis

Chromosome analysis of the growing epithelial cells is essential to confirm that endometrial carcinoma cells have been exactly cultured. As mentioned above the chromosome constitution of endometrial carcinoma is usually pseudo- or near-diploid in mode with some exceptions.[2] This chromosome constitution is also very convenient for showing the cultured cells to be of human origin.

Transplantation to Heterologous Animals

Transplantability of the cultured cells and histological findings of the tumor developed in heterologous animals such as nude mice are the most reliable evidences that prove a specific cell line has been established. The former capability in heterologous animals is a proof of malignancy of the cells. The histology of the transplanted tumor is to assure that the in vitro cells are undoubtedly cultured representing the character of the original endometrial carcinoma. The finding of adenocarcinoma developed in the cheek pouch of a hamster was unquestionable proof that a cell line HEC-1 was endometrial carcinoma.[6] HEC-6 cells[8] and HEC-88nu (FIG. 6) reconstructed adenoacanthomas the same as the originals. Ishikawa cells[9,11] developed well-differentiated (G1) adenocarcinoma in the tumor sustained in nude mice resembling to the original finding. HEC-50[10] and HEC-59 (FIG. 3)[7] reconstructed poorly differentiated adenocarcinomas. The histological findings of HEC-108 and HEC-116 transplanted to nude mice revealed endometrial carcinoma, but better differentiated than those of the original tumors (FIGS. 8 and 10).

Hormone Receptors

Endometrial adenocarcinoma is a carcinoma originating from the endometrial gland, which is a target of ovarian steroid hormones and possesses estrogen and progesterone receptors (ER and PR) in its own cells as the target. Although endometrial carcinoma cells do not always preserve estrogen and progesterone receptors, these functional traits are conclusive proof that a cell line of endometrial carcinoma is precisely established. Immunocytochemical staining of ER and PR by using monoclonal antibodies shows the evidence that Ishikawa cells are the functioning cell lines of the carcinoma (FIGS. 11 and 12).

HORMONE RESPONSIVENESS OF ENDOMETRIAL CARCINOMA CELLS

Clinical evidences suggest that estrogen either endogenous[12-16] or exogenous[17-20] plays an important role in the development of endometrial carcinoma. In contrast, progestin is effective in treating patients with endometrial carcinoma in approximately 30% of cases[21,22] and especially in over 50% of cases of G1 adenocarcinoma.[23] *In vitro* culture systems using the cell lines of human endometrial carcinomas should be one of the most valuable basic methods for clarifying the mechanism of action of these ovarian sex steroid hormones. Quite a few studies have been performed *in vitro* by using our cell lines and have been reported elsewhere.[24-38] Hormone responsiveness *in vivo* of the tumor developed in nude mice into which the carcinoma cells *in vitro* were transplanted is reported in the present paper.

The Responsiveness of HEC-88nu Cells in Vivo

HEC-88nu cells, an *in vitro* cell line established from a tumor transplanted into nude mice of human adenoacanthoma origin, show positive ER and negative PR. The tumor of HEC-88nu cells retransplanted to nude mice, however, induced PR when a 0.72 mg estradiol (E2) pellet (Innovative Research of America, Inc.) is injected subcutaneously to nude mice. Progesterone receptors started to appear after 2 weeks of the treatment and elevated up to the range of 170 to 220 fmol/mg protein after 5 weeks, as measured by radio receptor assay (TABLE 9). The growth curve of the tumor was stimulated by up to 160% of the untreated control after 6 weeks when the E2 pellet was given. On the contrary, when a pellet of 50 mg medroxyprogesterone acetate (MPA) was given to the mice, growth was suppressed to 50% within 2 weeks of the treatment. The result proves that MPA is effective for the PR-negative tumor. When E2 and MPA were given simultaneously, the growth curve was stimulated to the level of the single E2-treated tumor without showing the effect of MPA. The curve, however, was suppressed to 40% after 5 weeks, developing the effect from the third week, when MPA was given after priming with E2 previously for 4 weeks.[28] The result suggests MPA also acts through the induced progesterone receptor.

The Responsiveness of Ishikawa Cells in Vivo

Ishikawa cells, which possess both ER and PR, and which are responsive to estrogen *in vitro*[11,31-33] are transplantable to nude mice, and develop into well-differentiated

TABLE 9. Induction of Progesterone Receptor by E_2 in the Tumor Transplanted in Nude Mice (HEC-88nu)

Weeks after E_2 Administration	Case No.	PR (fmol/mg, P)
2	1	0
	2	0
	3	13.5
	4	32.8
3	1	21.7
	2	27.7
	3	39.8
4	1	25.1
	2	33.6
	3	34.4
5	1	166.0
	2	181.0
	3	220.0

adenocarcinoma.[11] The growth curve of the tumors was much sharper when a 0.72 mg E2 pellet was given to the host nude mice, and the converted tumor weights were revealed to be 2.8 times greater than those of the untreated animals (FIG. 1). When E2 was removed 2 weeks after the cells were transplanted, the growth curve reduced apparently to 24.8% of the E2-persistent tumor 6 weeks after the removal. On the contrary, when an E2 pellet was given 5 weeks after the transplantation the cells still preserved the ability to enhance their growth by the stimulation of estrogen (FIG. 1).

CONCLUSION

Our experiences in establishing the cell lines of human endometrial carcinomas and characterizing those *in vitro* cells have been reported here through the presentation of data on the culture trials of 210 cases. The success of culture trials was analyzed chronologically for the experience of 22 years. Overall, positive growth was obtained in 72.1% of cases and the success rate of the epithelial growth was 56.2%, although 47.6% were cultured with mixture of fibroblasts. The cells were able to transfer to the second passage generation in 19.5% of trials and to the third generation in 10.6%. The cell lines were established in 4.8% of all trials of the culture. The culture was analyzed according to the histological grades and types, with G3 adenocarcinomas showing the least success at the primary culture. It was, however, quite difficult to establish the cell line of G1 adenocarcinomas. The morphology and growth pattern of the epithelial carcinoma cells in addition to their chromosome constitution were analyzed in comparison with those of normal epithelial and fibroblastic cells. Ten cell lines established by our group were characterized through growth kinetics, morphology, and cytogenetics. Chromosome study on endometrial carcinoma cells, which is a convenient method to confirm their human origin, showed mainly near- and pseudo-diploidy. Transplantability and histology of the tumors transplanted to heterologous animals are worthwhile for detecting the malignancy of the cultured cells and for confirming that the exact cells of the original endometrial carcinoma have been cultured as

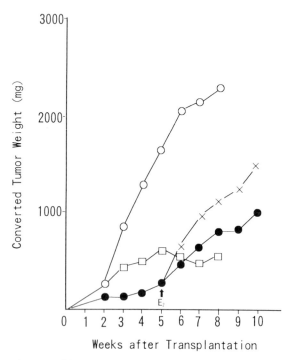

FIGURE 1. Growth curves of the tumor of Ishikawa cells transplanted into nude mice. —●— Control; —○— Treated with 0.72mg estradiol pellet; —□— E2 removed at 2nd week; —×— E2 added at 5th week.

well as for determining its histological stability. Some evidence for hormone responsiveness of the *in vitro* cell lines was evaluated in the tumor transplanted *in vivo* to nude mice.

It is really painful and time-consuming work to establish the cell lines. Those cell lines, however, are unquestionably worthwhile once they are established and immortal *in vitro*, even though established cell lines appear in about 5% of the culture trials. Use of culture system is unavoidable in clarifying the detailed character of endometrial carcinoma especially when human materials are used for the study. The cell lines of human endometrial carcinoma will be undoubtedly useful for the study on hormone responsiveness, either progressive or therapeutic of the carcinoma.

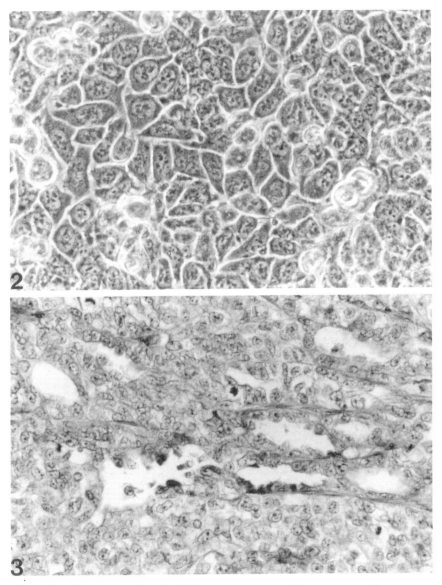

FIGURE 2. Growing cells of line HEC-59 showing a pavement-like arrangement. Phase-contrast; 2.5×40 (original magnification).

FIGURE 3. Histology of the tumor of HEC-59 cells transplanted into a nude mouse showing poorly differentiated adenocarcinoma. H-E stain. 2.5×40 (original magnification).

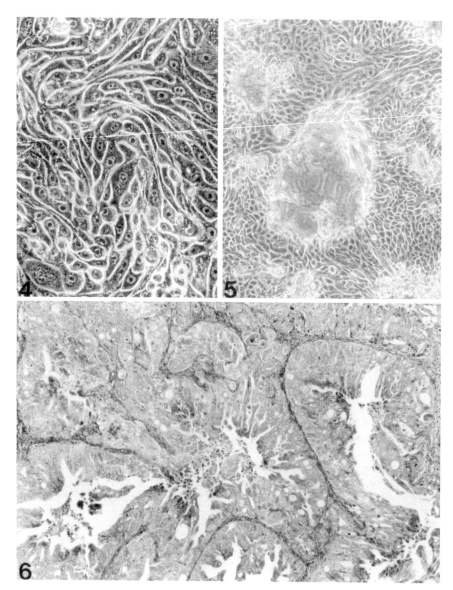

FIGURE 4. Growing cells of line HEC-88nu showing typical jigsaw puzzle–like pattern. Phase-contrast; 2.5×20 (original magnification).

FIGURE 5. HEC-88nu cells developing a dome- or hemicyst-like elevation in center from monolayer sheet. Phase contrast. 2.5×10 (original magnification).

FIGURE 6. Histology of the tumor of HEC-88nu cells transplanted in a nude mouse showing adenoacanthoma. H-E stain; 5×4 (original magnification).

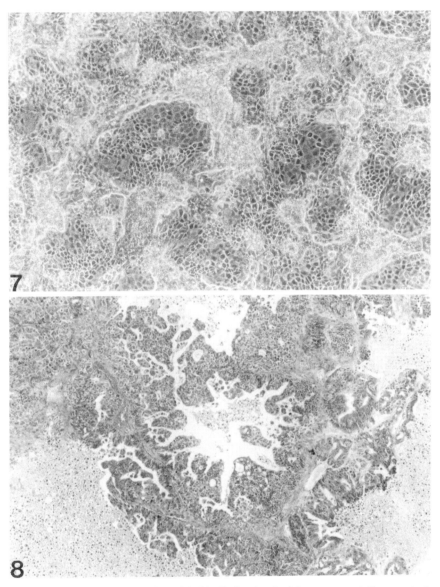

FIGURE 7. Confluent area of growing HEC-108 cells showing glandular arrangement. Phase-contrast; 2.5×10 (original magnification).

FIGURE 8. Histology of the tumor of HEC-108 cells transplanted in a nude mouse showing adeno-carcinoma moderately differentiated. H-E stain; 2.5×4 (original magnification).

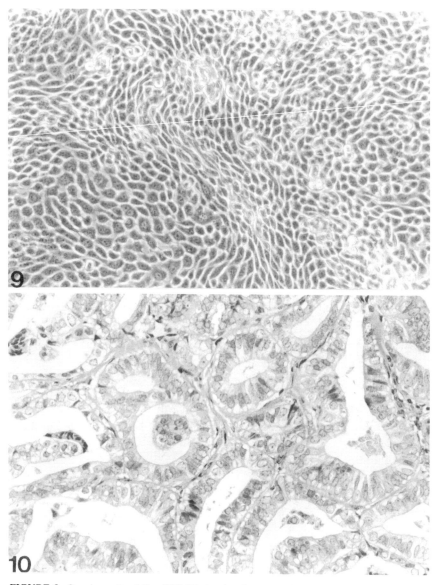

FIGURE 9. Growing cells of line HEC-116 showing jigsaw puzzle–like tendency of arrangement. Phase-contrast. 2.5×20 (original magnification).

FIGURE 10. Histology of the tumor of HEC-116 cells transplanted in a nude mouse showing well differentiated adenocarcinoma. H-E stain; 5×10 (original magnification).

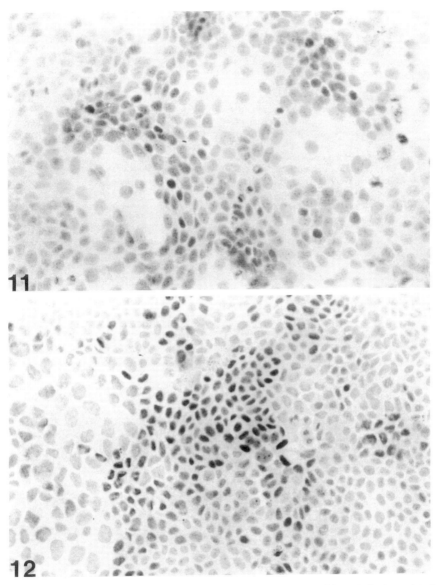

FIGURE 11. Immunocytochemistry of estrogen receptor showing the positive stain in the nuclei of Ishikawa cells. PAP stain; 5×20 (original magnification).

FIGURE 12. Immunocytochemistry of progesterone receptor localizing in the nuclei of Ishikawa cells. PAP stain; 5×20 (original magnification).

REFERENCES

1. KURAMOTO, H. 1988. Color atlas: Detection for endometrial cancer. Ishiyaku-syuppan. Tokyo.
2. KURAMOTO, H. & M. HAMANO. 1977. Cytogenetic studies of human endometrial carcinomas by means of tissue culture. Acta Cytol. **21:** 559–565.
3. HAYFLICK, L. & P. S. MOOREHEAD. 1961. The serial cultivation of human diploid cell strains. Exp. Cell Res. **25:** 585–621.
4. CHANG, R. S. 1961. A comparative study of the growth, nutrition and metabolism of the primary and the transformed human cells in vitro. J. Exp. Med. **113:** 405–417.
5. KURAMOTO, H. 1972. Studies of the growth and cytogenetic properties of human endometrial adenocarcinoma in culture and its development into an established line. Acta Obstet. Gynaecol. Jpn. **19:** 47–58.
6. KURAMOTO, H., S. TAMURA & Y. NOTAKE. 1972. Establishment of a cell line of human endometrial adenocarcinoma in vitro. Am. J. Obstet. Gynecol. **114:** 1012–1019.
7. MORISAWA, T. 1987. The results of primary culture of endometrial adenocarcinoma and characterization of its established cell lines. J. Jpn. Soc. Clin. Cytol. **26:** 433–442. (In Japanese.)
8. KURAMOTO, H. & M. HAMANO. 1977. Establishment and characterization of the cell-line of a human endometrial adenoacanthoma. Eur. J. Cancer **13:** 253–259.
9. NISHIDA, M., K. KASAHARA, M. KANEKO, H. IWASAKI & K. HAYASHI. 1985. Establishment of a new human endometrial adenocarcinoma cell line, Ishikawa cells, containing estrogen and progesterone receptors. Acta Obstet. Gynaecol. Jpn. **37:** 1103–1111. (In Japanese.)
10. KURAMOTO, H., M. HAMANO, M. NISHIDA, A. TAGUCHI, T. JOBO, M. SUZUKI & K. OSANAI. 1976. Establishment of a cell line of human endometrial carcinoma originated from ascitic fluid. Acta Obstet. Gynaecol. Jpn. **28:** 1405–1406. (In Japanese.)
11. HOLINKA, C. F., H. HATA, H. KURAMOTO & E. GURPIDE. 1986. Responses to estradiol in a human endometrial adenocarcinoma cell line (ISHIKAWA). J. Steroid Biochem. **24:** 85–89.
12. DOCKERTY, M. B., S. B. LOVELADY & G. T. FOUST, JR. 1951. Carcinoma of the corpus uteri in young women. Am. J. Obstet. Gynecol. **61:** 966–981.
13. SILVERBERG, S. G., E. L. MAKOWSKI & W. D. ROCHE. 1977. Endometrial carcinoma in women under 40 years of age. Comparison of cases in oral contraceptive users and non-users. Cancer **39:** 592–598.
14. KEMPSON, R. L. & G. E. POKORNY. 1968. Adenocarcinoma of the endometrium in women aged forty and younger. Cancer **21:** 650–662.
15. MacMAHON, B. 1974. Risk factors for endometrial cancer. Gynecol. Oncol. **2:** 122–129.
16. GUSBERG, S. B. 1967. Hormone-dependence of endometrial cancer. Obstet. Gynecol. **30:** 287–293.
17. ZIEL, H. K. & W. D. FINKLE. 1975. Increased risk of endometrial carcinoma among users of conjugated estrogens. N. Engl. J. Med. **293:** 1167–1170.
18. SMITH, D. C., R. PRENTICE, D. J. THOMPSON & W. L. HERMANN. 1975. Association of exogenous estrogen and endometrial carcinoma. N. Engl. J. Med. **293:** 1164–1167.
19. MACK, T., M. C. PIKE, B. E. HENDERSON, R. I. PFEFFER, V. R. GERKINS, M. ARTHUR & S. E. BROWN. 1976. Estrogens and endometrial cancer in a retirement community. New Engl. J. Med. **294:** 1262–1267.
20. COLLINS, J., et al. 1980. Oestrogen use and survival in endometrial cancer. Lancet (Nov. 1): 961–963.
21. KELLY, R. M. & W. H. BAKER. 1965. The role of progesterone in human endometrial cancer. Cancer Res. **25:** 1190–1192.
22. REIFENSTEIN, E. C. 1974. The treatment of advanced endometrial cancer with hydroxyprogesterone caproate. Gynecol. Oncol. **2:** 377–414.
23. KOHORN, E. I. 1976. Gestagens and endometrial carcinoma. Gynecol. Oncol. **4:** 398–411.
24. KURAMOTO, H. & K. SUZUKI. 1976. Effects of progesterone on the growth kinetics and the morphology of a human endometrial cancer cell-line. Acta Obstet. Gynaecol. Jpn. **23:** 123–132.
25. SUZUKI, M., H. KURAMOTO, M. HAMANO, M. ARAI, H. SHIRANE & K. WATANABE. 1978. Effects of sex steroid hormones on the alkaline phosphatase activity of a cultured endometrial carcinoma cell line. Acta Obstet. Gynaecol. Jpn. **30:** 509–510. (In Japanese.)
26. SUZUKI, M., H. KURAMOTO, M. HAMANO, T. MORISAWA, M. ARAI, H. SHIRANE & K. WATANABE. 1979. Effects of steroid hormones on the alkaline phosphatase activity of cultured corpus cancer cells. Acta Obstet. Gynaecol. Jpn. **31:** 577–582. (In Japanese.)
27. SUZUKI, M., H. KURAMOTO, M. HAMANO, H. SHIRANE & K. WATANABE. 1980. Effects of oestra-

diol and progesterone on the alkaline phosphatase activity of a human endometrial cancer cell-line. Acta Endocrinol. **93**: 108–113.

28. KURAMOTO, H. 1988. Cell culture—Its application in the study of hormone and endometrial carcinoma and feed-back to clinical medicine. Acta Obstet. Gynaecol. Jpn. **40**: 1050–1055. (In Japanese.)

29. KURAMOTO, H., H. HATA, Y. KATO, K. HATA, M. HAMANO, Y. ANZAI, J. WATANABE, C. F. HOLINKA & E. GURPIDE. 1989. Mechanism of action of endocrine therapy for endometrial carcinoma. Jpn. J. Cancer Chemother. **16**(Part-II): 1851–1857. (In Japanese.)

30. FLEMING, H., R. BLUMENTHAL & E. GURPIDE. 1982. Effects of cyclic nucleotides on estradiol binding in human endometrium. Endocrinology **111**: 1671–1677.

31. FLEMING, H., R. BLUMENTHAL & E. GURPIDE. 1983. Rapid changes in specific estrogen binding elicited by cGMP or cAMP in cytosol from human endometrial cells. Proc. Natl. Acad. Sci. USA **80**: 2486–2490.

32. GRAVANIS, A. & E. GURPIDE. 1986. Effects of estradiol on deoxyribonucleic acid polymerase alpha activity in the Ishikawa human endometrial adenocarcinoma cell line. J. Clin. Endocrinol. **63**: 356–359.

33. HOLINKA, C. F., H. HATA, A. GRAVANIS, H. KURAMOTO & E. GURPIDE. 1986. Effects of estradiol on proliferation of endometrial adenocarcinoma cells (Ishikawa line). J. Steroid Biochem. **25**: 781–786.

34. HOLINKA, C. F., H. HATA, H. KURAMOTO & E. GURPIDE. 1986. Effects of steroid hormones and antisteroids on alkaline phosphatase activity in human endometrial cancer cells (Ishikawa line). Cancer Res. **46**: 2771–2774.

35. HATA, H., C. F. HOLINKA, S. L. PAHUJA, R. B. HOCKBERG, H. KURAMOTO & E. GURPIDE. 1987. Estradiol metabolism in Ishikawa endometrial cancer cells. J. Steroid Biochem. **26**: 699–704.

36. ANZAI, Y., C. F. HOLINKA, H. KURAMOTO & E. GURPIDE. 1989. Stimulatory effects of 4-hydroxytamoxifen on proliferation of human endometrial adenocarcinoma cells (Ishikawa line). Cancer Res. **49**: 2362–2365.

37. HOLINKA, C. F., Y. ANZAI, H. HATA, N. KIMMEL, H. KURAMOTO & E. GURPIDE. 1989. Proliferation and responsiveness to estrogen of human endometrial cancer cells under serum-free culture conditions. Cancer Res. **49**: 3297–3301.

38. WATANABE, J., C. F. HOLINKA, Y. ANZAI, H. KURAMOTO & E. GURPIDE. 1989. Effects of serine and glycine on proliferation of an Ishikawa cell variant. J. Steroid Biochem. **34**: 165–168.

Effects of Hormones on Endometrial Cancer Cells in Culture

C. F. HOLINKA,[a,b] Y. ANZAI,[b] H. HATA,[c]
J. WATANABE,[b] H. KURAMOTO,[c]
AND E. GURPIDE[b]

[b] Department of Obstetrics, Gynecology and Reproductive Science
Mount Sinai School of Medicine
New York, New York 10029
[c] Department of Obstetrics & Gynecology
Kitasato University School of Medicine
Sagamihara 228, Japan

INTRODUCTION

Considerable advances have been made in identifying the effects of hormones in hormone-responsive tumors and elucidating the mechanisms by which they exert their actions. *In vivo* assessment of biochemical properties of endometrial cancer tissue has yielded valuable information, successfully employed to select endocrine treatment strategies and to estimate survival rates.[1] *In vivo* observations on hormone-tumor interactions are limited, however, by the lack of experimental controls, tumor heterogeneity, interfering host mechanisms that are not directly related to tumor biology, and a number of other factors. To circumvent some of those limitations, serial transplantation of endometrial cancer tissue in nude mice has been used as an experimental model and has yielded relevant results on hormone-tumor interactions.[2]

In order to distinguish specific hormonal actions on tumor cells from the effects contributed by the host, it is essential to have available hormone-responsive cancer cells. While tumor cells, once established as cell lines in culture, retain their constitutive growth-related biologic properties, such as enzymatic functions regulating cell replication, many characteristics of the differentiated state, such as responses to hormones, are lacking or have been lost during repeated passages in culture. As a result, *in vitro* experiments to investigate the relationship between hormones and endometrial cancer have been limited by the lack of hormone responsiveness of endometrial cancer cell lines. However, in recent years we have been able to conduct studies in a hormone-responsive endometrial cancer cell line, Ishikawa, established by Nishida and coworkers from a well differentiated adenocarcinoma.[3]

Experimental work using this cell line has yielded interesting information on the effects of estrogens and antiestrogens on growth, on steroid hormone receptors, and on enzymatic activities. Moreover, a variant of Ishikawa cells (Var-I) that lost responsiveness to estradiol regarding proliferation showed accelerated cell growth in culture when exposed to progesterone and to hydroxytamoxifen. These findings call attention

[a] *Present Address:* Clinical Development Department, Organon, Inc., West Orange, NJ 07052.

to the possibility that similar responses of particular clones of endometrial cancer cells may occur *in vivo*. These observations provide models for studies on the mechanisms of action of progesterone and hydroxytamoxifen on cell proliferation.

In this chapter we review and discuss our studies on the effects of hormones in Ishikawa cells.

MORPHOLOGIC CHARACTERISTICS OF ISHIKAWA CELLS

Ishikawa cells cultured at high density form multilayers with spotty single cell crater-shaped regions.[4] When subcutaneously inoculated into nude mice (BALB/c, nu/nu, female), Ishikawa cells form solid tumors exhibiting well-differentiated features.[4] Measurements of specific estradiol and progesterone binding by the hydroxylapatite method revealed the presence of receptors for both hormones in the solid tumor tissues.[4] When cultured under anchorage-independent conditions in soft agar, Ishikawa cells form colonies, as illustrated in FIGURE 1; the colony formation efficiency depends on the number of cells seeded.[5]

METHODOLOGIC CONSIDERATIONS FOR STUDIES OF HORMONAL EFFECTS IN CULTURED CELLS

Serum-free Cultures

It has been known for a number of decades that cultured cells require the presence of serum (usually bovine or fetal bovine serum added at 5–15% concentrations) for

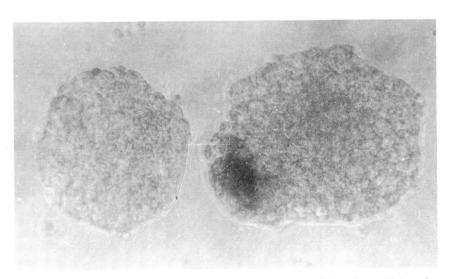

FIGURE 1. Phase contrast photomicrograph of colonies of Ishikawa cells in soft agar, 22 days after seeding (×480) (see ref. 4).

proliferation, and it is now evident that a variety of serum growth factors function as mitogenic agents to stimulate *in vitro* proliferation. We examined a series of commercially available media and their combinations to achieve proliferation of endometrial cancer cells in the absence of serum with the aim to distinguish the effects of hormones from those contributed by serum factors and to eliminate possible synergistic mechanisms between hormones and serum factors. We also considered the estrogenic effects of a contaminant of phenol red,[6] an indicator dye usually present in commercial media. Based on those considerations we developed a medium that supported rapid proliferation under serum-free conditions.[7] Most of the studies discussed below that were conducted under serum-free conditions employed a basal medium (BM) consisting of a phenol red–free mixture of equal volumes of DMEM and Ham's F-12, supplemented with glutamine, HEPES, penicillin, streptomycin, and Fungizone. Surprisingly, no additional growth factors, such as insulin or transferrin, were needed. Cells were routinely maintained in MEM plus 10% FBS prior to changing to serum-free conditions for experimental purposes.

Tumor cell growth under anchorage-independent conditions is often considered to be the experimental system that is most representative for *in vivo* tumor cell growth. Anchorage-independent growth is considered the most stringent index of neoplastic transformation and it is likely that only the more virulent cells, which may determine the *in vivo* course of the cancer, are capable of proliferating under these conditions. Several of the experiments described here were performed using a cell suspension in 0.3% soft agar which was placed over a bottom layer of 0.6% soft agar.

ESTROGEN EFFECTS ON PROTEINS

Progesterone Receptor

In vivo experiments in the animal uterus,[8] as well as studies in human endometrium, have demonstrated progesterone receptor induction by estrogens. Ishikawa cells showed a significant enhancement of specific progesterone binding when estradiol was added to the culture medium (FIG. 2). Maximal increases in binding, relative to control levels, occurred at a concentration of 10^{-8} M estradiol added to the medium, but increases were apparent at a concentration as low as 10^{-9} M.[4] If the rapid metabolism of estradiol by Ishikawa cells is considered, the net effective concentration of the hormone during the three-day culture period was considerably lower than the initial concentration. In experiments designed to determine estrogen metabolism by Ishikawa cells, Hata *et al.*[9] found that over 90% of the added estradiol was metabolized after 24 hours in culture. The metabolites isolated were estradiol-3-sulfate, estrone sulfate, and estrone.

These results also demonstrate the presence of functional estrogen receptors. We have repeatedly found measurable levels of specific estrogen binders in Ishikawa cells[10] (also, Holinka *et al.*, unpublished).

Alkaline Phosphatase

Our interest in examining responsiveness of alkaline phosphatase to estrogens in Ishikawa cells was based on earlier findings indicating that the activity of this enzyme appears to be highest in proliferative endometrium,[11] an observation which suggested

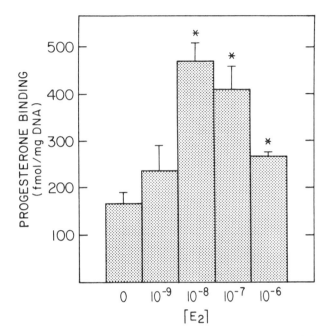

FIGURE 2. Enhancement of specific progesterone binding by estradiol (see ref. 4).

that alkaline phosphatase activity might be stimulated by estradiol. As illustrated in FIGURE 3, addition of 10^{-8} M estradiol significantly increased alkaline phosphatase activity.[12] When tested over a concentration range of 10^{-11} to 10^{-7} M, stimulation of enzyme activity, measured over a culture period of four days with one medium change after two days, was greatest at 10^{-8} M estradiol. As illustrated in FIGURE 4, maximal enzyme stimulation was achieved between 48–72 h.

Interestingly, the activity of the enzyme in Ishikawa cells was not influenced by cell density, in contrast to alkaline phosphatase activities in the estrogen-unresponsive endometrial cancer cell line HEC-50, which increased up to 10-fold at high density, relative to low density cultures. It is also noteworthy that another estrogen-unresponsive human endometrial cancer cell line, HEC-1, did not reveal any detectable alkaline phosphatase activity in the absence or presence of estradiol, an observation that illustrates the fundamental differences in biologic properties among cell lines derived from endometrial cancer.

Further analysis of alkaline phosphatase activity in Ishikawa cells by methods recognized to distinguish organ-specific alkaline phosphatase isoenzymes, such as those of intestine, liver, bone, or placenta,[13] yielded several interesting results. In the absence of estradiol, alkaline phosphatase activity was not inhibited on exposure to elevated temperatures and was resistant to homoarginine and phenylalanine. However, the estradiol-stimulated alkaline phosphatase activity was inhibited by about 40% in the presence of phenylalanine (TABLE 1). Comparisons of these results with those reported for other endometrial cancer cell lines and for normal endometrium permit a number of interesting conclusions: Ishikawa cells express the placental type alkaline

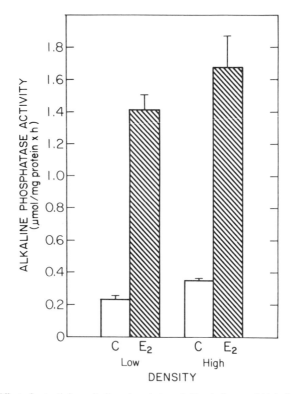

FIGURE 3. Effect of estradiol on alkaline phosphate activities in low- and high-density cultures of Ishikawa cells (see ref. 12).

phosphatase isoenzyme, in contrast to the nonplacental isoenzyme identified in normal endometrium and in endometrial glandular epithelial cells;[11] however, the expression of the placental-type alkaline phosphatase isoenzyme is not an invariant property of human endometrial adenocarcinoma cells, since HEC-50 cells show high activity of the nonplacental isoenzyme characteristic of normal endometrium. Furthermore, the estradiol-stimulated component of Ishikawa-cell alkaline phosphatase activity, but not the basal levels, appears to be sensitive to inhibition (TABLE 1), suggesting that estradiol stimulates an isoenzyme different from the alkaline phosphatase at basal levels. These observations offer interesting experimental possibilities to examine different mechanisms of neoplastic changes at the genetic level and to relate those changes to hormonal responsiveness.

GROWTH RESPONSES TO HORMONES

Responsiveness to Estrogen

FIGURE 5 illustrates marked growth promoting effects of estradiol in the parent Ishikawa cell line cultured in MEM + 15% ctFBS. After control cultures had reached

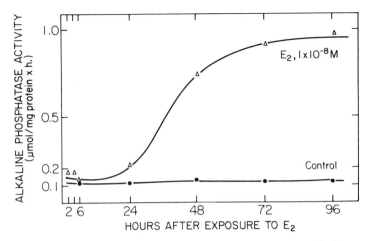

FIGURE 4. Time course of alkaline phosphate stimulation by estradiol (see ref. 12).

plateau densities, the cell numbers in estradiol-containing cultures continued to increase to approximately three times those of controls, an effect that was prevented by hydroxytamoxifen. When added to cells at high density plateau levels, estradiol overcame the density-dependent growth arrest and caused the resumption of proliferation (FIG. 6). These results indicate that growth arrest of cells in control cultures was not related to nutritional deprivation, since the same regimen of medium changes supported cell proliferation to threefold higher densities in the presence of estradiol.

No obvious estrogen effects on doubling times during the exponential phase of proliferation were apparent in the presence of ctFBS, possibly because serum growth factors exerted maximal stimulatory effects. However, when maintained under serum-free conditions in basal medium, marked increases in proliferation rates were noted during the exponential phase (FIG. 7).[7] From the proliferation rates in the presence and absence of E_2 it was calculated that the hormone shortened the doubling time of exponentially proliferating cells from 38 to 29 hours. The labeling index, deter-

TABLE 1. Alkaline Phosphatase Isoenzymes in Endometrial Cells

	Control Activity (μmol/mg protein/h)	% of Inhibition		
		Heat (57°C, 15 min)	Phenylalanine (5 mM)	Homoarginine (8 mM)
Ishikawa cells				
Control	0.140	8	0	0
Estradiol (10^{-8} M)	0.730	0	40	0
Endometrial glands				
Proliferative	5.8 ($n=4$)	78 ($n=1$)	30 ($n=2$)	85 ($n=2$)
Secretory	1.0 ($n=4$)	90 ($n=1$)	8 ($n=3$)	
Placenta	20.4	0	75	5

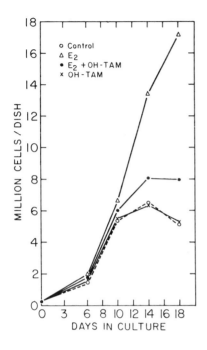

FIGURE 5. Growth-promoting deffect of estradiol in Ishikawa cells and its reversal by OHTam (see ref. 4).

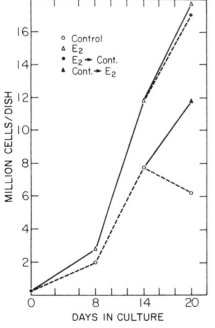

FIGURE 6. Resumption of cell proliferation after addition of estradiol to high-density cultures at a plateau level (see ref. 4).

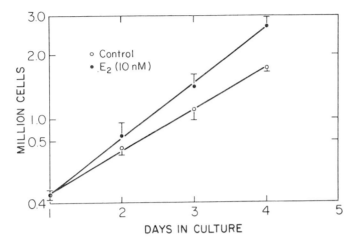

FIGURE 7. Estrogen effects on exponential growth rates of Ishikawa cells (see ref. 7).

mined after exposure to a pulse of [^{3}H]thymidine, and the mitotic index, both obtained in exponentially proliferating cells, allowed calculation of the duration of the S and M phases of the cell cycle, which were found to be about 11 and 1 hours, respectively. From these data it was estimated that E_2 shortened the G_1 phase by approximately 40%, from 22 to 13 hours.[7] Similar to our findings in the presence of serum, E_2 also affected the plateau densities under serum-free conditions. The mechanisms by which E_2 both shortens the cell cycle and overcomes density-dependent growth arrest remain to be identified although evidence is accumulating on the mediation of growth factors and oncogene expression in the effect of estrogens on cell proliferation. The mechanisms of growth regulation are likely to differ in exponentially proliferating cells, where the shortening of the cell cycle appears to reflect enhanced mitogenesis, and in high density cultures, where E_2 may predominantly affect factors related to controlled cell death.

A surprising observation emerging from our studies comparing cell proliferation in MEM with that in BM concerns the influence of the medium on growth responses to estrogen, as well as to serum. This point is illustrated by the finding that MEM failed to support colony formation in the absence of serum (FIG. 8). In the presence of comparable serum concentrations, colony formation was substantially lower in MEM than it was in BM. Furthermore, E_2 did not affect the colony formation efficiency of cells maintained in MEM, whereas the hormone significantly stimulated colony formation in BM, both in the absence and presence of serum (FIG. 9). In this context it is also noteworthy that cells growing attached to plastic culture dishes in the presence of comparable serum concentrations attained markedly higher densities in BM than they did in MEM.

The mechanisms by which E_2 enhances colony formation efficiency under anchorage-independent conditions remain to be elucidated. Our observation that the colony formation efficiency significantly increases as cells are seeded at higher densities (FIG. 10) suggests that Ishikawa cells secrete factors that may act as autocrine and paracrine

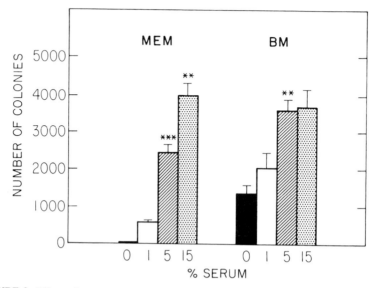

FIGURE 8. Effects of serum concentration on colony formation of Ishikawa cells (see ref. 7).

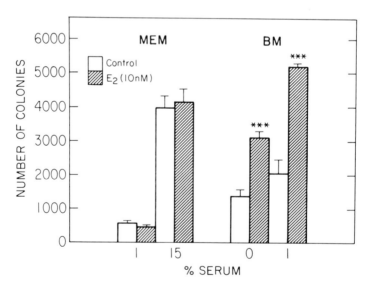

FIGURE 9. Stimulation by estradiol of colony formation of Ishikawa cells (see ref. 7).

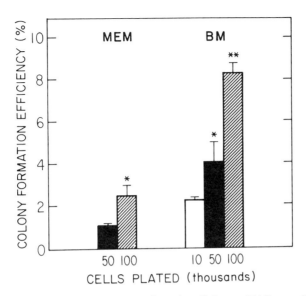

FIGURE 10. Effects of cell density on colony formation efficiency of Ishikawa cells (see ref. 7).

mitogens and that growth factor secretion is influenced by E_2. Evidence that E_2 stimulates IGF-1 expression in the immature rat uterus[14] supports the hypothesis that growth promotion by estrogens is linked to the action of autocrine and paracrine growth factors. A major role for polypeptide growth factors as mediators of estrogen-induced growth responses has also been demonstrated in MCF-7 human breast cancer cells.[15]

Responsiveness to Hydroxytamoxifen

Anzai *et al.*[16] have reported that addition of hydroxytamoxifen (OHTam) to Ishikawa cell cultures in BM did not antagonize the action of estrogen but, quite unexpectedly, significantly promoted cell growth (FIG. 11) at concentrations as low as 100 nM (FIG. 12). The growth promoting effects of OHTam also occurred in the presence of serum, but the effects were specific to BM. In MEM, OHTam did not stimulate cell growth and acted as an antiestrogen. In contrast, OHTam consistently exhibited antiestrogenic effects on alkaline phosphatase activity, regardless of the medium, and had only minor stimulatory effects when added by itself (FIG. 13).

It is significant that growth promoting effects of OHTam were also apparent in the estrogen-unresponsive variant cell line Ishikawa-Var I. The dissociation of the proliferative effects of OHTam from those of estrogen in this variant appears to contradict the general assumption that OHTam acts by competition with E_2 for a common receptor. Some variants of MCF-7 cells have also been shown to exhibit discrepancies between tamoxifen (Tam) and E_2, such as Tam resistance associated with responsiveness to E_2,[17] or growth inhibition by Tam in E_2-unresponsive cells. These observa-

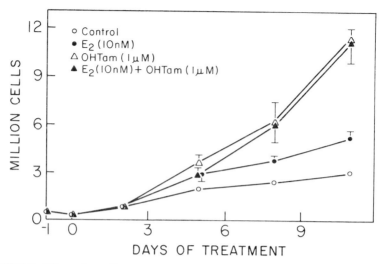

FIGURE 11. Effects of estradiol and OHTam on proliferation of Ishikawa cells in serum-free BM (see ref. 16).

tions suggest direct effects of Tam and OHTam by mechanisms that may not involve the estrogen receptor. The antiestrogenic effect of OHTam on estrogen-induced alkaline phosphatase activity further indicates that stimulation of cell growth by OHTam may occur by a different mechanism than its action on alkaline phosphatase and may not involve the estrogen receptor. The contribution of medium factors to the growth-promoting effects of OHTam remains to be elucidated.

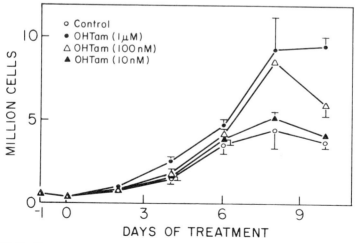

FIGURE 12. Concentration dependence of the effects of OHTam on proliferation of Ishikawa cells in BM (see ref. 16).

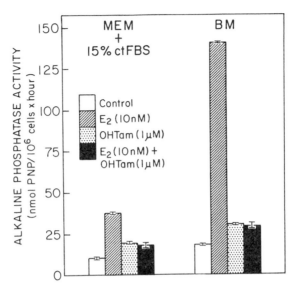

FIGURE 13. Effects of progesterone and estradiol and OHTam on alkaline phosphatase activity in Ishikawa cells (see ref. 16).

Responsiveness to Progesterone

A spontaneously arisen variant of Ishikawa cells, Var-I, exhibited significant growth responses to 10^{-6} M progesterone (P), added to basal medium (FIG. 14). In contrast, estradiol did not affect cell growth. The effects of P were apparent both on the rates of exponential proliferation and on maximal densities. The doubling time of expo-

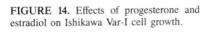

FIGURE 14. Effects of progesterone and estradiol on Ishikawa Var-I cell growth.

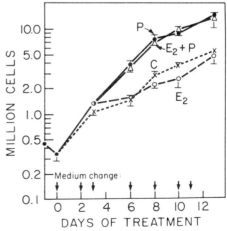

nentially proliferating cultures was shortened from 44 to 35.6 hours in the presence of P, which represents a statistically significant increase in proliferation rates ($p <$ 0.05). By calculations described above for exponentially proliferating Ishikawa cells in serum-free medium, we estimated that this reduction represents a 31% shortening of the G_1 phase. Maximal densities were consistently 2 to 3 times higher in the presence of P.

As indicated in FIGURE 15, P also enhanced colony formation of Ishikawa Var-I cells growing in soft agar under anchorage-independent conditions. Interestingly, the effects were usually higher in the presence of E_2. In contrast to the lack of E_2 effects on attached cells of this variant in liquid medium, addition of E_2 to soft agar cultures consistently produced small but significant increases in colony formation efficiency.

The observed stimulatory effects of P on the growth of Ishikawa-Var I cells are surprising but not without precedent. While progestins have been found to inhibit growth in several breast cancer cell lines by antagonizing the action of estrogen or by producing independent antimitogenic effects in the absence of estrogens,[18-22] growth-promoting effects of progestins have also been demonstrated in experimental mammary tumors *in vivo* and *in vitro*[23,24] and in human breast cancer cell lines.[25,26] Primary cultures of epithelial cells derived from breast cancer cells, but not from normal breast cells of the same patient, also exhibited significant growth responses to P.[27] In this context it is of interest that glandular epithelial cells in the lower ba-

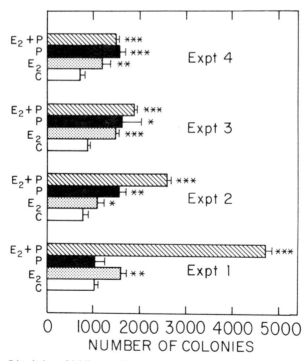

FIGURE 15. Stimulation of Ishikawa cell colony formation by ovarian steroids.

salis layer of the Rhesus monkey endometrium shows significantly increased levels of thymidine incorporation *in vivo* during the P-dominated luteal phase.[28] Taken together, these observations raise the question whether under certain conditions progestins may enhance growth, a possibility that warrants further experimental investigation.

DISCUSSION

The preceding sections provide clear evidence for hormonal responsiveness of human endometrial cancer cells under two different culture conditions, *viz.*, in cells growing attached in regular culture dishes and in cells growing under anchorage-independent conditions in soft agar. Comparable to *in vivo* conditions, hormonal responsiveness in cultured cells appears to be modulated by a number of as yet poorly understood factors. For example, relatively simple differences in medium composition, such as those between MEM and BM, fundamentally influenced the cellular responsiveness to hormones. Colony formation efficiency was significantly enhanced by estradiol in BM but not in MEM, and OHTam acted as a pure antiestrogen in MEM, whereas its addition to BM provoked significant growth responses both in the absence and presence of medium, but did not produce antiestrogenic effects. It is also noteworthy that proliferation rates were generally poor in serum-free MEM and significantly slower in the presence of a comparable serum conscentration when compared to BM. Watanabe *et al.*[29] have shown in recent experiments designed to identify specific medium factors that may have growth regulatory functions that proliferation rates were greatly enhanced when serine or glycine were added to serum-free MEM (FIG. 16).

Spontaneously arising variants, as described here for Ishikawa cells, have been found in a variety of cell lines. Interestingly, the loss of growth responsiveness to E_2 in the Ishikawa cell Var-I represents a selective loss of estrogen responsiveness. Our observation that alkaline phosphatase activity of Var-I cells remains remarkably responsive to estrogens suggests that the basic structural and functional characteristics of the estradiol-receptor interactions have remained intact and that the loss of growth responsiveness to the hormone is due to an alteration specific to growth regulation.

It is also noteworthy that Ishikawa Var-I cells growing under anchorage-independent conditions in soft agar clearly respond to E_2. Since only a small fraction of cells forms colonies in soft agar, one may speculate that this subpopulation has retained estrogen responsiveness which is masked in the presence of the majority of unresponsive cells examined in regular cultures. Alternatively, each of the two culture systems may provide unique conditions that inhibit or enhance hormonal effects on growth. For example, hormonal responsiveness in hepatocytes depends on certain properties of the substratum to which the cells are attached;[30] similarly, growth regulation of cells under anchorage-independent conditions is influenced by the extent of sulfurylation of the agar.[31]

The clinical implications of results derived from *in vitro* systems, and in particular from cultured endometrial cancer cells, can not be categorized. While basic mechanisms, such as hormone-target cell interactions, are likely to be common to all responsive cells, the regulation of more complex systems, such as growth, may differ considerably between cultured cells and *in vivo* systems. It is possible that the stimulation of growth by P in Ishikawa Var-I cells is limited to culture conditions. Nevertheless, the possibility also merits consideration that endometrial adenocarcinomas may express a progestin-responsive phenotype as a result of neoplastic changes. In

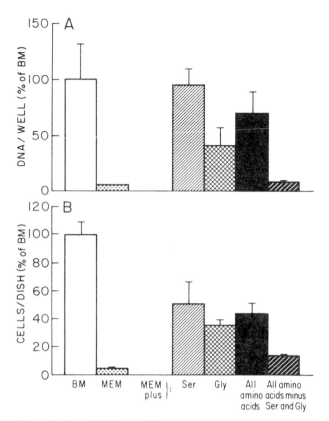

FIGURE 16. Effects of serine and glycine on cell population density in serum-free medium (see ref. 29).

light of this possibility it is interesting that primary cell cultures established from normal breast epithelial cells were unresponsive to progestins, whereas P significantly stimulated the growth of epithelial cells established from breast cancer tissues of the same patients.[27] The finding of mitogenic effects of P in an endometrial cancer cell line is of considerable importance since progestins are given to a significant proportion of endometrial cancer patients. While many patients respond favorably, the possibility must be considered that progestin treatment aggravates the course of the cancer in the non-responding patients.

REFERENCES

1. RICHARDSON, G. S. & D. T. McLAUGHLIN. 1986. The status of receptors in the management of endometrial cancer. Clin. Obstet. Gynecol. **29:** 628–637.
2. SATYASWAROOP, P. G., R. J. ZAINO & R. MORTEL. 1983. Human endometrial adenocarcinoma transplanted into nude mice: Growth regulation by estradiol. Science **219:** 58–60.
3. NISHIDA, M., K. KASAHARA, M. KANEKO & H. IWASAKI. 1985. Establishment of a new human

endometrial adenocarcinoma cell line, Ishikawa cells, containing estrogen and progesterone receptors. Acta Obstet. Gynaecol. Jpn. **37**: 1103–1111.

4. HOLINKA, C. F., H. HATA, H. KURAMOTO & E. GURPIDE. 1986. Responses to estradiol in a human endometrial adenocarcinoma cell line (Ishikawa). J. Steroid Biochem. **24**: 85–89.

5. HOLINKA, C. F., H. HATA, A. GRAVANIS, H. KURAMOTO & E. GURPIDE. 1986. Effects of estradiol on proliferation of endometrial adenocarcinoma cells (Ishikawa line). J. Steroid Biochem. **25**: 781–786.

6. BERTHOIS, Y., J. A. KATZENELLENBOGEN & B. S. KATZENELLENBOGEN. 1986. Phenol red in tissue culture media is a weak estrogen: Implications concerning the study of estrogen-responsive cells in culture. Proc. Natl. Acad. Sci. USA. **83**: 2496–2500.

7. HOLINKA, C. F., Y. ANZAI, H. HATA, N. KIMMEL, H. KURAMOTO & E. GURPIDE. 1989. Proliferation and responsiveness to estrogen of human endometrial cancer cells under serum-free culture conditions. Cancer Res. **49**: 3297–3301.

8. HOLINKA, C. F., R. S. BRESSLER, D. R. ZEHR & E. GURPIDE. 1980. Comparison of effects of estetrol and tamoxifen with those of estriol and estradiol on the immature rat uterus. Biol. Reprod. **22**: 913–926.

9. HATA, H., C. F. HOLINKA, S. L. OAHUJA, R. B. HOCHBERG, H. KURAMOTO & E. GURPIDE. 1987. Estradiol metabolism in Ishikawa endometrial cancer cells. J. Steroid Biochem. **26**: 699–704.

10. KASSAN, S. & E. GURPIDE. 1989. Altered estrogen receptor system in estrogen-unresponsive human endometrial adenocarcinoma cells. J. Steroid Biochem. **33**: 327–333.

11. HOLINKA, C. F. & E. GURPIDE. 1981. Hormone-related enzymatic activities in normal and cancer cells of human endometrium. J. Steroid Biochem. **15**: 183–192.

12. HOLINKA, C. F., H. HATA, H. KURAMOTO & E. GURPIDE. 1986. Effects of steroid hormones and antisteroids on alkaline phosphatase activity in human endometrial cancer cells (Ishikawa line). Cancer Res. **46**: 2771–2774.

13. FISHMAN, W. H. 1974. Perspectives on alkaline phosphatase isoenzymes. Am. J. Med. **56**: 617–650.

14. MURPHY, L. J. & A. GHAHARY. 1990. Insulin-like growth factor-1: Regulation of expression and its role in estrogen-induced uterine proliferation. Endocrine Rev. **11**: 443–453.

15. DICKSON, R. B. & M. E. LIPPMAN. 1987. Estrogenic regulation of growth and polypeptide growth factor secretion in human breast carcinoma. Endocrine Rev. **8**: 29–43.

16. ANZAI, Y., C. F. HOLINKA, H. KURAMOTO & E. GURPIDE. 1989. Stimulatory effects of 4-hydroxytamoxifen on proliferation of human endometrial adenocarcinoma cells (Ishikawa line). Cancer Res. **49**: 2362–2365.

17. KATZENELLENBOGEN, B. S., K. L. KENDRA, M. J. NORMAN & Y. BERTHOIS. 1987. Proliferation, hormonal responsiveness, and estrogen receptor content of MCF-7 human breast cancer cells grown in the short-term and long-term absence of estrogens. Cancer Res. **47**: 4355–4360.

18. VIGNON, F., S. BARDON, D. CHALBOS & H. ROCHEFORT. 1983. Antiestrogenic effect of R 5020, a synthetic progestin, in human breast cancer cells in culture. J. Clin. Endocrinol. Metab. **56**: 1124–1130.

19. IACOBELLI, S., G. SICA, C. NATOLI & D. GATTI. 1983. Inhibitory effects of medroxyprogesterone acetate on the proliferation of human breast cancer cell. *In* Role of Medroxyprogesterone in Endocrine-Related Tumors. L. Campio, G. Robustelli Della Cuna & R. W. Taylor, Eds.: 1–6. Raven Press, New York.

20. HORWITZ, K. B. & G. R. FREIDENBERG. 1985. Growth inhibition and increase of insulin receptors in antiestrogen-resistant T47D human breast cancer cells. Cancer Res. **45**: 167–173.

21. MAUVAIS-JARVIS, P., F. KUTTEN & A. GOMPEL. 1986. Antiestrogen action of progesterone in breast tissue. Breast Cancer Res. Treatment. **8**: 179–187.

22. SUTHERLAND, R. L., R. E. HALL, G. Y. N. PANG, E. A. MUSGROVE & C. L. CLARKE. 1988. Effect of medroxyprogesterone acetate on proliferation and cell cycle kinetics of human mammary carcinoma cells. Cancer Res. **48**: 5084–5091.

23. GOTTARDIS, M., E. ETURK & D. P. ROSE. 1983. Effects of progesterone administration on N-nitrosomethylurea-induced rat mammary carcinogenesis. Eur. J. Cancer Clin. Oncol. **19**: 1479–1484.

24. KISS, R., R. J. PARIDAENS, J-C. HEUSON & A. J. DANGUY. 1986. Effect of progesterone on cell proliferation in the MXT mouse hormone-sensitive mammary neoplasms. J. Nat. Cancer Institute **77**: 173–177.

25. BRAUNSBERG, H., N. G. COLDHAM & W. WONG. 1986. Hormonal therapies of breast cancer: Can progesterone stimulate growth? Cancer Lett. **30:** 213–218.

26. HISSOM, J. R. & M. R. MOORE. 1987. Progestin effects on growth in the human breast cancer cell line T-47D; possible therapeutic implications. Biochem. Biophys. Res. Commun. **145:** 706–711.

27. LONGMAN, S. M. & G. C. BUEHRING. 1987. Oral contraceptives and breast cancer. In vitro effect of contraceptive steroids on human mammary cell growth. Cancer **59:** 281–287.

28. PADYKULA, H. A., L. G. COLES, W. C. OKULICZ, S. I. RAPAPORT, J. A. McCRACKEN, N. W. KING, JR., C. LONGCOPE & I. R. KAISERMAN-ABRAMOF. 1989. The basalis of the primate endometrium: A bifunctional germinal compartment. Biol. Reprod. **40:** 681–690.

29. WATANABE, J., C. F. HOLINKA, Y. ANZAI, H. KURAMOTO & E. GURPIDE. 1989. Effects of serine and glycine on proliferation of an Ishikawa cell variant. J. Steroid Biochem. **34:** 165–168.

30. GOSPODAROWICZ, D. J. 1984. Extracellular matrices and the control of cell proliferation and differentiation in vitro. In New Approaches to the Study of Benign Prostatic Hyperplasia, F. A. Kimbel, A. E. Buhl & D. B. Carter, Eds.: 103–128. Alan Liss, New York.

31. KIRK, D., S. KANAGAWA & G. VENER. 1983. Comparable growth regulation of five human tumor cell lines by neonatal human lung fibroblasts in semisolid culture media. Cancer Res. **43:** 3754–3757.

Tamoxifen-stimulated Growth
of Human Endometrial Carcinoma

V. C. JORDAN AND M. M. GOTTARDIS

Department of Human Oncology
University of Wisconsin
Clinical Cancer Center
Madison, Wisconsin 53792

P. G. SATYASWAROOP

Department of Obstetrics and Gynecology
Milton S. Hershey Medical Center
Pennsylvania State University
Hershey, Pennsylvania 17033

INTRODUCTION

Tamoxifen (TAM) is the antihormonal treatment of choice for all stages of breast cancer. Since TAM appears to be a tumoristatic agent in laboratory models of breast cancer[1-3] long-term adjuvant therapy is being evaluated in clinical trials.[4-6]

TAM exhibits a mixture of estrogenic and antiestrogenic actions in laboratory animals.[7-9] The estrogen-like properties of TAM are well documented in patients;[10] however, relatively little is known about the actions of TAM in the human uterus. Although TAM has efficacy in the treatment of endometrial carcinoma,[11,12] the finding that this "antiestrogen" can facilitate the growth of human endometrial carcinoma transplanted into athymic mice[13-15] has raised concerns[16-19] about the activation of occult endometrial carcinoma during long-term adjuvant therapy for breast cancer.

This paper describes the biological and pharmacological responsiveness of the estrogen and progesterone receptor positive, human endometrial carcinoma EnCa101 transplanted into athymic mice.

MATERIALS AND METHODS

Tumors

EnCa101 tumors were continuously passaged in athymic mice with 5mg TAM pellets as previously described.[11] Tumors were transplanted into 4–5 week-old Balb/C ovariectomized athymic mice (Harlan Sprague Dawley, Indianapolis, IN). Mice were housed in laminar flow hoods with sterile cages and bedding. Tumors were measured using Vernier calipers at weekly intervals and mean cross-sectional area was calculated as length/2 × width/2 × π.

439

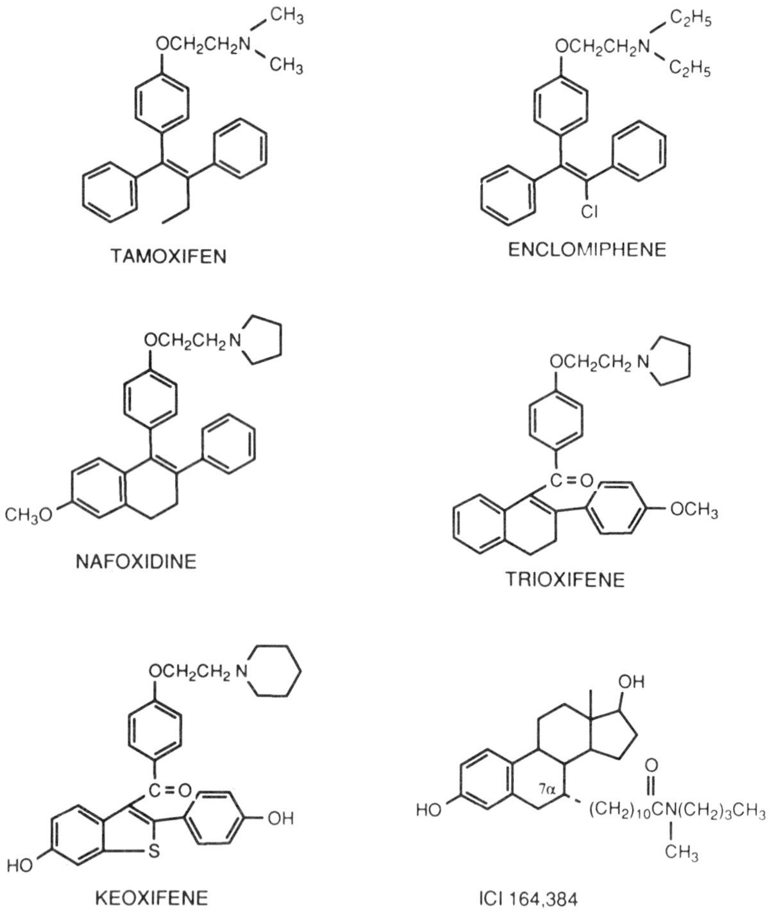

FIGURE 1. Chemical structures of the antiestrogens used in this study.

Drug Therapies

Compounds used in the experiments (FIG. 1) were gifts from the following sources: TAM free base, ICI Pharma, Wilmington, Delaware; ICI 164,384, Roussel Uclaf, Romainville, France; keoxifene (LY 156,758) and trioxifene mesylate (LY 133,314), Lilly Research Laboratory, Indianapolis, IN; enclomiphene, Merrill Dow Laboratories, Cincinnati, OH; nafoxidine, Upjohn Laboratories, Kalamazoo, MI.

Different methods were used for the administration of TAM during the experimental period. TAM free base (5mg, 4-week release) cholesterol pellets were custom made by Innovative Research of America, Toledo, OH. Silastic capsules used in the experiments were made from Silastic® tubing (Dow Corning, Midland, MI) 0.125 inches O.D. × 0.078 inches I.D. This was cut to 2.0cm and packed with TAM. The ends were plugged with Silastic cement (Dow Corning, Midland, MI). All capsules were sterilized by gamma irradiation. In experiments that injected TAM s.c., the compound was weighed, dissolved in 100% ethanol and mixed with peanut oil. The ethanol was evaporated under a gentle stream of nitrogen while mixing at 45°C.

Other antiestrogens were administered in similar ways. Keoxifene was made into cholesterol pellets containing 5mg by Innovative Research of America. Various antiestrogens were injected s.c. as 100g/0.1 ml peanut oil 3 times weekly. ICI 164,384 was injected s.c. every other day at a concentration of 1mg/0.1 ml peanut oil as a fine suspension. Preliminary experiments showed that ICI 164,384 was not released from silastic capsules.

Stimulatory Activity of Antiestrogens

The ability of various antiestrogens (TAM, trioxifene, enclomiphene, and nafoxidine) to promote the growth of EnCa101 implanted in athymic animals was studied by injecting compound (100µg s.c.) 3 times weekly (Mon, Wed, Fri).

Inhibitory Activity of Antiestrogens

Several experiments were conducted to inhibit TAM-stimulated growth of EnCa101. Keoxifene (5mg cholesterol pellet) was co-administered with TAM (5mg cholesterol pellet) to determine the inhibitory activity of the compound. ICI 164,384 (1mg suspension in 0.1 ml peanut oil s.c. every other day) was studied to determine the inhibition of TAM (2.0 cm silastic capsule) stimulated tumor growth. The injection method of administration of the steroidal antiestrogens was used because ICI 164,384 cannot be administered by silastic capsule.

Statistical Analysis

Differences in mean tumor area were measured using analysis of variance followed by unpaired Student's *t*-test.

RESULTS

TAM increased the growth rate of human endometrial carcinoma EnCa101 implanted into athymic mice (FIG. 2). The tumors were estrogen receptor (ER) positive and TAM treatment increased progesterone receptor (PgR) content. We also evaluated a range of antiestrogens to determine whether the increase in growth rate of EnCa101 produced by TAM was unique to this antiestrogen or whether compounds were available to inhibit growth.

The administration of enclomiphene, trioxifene or nafoxidine to athymic mice produced an increase in the growth of EnCa101 comparable to that observed with TAM (FIG. 3). In contrast the antiestrogen keoxifene only partially stimulated the growth of EnCa101 and this was associated with the ability to block TAM-stimulated growth (FIG. 4). The result encouraged us to test the ability of a new pure antiestrogen ICI 164,384 to inhibit TAM-stimulated growth. Unfortunately ICI 164,384 is not very

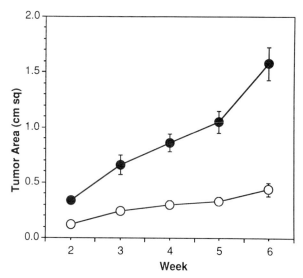

FIGURE 2. Growth curves for EnCal01 endometrial carcinoma with (●) and without (○) a sustained release 5 mg TAM pellet. Tumor was taken to measure estrogen (ER) and progesterone (PgR) receptor by methods previously described.[15] Control tumor had values for ER of 36 ± 5 fmol/mg cytosol protein and PgR of 49 ± 10 fmol/mg cytosol protein. The TAM-stimulated tumor had values for ER of 140 ± 10 fmol/mg cytosol protein and PgR of 217 ± 19 fmol/mg cytosol protein.

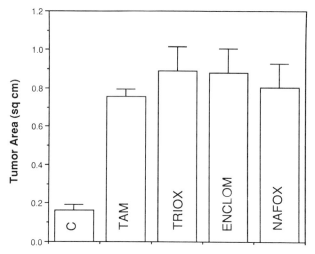

FIGURE 3. Growth of EnCal01 endometrial carcinoma (n=4) in athymic mice after 4 weeks of treatment (100μg compound s.c. injection every other day in 0.1ml peanut oil) with vehicle (c), tamoxifen (TAM), trioxifene (Triox), enclomiphene (enclom) or nafoxidine (Nafox). Bars SE.

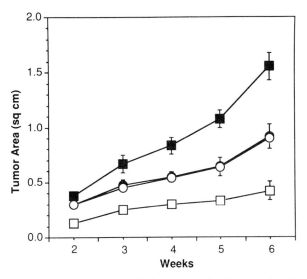

FIGURE 4. Growth of EnCal01 tumors (n = 12) in athymic mice after 6 weeks of treatment in 5mg TAM pellet (■); 5mg TAM pellet + 5mg keoxifene pellets (●); 5mg keoxifene pellets (○); or placebo (□). Bars SE.

active on oral administration and the compound cannot be administered in silastic capsules or in a cholesterol pellet. Injection (subcutaneous) of ICI 164,384 (1 mg) every other day was unable to stimulate the growth of EnCal01 but inhibited TAM-stimulated growth (FIG. 5).

DISCUSSION

The human endometrial carcinoma EnCal01 is extremely sensitive to the growth-promoting effects of TAM and other related antiestrogens, e.g., clomiphene, trioxifene, nafoxidine. Overall the ability to facilitate growth in the athymic mouse appears to be related to the intrinsic estrogenicity of the non-steroidal antiestrogens. The estrogen-like activity of the triphenylethylenes is well documented[9] however antiestrogens with less estrogenic activity are available for evaluation in the laboratory. Keoxifene[20] and its related compound LY117018[21,22] are potent inhibitors of the binding of [^{3}H]estradiol to the estrogen receptor and appear to exhibit only weak estrogen-like properties. The reduced estrogenicity is reflected in the results from the current investigation. Keoxifene is only a weak stimulator of EnCal01 growth and can prevent the growth observed with TAM. This is further illustrated with the pure antiestrogen[23] ICI 164,384 which did not promote EnCal01 growth at all. Unfortunately, the poor bioavailability of ICI 164,384 may in fact be a limiting factor for its ability to inhibit TAM-stimulated growth completely. However, these studies clearly demonstrate that agents can be developed to control TAM-stimulated growth should it occur in the clinic. In fact the principles illustrated here may also be relevant to the development of TAM-stimulated breast cancer growth in the clinic. Although there are only anecdotal reports[24] to demon-

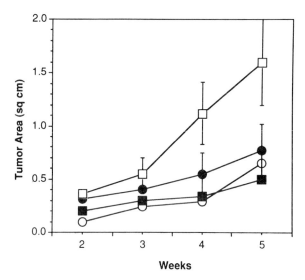

FIGURE 5. Effect of the pure antiestrogen ICI 164,384 on TAM-stimulated growth of endometrial tumor EnCa101 in the athymic mouse. Animals were treated with a sustained release preparation of TAM (2 cm silastic capsule) (□), a control capsule (○), or ICI 164,384 1mg/0.2 ml peanut oil s.c. 3× weekly (■) or TAM + ICI 164,384 (●).

strate TAM-stimulated growth of breast cancer after long-term treatment, this is not true in the laboratory. The breast cancer cell line MCF-7 can be "educated" to grow in response to TAM when tumors are implanted into athymic mice.[25,26] Clearly pure antiestrogens, which inhibit TAM stimulated MCF-7 breast tumor growth,[27] could be a valuable second-line therapy if TAM-stimulated breast cancer recurrence occurs during long-term adjuvant therapy.

In contrast to the clinical situation with breast cancer, Fornander[28] has described an increase in endometrial carcinoma in women receiving long-term (up to 5 years) of adjuvant TAM therapy for breast cancer. Obviously women should not be denied the benefits of TAM therapy because of a potential complicating disorder like endometrial carcinoma: endometrial carcinoma has a good prognosis whereas breast cancer is invariably fatal, but physicians should be aware of the clinical possibility of endometrial stimulation. Fornander and coworkers[28] have suggested that a progestin could be integrated into the treatment plan to avoid endometrial carcinoma but this strategy may, for the moment, be unwise since we are ignorant about the interaction of low dose progestins and TAM in the breast. There are reports[29,30] to show that progestins can reverse the beneficial antitumor actions of TAM both in the clinic and the laboratory.

The antiestrogen TAM which exhibits some estrogen-like properties in patients is now widely available for the treatment of all stages of breast cancer. The use of long-term therapy may result in continuous estrogen-like stimulation of the uterus which might activate occult endometrial carcinoma. We have found that, in the laboratory, a human endometrial carcinoma EnCa101 will grow in athymic mice in response to antiestrogens that also exhibit estrogen-like properties. Physicians should remain vigilant to the possibility that endometrial carcinoma may occur in breast cancer patients treated with TAM. Routine gynecological investigations will provide adequate reassurance during long-term TAM therapy.

SUMMARY

An estrogen receptor and progesterone receptor positive endometrial carcinoma (EnCal01) will grow in response to either estradiol or tamoxifen when transplanted into athymic mice. We have tested several antiestrogens with different properties to determine their ability to support endometrial tumor growth. Trioxifene, enclomiphene and nafoxidine are all as active as tamoxifen whereas the antiestrogen keoxifene, that has reduced estrogen-like properties, will partially inhibit tamoxifen-stimulated growth. Furthermore, the pure antiestrogen ICI 164,384 will block tamoxifen-stimulated growth without having any effect itself on tumor growth rate. Overall, the ability of antiestrogens to stimulate the growth of human endometrial carcinoma EnCal01 appears to be related to their intrinsic estrogenic activity.

ACKNOWLEDGMENTS

We would like to thank Doug Wolf and Bonnie Rayho for their help with the preparation of this manuscript.

REFERENCES

1. JORDAN, V. C., ALLEN, K. E. & DIX, C. J. 1980. The pharmacology of tamoxifen in laboratory animals. Cancer Treat. Rep. **64**: 745–759.
2. JORDAN, V. C. 1988. Chemosuppression of breast cancer with tamoxifen: Laboratory evidence and future clinical investigations. Cancer Invest. **6**: 5–11.
3. JORDAN, V. C. 1990. Long-term adjuvant tamoxifen therapy for breast cancer. Breast Cancer Res. Treat. **15**: 125–136.
4. BREAST CANCER TRIALS COMMITTEE, SCOTTISH CANCER TRIALS OFFICE (MRC). 1987. Adjuvant tamoxifen in the management of operable breast cancer: The Scottish Trial. Lancet **ii**: 171–175.
5. FISHER, B., J. CONSTANTINO, C. REDMOND & OTHER MEMBERS OF THE NSABP. 1989. A randomized clinical trial evaluating tamoxifen in the treatment of patients with node-negative breast cancer who have estrogen-receptor positive tumors. N. Engl. J. Med. **320**: 479–484.
6. FALKSON, H. C., R. GRAY, W. H. WOLBERG, K. W. GILCHRIST, J. E. HARRIS, D. C. TORMEY & G. FALKSON. 1990. Adjuvant trial of 12 cycles of CMFPT followed by observation or continuous tamoxifen versus four cycles of CMFPT in postmenopausal women with breast cancer: An ECOG Phase III study. J. Clin. Oncol. **8**: 599–607.
7. HARPER, M. J. K. & A. L. WALPOLE. 1966. Contrasting endocrine activities of *cis* and *trans* isomers in a series of substituted triphenylethylenes. Nature (Lond) **212**: 87.
8. HARPER, M. J. K. & A. L. WALPOLE. 1967. A new derivative of triphenylethylene: Effect on implantation and mode of action in rats. J. Reprod. Fertil. **13**: 101–119.
9. JORDAN, V. C. 1984. Biochemical pharmacology of antiestrogen action. Pharm. Rev. **36**: 245–276.
10. FURR, B. J. A. & V. C. JORDAN. 1984. The pharmacology and clinical uses of tamoxifen. Pharm. Ther. **25**: 127–205.
11. SWENTERTON, K. D. 1980. Treatment of advanced endometrial adenocarcinoma with tamoxifen. Cancer Treat. Rep. **64**: 7–16.
12. BONTE, J., P. IDE, G. BILLET & P. WYRENTS. 1981. Tamoxifen as a possible chemotherapeutic agent in endometrial adenocarcinoma. Gynecol. Oncol. **11**: 140–161.

13. SATYASWAROOP, P. G., R. J. ZAINO & R. MORTEL. 1984. Estrogen-like effects of tamoxifen on human endometrial carcinoma transplanted into nude mice. Cancer Res. **44**: 4006–4010.

14. CLARK, C. L. & P. G. SATYASWAROOP. 1985. Photoaffinity labeling of the progesterone receptor from human endometrial carcinoma. Cancer Res. **45**: 5417–5420.

15. GOTTARDIS, M. M., S. P. ROBINSON, P. G. SATYASWAROOP & V. C. JORDAN. 1988. Contrasting actions of tamoxifen on endometrial and breast tumor growth in the athymic mouse. Cancer Res. **48**: 812–815.

16. KILLACKEY, M. A., T. B. HAKES & V. K. PIERCE. 1985. Endometrial adenocarcinoma in breast cancer patients receiving tamoxifen. Cancer Treat. Rep. **69**: 237–238.

17. HARDELL, L. 1988. Tamoxifen as risk factor for carcinoma of corpus uteri. Lancet **ii**: 563.

18. HARDELL, L. 1988. Pelvic irradiation and tamoxifen as risk factors for carcinoma of corpus uteri. Lancet **ii**: 1432.

19. GUSBERG, S. 1990. Tamoxifen for breast cancer: Associated endometrial cancer. Cancer **65**: 1463–1464.

20. BLACK, L. J., C. D. JONES & J. F. FALCONE. 1983. Antagonism of estrogen action with a new benzothiophene-derived antiestrogen. Life Sci. **32**: 1031–1036.

21. BLACK, L. J. & R. L. GOODE. 1980. Uterine bioassay of tamoxifen, trioxifene and a new estrogen antagonist (LY117018) in rats and mice. Life Sci. **26**: 1453–1458.

22. BLACK, L. J., C. D. JONES & R. L. GOODE. 1981. Differential interaction of antiestrogens with cytosol estrogen receptors. Mol. Cell. Endocrinol. **22**: 95–103.

23. WAKELING, A. E. & J. BOWLER. 1987. Steroidal pure antioestrogens. J. Endocrinol. **112**: R7-R10.

24. LEGAULT-POISSON, S., J. JOLIVET, R. POISSON, M. PERETTA-PICCOLI & P. R. BAND. 1979. Tamoxifen-induced tumor stimulation and withdrawal response. Cancer Treat. Rep. **63**: 1839–1841.

25. GOTTARDIS, M. M. & V. C. JORDAN. 1988. Development of tamoxifen-stimulated growth of MCF-7 tumors in athymic mice after long-term antiestrogen administration. Cancer Res. **48**: 5183–5187.

26. GOTTARDIS, M. M., R. J. WAGNER, E. C. BORDEN & V. C. JORDAN. 1989. Differential ability of antiestrogens to stimulate breast cancer cell (MCF-7) growth *in vivo* and *in vitro*. Cancer Res. **49**: 4765–4769.

27. GOTTARDIS, M. M., S. Y. JIANG, M. H. JENG & V. C. JORDAN. 1989. Inhibition of tamoxifen-stimulated growth of an MCF-7 tumor variant in athymic mice by novel steroid antiestrogens. Cancer Res. **49**: 4090–4093.

28. FORNANDER, T., L. E. RUTQUIST, B. V. CEDERMARK, U. GLAS, A. MATTSON, J. D. SILVERSWARD, L. SKOOG, A. SOMELL, T. THEVE, N. WILKING, J. ASKERGREN & M. L. HJOLMAR. 1989. Adjuvant tamoxifen in early breast cancer: Occurrence of new primary cancers. Lancet **i**: 117–120.

29. MOURIDSEN, H. T., K. ELLEMANN & W. MATTSSON. 1979. Therapeutic effect of tamoxifen versus tamoxifen combined with medroxy progesterone acetate in advanced breast cancer in post-menopausal women. Cancer Treat. Rep. **63**: 171–175.

30. ROBINSON, S. P. & V. C. JORDAN. 1987. Reversal of the antitumor effect of tamoxifen by progesterone in the 7,12 dimethylbenz-anthracene-induced rat mammary carcinoma model. Cancer Res. **47**: 5386–5390.

Natural History of Endometrial Carcinoma

G. DE PALO

Istituto Nazionale per lo Studio e la Cura dei Tumori
Via G. Venezian, 1
20133 Milano, Italy

Endometrial carcinoma is the "Cinderella" of gynecologic oncology. Being the gynecologic tumor with the most favorable prognosis and the highest survival rate, the interest among clinicians has always been low. Had it not been for the studies related to endocrine genesis and the increase in countries where estrogens are widely used for replacement therapy around and after menopause, the specialized and nonspecialized literature would have been completely without contributions. Nevertheless, the natural history of endometrial carcinoma was not known for many years.

Although many authors had established the prognostic significance of myometrial invasion and histological grade, it has taken over 15 years since the FIGO classification of 1971 for old concepts such as the prognostic importance of the length of the uterine cavity to be abandoned and for it to be understood that myometrial invasion, histological grade, retroperitoneal involvement, and postitive peritoneal cytology were relevant prognostic factors.

In 1988, the FIGO Staging Committee revised the classification of corpus cancer and introduced some concepts that are tied to the pathological extension of disease and that are of real prognostic value.

Further background to this classification may be offered by the data of the study performed in Italy under the aegis of the CNR, a study started in February 1980 with 21 university gynecology departments, closed to accrual of patients on December 31, 1983, and still unpublished.

The objectives of the study were to perform in FIGO stage I a surgical-pathological staging, to establish a treatment plan on the basis of pathological extension of the disease, and to establish the effectiveness of adjuvant medroxyprogesterone acetate treatment when administered at low doses *per os* for 1 year.

The design of the study was the following. All patients with FIGO stage I were registered. Ineligible cases were those with age >75 years; previous or synchronous neoplastic disease; severe concomitant disease; previous treatment; surgery impossible because of high operative risk; geographic inaccessibility, and patients refusing work-up or post-surgical treatment. All eligible cases were subjected to presurgical staging with chest x-ray, intravenous urography, lymphography, x-ray of the pelvic bones, rectosigmoidoscopy and/or double contrast enema. Surgical staging consists in inspection of omentum and abdominal viscera with biopsies on suspicious lesions; selective lymphadenectomy on pelvic and para-aortic nodes in presence of abnormal lymphography or enlarged anatomosurgical nodes. Peritoneal cytology (free fluid or washing) performed during laparotomy was optional. Surgical treatment consists in total abdominal hysterectomy, bilateral salpingoovariectomy, and colpectomy of the superior third of the vagina. Pathological staging consists in three sections from the ovaries, three sections from the tubes (intramural tract, isthmus, ampulla), one section transversal about 2 cm above the internal uterine orifice, three longitudinal segments of the upper two-thirds (anterior and posterior) and three longitudinal segments of the lower third of the corpus uteri and the cervix (anterior and posterior aspects).

On the basis of pathological extension of the disease, histological grade, myometrial invasion, and histological lymph node metastases, patients were classified in five risk groups:

R0: no myometrial invasion, any G.
R1: one-third myometrial invasion (M1) and high (G1) or medium (G2) degree of differentiation.
R2: two (M2) or three-thirds (M3) myometrial invasion, G1 or G2. M1-M2-M3 and low degree of differentiation (G3).
R3: retroperitoneal involvement, G1-G2-G3, M1-M2-M3.
RE: pathological stage II (occult involvement of the cervix), III (involvement of ovaries, free tract of fallopian tubes, pelvic peritoneum, parametrium, with exclusion of retroperitoneal involvement), IV (involvement beyond the true pelvis).

According to these parameters 1476 cases were registered: 379 were ineligible cases and 42 protocol violations for various reasons, the most frequent being incomplete work-up. One-hundred-sixty-three were in R0 group; 382 in R1; 341 in R2; 23 in R3; and 146 patients in the RE group. The reclassification of the 1055 FIGO (1971) stage I cases in FIGO (1988) shows that 163 were stage IA; 382 stage IB-C; and 341 stage IC. Thirty-five patients had stage IIA, and 57 stage IIB. Thirty-five patients had stage IIIA, 3 stage IIIB, and 34 stage IIIC. Finally, 5 patients had stage IVB. All patients were followed every 3 months for the first two years, every 6 months from years 3 to 5 and every 12 months thereafter. Data from our analysis, performed in April 1990, on the extent of disease, sites of relapse, overall and relapse-free survival have been reported.

Preinvasive Lesions
of the Endometrium

SERGIO PECORELLI, LUCA FALLO,
ENRICO SARTORI, AND ATTILIO GASTALDI

Cattedra di Oncologia Ginecologica
e di Clinica Ostetrica e Ginecologica
Università degli Studi di Brescia
Brescia, Italy

INTRODUCTION

Endometrial glandular proliferation appears to form a morphological and biological continuum ranging from focal glandular crowding, through a variety of lesions, to subsequent development of cancer.[1,2] Whitehead defined endometrial hyperplasia (EH) as an abnormal increase in the amount of proliferative endometrium which exhibits varying degrees of cytological and architectural atypia.[3] The association of EH with adenocarcinoma of the endometrium has been amply documented;[4-8] some of these lesions revert to normal, eventually with medical therapy, some persist as hyperplasia, and a few progress to endometrial adenocarcinoma.[9] More recently the continuum concept has been amply discussed and now it appears that there are two endometrial alterations not directly related, hyperplasia and neoplasia, and that cytologic atypia is the most important feature to distinguish endometrial benign lesions from those with invasive potential.

Until recently the controversies about the existing terminology and classifications and the shortage of criteria which can accurately predict the outcome of the disease were the major causes of misleading diagnoses and overtreatment of these patients. It is now apparent that the presence of cytological atypia in a preinvasive lesion identifies a high risk for development of carcinoma, thereby providing the basis for patients' management.[2] Thus the distinction between non-atypical and atypical hyperplasia is important to make differences in the premalignant potential; with simple hyperplasia the subsequent conversion to carcinoma is approximately 1%, whereas with atypical forms of hyperplasia the rate increases to 10–23%[11,12] of progression.

There is ample evidence that hormonal imbalance creates an environment favorable for the development of both EH and carcinoma, mostly linked to the excess of endogenous estrogens or to unopposed exogenous estrogens, in the absence of progesterone or progestagens.

The present paper attempts to summarize the different points of view on preneoplastic lesions considering: 1) a brief review of nomenclature and classifications; 2) some procedures to better characterize hyperplasia; 3) the diagnostic tools; 4) the premalignant significance of EH; and 5) some therapeutic considerations.

CLASSIFICATION OF ENDOMETRIAL HYPERPLASIA

The classification of EH have been amply discussed over the past years until recently because of the need of a uniform terminology to consider the behavior of the various forms of hyperplasia. According to Welch and Scully[13] and Winkler et al. in fact "these differences in terminology must be kept in mind not only in evaluating the various studies in the literature but also in communicating with gynecologists and other pathologists," and "the clinician is faced with a seemingly endless number of variations in terminology that almost preclude a rational approach to management."[14]

In TABLE 1 the different authors who suggested a histopathological classification in past years are reported until the proposal of the International Society of Gynecological Pathologists. The classification by F. Vellios, for the Armed Forces Institute of Pathology, considers the adenocarcinoma in situ as a precursor of invasive endometrial carcinoma (TABLE 2).

The term "carcinoma in situ" was introduced by Hertig in 1949;[15] Welch and Scully used it to denote small focal lesions involving no more than five or six glands in which the cytologic features of carcinoma are present but there is no evidence of invasion of the stroma: so the term has been applied to any adenocarcinoma confined to the endometrium with no invasion of the myometrium. On the other hand, Fox asserts that "a true adenocarcinoma in situ of the endometrium is one in which the glands have undergone neoplastic change but in which there is no invasion of the endometrial stroma. It is doubtful if an adenocarcinoma of this type exists or if it could be recognized even if it did exist."[16]

In 1982 Fox proposed a classification distinguishing three forms of EH (TABLE 3). Fox believes that the neoplastic nature of glandular hyperplasia with cellular atypia leads to a comparison with cervical intraepithelial neoplasia and for this reason a similar classification can be identified for endometrium too. Thus, glandular hyperplasia with mild cellular atypia could be classified as "intraendometrial neoplasia" (IEN) grade I, cases with moderate atypia as IEN grade II, and both glandular hyperplasia

TABLE 1. Different Histopathological Classifications

1951	Dockerty	1979	Koss
1963	Gusberg	1980	Bonk
1967	Campbell	1981	Robertson
1971	Gore	1981	Dallenbach-Hellweg
1972	Vellios (A.F.I.P.)	1981	Cove
1977	Dargent	1982	Fox
1977	Welch-Scully	1984	I.S.G.P.
1978	Tavassoli		

TABLE 2. Precursor Lesions of Invasive Endometrial Carcinoma[a]

1. Cystic hyperplasia
2. Adenomatous hyperplasia
3. Atypical hyperplasia
4. Carcinoma in situ

[a] F. Vellios, 1972.

TABLE 3. Classifications of Endometrial Hyperplasia[a]

1. Simple endometrial hyperplasia
2. Simple glandular hyperplasia
3. Intraendometrial neoplasia (IEN)
• grade I
• grade II
• grade III

[a] H. Fox, 1982.

with severe cellular atypia and intraendometrial adenocarcinoma could be classified as IEN grade III.[16]

In 1984 the International Society of Gynecological Pathologists presented a classification (TABLE 4) which primarily takes into account cytologic abnormalities. Proliferations showing no evidence of cytologic atypia are classified as either simple or complex hyperplasia depending on the extent of glandular complexity and crowding, whereas those displaying cytologic atypia regardless of the architectural pattern are classified as atypical hyperplasia.[1]

CLINICAL PRESENTATION

The most common symptom associated with the presence of EH is irregular, abnormal uterine bleeding.[17] This is sometimes accompanied by lower abdominal pains caused by accumulation and subsequent expulsion of blood from the uterine cavity. In younger patients hyperplasia is diagnosed for its association with anovulatory cycles, as in the perimenopausal women. Postmenopausal women treated with estrogens for prolonged periods, if bleeding does not appear, may have the diagnosis because of the biopsy performed as a precautionary measure. EH can also be associated to polycystic ovarian syndrome, estrogen-secreting tumors, and adrenocortical hyperplasia. The typical history of this group of patients reveals an interruption in cyclic menses, usually with skips and delays of menstrual flow or with a prolonged period of amenorrhea.[9]

CHARACTERIZATION OF HYPERPLASIA

Atypical hyperplasia of the endometrium forms a continuum with invasive cancer and may be difficult to distinguish it from well-differentiated carcinoma. In the present years a lot of studies have been undertaken to help the pathologists and the clinician

TABLE 4. Classification of Endometrial Hyperplasia[a]

1. Simple hyperplasia
2. Complex hyperplasia (Adenomatous hyperplasia without atypia)
3. Atypical hyperplasia (Adenomatous hyperplasia with atypia)

[a] International Society of Gynecological Pathologists, 1984.

to better define and characterize preneoplastic lesions of endometrium. In spite of the efforts of many pathologists there are in fact several cases of misdiagnoses between endometrial hyperplasia and carcinoma. In a Swedish cancer registry study,[18] 12% of the lesions initially diagnosed as cancer were reclassified as premalignant by an independent reviewer; a second reviewer reinstated as carcinoma 14 of the 44 that had been downgraded by the first reviewer and a third reviewer examined 21 of these cases and reinstated 14 of them.

As regards the diagnostic problem of hyperplasia Winkler *et al.* reviewed 100 consecutive consultation cases that had been referred with the diagnosis of endometrial hyperplasia, and failed to confirm the diagnosis in 69% of the cases.[14] This general agreement concerning frequent misdiagnoses points out the need for a standardized and reproducible classification system.

Evidence supporting these concepts came from a number of studies on experimental techniques applied to increase the sensibility and specificity of diagnosis. The goal of these different methods is to identify more objective criteria, translating the qualitative impression into quantitative terms, to reach a valid acceptance of characterization of various forms of EH, especially in the clinical practice.

Scanning and transmission electron microscopic studies[19-21] evidence that the non atypical forms of EH have an increase in the number of estrogen-related organelles (cilia, microvilli, free ribosomes, RER, *etc.*) in the glandular epithelial cells. However, these appear to be non-specific features and it's impossible to distinguish between normal proliferative and non-atypical endometrium.

The concentration of estrogen-related organelles decreases as the lesion approaches carcinoma, but because the heterogeneous population of cells in the forms of atypical hyperplasia and the limited size of endometrial samples this technique could fail in the characterization of endometrial hyperplasias.

Quantitative microscopy could offer an objective and reproducible method to identify degrees of architectural and cytological atypia.[22-24] Glandular form, nuclear size, stromal volume and nuclear shape can be quantitatively measured to reach an objective diagnosis. According to Colgan *et al.* measurements of nuclear size were demonstrated to predict, with 83% accuracy, the outcome of atypical hyperplasia.[23] However, morphometric analysis is not routinely available in most pathologic laboratories, and in any event they seem to be valid only in predicting the behavior of atypical hyperplasias[23,25] or in grading known carcinomas,[26] but it appears not to be useful in distinguishing EH and carcinoma.

The demonstration of an aneuploid distribution in some EH,[27,28] because of the assumption that aneuploidy is a feature of malignant cells, except some endocrine tumors, suggested DNA microspectrophotometry as a method to identify the forms of EH evolving to carcinoma. However, it has been demonstrated that a significant number of well-differentiated endometrial carcinomas may be diploid or peridiploid[27,29] preventing the recognition of high risk lesions.

Actually the studies concerning flow cytometry using comparison between endometrial proliferative and S-phase labeling indices, have demonstrated that *in vitro* DNA labeling shows a prolonged S-1 phase (kinetic parameter of DNA synthesis) coupled with a shorter cell doubling time, as in carcinoma.[19,30] Flow cytometric proliferative indices may be useful to recognize severe forms of atypical hyperplasia and carcinoma, non-DNA aneuploid, predicting the likelihood of progression.

It is well established that normal endometrial growth is estradiol-dependent and that progesterone can inhibit estradiol-mediated endometrial cell proliferation.[31] For this reason, according to the hypothesis that the presence of steroid hormone receptors is a prerequisite for steroid hormones to mediate their efforts in target tissues,[32,33] estrogen and progesterone receptors have been identified and studied.[34] Their content is usually high in proliferative endometrium as in EH, decreases in the forms of atypical hyperplasia as well as in carcinoma.[35]

Estrogen receptors may predict response to endocrine treatment,[36] but according to Thornton the receptor level is important in the glandular component of endometrium, where the most important variations in estrogen receptor content appear.[35,37]

Controversies have developed concerning the role of immunocytochemistry in distinguishing atypical hyperplasia from carcinoma: α-feto-protein, luteinizing hormone, human chorionic gonadotropin, carcinoembryonic antigen, and casein have been analyzed in endometrial hyperplasia and carcinoma, but the number of cases studied is too small to be conclusive. Consequently, electron microscopic studies, quantitative microscopy, DNA microspectrophotometry, and steroid hormone receptor analysis are unable to discriminate between atypical forms of endometrial hyperplasia and adenocarcinoma in all cases.[38]

DIAGNOSTIC TOOLS

Many techniques have been used for the diagnosis of EH, and each of them must satisfy several criteria: it's fundamental to decrease both false negatives and false positives; the technique has to be widely adopted to decrease the costs and it has to be safe and well accepted by the patients (TABLE 5).

The first step is a correct anamnesis coupled with a thorough objective examination of the patient, to detect in particular if the patient belongs to high risk categories. Then the most important diagnostic tools can be divided into 4 categories: cytology, histology, ultrasound, and hysteroscopy.

There has always been a need for a simple and painless method to detect endometrial abnormalities and actually cytology becomes more important than ever. For this reason various simple procedures to obtain endometrial specimens for cytological diagnosis have been proposed and developed.[39-46] These techniques are divided into two groups: those which request intrauterine manipulation and those which don't. The latter method is represented by the investigation of the presence of normal endometrial cells in vaginal and cervicovaginal smears, executed in the second half of the menstrual cycle or in the postmenopausal period: the association of these findings with endometrial diseases in women over 40 years range from 20–60%, and the correlation with adenocarcinoma of the endometrium from 1–13%;[47] in EH this correlation appears to be even less reliable owing to the rare exfoliations.

TABLE 5. Diagnostic Tools

■ Cytology	■ Histology
a. Intrauterine	a. D&C
• Aspiration	b. Vabra aspiration
• Scraping	c. CIEC
• Washing	■ Ultrasound
b. Non-intrauterine	■ Hysteroscopy
• Pap smear	

In order to obviate these problems, methods are used to obtain samples directly from the uterine cavity; this can be done in three ways: 1) washing, 2) aspiration, 3) scraping. Nevertheless, washing systems appear to be not as useful in EH and in benign lesions as in carcinoma, whereas aspiration systems (Vakutage, Curity Isaacs Cell Sampler) turned out to be more sensible for histologic techniques. Endometrial cytology obtained with scraping of intrauterine walls appears a simple, painless, and cheap diagnostic method, especially after the introduction of the Endo-Pap endometrial sampler.

The investigation of useful parameters for cytologic diagnosis of endometrial samples obtained with the Endo-Pap showed that: 1) there is no useful parameter differentiating between normal proliferative endometrium and simple hyperplasia; 2) complex hyperplasia is characterized by cellular aggregates, dilated glandular borders in cellular sheets, nuclear clearing, clumped chromatin, and anysokaryosis; 3) enlargement of nucleoli and eosinophilic cytoplasm alone are not sufficient for the diagnosis of intraendometrial neoplasia.[48]

In a comparative study between normal endometrium, well-differentiated endometrial adenocarcinoma, and EH, differences in tumor diathesis, hypercellularity, uneven internuclear distance, severe piling up of nuclei, anisokaryosis, nuclear size and macronucleoli were the main cytologic findings varying among the three conditions. However, these features, as in particular, the identification of tumor diathesis, internuclear distance and piling up of nuclei are subjective criteria, and thus may vary for different pathologists.[49]

In another study on 318 symptomatic women, among whom were 42 with malignant uterine tumors, satisfactory material for cytological diagnosis was obtained in 96% (92% in a 1984 Ferenczy study). Forty of 42 women with endometrial cancer (sensitivity 97%), all 5 cases of high grade cytological atypia in endometrial polyps or endometrial hyperplasia, 4 of 5 patients with adenomatous endometrial hyperplasia (sensitivity 80%) had atypical endometrial cytology.[50] Ferenczy reported 80.5% sensitivity for endometrial hyperplasia and 100% for carcinoma.[51] The findings of Hansen were not so encouraging: the cytological investigation detected all 16 cases of endometrial cancer but none of 6 cases of atypical hyperplasia.[52] Schneider, determined the location, using histologic specimens and nuclear patterns, of endometrial hyperplasias, reporting that 8.6% of the precancerous endometrial hyperplasias are situated exclusively in deeper mucous layers and thus escape detection by cytologic instruments; no nuclear enlargement was shown in 22.9% of precancerous cells, 14.2% showed no changes in chromatin pattern and 8.6% of precancerous cells revealed neither nuclear enlargement nor changes in chromatin.[53] Skaarland reported that diagnosis of adenomatous hyperplasia shows a low sensitivity: only 10 of 50 histologically controlled cases could be verified after curettage.[54] Other studies reported concordance between cytology and histology respectively in 68.7% (55) and 78% cases of preneoplastic pathology.[56]

In conclusion, cytologic evaluation of endometrial pathology appears to be very difficult and needs experienced pathologists; recognizing the validity of cytology for malignant disease, a detailed histologic enquiry of the state of the endometrium, especially in doubtful or positive cases and in subjects at high risk, should necessarily be made.

Histologic techniques allow recognition in a more exhaustive and uniform manner of endometrial pathology, both hyperplastic and neoplastic. Women with postmenopausal and premenopausal abnormal uterine bleeding are traditionally investigated with dilatation and curettage (D&C). Nevertheless D&C represents a very expensive test[57] and, furthermore, its accuracy is debatable.

An alternative method has been introduced with aspiration techniques as Vabra aspiration or Curity Isaacs Endometrial Cell (CIEC) sampler. The advantages of Vabra are its absolute simplicity and speed of execution, patients' acceptance, the extremely low risk of adverse reactions and severe uterine lesions, and the negligible post-exam bleeding. The disadvantages are the possibility of sampling in not specifically pathologic areas, the necessity of a skilled pathologist and sometimes, the impossibility of performing the exam because of anatomic obstacles (narrow cervical canal or uterine myoma). In the Gynaecologic Department at the University of Brescia we reported a 97.7% accuracy. Comparing Vabra aspiration with uterine curettage Alberico *et al.* established a concordance in 80.8% of the cases; only in 1.2% of the specimens did the Vabra curettage not allow exclusion of endometrial pathology for lack of material.[58] The CIEC sampler, in a comparative study with D&C on 230 patients was found to be safe and without complications, easy to insert in 92% of patients without causing discomfort in 88.9% of them. Using histopathological diagnostic techniques there was 100% accuracy in detecting carcinomas but only 33.3% in diagnosing EH.[59]

A lot of reports have suggested that hysteroscopy is superior to D&C and is the most appropriate method for evaluating abnormal uterine bleeding.[60,61] Several techniques can be adopted: 1) panoramic hysteroscopy; 2) contact hysteroscopy; and 3) microhysteroscopy. These techniques permit direct vision, by using vital coloring agents, of suspicious or malignant lesions, allowing a direct and selected tissue sampling. In comparison with D&C, hysteroscopy appears to be more accurate in 9.1% and less accurate in only 0.5% of the patients; specificity of both techniques was 100%, but the sensitivity of hysteroscopy was greater (98%) than that of D&C (65%).[62] Another study performed on 618 women, 45 years of age or older, with abnormal uterine bleeding, showed a 100% accuracy of hysteroscopy in detecting endometrial adenocarcinomas, 87.5% for high-risk hyperplasia, and 65.2% for low-risk hyperplasia.[63]

Echotomographic investigation offers a morphologic and anatomic assessment of endometrium, allowing the measurements of endometrial thickness. In comparison with hysteroscopy and tissue sampling sonographic investigation has an accuracy reaching 87% in premenopausal women and 94% in postmenopausal. Vaginosonographic measurement was reported to reach a 89% specificity and a 81% sensitivity.[64] It's therefore important to remember that this is a non-invasive, simple and relatively cheap technique and is suitable for other diagnostic necessities as the evaluation of a possible ovarian pathology.

PREMALIGNANT SIGNIFICANCE OF ENDOMETRIAL HYPERPLASIA

At present there is a general agreement that this kind of lesion has at least some premalignant potential. According to the continuum concept, initially several authors estimated that most, if not all, endometrial adenocarcinoma arose in hyperplastic areas, and, on the other side, most hyperplasia had precancerous potential. Gradually the concept became similar to that for cervical intraepithelial neoplasia where the discriminating feature is presence of cytologic atypia. The atypical forms of EH are more likely to develop carcinoma than non-atypical ones, although their potential is difficult to quantitate. Nevertheless, if simple hyperplasia becomes malignant, it would only do so after it had passed through the steps of complex and atypical hyperplasia.[28]

Many studies evidenced the simultaneous presence of EH and carcinoma but the relative incidence of these lesions was different according to the diagnostic pathologic criteria. Prospective studies, in which known hyperplasias are followed for a number of years to determine the subsequent incidence of carcinoma, may provide better evidence but their number is small because most patients usually undergo hysterectomy, which abruptly ends the investigations, or other forms of therapy, including irradiation, which obscure the true natural history of the lesion.

Wentz,[65] using the criteria of Vellios and including only women who did not undergo hysterectomy or hormonal therapy, reported a 26.7% progression to carcinoma for adenomatous hyperplasia, 81.8% for atypical hyperplasia and 100% for carcinoma *in situ*.

Sherman and Brown[66] (excluding patients treated with hormones prior to diagnosis) reported 204 women with precursor lesions followed for 1 to 18 years and noted that there was a high rate of subsequent carcinoma: 10% for cystic, 22% for adenomatous, 57% for atypical hyperplasia, and 58% for CIS.

Kurman[12] followed 170 patients with all grades of EH without a hysterectomy being performed for at least 1 year and with no anamnestic irradiation. One third of the patients with both types of hyperplasia (non-atypical and atypical) were asymptomatic after the diagnostic curettage and required no other treatment; 2% of the patients with non-atypical EH and 23% with atypical EH progressed to carcinoma ($p = 0.001$). The 2 cases of hyperplasia that progressed underwent an alteration to atypical hyperplasia before developing carcinoma.

In summary, these studies provide evidence that cytologic atypia is the most useful feature in identifying a lesion that can and does progress to carcinoma. The quoted incidence of such progression has, however, varied widely and there are few reliable guidelines for assessing the true malignant potential of this form of hyperplasia. Welch and Scully[13] came to the conclusion that "it is impossible to render even a scientific estimate of the proportion of cases of precancerous hyperplasia that are destined to progress to cancer if untreated." Ferenczy[67] suggested that approximately 10% of women with glandular hyperplasia and cellular atypia will eventually develop an adenocarcinoma: however it must be emphasized that this is a guess rather than a hard or proven fact.[16] Kurman suggested a percentage varying from 11% to 23% of progression if hysterectomy is not performed.[11,12] In contrast to this kind of EH, simple hyperplasia shows a very low likelihood of progression to carcinoma: this is confirmed by McBride in a study with a follow-up period of up to 24 years, in which cancer developed in less than 0.4% of the patients.[10]

The mean duration of progression from EH to carcinoma is about 10 years for non-atypical lesions and 4 years for atypical.[12] The risk of progression appears to be greater for postmenopausal than for premenopausal women: it is reported a 3% risk for premenopausal and 25% for postmenopausal women.[68] Furthermore, Corscaden interpreted the risk for menopausal women with EH to be 10 times that of women without hyperplasia.[69]

THERAPEUTIC CONSIDERATIONS

The selection of treatment for these types of lesions depends on many considerations, the most important being the histologic type of EH with its malignant potential, and the age and childbearing desire of the patients. A woman with EH can be treated with medical and/or surgical therapeutic modalities: medical approach consists in progestin therapy or ovulation induction, while surgical procedures may be conservative (endometrial ablation) or demolitive (hysterectomy).

Progestin therapy has been reported to be effective in treating EH in various studies.[70-72] The majority receives progestational compounds but combinations of estrogens and progesteron have sometimes been utilized as well.[73]

The possible therapeutic role of progesterone is justified both by its antimitotic effect (due to mitotic activity blockage in G1-phase, DNA synthesis inhibition, decreased synthesis of estrogen receptors and induction of 17-β-dehydrogenase activity) and by its androgenic action, which has a direct hemostatic effect.

Ferenczy recently conducted a prospective study on 85 post-menopausal women with EH, with or without cytologic atypia, to evaluate the response to oral medroxyprogesterone acetate (MPA) therapy. In non-atypical lesions, 20% of the patients had persistence or recurrence and none developed carcinoma, whereas in atypical forms 10 of 20 patients had persistence, 5 had recurrence, and 5 developed carcinoma.

In contrast to EH without cytological atypia these data suggest a low response rate to MPA therapy for cytologically atypical lesions.[74] These results contrast with some previously reported series in which a complete response to MPA therapy as high as 84% by Gal[75] to 100% by Wentz[76,77] has been achieved.

Our experience in the treatment of EH consists in 151 cases followed for 1 to 6 years after initial diagnosis. The ISGP classification was adopted, and the patients were either untreated (group 1 = 38 cases) or treated with MPA (group 2 = 113 cases). The therapeutic regimen for atypical forms was 500 mg/day i.m. for 1 month and then 150 mg/day orally. Non-typical forms were treated *ab initio* with 150 mg/day administered orally. The regression rates for non-atypical and atypical forms were, respectively, 54% and 0/5 in group 1 versus 76% and 58% in group 2.

The different reported results may be interpreted because of the varying follow-up periods considered and the different doses of MPA employed. Although high doses of progestogens provoke side effects that lead to poor patient compliance for long-term therapy it seems necessary to use medium-high doses of MPA to get a prolonged therapeutic effect. In fact Dallenbach *et al.* reported that regression occurred with 50 mg/day for women with adenomatous EH grade I and with 100 mg/day for grade II, while 150 mg/day was required to obtain a similarly good result in grade III lesions.[78]

Progestogens had been administered also locally using the so-called "Intrauterine Contraceptive Progesterone System" (ICPS), capable of releasing continuously therapeutic doses of hormones (progesteron or levonorgestrel).[79,80]

Since some authors recently reported that Danazol (an isoxazol derivative of 17-α-ethinyltestosterone) inhibits the growth of human endometrial cancer cells *in vitro*,[81] the use of this drug has been suggested for the treatment of non-invasive endometrial proliferations. Preliminary data show that Danazol has a potential application in the treatment of endometrial adenomatous hyperplasia.[82]

In younger patients the reinstatement of ovulatory cycles can be attempted, but it should be emphasized that, if non-operative management is to be used, the patients must be carefully followed at frequent intervals and the endometrium sampled periodically.

A useful alternative to medical therapy is represented by hysteroscopic endometrial ablation. The goal of this treatment is to excise totally the basal layer of endometrium, causing a Ascherman-like syndrome, to inhibit the possibility of tissue regeneration. This effect can be obtained using two different techniques: Nd:Yag laser photocoagulation or electroresection. The Nd:Yag laser is used because of its ability to penetrate tissue, provoking a deep coagulation with self-limiting penetration to get a penetration up to 3–4 mm, acting as a proteic coagulator.

Two procedures can be adopted: the "dragging technique," described by Goldrath,[83] which permits a deeper level to be reached (but with more risks of side-effects) and the "non-touching technique" in which the laser does not come in contact with endometrium. According to Loffer this nontouching technique caused no complications in his series and may prevent the problems of fluid overload and postoperative bleeding found when contact is made with the mucosa.[84]

The electroresection technique has been described by Neuwirth:[85] it takes less time for a complete resection (about 30 minutes) while at least 1 hour is requested by laser. Recently Hamou et al. suggested the "surgical partial resection" technique, saving the lower third of the uterine cavity and the uterine isthmic zone.[86]

Finally hysterectomy has been the most common therapeutic modality in the treatment of EH, especially in complex and atypical forms. However, this demolitive approach should be indicated in selected cases depending on the histologic type of hyperplasia, the age and the compliance of the patient or after the failure of medical therapy. Furthermore, hysterectomy requires at least 1 week hospitalization and its total cost is quite high (10 thousand dollars in the USA; 5 million lire in Italy).

Management of patients with noninvasive endometrial proliferations is based on consideration of age and compliance of the patient in addition to the histologic type of the lesion. Women less than 40 years old, with non-atypical forms of EH should be treated with a progestin treatment or, if they plan childbearing, with ovulation induction therapy (clomiphene or menotropins). Otherwise they can be followed: both the medically treated and the untreated cases must be investigated performing an endometrial biopsy in 3–6 months, or earlier if symptoms recur, to ensure reversion to a benign pattern. Women with atypical hyperplasia who wish to retain their fertility can have hormonal treatment, either with progestin or induction of ovulation, but

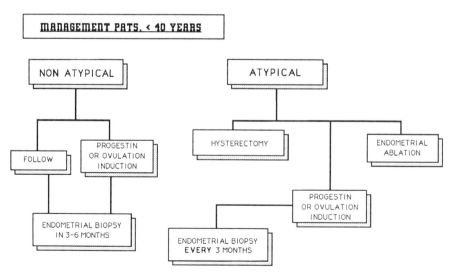

FIGURE 1. Management in women less than 40 years of age.

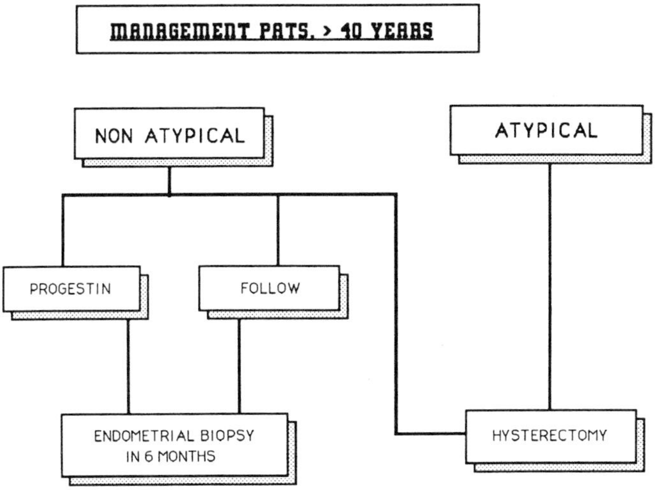

FIGURE 2. Management in women more than 40 years of age.

close follow-up and periodical endometrial sampling is necessary. Otherwise an endometrial ablation or a hysterectomy can be performed.

Women older than 40 years without atypical form of EH can be treated with progestins or followed and sampled after 3–6 months. In these women, hysterectomy can also be performed, if symptoms keep recurring. If there is atypical hyperplasia, hysterectomy must be performed.

FIGURES 1 and 2 show the general guidelines for management of EH both in young and older patients.

REFERENCES

1. KURMAN, R. J. & H. J. NORRIS. 1987. Endometrial hyperplasia and metaplasia. *In* Blaustein's Pathology of the Female Genital Tract. R. J. Kurman, Ed.: 322. Springer Verlag, New York.
2. NORRIS, H. J., M. P. CONNOR & R. J. KURMAN. 1986. Preinvasive lesions of the endometrium. Clin. Obstet. Gynaecol. **13**(4): 725.
3. WHITEHEAD, M. I. 1986. Prevention of endometrial abnormalities. Acta Obstet. Gynecol. Scand. **134**(Suppl): 81.
4. BAMFORTH, J. 1956. Carcinoma of body of uterus and its relationship to endometrial hyperplasia: Histological study. J. Obstet. Gynaecol. Br. Commonw. **63**: 415.
5. CAMPBELL, P. E. & R. A. BARTER. 1961. The significance of atypical hyperplasia. J. Obstet. Gynaecol. Br. Commonw. **68**: 668.
6. GRAY, L. A. & M. L. BARNES. 1964. Histogenesis of endometrial carcinoma. Ann. Surg. **159**: 976.
7. NOVAK, E. & E. YUI. 1936. Relation of endometrial hyperplasia to adenocarcinoma of the uterus. Am. J. Obstet. Gynecol. **32**: 674.
8. TELINDE, R. W., H. W. JONES & G. A. GALVIN. 1953. What are the earliest endometrial changes to justify diagnosis of endometrial cancer? Am. J. Obstet. Gynecol. **66**: 953.
9. DISAIA, P. J. & W. T. CREASMAN. 1989. Endometrial hyperplasia. *In* Clinical Gynecologic Oncology, 3rd edit.: 133–160. C. V. Mosby Co., St. Louis, MO.
10. MCBRIDE, J. M. 1959. Premenopausal cystic hyperplasia and endometrial carcinoma. J. Obstet. Gynaecol. Br. Commonw. **66**: 288.
11. GUSBERG, S. B. & A. L. KAPLAN. 1963. Precursors of corpus cancer. IV. Adenomatous hyperplasia as stage 0 carcinoma of the endometrium. Am. J. Obstet. Gynecol. **87**: 662.

12. KURMAN, R. J., P. F. KALMINSKI & H. J. NORRIS. 1985. The behavior of endometrial hyperplasia. A long-term study of "untreated" hyperplasia in 170 patients. Cancer 56: 403.
13. WELCH, W. R. & R. E. SCULLY. 1977. Precancerous lesions of endometrium. Hum. Pathol. 8: 503.
14. WINKLER, B., S. ALVAREZ, R. M. RICHART & C. P. CRUM. 1984. Pitfalls in the diagnosis of endometrial neoplasia. Obstet. Gynecol. 64: 185–194.
15. HERTIG, A. T. & S. C. SOMMERS. 1949. Genesis of endometrial carcinoma. Study of prior biopsy. Cancer 2: 946.
16. FOX, H. & C. H. BUKLEY. 1982. The endometrial hyperplasias and their relationship to endometrial neoplasia. Histopathology 6: 493.
17. HERTIG, A. T., S. C. SOMMERS & H. BENGLOFF. 1949. Genesis of endometrial carcinoma. Carcinoma in situ. Cancer 2: 964.
18. PERSSON, I., H. O. ADAMI & A. B. LINDGREN. 1986. Reliability of endometrial cancer diagnoses in a Swedish cancer registry, with special reference to classification bias related to exogenous oestrogens. Acta Pathol. Microbiol. Immunol. Scand. 94: 187.
19. FERENCZY, A. 1982. Cytodynamics of endometrial in hyperplasia and neoplasia. I. Histology and ultrastructure. In Progress in Surgical Pathology, Vol. 4: 95. C. M. Fenoglio & M. Wolff, Eds. Masson Publishing, USA, New York.
20. KLEMI, P. J., M. GRONROOS, L. RAURAMO & R. PUNNONEN. 1980. Ultrastructural features of endometrial atypical adenomatous hyperplasia and adenocarcinomas and the plasma levels of estrogens. Gynecol. Oncol. 9: 162.
21. RICHART, R. M. & A. FERENCZY. 1974. Endometrial morphologic response to hormonal environment. Gynecol. Oncol. 2: 180.
22. BAAK, J. P. A., P. H. J. KURVER, P. C. DIEGENBACH, J. F. M. DELEMARRE, E. C. M. BREKELMANS & J. E. NIEUWLAAT. 1981. Discrimination of hyperplasia and carcinoma of endometrium by quantitative microscopy: A feasibility study. Histopathology 5: 61.
23. COLGAN, T. J., H. J. NORRIS, W. FOSTER, R. J. KURMAN & C. H. FOX. 1983. Predicting the outcome of endometrial hyperplasia by quantitative analysis of nuclear features using a linear discriminant function. Int. J. Gynecol. Pathol. 1: 347.
24. NORRIS, H. J., F. A. TAVASSOLI & R. J. KURMAN. 1983. Endometrial hyperplasia and carcinoma. Am. J. Surg. Pathol. 7: 839.
25. AUSEMS, E. W. M. A., J. K. VAN DER KAMP & J. P. A. BAAK. 1985. Nuclear morphometry in the determination of the prognosis of marked atypical endometrial hyperplasia. Int. J. Gynecol. Pathol. 4: 180.
26. BAAK, J. P. A. 1984. The use and disuse of morphometry in the diagnosis of endometrial hyperplasia and carcinoma. Pathol. Res. Pract. 179: 20.
27. KATAYMA, K. P. & H. W. JONES. 1967. Chromosomes of atypical (adenomatous) hyperplasia and carcinoma of the endometrium. Am. J. Obstet. Gynecol. 97: 978.
28. WAGNER, D., R. M. RICHART & J. Y. TERNER. 1967. Deoxyribonucleic acid content of presumed precursors of endometrial carcinoma. Cancer 20: 2067.
29. HUSTIN, J. 1976. Morphology and DNA content of endometrial cancer nuclei under progestogen treatment. Acta Cytol. 20: 556.
30. FERENCZY, A. 1983. Cytodynamics of endometrial hyperplasia and neoplasia. Part II: In vitro DNA histoautoradiography. Hum. Pathol. 14: 77.
31. FERENCZY, A., G. BERTRAND & M. M. GELFAND. 1979. Proliferation kinetics of human endometrium during the normal menstrual cycle. Am. J. Obstet. Gynecol. 133: 859.
32. GORSKI, J., D. TOFT, G. SHYAMALA, D. SMITH & A. NOTIDES. 1968. Hormone receptors: Studies on interaction of estrogens with the uterus. Recent Prog. Horm. Res. 29: 45.
33. JENSEN, E. V., G. L. GREENE, L. E. CLOSS, E. R. DE SOMBRE & M. NADJI. 1982. Receptors reconsidered: A 20 year perspective. Recent Prog. Horm. Res. 38: 1.
34. SHYAMALA, G. & A. FERENCZY. 1981. The effect of sodium molybdate on the cytoplasmic estrogen and progesterone receptors in human endometrial tissues. Diagn. Gynecol. Obstet. 3: 277.
35. BERGERON, C., A. FERENCZY & G. SHYAMALA. 1988. Distribution of estrogen receptors in various cell types of normal, hyperplastic, and neoplastic human endometrial tissues. Lab. Invest. 58: 338.
36. KAUPILLA, A. & L. FRIBERG. 1981. Hormonal and cytotoxic chemotherapy for endometrial carcinoma steroid receptor in the selection of appropriate therapy. Acta Obstet. Gynecol. Scand. 101: 59.

37. THORNTON, J. G. & M. WELLS. 1987. Oestrogen receptor in glands and stroma of normal and neoplastic human endometrium: A Combined biochemical, immunohistochemical, and morphometric study. J. Clin. Pathol. **40**: 1437.
38. SILVERBERG, S. G. 1988. Hyperplasia and carcinoma of endometrium. Semin. Diag. Pathol. **2**: 135.
39. COHEN, J. 1978. La cytologie endométriale par grattage. Intéret de l'endocyte dans le dépistage du cancer de l'endométre. Rev. Franc. Gynécol. Obstèt. **73**: 413.
40. GRAVLEE, L. C. 1969. Jet-irrigation method for the diagnosis of endometrial adenocarcinoma: Its principle and accuracy. Obstet. Gynecol. **34**: 168.
41. ISAACS, J. H. & F. H. ROSS. 1978. Cytologic evaluation of the endometrium in women with postmenopausal bleeding. Am. J. Obstet. Gynecol. **131**: 410.
42. MILAN, A. R. & R. L. MARKLEY. 1973. Endometrial cytology by a new technique. Obstet. Gynecol. **42**: 469.
43. MEISELS, A. & C. JOLICOEUR. 1985. Criteria for the cytologic assessment of hyperplasias in endometrial samples obtained by the Endo-Pap endometrial sampler. Acta Cytol. **29**: 297.
44. PALERMO, V. 1985. Interpretation of endometrium obtained by the Endo-Pap sampler and a clinical study of its use. Diagn. Cytopathol. **1**: 5.
45. IVERSEN, O. & E. SEGEDAL. 1985. The value of endometrial cytology. A comparative study of the Gravlee Jet-washer, Isaacs cell sampler, and endoscann versus curettage in 600 patients. Obstet. Gynecol. **40**: 14.
46. SCHNEIDER, M. 1985. Potential and limitations of a cytological early diagnosis program for endometrial carcinoma. Geburtsch. Frauenheilkd. **45**: 831.
47. ZUCKER, P. K., E. J. KASDON & M. L. FELSTEIN. 1985. The validity of Pap smear parameters as predictors of endometrial pathology in menopausal women. Cancer **56**: 2256.
48. COSCIA-PORRAZZI, L. O. 1988. Cytologic criteria of hyperplastic lesions in endometrial samples obtained by the endocyte sampler. Diagn. Cytopathol. **4**: 283.
49. KASHIMURA, M., S. BABA, M. SHINOHARA, Y. KASHIMURA, T. SAITO & T. HACHISUGA. 1988. Cytologic findings in endometrial hyperplasia. Acta Cytol. **32**: 335.
50. BISTOLETTI, P., A. HJERPE, & G. MOLLERSTROM. 1988. Cytological diagnosis of endometrial cancer and preinvasive endometrial lesions. Acta Obstet. Gynecol. Scand. **67**: 343.
51. FERENCZY, A. & M. M. GELFAND. 1984. Outpatient endometrial sampling with Endocyte: Comparative study of its effectiveness with endometrial biopsy. Obstet. Gynecol. **63**: 295.
52. HANSEN, P. K., J. JUNGE, H. ROED, W. FISCHER-RASMUSSEN & K. HJGAARD. 1986. Endoscann cell sampling for cytological assessment of endometrial pathology. Acta Obstet. Gynecol. Scand. **65**: 397.
53. SCHNEIDER, M. L. 1986. Localization of endometrial hyperplasias and their nuclear morphology. Geburt. Frauenheilkd. **46**: 381.
54. SKAARLAND, E. 1986. New concept in diagnostic endometrial cytology: Diagnostic criteria based on composition and architecture of large tissue fragments in smears. J. Clin. Pathol. **39**: 36.
55. CAROTI, S. & F. SILIOTTI. 1987. Comparison between the diagnostic validity of cytology and histology in preneoplastic and neoplastic endometrial pathology. Clin. Exp. Obstet. Gynecol. **14**: 193.
56. POLSON, D. W., A. MORSE & R. W. BEARD. 1984. An alternative to the diagnostic dilatation and curettage endometrial cytology. Br. Med. J. **288**: 981.
57. GRIMES, D. A. 1982. Diagnostic dilatation and curettage: A reappraisal. Am. J. Obstet. Gynecol. **42**: 1.
58. ALBERICO, S., A. ELIA, L. DAL CORSO, G. P. MANDRUZZATO, L. DI BONITO & S. PATRIARCA. 1986. Diagnostic validity of the Vabra curettage. Compared study on 172 patients who underwent Vabra Curettage and the fractional curettage of the uterine cavity. Eur. J. Gynaecol. Oncol. **7**: 135.
59. NGAN, H. Y., C. HSU & H. K. MA. 1987. Diagnosis of endometrial carcinoma by histopathological examination of the endometrial aspirate by the Curity-Isaacs sampler. Aust. N. Z. J. Obstet. Gynaecol. **27**: 234.
60. VALLE, R. F. 1981. Hysteroscopic evaluation of patients with abnormal uterine bleeding. Surg. Gynecol. Obstet. **153**: 521.
61. GIMPELSON, R. J. 1984. Panoramic hysteroscopy with directed biopsies vs. dilatation and curettage for accurate diagnosis. J. Reproduc. Med. **29**: 575.
62. LOFFER, F. D. 1989. Hysteroscopy with selective endometrial sampling compared with D&C

for abnormal uterine bleeding: The value of a negative hysteroscopic view. Obstet. Gynecol. **73**: 16.

63. MENCAGLIA, L., A. PERINO & J. HAMOU. 1987. Hysteroscopy in perimenopausal and postmeno-pausal women with abnormal uterine bleeding. J. Reprod. Med. **32**: 577.

64. OLMERS, R., M. VOLKSEN, W. RATH, A. TEICHMANN & W. KUHN. 1989. Vaginosonographic measurements of the postmenopausal endometrium in the early detection of endometrial cancer. Geburt. Frauenheilkd. **49**: 262.

65. WENTZ, W. B. 1974. Progestin therapy in endometrial hyperplasia. Gynecol. Oncol. **2**: 362.

66. SHERMAN, A. I. & S. BROWN. 1979. The precursors of endometrial carcinoma. Am. J. Obstet. Gynecol. **135**: 947.

67. FERENCZY, A. 1980. The ultrastructural dynamics of endometrial hyperplasia and neoplasia. *In* Advances in Clinical Cytology. L. G. Koss & D. V. Coleman, Eds.:1. Butterworths, London.

68. KUCERA, F. 1957. The histogenesis of carcinoma of the body of the uterus. Zentralb. Gynaekol. **79**: 345.

69. CORSCADEN, J. A., J. W. FERTIG & S. B. GUSBERG. 1946. Carcinoma subsequent to the radio-therapeutic menopause. Am. J. Obstet. Gynecol. **51**: 1.

70. KISTNER, R. W. 1970. The effects of progestational agents on hyperplasia and carcinoma of the endometrium. Int. J. Gynaecol. Obstet. **8**: 561.

71. STEINER, G. J., R. W. KISTNER & J. M. CRAIG. 1965. Histological effects of progestins on hyper-plasia and carcinoma in situ of the endometrium: Further observation. Metabolism **14**: 356.

72. WENTZ, W. B. 1966. Treatment of persistent endometrial hyperplasia with progestins. Am. J. Obstet. Gynecol. **96**: 999.

73. CHRISTOPHERSON, W. M. & L. A. GRAY. 1981. Premalignant lesions of the endometrium: endo-metrial hyperplasia and adenocarcinoma in situ. *In* Gynaecologic Oncology. M. Coppleson, Ed.: 531. Churchill-Livingstone, New York.

74. FERENCZY, A. & M. GELFAND. 1989. The biologic significance of cytologic atypia in progestogen-treated endometrial hyperplasia. Am. J. Obstet. Gynecol. **160**: 126.

75. GAL, D. 1986. Hormonal therapy for lesions of the endometrium. Semin. Oncol. **13**: 33.

76. WENTZ, W. B. 1964. Effect of a progestional agent on endometrial hyperplasia and endometrial cancer. Obstet. Gynecol. **24**: 370.

77. WENTZ, W. B. 1966. Treatment of persistent endometrial hyperplasia with progestagen. Am. J. Obstet. Gynecol. **96**: 999.

78. DALLENBACH-HELLWEG, G., B. CZERNOBILSKY & J. ALLEMANN. 1986. Medroxyprogesterone acetate in adenomatous hyperplasia of the uterine endometrium. Clinical and morphologic studies on the duration and dosage of gestagen therapy. Geburt. Frauenheilkd. **46**: 601.

79. PERINO, A., P. QUARTARARO, E. CATINELLA, G. GENOVA & E. CITTADINI. 1987. Treatment of endometrial hyperplasia with levonorgestrel releasing intrauterine devices. Acta Eur. Fertil. **18**: 137.

80. SCARSELLI, G., C. TANTINI, M. COLAFRANCESCHI, G. L. TADDEI, G. BARGELLI, N. VENTURINI & F. BRANCONI. 1988. Levo-nor-gestrel-nova-T and precancerous lesions of the endometrium. Eur. J. Gynaecol. Oncol. **9**: 284.

81. IKEGAMI, H., N. TERAKAWA & I. SHIMIZU. 1986. Danazol binds to progesterone receptors and inhibits the growth of human endometrial cancer cells in vitro. Am. J. Obstet. Gynecol. **155**: 857.

82. TERAKAWA, N., M. INOUE, I. SHIMIZU & H. IKEGAMI. 1988. Preliminary report on the use of Danazol in the treatment of endometrial adenomatous hyperplasia. Cancer **62**: 2618.

83. GOLDRATH, M. H. 1986. Hysteroscopic laser obliteration of the endometrium. *In* Gynecologic Laser Surgery. F. Sharp & M. A. Jordan, Eds.: 357. Perinatology Press, Ithaca, NY.

84. LOFFER, F. D. 1987. Hysteroscopic endometrial ablation with the Nd:Yag using a nontouch tech-nique. Obstet. Gynecol. **69**: 679.

85. NEUWIRTH, R. S., A. R. HUSSEIN, B. M. SCHIFFMAN & H. K. AMIN. 1982. Hysteroscopic re-section of intrauterine scars using a new technique. Obstet. Gynecol. **60**: 111.

86. HAMOU, J., L. MENCAGLIA, A. PERINO & G. GILARDI. 1988. L'electrocoaulation en hysteros-copie et microcolpohysteroscopie operatoire. *In* Isteroscopia Operativa e Laser Chirurgia in Ginecologia. E. Cittadini, G. Scarselli, L. Mencaglia & A. Perino, Eds.: 31. CIC Interna-tional Ed., Roma.

The Effect of Progestin on Factors Influencing Growth and Invasion of Endometrial Carcinoma

V. M. JASONNI,[a,b] C. BULLETTI,[b] M. BALDUCCI,[b]
S. NALDI,[b] G. MARTINELLI,[c] A. GALASSI,[d]
AND C. FLAMIGNI[b]

[b]Reproductive Medicine Unit
Department of Obstetrics and Gynecology
University of Bologna
40138 Bologna, Italy

[c]Department of Pathology
University of Bologna
Via Massarenti 9
40138 Bologna, Italy

[d]Department of Pathology
Bassano del Grappa General Hospital
Via delle Fosse 43
36025 Bassano del Grappa (VI), Italy

INTRODUCTION

Progesterone (P) and synthetic progestins play an important role in the control of endometrial growth. These steroids exert their action mainly via a "down regulation" of cellular estradiol receptors (E_2R). However this mechanism is not sufficient to explain fully the control of estrogenicity in the endometrium. Other factors such as increased sensitivity of endometrium to estrogen and variations in estrogen influx may be involved. Furthermore there is increasing evidence that the endometrium has the ability to synthesize its own hormones thereby becoming independent of hormones from the blood stream. In the present paper we will attempt to examine the effect of P and progestins on the estrogen endometrial uptake, basement membranes (BMs) and some growth factors such as epidermal growth factor receptor (EGFr) and transforming growth factor-alpha (TGF-α).

MATERIALS AND METHODS

The studies on estrogen influx into the endometrium were done using isolated human uteri maintained with extracorporeal perfusion as previously described.[1] Immunohisto-

[a] Address for correspondence: Valerio M. Jasonni, MD, Reproductive Medicine Unit, Dept. Ob/Gyn, University of Bologna, Via Massarenti, 13, 40138 Bologna, Italy (Tel. 051-343934; Fax 051-342820).

chemical detection for laminin and collagen type IV were carried out as previously described.[2]

Endometrial samples were obtained at the S. Orsola General Hospital of the University of Bologna, Italy, by curettage or hysterectomy during routine diagnostic or therapeutic procedures from 19 patients ranging from 21 to 64 years of age. All patients gave free consent to participate in this study and did not take exogenous therapy for at least 2 years before the study. Three women were in the proliferative (days 6 to 14) and three in the secretory phase. Endometrial biopsies of typical adenomatous hyperplasia were obtained from 6 women (age 38–51) with menstrual irregularities, four of atypical adenomatous hyperplasia (age 38–59), one of these evolved to adenocarcinoma. Three well-differentiated adenocarcinoma tissue samples were obtained from postmenopausal women aged 51–64. Specimens were fixed in 10% buffered formalin, embedded in paraffin and cut in serial section about 6μm thick and stained with hematoxylin-eosin for histological diagnosis. Menstrual dating was effected using the method of Noyes *et. al.*,[3] while endometrial hyperplasia and carcinoma were evaluated according to Di Saia and Creasman.[4]

Paraffin sections were attached to slides with polylysine for immunohistochemistry, deparaffinized in xylene, and rehydrated in graded alcohols and distilled water. Primary antisera used were: monoclonal mouse anti-EGFr (Cambridge Res., Lab; Cambridge, UK);[5] polyclonal rabbit anti-TGF-α (Oncogene Science, Inc., USA); Dilutions were 1/400, 1/10, 1/400 respectively for EGFr, TGF-α. The secondary antiserum, Biotinilated rabbit anti-mouse and goat anti-rabbit, were purchased from Sclavo (Siena, Italy) and were used diluted 1/50 for 30 minutes. ABC alkaline phosphatase were purchased from Dako, Copenhagen, Denmark.

The slides were flooded with Fast-Red GBC salt naftol AS-BI phosphatase plus 0.01% levamisole, and subsequently rinsed in tap water before dehydration in ethanol and xylene and mounting with Permount (Fisher Scientific, Fairlawn, NJ).

RESULTS AND DISCUSSION

The estrogen influx into endometrium was significantly different in the proliferative and secretory phase, the estradiol (E_2) and estrone (E_1) uptake being lower in the latter.[6]

On the other hand, this difference was not observed when E_2 and E_1 were administered using Ringer's solution instead of human plasma (FIG. 1).

Since the biological effects of steroids are functions of their availability in the tissues, this different uptake is important. Probably alterations in BM structure and functions can increase the permeability to proteins such as albumin. When the neovascularization is forming, as occurs in the proliferative phase, the BM structure may not be completed and their functions may not mature. Moreover, in secretory endometrium the BM are also present around stromal cells.[2] This presence appears specific for P action and could be regarded as a barrier that is encountered by steroids in their diffusion into the tissue. Considering the role of stromal-epithelial interaction, the stromal BMs might play a role in mediating the estrogen action in the endometrium. The BMs, besides the boundary function also have the function of a substratum that acts as a solid support anchoring cells and integrating cellular events into outcomes at tissue level. Therefore BMs around stromal cells induced by P and progestins, might be more than just a simple barrier. The substratum function of BMs can coordinate

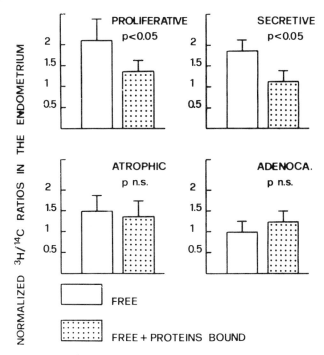

FIGURE 1. ^{3}H-Estradiol/^{14}C-estrone administration in human perfused uteri.

the cell movements, their proliferation and protein synthesis modulating the paracrine signals between stroma and epithelium. Progestin as Danazol was able to induce BMs in stromal cells even in cases of endometrial carcinoma (TABLE 1) and to restore the defective and discontinued BMs around epithelial glands in case of hyperplasia. The visual evidence of BM fragmentation does not prove an increase of estrogen influx into epithelial glands. However the loss of these barriers between interstitium and glands suggests this hypothesis.

Estrogens are known mitogens for estrogen-sensitive cells and evidence is accumulating that these steroids are able to induce the synthesis of auto-stimulatory growth factors and their receptors.[7] Estrogen administration stimulates the EGFr levels in uterine tissue as well as breast cancer cells.[7,8] The EGFr provided the first direct support for a relation between growth factors and oncogenes. The v-erb B protein is a truncated version of the EGFr that lacks most of the extracellular binding domain but shares most homology in the tyrosine protein kinase domain. Furthermore, EGFr are able to bind closely related EGF growth factors such as TGF-α. The latter is present in tumor cells and cells transformed by retroviruses, oncogenes and chemicals. Estrogens may also cause the release of TGF-α from hormone-sensitive, breast-cancer cell lines, and this peptide may mediate the growth response.[9]

In this preliminary study we investigated using immunochemistry EGFr and TGF-α staining in normal and pathologic endometrium. The data are summarized in TABLES 2–5.

TABLE 1. Basement Membrane Immunoreactivity of Hyperplastic and Carcinomatous Endometrium

| | Number of Cases Tested | Number of Anti-lamin Cases Positive (%) | | | | | |
| | | Before Treatment[a] | | | After Treatment[a] | | |
		Vessels	Glands	Stromal Cells	Vessels	Glands	Stromal Cells
Adenomatous hyperplasia	43	43 (100%)	43 (100%) defective and discontinued	19 (44%)	43 (100%)	43 (100%)	43 (100%)
Endometrial adenocarcinoma	23	20 (87%)	3 (13%) defective and discontinued	0 (0%)	22 (96%)	3 (13%)	19 (83%)

[a] Danazol 600 mg/day for 20–30 days.

TABLE 2. EGFr and TGF-α During Normal Cycles (6 Cases)

	Mid-Proliferative	Mid-Secretive
EGFr	+ + + (Ep. cells)	− − −
TGF-α	− − −	− − −

TABLE 3. EGFr and TGF-α in Typical Endometrial Hyperplasia Treated with Danazol 400 mg/day for 6 Months (6 Cases)

	Before	After
EGFr		
Glandular cells	+ + +	− − −
Endothelial cells	+ + +	+ + +
Stromal cells	− − −	− − −
TGF-α		
Glandular cells	+ + −	− − −
Endothelial cells	− − −	− − −
Stromal cells	− − −	− − −

The disappearance of EGFr positivity is evident during the luteal phase. The same was observed after Danazol treatment in cases of endometrial hyperplasia, TGF-α staining also disappeared.

These results strongly suggest that progestins may act by inhibiting the growth factors induced by estrogens, obtaining the control of endometrial growth. However, in one case of atypical adenomatous hyperplasia which evolved to endometrial cancer, despite Danazol treatment, as well as in cancer, the therapy was unable to suppress the presence of EGFr while TGF-α disappeared. Considering the role of TGF-α in

TABLE 4. EGFr and TGF-α in Atypical Endometrial Hyperplasia Treated with Danazol 400 mg/day for 3 Months (4 Cases)

	Before	After
EGFr		
Glandular Cells	+ + +	− − −
		+ + + (1 case[a])
Endothelial cells	+ + +	+ + +
Stromal cells	− − −	− − −
TGF-α		
Glandular cells	+ + −	− − −
Endothelial cells	− − −	− − −
Stromal cells	− − −	− − −

[a] Evolved to adenocarcinoma.

TABLE 5. EGFr and TGF-α in Well-Differentiated Adenocarcinoma Treated with Danazol 400 mg/day for 20 Days (3 Cases)

	Before	After
EGFr	+ + +	+ + +
TGF-α	+ − −	− − −

angiogenesis, responsible for vessels invasion of tumors. The suppressive effect of Danazol might be regarded as one of the inhibitory action of progestins in pathologic endometrium. The length of treatment was, of course, short, just twenty days, as compared to the cases where the control biopsies showed the morphological regression of endometrial hyperplasia. Therefore this lack of suppressive effect of Danazol on EGFr staining could be due to this shorter duration of therapy. However, it is reasonable to suppose that EGFr could become autonomous and then not respond to exogenous steroids under these pathologic conditions. The relatively small number of cases does not permit an explanation to be made of why the TGF-α staining is inhibited by Danazol in all conditions whereas EGFr are unaffected when the treatment is unable to suppress the hyperplasia or in case of cancer. Obviously it is hazardous on the basis of these data to conclude that EGFr staining is a marker of progestin effect in the endometrium and further studies are needed.

However these aspects of steroids action on tissues should be regarded as a possible way to throw new light on the problem of endometrial growth control.

SUMMARY

Progesterone (P) and progestins play an important role in the control of endometrial growth. We have investigated P and progestin effects on endometrial estrogen extraction, on basement membrane (BM) synthesis and on the presence of the epidermal growth factor receptor (EGFr) in normal and pathologic endometrium. E2 uptake, evaluated in human isolated perfused uteri is significantly decreased by P. BMs investigated using immunohistochemistry, with antisera to collagen IV and laminin, were found around stromal cells only in the luteal phase or during P or progestin administration. Glandular BM, discontinuous in hyperplastic and carcinomatous endometria, were restored to integrity only in typical hyperplasia after therapy with progestin. Endometrial EGFr is modified by P: revelation of this antigen is increased in proliferative phase and decreased in secretory phase. Similarly this molecule was present in hyperplastic and carcinomatous endometria. Only in benign hyperplasia did we observe no staining for the same antigen after progestinic therapy. These data suggest that P or progestins may also have an indirect influence through mechanisms such as estrogen uptake and tissue factor activity with important differences between normal and pathologic endometrium.

REFERENCES

1. BULLETTI, C., V. M. JASONNI, S. LUBICZ, C. FLAMIGNI & E. GURPIDE. 1986. Extracorporeal perfusion of the human uterus. Am. J. Obstet Gynecol. **154:** 683–688.
2. BULLETTI, C., A. GALASSI, V. M. JASONNI, G. MARTINELLI, S. TABANELLI & C. FLAMIGNI. 1988. Basement membrane components in normal, hyperplastic and neoplastic endometrium. Cancer **62:** 142–149.
3. NOYES, R. W., A. T. HERTIG & J. ROCK. 1950. Dating the endometrial biopsy. Fertil. Steril. **1:** 3–15.
4. DISAIA, P. J. & W. T. CREASMAN, Eds. 1989. Clinical Gynecologic Oncology, 3rd Edit. St. Louis, Washington D.C., Toronto, The C. V. Mosby Company.
5. PARKER, T. J., S. YOUNG, W. J. GULLICH, E. L. MAYES, P. BENNET & M. D. WATERFIELD. 1984. Monoclonal antibody against the human epidermal growth factor receptor from A 431 cells. J. Biol. Chem. **259:** 9906–9910.
6. BULLETTI, C., V. M. JASONNI, P. M. CIOTTI, S. TABANELLI, S. NALDI & C. FLAMIGNI. 1988. Extraction of estrogens by human perfused uterus. Am. J. Obstet. Gynecol. **159:** 509–515.
7. DICKSON, R. B. & M. E. LIPPMAN. 1987. Estrogenic regulation of growth and polypeptide growth factor secretion in human breast carcinoma. Endocrinol. Rev. **8:** 29–43.
8. MUKKU, V. R. & G. M. STANCEL. 1985. Regulation of epidermal growth factor receptor by estrogen. J. Biol. Chem. **260:** 9820–9824.
9. LIPPMAN, M. E., R. B. DICKSON & S. BATES. 1986. Autocrine and paracrine growth regulation of human breast cancer. Breast Cancer Res. Treat. **7:** 59–70.

Effects of Tamoxifen on the Female Genital Tract

TOMMY FORNANDER,[a] LARS E. RUTQVIST,
AND NILS WILKING

Radiumhemmet
Karolinska Hospital
S-104 01 Stockholm, Sweden

INTRODUCTION

Tamoxifen is one of several triphenylethylene derivatives, all of which are partial estrogen agonists/antagonists. These agents are non-steroidal and show many structural similarities to one another.[1] In human breast cancer the anti-tumor effect has been suggested to be mainly anti-estrogenic through a competitive blockade of the estrogen receptors (ER).[2,3] Other mechanisms, however, have been suggested to explain the objective response that occasionally can be seen in ER-negative tumors.[4-9] Other anti-estrogens with different estrogen and anti-estrogen properties than tamoxifen may give an increased knowledge about the control of the normal or malignant breast cell growth and may possibly be more useful in the clinical setting. The research for new such agents is intense and follows two directions: the development of other triphenylethylene agents with less prominent estrogenic effects or the development of steroid-based molecules without estrogenic properties.[10,11]

In animal studies the balance between the antiestrogenic and estrogenic effect of tamoxifen has been shown to be both organ- and species specific.[4,12] In premenopausal women tamoxifen is mainly an anti-estrogenic compound. This mode of action is probably due to the blockade of the high endogenous estrogen levels in young women. In post-menopausal women, however, there are substantial evidence for a predominantly estrogenic effect of tamoxifen in several organ systems, *e.g.*, the pituitary, the liver and the skeleton.[13-18]

The acute side effects of tamoxifen are few and usually mild, which have made the substance extremely useful for adjuvant treatment of breast cancer.[12] An overview of all available trials of adjuvant tamoxifen in early breast cancer indicated a significant improvement of both recurrence-free survival and overall survival in postmenopausal patients.[19] Animal data suggest that long-term treatment might be superior to short-term treatment. Five years or even lifelong treatment has been suggested, but the optimal duration is currently not known.[20] Tamoxifen may possibly be of benefit for chemoprevention of breast cancer and there now are on-going controlled trials in healthy high-risk women.[21-23] The benign indications that have been suggested include prevention of arteriosclerosis and osteoporosis. These circumstances emphasize the need to monitor on-going adjuvant tamoxifen trials for long-term adverse effects, partic-

---

[a] Author to whom correspondence should be addressed.

ularly with regard to certain target tissues for estrogenic action, *e.g.*, the endometrium, the liver, and bone.

CLINICAL OBSERVATIONS

The Stockholm trial of adjuvant tamoxifen in early breast cancer was initiated in 1976.[24] After surgery, postmenopausal women were randomized between adjuvant tamoxifen 40mg daily for 2 years versus no adjuvant endocrine therapy. Patients from the tamoxifen group who were disease-free at two years were randomized to stop treatment after 2 years or to continue for 3 more years — *i.e.*, a total treatment period of 5 years (FIG. 1). From 1976 through 1986 a total of 1846 patients were included in the trial. The median follow-up time was 4.5 years. At present the median duration of tamoxifen therapy in the 5-year group was 3.8 years. The frequency of hysterectomy was similar, about 2%, in the tamoxifen group and in the controls.

TABLE 1 presents preliminary data from a study of hospital admissions among the patients included in the trial. The study was based on a register of hospital admissions including discharge diagnoses. This register covers about 95% of all admissions in the Stockholm region.[25,26] The difference in the number of admissions due to uterine bleeding among treated and control patients was small, but admissions because of endometrial cancer and miscellaneous gynecologic disorders was increased in the tamoxifen-treated group. TABLE 2 shows a more detailed analysis of the gynecologic diagnoses. At least 8 of the tamoxifen patients were treated for disorders which can be related to estrogenic stimulation of the endometrial or vaginal epithelium compared to none in the control group. It should be emphasized that these numbers only represent hospitalized patients, *i.e.*, patients with severe symptoms. Patients treated on an out-patient basis were not included in the analysis.

These data indicate that tamoxifen has predominantly estrogenic effects on the female genital tract. This observation accords with previous reports. In 1980, Clark showed that clomiphene (a triphenylethylene derivative) had estrogenic effects in the uterine epithelium of the baboon and concluded that this might have implications for

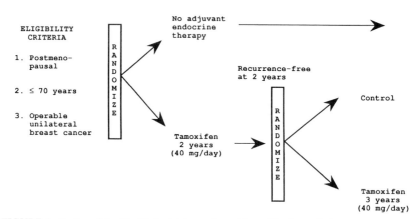

FIGURE 1. Design of the Stockholm trial on adjuvant tamoxifen for early breast cancer.

TABLE 1. Number of First Hospital Admissions for Gynecologic Disease According to Allocated Treatment and Main Diagnosis

Diagnosis	Tamoxifen (n=931)	Control (n=915)	RR of Admission TAM vs. Control (95% C. I.)
Uterine cancer	10	3	2.7 (0.9–8.1)
Benign gynecologic disorders			
Uterine prolapse	14	12	1.0 (0.5–2.2)
Uterine bleeding	28	23	1.1 (0.7–1.9)
Miscellaneous	13	3	3.2 (1.2–8.6)

the risk of endometrial tumors with both clomiphene and tamoxifen in humans.[27] In contrast, Kauppila found that clomiphene in cyclical treatment of postmenopausal women receiving estrogen replacement treatment reduced vaginal cornification and endometrial hypertrophy.[28] However, these results are difficult to interpret because clomiphene is a mixture of the estrogenic *cis*-isomer and the anti-estrogenic *trans*-isomer. Tamoxifen, on the other hand has mainly estrogenic effects on the vaginal epithelium, and has been associated with intrauterine polyps and hyperplasia.[29-32]

SECOND CANCERS

Estrogens are known to increase the risk for certain cancers. It is thus warranted to study the cancer incidence during long-term tamoxifen therapy.[33] Information on second cancers among patients included in the mentioned Stockholm trial was obtained from the Swedish Cancer Registry. The completeness of this register has been estimated at about 96%.[34,35]

TABLE 3 shows the total number of new primary cancers, the number of second breast cancers and uterine cancers by allocated treatment. The total number of new primary cancers in any site was decreased in the tamoxifen group, but the difference was not statistically significant. The number of second breast cancers was significantly decreased and the number of uterine cancers was significantly increased in the tamoxifen

TABLE 2. Number of First Hospital Admissions for Miscellaneous Benign Gynecological Disorders According to Allocated Treatment

Diagnosis	Tamoxifen (n=931)	Control (n=915)
Leukorrhea	4	
Intrauterine polyps	3	
Endometrial hyperplasia	1	
Dysplasia of uterine cervix	2	2
Polyps of uterine cervix	1	1
Ovarian cyst	1	
Pelvic adhesions	1	
TOTAL	13	3

TABLE 3. Number of New Primary Cancers According to Allocated Treatment

Site	TAM (n=931)	Control (n=915)	p^a
Breast	18	32	0.05
Uterus			
Cervix	1	2	n.s.
Corpus	13	2	<0.01
Any site	57	70	n.s.

^{a} n.s., $p > 0.05$.

group. The greatest cumulative frequency of endometrial cancer was observed among those who were allocated to 5 years of tamoxifen (data not shown). The histopathological specimens for all cases of uterine cancer were reviewed by a senior pathologist. All tumors were infiltrative and the tumors in the tamoxifen group were all found to be endometrial epithelial malignancies. These observations were not confirmed by the Scottish adjuvant tamoxifen trial, but the number of second cancers in that study was small and the results were inconclusive.[36-38]

EXPERIMENTAL RESULTS

In addition to the reports from the Stockholm and Scottish trials and a few case reports, there are still few reports about second cancers with long-term adjuvant tamoxifen for early breast cancer.[39-41] Animal and *in vitro* data support the hypothesis of a clinically important stimulation of the endometrium by tamoxifen and other putative anti-estrogens. In 1984, Satyaswaroop *et al.*[42] reported estrogen-like effects of tamoxifen on human endometrial carcinoma transplanted into nude mice. This observation was confirmed by Gottardis *et al.* (1988)[43] who also reported contrasting actions of tamoxifen on endometrial tumor growth and hormone dependent breast tumor growth in athymic mice. Furthermore, they observed that the growth stimulation of endometrial cancer was higher with the combination of tamoxifen and estradiol than with estradiol alone. These effects have also been studied *in vitro*. Friedl *et al.*[44] reported an increased growth of ER-positive endometrial cancer with the combination of estradiol and tamoxifen, compared to estradiol or no treatment. Tamoxifen appears to stimulate growth in ER-negative endometrial cancer, although tamoxifen may inhibit the growth stimulation obtained with estradiol. Anzai *et al.*[45] studied the effect of the active 4-hydroxylated tamoxifen metabolite on the growth of Ishikawa human endometrial adenocarcinoma cells. They found a greater growth stimulation with 4-hydroxytamoxifen alone or 4-hydroxytamoxifen plus estradiol than with estradiol alone. The effect was dose dependent. Tamoxifen was less potent than estradiol at low concentrations, but had twice the effect obtained with estradiol at high concentrations. 4-Hydroxytamoxifen was also found to have a proliferative effect on an estradiol unresponsive cell line.

The mechanism of tamoxifen effects on the endometrium is not known. Although a direct estrogenic agonistic effect at the tissue level seems obvious, the effect may also be mediated through secretion of growth factors or through an androgenic effect. Previous reports indicate that endometrial pathology may be correlated to androgenic influences.[46-48] Androgenic effects of tamoxifen may be secondary to effects on sex hormone–binding globulin, i.e., the levels of unbound, biologically active androgens may be increased.

Another possibility is an influence of tamoxifen on the intra-adrenal steroidogenic pathways.[46,49] Unfortunately, the effect of tamoxifen on adrenal steroid synthesis in postmenopausal women is not well known.[50] Preliminary data on the effects of tamoxifen on, for example, IGF-1 (somatomedin C) levels and corticotropin-induced steroid levels indicate that such effects may be of clinical significance (Fornander, unpublished data).

TREATMENT OF ENDOMETRIAL CANCER

Tamoxifen has been reported to be useful for second line treatment of endometrial cancer.[51,52] The benefit can possibly be further increased if the drug is given in combination or sequence with progesterone.[53] Therefore, the clinical observation of an increased risk of endometrial cancer with tamoxifen seems like a paradox. However, both experimental and clinical data support the possibility of a proliferative action of tamoxifen on the endometrial epithelium and certain subclones of endometrial cancer. Potential hazards of tamoxifen treatment of endometrial cancer therefore warrant further investigations.

CONCLUSIONS

In summary, the increased incidence of endometrial cancer with long-term tamoxifen limits the usefulness of the drug for benign indications. However, in the adjuvant setting, the improvement of both recurrence-free survival and overall survival among patients with breast cancer, probably outweighs the potential hazards. The possibility of growth stimulation of tumor subclones should be considered when tamoxifen is used for treatment of endometrial cancer.

SUMMARY

Tamoxifen is a widely used drug in medical oncology, mainly for treatment of breast cancer, but also for second line treatment of endometrial cancer. We recently reported an increased incidence of endometrial cancer associated with long-term adjuvant tamoxifen. This observation, previous reports of stimulatory effects of tamoxifen in the female genital tract, and experimental data are in accordance with a mainly estrogenic effect of tamoxifen in these tissues. An increased incidence of endometrial cancer may limit the usefulness of tamoxifen for benign indications. For adjuvant treatment of early breast cancer, however, the improvement of both recurrence-free survival and overall survival probably outweighs the increased frequency of uterine tumors. However, the possibility of growth stimulation of tumor subclones should be considered when tamoxifen is used in the treatment of endometrial cancer.

REFERENCES

1. SUTHERLAND, R. L. & V. C. JORDAN. 1981. Non-steroidal antioestrogens. Sydney, Academic Press.
2. JORDAN, V. C. 1974. Antitumor activity of antiestrogen ICI 46, 474 (tamoxifen) in dimethyl-benzantracene (DMBA)-induced rat mammary carcinoma model. J. Steroid Biochem. 4: 354.
3. LIPPMAN, M., G. BOLAN & K. HUFF. 1976. Interactions of antiestrogen with human breast cancer in long-term tissue culture. Cancer Treat. Rep. 60: 1421–1429.
4. PATTERSON, M. B., B. FURR, A. WAKELING, et al. 1982. The biology and physiology of "Nolvadex" (tamoxifen) in the treatment of breast cancer. Breast Cancer Res. Treat. 2: 363–374.
5. O'BRIAN, C. A., R. M. LISKAMP, D. H. SOLOMON, et al. 1985. Inhibition of protein kinase C by tamoxifen. Cancer Res 45: 2462–2465.
6. HORGAN, K., E. COOKE, M. B. HALLETT, et al. 1986. Inhibition of protein kinase C mediated signal transduction by tamoxifen. Biochem. Pharmacol. 35: 4463–4465.
7. GULINO, A., G. BARRERA, A. VACCA, et al. 1986. Calmodulin antagonism and growth-inhibiting activity of triphenylethylene antiestrogens in MCF-7 human breast cancer cells. Cancer Res. 46: 6274–6278.
8. SUTHERLAND, R. L., C. K. W. WATTS, R. E. HALL, et al. 1987. Mechanisms of growth inhibition by nonsteroidal antioestrogens in human breast cancer cells. J. Steroid Biochem. 27: 891–897.
9. JORDAN, V. C. 1989. Resistance to antioestrogen therapy: A challenge for the future. In Endocrine Therapy of Breast Cancer III. F. Cavalli, Ed. European School of Oncology-Monographs. U. Vermesi, Series Ed. Springer-Verlag.
10. WAKELING, A. E. & J. BOWLER. 1988. Biology and mode of action of pure antioestrogens. J. Steroid Biochem. 30: 141–147.
11. WAKELING, A. E. 1989. New antioestrogens without oestrogenic activity. In Endocrine Therapy of Breast Cancer III. F. Cavalli, Ed. European School of Oncology-Monographs. U. Vermesi, Series Ed. Springer-Verlag.
12. FURR, B. & V. C. JORDAN. 1984. The pharmacology and clinical uses of tamoxifen. Pharmacol. Ther. 25: 127–205.
13. HELGASON, S., N. WILKING, K. CARLSTRÖM, et al. 1982. A comparative study of the estrogenic effects of tamoxifen and 17beta-estradiol in postmenopausal women. J. Endocrinol. Metab. 54: 404–408.
14. RÖSSNER, S. & A. WALLGREN. 1984. Serum lipoproteins and proteins after breast cancer surgery and effects of tamoxifen. Atherosclerosis 52: 339–346.
15. BRUNING, P. F., J. M. G. BONFRER, A. A. M. HART, et al. 1988. Tamoxifen, serum lipoproteins and cardiovascular risk. Br. J. Cancer 58: 497–499.
16. BOCCARDO, F., D. GUARNERI, A. RUBAGOTTI, et al. 1984. Endocrine effects of tamoxifen in postmenopausal breast cancer patients. Tumori 70: 61–68.
17. TURKEN, S., E. SIRIS, D. SELDIN, et al. 1989. Effects of Tamoxifen on spinal bone density in 10 postmenopausal women with breast cancer. J. Natl. Cancer Inst. 81: 1086–1088.
18. FORNANDER, T., L. E. RUTQVIST & H.-E. SJÖBERG. 1989. Long-term adjuvant tamoxifen in early breast cancer: Risk of accelerated bone loss? Twenty-Fifth Annual Meeting of the American Society of Clinical Oncology. San Francisco, CA (meeting abstract).
19. EARLY BREAST CANCER TRIALISTS' COLLABORATIVE GROUP. 1988. Effects of tamoxifen and of cytotoxic therapy on mortality in early breast cancer: An overview of 61 randomized trials among 28,896 women. N. Engl. J. Med. 319: 1681–1692.
20. WALLGREN, A., E. BARAL, J. CARSTENSEN, et al. 1984. Should adjuvant tamoxifen be given for several years in breast cancer? In Adjuvant Therapy of Breast Cancer. S. E. Jones & S. E. Salmon, Eds. :331–337. Grune and Stratton, New York.
21. FENTIMAN, I. S. 1989. The endocrine prevention of breast cancer. Br. J. Cancer 60: 12–14.
22. CUZICK, J., D. Y. WANG & R. D. BULBROOK. 1986. The prevention of breast cancer. Lancet i: 83–86.
23. POWLES, T. J., J. R. HARDY, S. E. ASHLEY, et al. 1989. Chemoprevention of breast cancer. Breast Cancer Res. Treat. 14: 23–31.
24. RUTQVIST, L. E., B. CEDERMARK, U. GLAS, et al. 1987. The Stockholm trial on adjuvant tamoxifen in early breast cancer. Br. Cancer Res. Treat. 10: 255–266.
25. STOCKHOLMS LÄNS LANDSTING. 1987. Hälso- och sjukvårdsstatistik 1976–88. Stockholms läns landsting Stockholm 1977–89. (In Swedish.)

26. LEIMANIS, A. 1989. Personal communication. Stockholms läns landsting, HSN/GEMI Box 9099, S-102 72 Stockholm, Sweden.

27. CLARK, J. H., S. A. MCCORMACK, R. KLING, *et al.* 1980. Effect of Clomiphene and other triphenylene derivates on the reproductive tract in the rat and baboon. *In* Hormones and Cancer. S. Iacobelli, Ed. :295–307. Raven Press, New York.

28. KAUPPILA, A., O. JÄNNE, S. KIVINEN, *et al.* 1981. Postmenopausal hormone replacement therapy with estrogen periodically supplemented with antiestrogen. Am. J. Obstet. Gynecol. **140:** 787–792.

29. FERRAZZI, E., G. CARTEI, R. MATTARAZO, *et al.* 1977. Oestrogen-like effect of tamoxifen on vaginal epithelium. Br. Med. J. **i:** 1351–1352.

30. BOCCARDO, F., P. BRUZZI, A. RUBAGOTTI, *et al.* 1981. Estrogen-like action of tamoxifen on vaginal epithelium in breast cancer patients. Oncology **38:** 281–285.

31. NUOVO, M. A., G. J. NUOVO, R. M. MCCAFFREY, *et al.* 1989. Endometrial polyps in postmenopausal patients receiving tamoxifen. Int. J. Gynecol. Pathol. **8:** 125–131.

32. NEVEN, P., X. DEMUYLDER, Y. VANBELLE, *et al.* 1989. Tamoxifen and the uterus and endometrium. Lancet **i:** 375.

33. HENDERSON, B. E., R. ROSS & L. BERNSTEIN. 1988. Estrogens as a cause of human cancer: The Richard and Hinda Rosenthal Foundation Award Lecture. Cancer Res. **48:** 246–253.

34. MATTSSON, B. & A. WALLGREN. 1984. Completeness of the Swedish Cancer Register. Nonnotified cancer cases recorded on death certificates in 1978. Acta Radiol. Oncol. **23:** 305–313.

35. MATTSSON, B. 1984. Cancer registration in Sweden: Studies on completeness and validity of incidence and mortality registers. University of Stockholm.

36. FORNANDER, T., L. E. RUTQVIST, B. CEDERMARK, *et al.* 1989. Adjuvant tamoxifen in early breast cancer: Occurrence of new primary cancers. Lancet **i:** 117–120.

37. STEWART, H. J. & G. M. KNIGHT. 1989. Tamoxifen and the uterus and endometrium. Lancet **i:** 375–376.

38. FORNANDER, T. & L. E. RUTQVIST. 1989. Adjuvant tamoxifen and second cancers. Lancet **i:** 616.

39. RIBEIRO, G. & R. SWINDELL. 1988. The Christie hospital adjuvant tamoxifen trial: Status at 10 years. Br. J. Cancer **57:** 601–603.

40. FISHER, B., J. COSTANTINO, C. REDMOND, *et al.* 1989. A randomized clinical trial evaluating tamoxifen in the treatment of patients with node-negative breast cancer who have estrogen-receptor-positive tumors. N. Engl. J. Med. **320:** 479–484.

41. CASTIGLIONE, M., R. D. GELBER & A. GOLDHIRSCH. 1990. Adjuvant systemic therapy for breast cancer in the elderly: Competing causes of mortality. J. Clin. Oncol. **8:** 519–526.

42. SATYASWAROOP, P. G., R. J. ZAINO & R. MORTEL. 1984. Estrogen-like effects of tamoxifen on human endometrial carcinoma transplanted into nude mice. Cancer Res. **44:** 4006–4010.

43. GOTTARDIS, M. M., S. P. ROBINSON, P. G. SATYASWAROOP, *et al.* 1988. Contrasting action of tamoxifen on endometrial and breast growth in the athymic mouse. Cancer Res. **48:** 812–815.

44. FRIEDL, A., M. M. GOTTARDIS, J. PINK, *et al.* 1989. Enhanced growth of an estrogen receptor-negative endometrial adenocarcinoma by estradiol in athymic mice. Cancer Res. **49:** 4758–4764.

45. ANZAI, Y., C. F. HOLINKA, H. KURAMOTO, *et al.* 1989. Stimulatory effects of 4-hydroxytamoxifen on proliferation of human endometrial adenocarcinoma cells (Ishikawa Line). Cancer Res. **49:** 2362–2365.

46. BRODY, S., K. CARLSTRÖM, A. LAGRELIUS, *et al.* 1982. Adrenocortical steroids, bone mineral content and endometrial condition in post-menopausal women. Maturitas **4:** 113–122.

47. GRATTAROLA, R. 1982. Increased androgenic activity in well-differentiated endometrial adenocarcinoma. Gynecol. Oncol. **14:** 40–48.

48. MARKIEWICZ, L. & E. GURPIDE. 1988. C19-adrenal steroids enhance prostaglandin F2-alpha output by human endometrium in vitro. Am. J. Obstet. Gynecol. **159:** 500–504.

49. BRODY, S., K. CARLSTRÖM, A. LAGRELIUS, *et al.* 1987. Serum sex hormone binding globulin (SHBG), testosterone/SHBG index, endometrial pathology and bone mineral density in postmenopausal women. Acta Obstet. Gynecol. Scand. **66:** 357–360.

50. WILKING, N., K. CARLSTRÖM, H. SKÖLDEFORS, *et al.* 1982. Effects of tamoxifen on the serum levels of oestrogens and adrenocortical steroids in postmenopausal breast cancer patients. Acta Chir. Scand. **148:** 345–349.

51. SWENERTON, K. D. 1980. Treatment of advanced endometrial adenocarcinoma with tamoxifen. Cancer Treat. Rep. **64:** 805–811.

52. BONTE, J., P. IDE, G. BILLIET, *et al.* 1981. Tamoxifen as a possible chemotherapeutic agent in endometrial adenocarcinoma. Gynecol. Oncol. **11:** 140–161.
53. BONTE, J., J. P. JANSSENS & P. IDE. 1986. Modalities and results of a combined anti-estrogenic therapy by means of tamoxifen and medroxyprogesterone in gynecologic cancerology. Eur. J. Gynecol. Oncol. **7:** 45–50.

Does Today's Vaginal Surgery Still Have a Specific Role in the Treatment of Endometrial Cancer?

L. CARENZA, C. VILLANI, F. NOBILI,
M. G. PORPORA, A. LUKIC, AND L. FALQUI

Department of Obstetrics and Gynecology
University of Rome, "La Sapienza"
Viale del Policlinico, 155
00161 Rome, Italy

Because of some assumptions which caused delays and confusion in acquiring a more specific knowledge of its natural history, for many years endometrial carcinoma has been considered as a low malignancy neoplasm.

Four so-called "myths"[1] have been dispelled over the years:

Endometrial cancer is a benign disease. Since hysterectomy is the cornerstone of management and in some institutions the only treatment used, this approach suggested that endometrial cancer, along with many other benign gynecologic diseases, should be considered a "milder" tumor among the gynecologic ones. Moreover, since in some reports the 5-year survival rates were particularly high (90–95%), many investigators have suggested that little could be done to improve treatment results in early endometrial cancer. This reinforced the idea that this tumor was a low malignancy neoplasm.

Contemporary gynecologic impressions suggested that endometrial cancer had a better prognosis than cervical cancer. The overall corpus cancer salvage rate is indeed better than that of cervical cancer, but the data analyzed reflect the fact that stage I endometrial cancer was diagnosed considerably more frequently (approx. 75% of the cases) than stage I cervical cancer.

The best way to treat endometrial cancer has been defined. The standard treatment consisted, and still consists of an extrafascial hysterectomy and upper colpectomy, with or without pre- or post-operative radiotherapy (radium or external beam). Although surgery was the first major modality to significantly control endometrial cancer, its general applicability, especially as a single procedure, was very restricted until the 1950s, when adequate blood banking, improved anesthesia, antibiotics and other supportive measures changed the picture. When intracavitary radiation was introduced in 1919, it was apparent that surgery alone could not deal with all problems, and that another treatment modality needed to be involved.

Radiation therapy from the early 1920s on has grown to play a major role: indeed, in many institutions it reduced surgery's role to little more than diagnosis and application of intracavitary radioactive sources.

By the mid 1950s, chemotherapy and hormonal therapy had come into the picture, thus further reducing the role of surgery. The interaction of 90 years of development for both radiation and surgery (even radical hysterectomy) led to the appearance of quite a number of programs involving single or multimodality approaches.

There were those who supported the simplest of procedures and those who supported the fairly complex evaluation. The Mayo Clinic's advocacy of vaginal hysterectomy (with at least half the patients having adnexal removal by the vaginal route) was supported by excellent results (overall 5-year survival rate: 84%). A more extensive surgery was not required, since less than 20% of the patients (lesions with low-grade malignancy, cervical involvement and large palpable lymph-nodes) would benefit, and even if malignancy were found in nodes, their removal and subsequent modification of therapy probably would not lead to better results than those achieved by less radical surgery.[2]

Vaginal hysterectomy has been used by a number of physicians whose results have supported the Mayo Clinic's work. The other extreme was represented by Stallworthy,[3] who stressed the importance of thorough exploration including the evaluation of pelvic and para-aortic nodes. He noted that deep myometrial penetration could mean higher incidence of positive nodes and metastases to other structures. He removed nodes whenever the inspection of the opened specimen indicated deep muscle penetration.

More recently, considerable data have been collected on the treatment of endometrial cancer. Jones[4] extensively reviewed the literature of the 1950s, 1960s and 1970s and noted that the 5-year survival rate for patients treated with surgery alone was essentially the same as for those who were treated with radiation plus surgery. Unfortunately, the vast majority of those reports were not evaluated in regard to the grade of the tumor or myometrial involvement. It is anticipated that many of the patients who were found to have poorly differentiated lesions were more likely to be treated in the combined group and, as a result, would bias the overall survival rate in the combined therapy category.

Furthermore, comparing the 5-year survival rates of the patients with FIGO stage I endometrial carcinoma, it is clear that over the years the differences are not statistically significant.[5,6] This is also confirmed in the overall survival rates: 60%[5] vs. 67.7.[6]

In a recent FIGO Annual Report[7] the 5-year survival rate (all stages) referring to the years 1979–1981 is 72.3%, showing once again that, in spite of the knowledge of its natural history, endometrial carcinoma cannot always be considered as a low malignancy neoplasm. Thus, surgery should be intended: a) to "cure" the patient, b) to outline diagnosis, and c) to delineate prognosis. Although the last two items have undoubtedly improved over the years, it seems that, concerning early stage endometrial carcinoma, nothing has changed in terms of cure from the results of 15 years ago.

The prognostic factors have been sufficiently elucidated. In 1962 Gusberg anticipated that "studies of the biology of this tumor have afforded us greater insight into its histogenesis, vitality and spread, but lack of agreement about coding these facts into an acceptable pattern of classification has deprived gynecologists of the clinical benefits of this knowledge."[8]

Over the years this fact caused delays in the comparison of various treatment modalities and a tendency to treat all patients with this disease in a standard manner, rather than selecting the most effective treatment with possible diminution in complication rate, thereby improving the recovery state. There was a widespread illusion that treatment of endometrial cancer conferred good results almost universally, but this fallacy is demonstrated when analyzing data from a sufficiently large series of unselected cases.

Over the years great emphasis has been placed on the correlation between the different biologic tumoral parameters and prognosis. These are now considered as real "markers" of aggressiveness and tumor spread.

A large amount of data on this subject[9] clearly shows the importance of pathologic features for a better definition of the tumor extent and possible clues for improving therapy. It is well-established that surgery, besides representing in most instances an adequate therapy (according to Boronow about 75% of cases are at low prognostic risk after surgical staging), allows intensive pathological staging. Indeed all tumoral parameters (TABLE 1) necessary for an accurate prognosis and for a rational use of therapeutic integrations can be obtained through surgery.

Staging criteria recommended by FIGO and universally accepted as methods of evaluation represented an international language for the exchange of data and results, but because of some limitations (*i.e.*, clinical staging instead of a pathological one) they could not select patients in risk categories and did not lead to targeted and individualized treatment programs. Subjective evaluations and inaccurate clinical staging (this was modified in 51% of the patients after surgery in the study by Cowles[10]) undermine the meaning of such a system. In effect the tumor extension, the only parameter taken into consideration, could not fully identify the biologic complexity of the tumor.

During the 1970s and 1980s the growing knowledge of the natural history of endometrial cancer and understanding of the propensity of certain sub-groups for a more aggressive clinical course led to improved pre-surgical diagnostic procedures and therapeutic results.

This influenced the staging system adopted so far. In 1988 such important factors as myometrial invasion, cervical involvement, peritoneal cytology and lymph-node metastases have been introduced in the staging system recommended by FIGO.

Pelvic and aortic nodes are of little or no consequence in endometrial cancer. It is now well-established that about 10% of patients with stage 1 disease show pelvic lymph-node metastases.[9] This incidence, however, is highly affected, both positively or negatively by other prognostic factors (TABLES 2–4). Because of this important observation, lymph-node involvement can be predicted by the assessment of other tumoral parameters such as grade of differentiation, depth of myometrial invasion and less significantly by the stage of the tumor. The therapeutic role of lymphadenectomy has always been very controversial: it did not improve survival rates and the incidence of relapses, it was of little applicability and entailed a high morbidity, especially in obese patients. A para-aortic lymphadenectomy—a very high risk procedure in obese

TABLE 1. Prognostic Factors in Endometrial Carcinoma

• Age	• Capillary-like spaces
• Histologic type	• Tumor size
• Grade	• Adnexal metastases
• Myometrial invasion	• Peritoneal cytology
• Stage	• Tumor ploidy
• Lymph-node metastases	• Growth factors
• Hormonal receptors	

TABLE 2. Grade versus Positive Pelvic and Aortic Nodes: Stage I[a]

Grade	Pelvic	Aortic
G1	3%	2%
G2	9%	5%
G3	18%	11%

[a] Based on Creasman.[13]

TABLE 3. Myometrial Invasion versus Positive Pelvic and Aortic Nodes: Stage I[a]

Myometrial Invasion	Pelvic	Aortic
M0	1%	1%
M1	5%	3%
M2	6%	1%
M3	25%	17%

[a] Based on Creasman.[13]

TABLE 4. Stage versus Positive Pelvic and Aortic Nodes[a]

Stage	Pelvic	Aortic
IA	7%	3%
IB	13%	8%

[a] Based on Creasman.[13]

patients — is recommended only when poor prognostic factors are found: in fact, para-aortic lymph-node metastases in early stages are restricted to poorly differentiated tumors with deep invasion of the myometrium, with a respective incidence of 11% and 17%.

Moreover, other parameters are well correlated to lymph-node involvement: tumor size, capillary-like spaces involvement, and peritoneal cytology. Schink et al.[11] found that the incidence of lymph-node metastases in patients with tumor size <2 cm was only 5.7%. If the tumor was >2 cm in diameter, there were nodal metastases in 21% of cases. If the entire endometrium was involved, the incidence was 40%.

Hanson et al.[12] found capillary-like spaces involvement in patients with poorly differentiated tumors with deep invasion. The incidence of pelvic and para-aortic node metastases, was 27% and 75% respectively. This compares with a 19% occurrence of pelvic node metastases, and 3% occurrence of periaortic node metastases when there is no capillary-like spaces involvement.

Therefore, on the strength of all these data, we think that in order to evaluate the real applicability of vaginal surgery in the treatment of stage I endometrial carcinoma we cannot fail to take into consideration the following elements:

- Endometrial carcinoma is not always a benign disease.
- The best way to treat it has not been completely defined for each individual case.

- Prognostic factors represent the major indicators for planning therapy.
- Pelvic and para-aortic lymph-nodes can be of great consequence in particular high-risk categories.

THE AUTHORS' EXPERIENCE

In the light of recently acquired information on prognostic risk factors, we present a review of our personal experience using the vaginal approach with the purpose of establishing the exact role of vaginal hysterectomy in the management of endometrial carcinoma. Between 1968 and 1985 we performed vaginal hysterectomy in 160 patients with stage I endometrial carcinoma. However, over the years greater selectivity of patients to be treated brought us to use this surgical procedure less frequently. Obesity or major medical problems, such as hypertension, placed these patients at high morbidity risk from an abdominal surgery operation (TABLE 5).

Patients underwent a standard pre-treatment evaluation and were staged according to FIGO staging criteria. All histologic specimens were evaluated, before and after surgery, by a pathologist experienced in gynecologic pathology. We performed a simple vaginal hysterectomy with salpingo-oophorectomy and dissection of the upper third of the vagina. The Schuchardt incision was used in most cases and the margins of the vaginal cuff clamped together with Chrobak clamps in order to envelop the cervix and avoid further neoplastic contamination during hysterectomy.

Vaginal hysterectomy was the only therapeutic modality in about half of the patients (TABLE 6). Adjuvant hormonal or radiation therapy followed in almost half of the other patients, depending on prognostic factors.

The 5-year survival rate as a function of age (TABLE 7) can be explained by the finding that younger women tend to have well-differentiated cancer more frequently than older women, and when corrected for grade, age does not seem to be an independent prognostic factor.

Histologic subtypes were: adenocarcinoma (81.25%), papillary adenocarcinoma (12.5%) and adenoacanthoma (6.25%). Grade provides one of the major prognostic

TABLE 5. Endometrial Carcinoma: Patients Treated by Vaginal Surgery (1968–1985)[a]

• 160 Patients
• Obesity 62.34%

[a] Data from the II Dept. Ob/Gyn, Rome.

TABLE 6. Endometrial Carcinoma: Vaginal Surgery and Combined Treatment[a]

Treatment	Number of Patients (%)
Vaginal hysterectomy only	81 (50.6)
+ hormonal therapy	50 (31.25)
+ radiotherapy	25 (15.6)
+ chemotherapy	4 (2.5)

[a] Data from the II Dept. Ob/Gyn, Rome.

TABLE 7. Endometrial Carcinoma Vaginal Surgery – Survival Rate and Prognostic Factors[a]

Prognostic Factors	5-Year Survival Rate (%)
Age	
<50 ys	94.2
<70 ys	63.8
Grade	
G1	95
G2	86.7
G3	63.3
Myometrial invasion	
M_0–M_1	96–87
M_2	70.2
M_3	67.5
Stage	
IA	81.7
IB	79.4

[a] Data from the II Dept. Ob/Gyn, Rome.

factors even in our series, but, fortunately, poorly differentiated tumors only account for a small percentage of cases (TABLE 7).

Myometrial invasion modifies 5-year survival rates (TABLE 7), but deep invasion is observed in a small number of patients. The sub-division in stage IA and IB does not seem to significantly affect survival rates as observed by other authors. In all patients lymphangiography was negative and computerized tomography (CT) and magnetic resonance imaging (MRI), when used, did not show lymph-node invasion.

Tumors recurred in eight patients (5%). Of these, two (25%) had tumor on the vaginal vault, which is the most common recurrence site. The reason why there were so few recurrences at this site was that the vaginal approach enabled us to dissect the upper third of the vagina. In the other six patients, a recurrent tumor was found in the pelvis in four (50%) and in multiple sites in two (25%).

Our experience with vaginal hysterectomy showed a 5-year survival rate in stage I endometrial carcinoma of 85.5%, similar to that of patients who underwent abdominal surgery (86.8%). Moreover, we believe that in selected cases the vaginal approach has several advantages compared with the abdominal one:

- it may be performed easily and rapidly by a skilled surgeon;
- it is not particularly traumatic for the patient;
- it provides better access for dissection of the vagina's upper and middle thirds;
- convalescence is frequently easier for the patient than after abdominal hysterectomy; moreover, lower morbidity and shorter hospitalization also contribute to bring costs down.

In our extensive experience with vaginal surgery, we never encountered technical difficulties caused by mistaken evaluations of uterine and adnexal dimensions. Thus, when we perform vaginal hysterectomy in patients who cannot undergo an abdominal operation, we feel confident in treating these high surgical risk patients with primary surgery.

CONCLUSIONS

Data from the literature and those from our personal case material of vaginal surgery in the treatment of endometrial carcinoma lead us to the following conclusions:

Although vaginal hysterectomy is not the treatment of choice for stage I endometrial cancer, this procedure may be performed in some categories of patients assuring a good tumoral control.

Even if in the past vaginal hysterectomy was restricted to high surgical risk patients, this indication is no longer sufficient: a low prognostic risk is now required if this kind of surgery is to be performed.

Since most pathological features can be ascertained by vaginal surgery, with an accurate pre-surgical study of the patient and by the assessment of grade, myometrial invasion, tumor size, and capillary-like spaces invasion, therefore, a selection of the patients to be treated with vaginal hysterectomy is mandatory.

The following findings define a low-risk subgroup:

- well-differentiated tumor (G1);
- myometrial invasion reaching the inner third (M1);
- tumor size less than 2 cm in diameter;
- negative peritoneal cytology;
- positive hormonal receptors (ER+/PR+);
- histotype: adenocarcinoma, adenoacanthoma;
- negative capillary-like spaces involvement (CLS);
- age below 60;
- negative lymphangiography (or negative RMI and TC)

Many surgeons have been reluctant to perform vaginal hysterectomy in patients with endometrial carcinoma because of a belief that they would jeopardize the patient's chances of survival. We believe that vaginal hysterectomy has a definite place in the therapeutic tool kit of the gynecological oncologist. Although we do not recommend that this procedure should be utilized routinely or indiscriminately, its use adds flexibility to the management of selected patients with stage I endometrial carcinoma, without being detrimental to their chances of total eradication of the tumor. It is also true that, if vaginal hysterectomy is so seldom used today in the management of endometrial cancer, it will unfortunately be used ever less frequently in the future.

REFERENCES

1. BORONOW, R. C. 1976. Endometrial cancer not a benign disease. Obstet. Gynecol. **47**(5): 630–634.
2. PRATT, J. H., R. E. SYMMONDS & J. S. WELCH. 1964. Vaginal hysterectomy for carcinoma of fundus. Am. J. Obstet. Gynecol. **88**: 1063–1071.
3. STALLWORTHY, J. A. 1971. Surgery of endometrial cancer in the Bonney tradition. Ann. R. Coll. Surg. Engl. **48**: 293–295.
4. JONES, H. W. 1975. Treatment of adenocarcinoma of the endometrium. Obstet. Gynecol. Surv. **30**: 147–152.
5. KOTTMEIER, H. & P. KOLSTAD. 1976. Annual report on the results of treatment of carcinoma of the uterus, vagina and ovary. Vol. 16, Stockholm, FIGO.
6. PETTERSSONN, F. 1985. Annual report on the results of treatment in gynecological cancer. Vol. 19, Stockholm, FIGO.
7. PETTERSSONN, F. 1988. Annual report on the results of treatment in gynecological cancer. Vol. 20, Stockholm, FIGO.

8. GUSBERG, S. B. & D. YANNOPOULOS. 1964. Therapeutic decisions in corpus cancer. Am. J. Obstet. Gynecol. **88**(2): 157–161.
9. BORONOW, R. C. 1984. Surgical staging in endometrial cancer: Clinical-pathological findings of a prospective. Obstet. Gynecol. **63**: 825–832.
10. COWLES, T. A. 1985. Comparison of clinical and surgical staging in patients with endometrial cancer. Obstet. Gynecol. **66**(3): 413–416.
11. SCHINK, L. C. 1987. Tumor size in endometrial cancer: a prospective factor for lymph-node metastases. Obstet. Gynecol. **70**: 216.
12. HANSON, M. B. 1985. Prognostic significance of lymph-vascular space invasion in stage I endometrial cancer. Cancer **55**: 1753.
13. CREASMAN, W. T., C. P. MORROW, B. N. BUNDY, H. D. HOMESLEY, J. E. GRAHAM & P. B. HELLER. 1987. Surgical pathologic spread patterns of endometrial cancer. Cancer **60**: 2035–2041.

Prognostic Significance of Ornithine Decarboxylase (ODC) Activity in Endometrial Adenocarcinoma

A. LANZA,[a] S. COLOMBATTO,[b] A. RE,[a]
R. BELLINO,[a] M. TESSAROLO,[a] AND L. LEO[a]

[a] Cattedra "B"
Istituto di Ginecologia ed Ostetricia
Università di Torino
Torino, Italy

[b] Sezione di Biochimica
Dipartimento di Medicina Oncologica Sperimentale
Università di Torino
Torino, Italy

Changes in ornithine decarboxylase (ODC) activity in the human endometrium in situations ranging from normal to hyperplasia and carcinoma were investigated in this study. Since ODC is known to increase in tumor tissues, possible correlation between ODC activity and recurrences in patients with endometrial adenocarcinoma before and after medroxyprogesterone acetate (MPA) treatment was also evaluated. ODC activity was determined in normal (32 cases), dysfunctional (30 cases), hyperplastic (13 cases), and neoplastic endometrium before (25 cases) and after MPA (Provera-Upjohn) treatment (30 cases) (1g/day *per os* for 30 days) (TABLES 1 and 2). Among these 30 patients, 16 were followed for periods of 18 to 29 months and 14 for 1–15 months. In the first group two recurrences were observed; in the second group there was one death by diffuse metastatization. The ODC activity increased significantly in the mid- and advanced proliferative phase, then gradually decreased to the menopausal endometrium. In the weakly proliferative endometrium, ODC activity was low. Values are comparable with those in the menopausal and lower (though no significantly) than in the proliferative endometrium. In the disordered endometrium and in endometria with histological signs of estrogen stimulation, ODC activity was very high. It is interesting to note that in the disordered endometrium two histologically similar, but metabolically different types of tissue are observed, probably due to different estrogen stimulation. In one of these types, ODC activity is comparable to that measured in hyperplasia. In view of the possible malignant progression of endometrial hyperplasia, these particular cases of dysfunction should be monitored and treated with progestins. ODC activity increased progressively in simple and atypical hyperplasia and in all carcinoma grades (32-fold in G1 and G2, 79-fold in G3 compared with menopausal endometrium). All G1 patients and the responders to the MPA treatment (tumor disappearance) displayed a significant ODC reduction. The patients with high endome-

TABLE 1. ODC Activity in the Human Endometrium (nmoles CO_2/g/h/37°C)

Normal Endometrium	No. Cases	ODC
Mid-proliferative	6	7.2 ± 6.2
Advanced proliferative	6	50 ± 2.4
Early secretory	6	16.2 ± 3.4
Advanced secretory	6	7.6 ± 3.1
Normal menopausal	8	4.1 ± 3.3

Dysfunctional Endometrium	No. Cases	ODC
Weakly proliferative	8	3.5 ± 2.7
Normal proliferative	6	11.2 ± 6.1
Disordered proliferative 1st group	5	26.1 ± 7.9
2nd group	6	40.9 ± 9.1
Perimenopausal with signs of estrogen stimulation	5	46.8 ± 3.5

Neoplastic Endometrium	No. Cases	ODC
Simple hyperplasia	7	39.6 ± 9.6
Hyperplasia with atypical features	6	62.2 ± 6.4
1st Degree adenocarcinoma	10	119 ± 18
2nd Degree adenocarcinoma	10	143 ± 42
3rd Degree adenocarcinoma	5	315 ± 25

TABLE 2. ODC Activity (nmoles CO_2/g/hr/37°C) in Endometrial Adenocarcinoma after Treatment with High Doses of MPA: Relationship between Biochemical Responders and Relapses

	G1	G2	G3	G1 or G2 with Tumor Disappearance	Total Number of Cases	Relapses
Responders	11.5 ± 4.9 (10)	11.6 ± 4.0 (6)	–	7.6 ± 1.9 (6)	22	0
Non-responders	–	235 (2)	425.8 ± 58.9 (6)	–	8	3

trium ODC activity who were non-responders to MPA were all G3. It follows that tumors of this histological grade do not respond to MPA treatment. However, high ODC activity after MPA does not necessarily point to an unfavorable prognosis, as three patients of one group and two of another one had high ODC activity without evidence of disease. Therefore, ODC activity is undoubtedly an important indicator of the proliferative capacity of endometrial tissue and of its ability to respond to progestins.

Management of Early Adenocarcinoma of the Endometrium with Surgical Staging Followed by Tailored Adjuvant Radiation Therapy

PHILIP J. DiSAIA

Department of Obstetrics and Gynecology
University of California, Irvine
101 The City Drive, Building 26
Orange, California 92668

Adenocarcinoma of the endometrium is the most commonly diagnosed invasive cancer of the female genital tract in the United States at present. Fortunately, 75% of the cases are clinically Stage I and survivals have been relatively good. This success has fostered a number of treatment methods utilizing surgery, and at times adjuvant radiotherapy in varying combinations. There has been a perception that patients with early stage endometrial adenocarcinoma, in general, do better with combination therapy, but careful study of the issues has been lacking. Several questions arise: 1) Do all patients with endometrial cancer need some sort of adjuvant radiation therapy? 2) Can some patients be adequately treated with hysterectomy and bilateral salpingo-oophorectomy alone? 3) If radiation therapy is to be used, should it be preoperative of postoperative? 4) What type of radiation therapy is appropriate, intracavitary or external?

A review of the literature suggests that there are a great many pathological features of prognostic significance in patients with Stage I lesions. Among these features are depth of myometrial invasion, occult involvement of the adnexa or cervix and evidence of lymph node metastasis. Absence of these features appears to define a very low-risk group with a good prognosis. Preoperative administration of intracavitary or external irradiation causes shrinkage of the lesion and a distortion of these pathologic risk factors. Rather than contending with these distortions, it seems more reasonable to adopt a philosophy which calls for all patients with Stage I endometrial cancer to receive surgery first. The surgical-pathological findings can then be used to select out the high-risk group, and that subset should receive irradiation therapy. Those patients at low risk would receive no further therapy with the resulting economy of morbidity and cost.

In order to firmly establish the existence of these pathological factors of prognostic significance, the Gynecologic Oncology Group (GOG) conducted two studies of apparent Stage I endometrial adenocarcinoma. Every effort was made to exclude cervical involvement (Stage II disease) by formal endocervical curettage. A bilateral pelvic lymph node sampling was performed on all cases, and, where the patient's condition permitted, a para-aortic lymphadenectomy was also done along with extrafascial hysterectomy and bilateral salpingo-oophorectomy. Peritoneal cytology was obtained from a pelvic washing on all cases. A report of the pathologic findings of 621 patients was reported by Creasman.[1] Among these 621 patients with clinical Stage I carcinoma of the endometrium, no form of pre-operative irradiation was permitted.

The distribution of study parameters were detailed by Creasman and are reprinted here (TABLE 1). Twenty-five percent of the patients had poorly differentiated lesions and 41% had significant myometrial invasion (invasion to middle or outer third of myometrium). Malignant cells were detected in the peritoneal cytology of 12% of the patients. Sixteen percent of the patients were found to have disease in the isthmus of the uterus on pathological review of the specimen. Five percent of the patients had metastasis to one or both of the adnexa and 58 patients (9%) had pelvic node metastasis. Only 34 patients (6%) had para-aortic node metastasis. Thirty-five patients (6%) had other extra-uterine intraperitoneal metastasis identified at the time of surgery.

Creasman compared the grade of tumor with depth of invasion and his findings are illustrated in TABLE 2. In general, the depth of invasion increased as the grade became less differentiated. Seventy-eight percent of the grade 1 lesions had endometrial or superficial muscle involvement only. In contrast, 58% of the grade 3 lesions had middle or deep muscle invasion. It should be noted, however, that there were some notable exceptions. Eleven patients (7%) with grade 3 lesions had no myometrial invasion, while 18 patients (10%) with grade 1 tumors had deep myometrial invasion. Seventy patients (11%) had metastasis either to the pelvic and/or pelvic-aortic nodes. Only 22 patients (3%) had metastasis to both pelvic and para-aortic nodes. Twelve

TABLE 1. Surgical-Pathologic Findings[a]

Stage		Adnexa Involvement	
IA	346 (56%)	Positive	34 (5%)
IB	275 (44%)	Negative	587 (95%)
Histology		Pelvic Node Metastasis	
Adenocarcinoma	459 (74%)	Positive	58 (9%)
Adenocanthoma	41 (7%)	Negative	563 (91%)
Adenosquamous	99 (16%)	Aortic Node Metastasis	
Others	22 (4%)	Positive	34 (6%)
Grade		Negative	587 (94%)
1 Well	180 (29%)	Other Extrauterine Metastasis	
2 Moderate	288 (46%)	Positive	35 (6%)
3 Poor	153 (25%)	Negative	586 (94%)
Myometrial Invasion		Capillary-Like Space Involvement	
Endometrium only	86 (14%)	Positive	93 (15%)
Inner 1/3	281 (45%)	Negative	528 (85%)
Middle 1/2	115 (19%)	Menopausal status	
Deep 1/3	139 (22%)	Premenopause	58 (10%)
Peritoneal Cytology		Postmenopause	549 (90%)
Positive	76 (12%)	(14 patients, status unknown)	
Negative	545 (88%)		
Site of Tumor Location			
Fundus	524 (84%)		
Isthmus	97 (16%)		

[a] From W. T. Creasman, et al.[1]

TABLE 2. Histologic Grade and Depth of Invasion[a]

Depth	Grade			
	G1	G2	G3	TOTAL
Endometrium only	44 (24%)	31 (11%)	11 (7%)	86 (14%)
Superficial	96 (53%)	131 (45%)	54 (35%)	281 (45%)
Middle	22 (12%)	69 (24%)	24 (16%)	115 (19%)
Deep	18 (10%)	57 (20%)	64 (42%)	139 (22%)
TOTAL	180 (100%)	288 (100%)	153 (100%)	621 (100%)

[a] From W. T. Creasman, et al.[1]

TABLE 3. Relationship of Positive Pelvic Nodes to Aortic Nodes[a]

Pelvic	Negative	Positive	TOTAL
Negative	551 (89%)	12 (2%)	563 (91%)
Positive	36 (6%)	22 (3%)	58 (9%)
TOTAL	587 (95%)	34 (5%)	621 (100%)

[a] From W. T. Creasman, et al.[1]

patients (2%) had metastasis to the para-aortic nodes only. TABLE 3 from Creasman's article summarizes the relationship of positive pelvic nodes to aortic node status.

A close correlation exists between depth of invasion and nodal metastasis. Only 1% of patients with involvement of the endometrium only, had metastasis to either pelvic or para-aortic nodes. The relative frequency of positive pelvic and para-aortic nodes increased to 25% and 17%, respectively, for deep muscle invasion. The same was noted with grade of tumor. Only 3% of well differentiated tumors have pelvic node metastasis. This increased to 18% in poorly differentiated cancers. The same correlation is noted with regards to para-aortic metastasis.

Seventy-five patients (12%) had positive peritoneal cytology. The incidence of pelvic node metastasis in this group was 25%. As one would expect, 35% of patients with extra-uterine disease (adnexa, lymph nodes or intraperitoneal metastasis) had positive cytology. Thirty-nine patients (52%) of patients with positive washings had no other evidence of extra-uterine disease. Gross intraperitoneal spread (exclusive of adnexal metastasis) was highly correlated with metastasis to both pelvic and para-aortic nodes. Fifty-one of those patients with gross intraperitoneal spread had positive pelvic nodes, whereas only 7% without gross spread had positive pelvic nodes. The relative frequencies of positive para-aortic nodes in patients with and without intraperitoneal spread were 23 and 4%, respectively.

DiSaia[2] reported on a similar group of patients studied in a comparable manner from 1973 to 1977 under the auspices of the GOG. His 1985 report allowed a study of risk factors and recurrence patterns in these Stage 1 patients. The study was conducted by four institutions within the Gynecologic Oncology Group and was under the direction of four investigators. Therapy based on the pathological findings was individualized based on physician preference. Data were available on outcome of 222 patients utilizing both surgery alone and various combinations of radiation therapy used preoperatively and postoperatively. Among these 222 patients 68 (31%) had surgery only. In an additional 97 patients (44%), cesium or radium therapy was used in either the preoperative or postoperative period. Individuals treated preoperatively with cesium or radium received 3,000 mg hours with tandem and ovoids and then underwent operation within the same hospitalization, usually within one to two days after removal of isotope. Sixteen percent of the patients were treated with operation plus cesium irradium and external irradiation, and an additional 9% of patients had surgery plus external irradiation (TABLE 4). External irradiation existed of 50 g whole pelvis given in the post-operative period. In most instances external irradiation was prescribed for patients with poor prognostic factors, extra-uterine disease, deep myometrial invasion (greater than 1/3 the thickness of the myometrium), or extension of the disease to the lower uterine segment. In 15 patients whole pelvis and para-aortic irradiation (45 g) was used. At the time of the review all patients had been followed from 36 to 72 months after completion of therapy. Recurrence had developed in a total of 34 patients (15%) and 24 (11%) had died of their disease. An additional 4 patients were never without evidence of disease and had also succumbed to their neoplasm. That brought to 28 (12%) the number of patients who had died of disease at the time of the report.

THERAPY AND RECURRENCE

Review of TABLE 4 suggests that external irradiation might be less efficacious than intracavitary therapy in preventing recurrences. However, those patients who receive external irradiation have a much poorer prognosis as manifested by the surgical/pathologic evaluation. Keeping this in mind, it is difficult to draw firm conclusions from the outcome of this patient group or any patient group where therapy is not dictated by the protocol. However, certain impressions can be drawn.

When the sites of recurrence were analyzed, it was noted that the control of local disease had been excellent despite the fact that 31% of the patients had surgery only (TABLE 5). Only 7 patients (3%) had recurrence in the vagina or pelvis alone. Twenty-seven patients (12%) had recurrence at a distant site, at times concomitive with the pelvic recurrence. When patterns of recurrence were compared to treatment, there were not statistically significant differences and the rate of local control was high regardless of therapy. When distant recurrences were evaluated and compared with therapy, those individuals who were treated with operation only or operation plus cesium or radium were found to have a recurrence rate of only 5%. On the other hand, when

TABLE 4. Treatment and Recurrences of Stage I Endometrial Adenocarcinoma[a]

	Patients		Recurrences	
Treatment	n	%	n	%
Operation only	68	31	6	9
Operation plus radium	97	44	8	8
Operation plus radium plus external irradiation	37	16	14	38
Operation plus external irradiation	20	9	6	30

[a] From P. J. DiSaia et al.[2]

TABLE 5. Recurrences by Site of Stage I Endometrial Adenocarcinoma[a]

	Recurrences	
Site	n	%
Vagina only	2	1
Pelvis	5	2
Pelvis plus distant	5	2
Distant	22	10

[a] From P. J. DiSaia et al.[2]

poor prognostic factors were present, and external irradiation to either the pelvic and/or para-aortic area was given, the distant failure was considerably higher with only 1/3 of these individuals having a recurrence. When all the data was analyzed with regards to treatment, location and site of recurrence, patient groupings seemed appropriate. The outcomes for patients treated with operation alone or operation plus cesium or radium were essentially the same and the recurrences on all sites were also the same; therefore, these two groups were combined. All of the patients who received external irradiation, whether or not radium was used, were also combined for data analysis since evaluation of these modalities separately showed no difference in their effectiveness. All patients who had recurrent disease present only in the vagina or pelvis were combined into a "local" recurrence group, and patients who had distant disease were combined into a "distant" recurrence category.

TABLE 6 illustrates the recurrences and depths by depth of invasion. Only 8% of the patients who had involvement of the endometrium only experienced a recurrence and 5% died of the disease. This increases to 46% recurrence and 36% deaths in patients with deep muscle involvement.

The pattern of recurrences was compared to pelvic node metastasis and good correlations were obtained. If the pelvic lymph nodes were not involved with tumor, 11% of the patients had a recurrence; however, if the lymph nodes were involved, 57% of the patients had a recurrence (TABLE 7). This was also the finding when para-aortic node involvement was evaluated. Eleven percent of patients without metastasis to the para-aortic area had recurrence compared with 59% of those who had metastasis to these areas. A more specific analysis was made comparing prognostic factors with specific treatments and sites of failure. When grade was analyzed, it was noted that patients with grade 1 or grade 2 lesions who were treated with operation, with or

TABLE 6. Recurrences and Deaths by Depth of Invasion of Stage I Endometrial Adenocarcinoma

	Recurrences		Deaths	
Depth of Invasion	n	%	n	%
Endometrium only	7	8	5	5
Inner myometrium	10	13	9	11
Middle myometrium	2	12	2	12
Deep myometrium	15	46	12	36

[a] From P. J. DiSaia et al.[2]

TABLE 7. Recurrences and Deaths by Pelvic and Para-aortic Node Involvement of Stage I Endometrial Adenocarcinoma[a]

	Recurrences		Deaths	
Involvement	n	%	n	%
Pelvic nodes				
Negative	21	11	16	5
Positive	13	57	12	52
Para-aortic nodes[b]				
Negative	15	11	12	8
Positive	10	59	9	53

[a] From P. J. DiSaia et al.[2]
[b] Para-aortic nodes were not sampled in 66 cases.

without cesium or radium, had a recurrence rate of either local or distant sites of less than 5%. In the grade 3 category, although local recurrences were low, distant recurrences were 21%. In evaluating treatment with operation plus external irradiation, a high failure rate was found in grade 2 and 3 cancers at distant sites (TABLE 8).

DISCUSSION

Therapy for endometrial carcinoma has been quite varied, especially with regard to the use and timing of radiation therapy. The new (1988) staging of endometrial carcinoma (TABLE 9) has placed the emphasis on surgical staging of this disease. Certainly this will accelerate the abandonment of treatment protocols that imply preoperative irradiation therapy. Individualization of therapy based on prognostic factors does seem to be safe and cogent. In the majority of patients, surgery with or without radium or cesium was the total treatment and in this group of patients the recurrence rate was quite low. The reports of Creasman and others[3,4] allows some suggestions for

TABLE 8. Local and Distant Recurrences by Grade and Treatment of Stage I Endometrial Adenocarcinoma[a]

	Recurrences							
	Operation ± RA[b] (n = 165)				Operation + XRT (n = 57)			
	Local		Distant		Local		Distant	
Grade	n	%	n	%	n	%	n	%
1 (n = 93)	2	2	2	2	0	0	0	0
2 (n = 88)	2	3	3	5	2	8	6	24
3 (n = 41)	1	5	4	21	0	0	12	41
TOTAL	5	3	9	5	2	3	18	31

[a] From P. J. DiSaia et al.[2]
[b] RA = Intracavitary radium or cesium; XRT = external irradiation.

TABLE 9. FIGO Staging of Corpus Cancer[a]

Stage IA	G123[b]	Tumor limited to endometrium
Stage IB	G123	Invasion to less than one-half the myometrium
Stage IC	G123	Invasion to more than one-half the myometrium
Stage IIA	G123	Endocervical glandular involvement only
Stage IIB	G123	Cervical stromal invasion
Stage IIIA	G123	Tumor invades serosa and/or adnexa, and/or positive peritoneal cytology
Stage IIIB	G123	Vaginal metastases
Stage IIIC	G123	Metastases to pelvic and/or para-aortic lymph nodes
Stage IVA	G123	Tumor invasion of bladder and/or bowel mucosa
Stage IVB		Distant metastases including intra-abdominal and/or inguinal lymph nodes

[a] FIGO, 1988.

[b] Within each stage, cases of carcinoma of the corpus should be classified (or graded) according to the degree of histologic differentiation.

future approaches. It appears that patients can be divided into three risk groups as suggested by Creasman (TABLE 10). His analysis was restricted to factors which were predictive of lymph node metastasis. Low risk patients were grade 1 patients with no myometrial invasion and no intraperitoneal disease. Moderate risk patients had grade 2 or 3 lesions with inner or middle third myometrial invasion and no intraperitoneal disease. High risk patients had intraperitoneal disease or deep myometrial invasion. Total abdominal hysterectomy with bilateral salpingo-oophorectomy and a peritoneal cytology appears to be adequate therapy for low risk patients. High risk patients seem to warrant the addition of pelvic and para-aortic lymphadenectomy followed by tailored radiation therapy to the involved areas. The high failure rate at distant sites begs the question of adjuvant chemotherapy, but clinical trials are not as yet forthcoming as the efficacy of such therapy. Treatment of moderate risk patients is somewhat less clear. Whether or not these patients need pelvic and para-aortic lymphadenectomy remains controversial. Some have based the decision for lymphadenectomy

TABLE 10. Determination of Risk Factors for Nodal Metastasis Using Multivariant Analysis[a]

Risk Factor	Pelvic	Aortic
Low Risk (No moderate or high risk factors) Grade 1, endometrium only, no intraperitoneal disease	0/44 (0%)	0/44 (0%)
Moderate Risk (Inner mid invasion, Grade 2 or 3, no intraperitoneal disease) Only one factor	4/158 (3%)	3/158 (2%)
Both factors	15/268 (6%)	6/268 (2%)
High Risk (Intraperitoneal disease, deep invasion only)	21/116 (18%)	17/116 (15%)
Intraperitoneal disease only	4/12 (33%)	1/12 (8%)
Both	14/23 (61%)	7/23 (30%)

[a] From W. T. Creasman et al.[1]

on the depth of myometrial invasion determined intraoperatively with frozen section assistance. Each physician will have to make his own therapy decisions and await further data from treatment trials ongoing at this time by the Gynecologic Oncology Group.

Concerning lymphadenectomy, two issues need discussion. First, adequate sampling must be done in order to have sufficient information upon which a treatment decision can be made. Especially in the pelvis, all lymph nodes should be removed without undue concern being given to remove all lymphatic channels. Palpation of the lymph node bearing areas is not adequate for deciding which nodal areas might be positive. Less than 15% of patients with metastasis to lymph nodes have grossly enlarged nodes palpable *in situ*. In many instances an enlargement can only be determined after the retroperitoneal spaces have been opened and the lymph nodes removed.

Factors such as grade, depth of myometrial invasion, extra-uterine disease and involvement of the lower uterine segment are inter-related. The value of whole pelvic irradiation in patients with extra-uterine disease remains unanswered by the analysis of these studies. The potential prevention of distant recurrences was not addressed. Prospective randomized treatment trials are necessary and will shape our treatment decisions in the future.

REFERENCES

1. CREASMAN, W. T., C. P. MORROW, B. N. BUNDY, H. D. HOMESLEY, J. E. GRAHAM & P. B. HELLER. 1987. Surgical pathologic spread patterns of endometrial cancer. Cancer **60:** 2035-2041.
2. DiSAIA, P. J., W. T. CREASMAN, M. D. BARONOW & J. A. BLESSING. 1985. Risk factors and recurrent patterns in Stage I endometrial cancer. Am. J. Obstet. Gynecol. **151:** 1009-1015.
3. LEWIS, G. C., JR. & B. BUNDY. 1981. Surgery for endometrial cancer. Cancer **48:** 568-374.
4. BORONOW, R. C., C. P. MORROW, W. T. CREASMAN, P. J. DiSAIA, S. G. SILVERBERG, A. MILLER & J. A. BLESSING. 1984. Surgical staging in endometrial cancer. 1. Clinical-pathologic findings of a prospective study. Obstet. Gynecol. **63:** 825-32.

Index of Contributors